Water-Soluble Vitamins							Minerals					
Ascorbic Acid mg	Folacin[f] μg	Niacin[g] mg	Riboflavin mg	Thiamin mg	Vitamin B₆ mg	Vitamin B₁₂ μg	Calcium mg	Phosphorus mg	Iodine μg	Iron mg	Magnesium mg	Zinc mg
35	50	5	0.4	0.3	0.3	0.3	360	240	35	10	60	3
35	50	8	0.6	0.5	0.4	0.3	540	400	45	15	70	5
40	100	9	0.8	0.7	0.6	1.0	800	800	60	15	150	10
40	200	12	1.1	0.9	0.9	1.5	800	800	80	10	200	10
40	300	16	1.2	1.2	1.2	2.0	800	800	110	10	250	10
45	400	18	1.5	1.4	1.6	3.0	1,200	1,200	130	18	350	15
45	400	20	1.8	1.5	2.0	3.0	1,200	1,200	150	18	400	15
45	400	20	1.8	1.5	2.0	3.0	800	800	140	10	350	15
45	400	18	1.6	1.4	2.0	3.0	800	800	130	10	350	15
45	400	16	1.5	1.2	2.0	3.0	800	800	110	10	350	15
45	400	16	1.3	1.2	1.6	3.0	1,200	1,200	115	18	300	15
45	400	14	1.4	1.1	2.0	3.0	1,200	1,200	115	18	300	15
45	400	14	1.4	1.1	2.0	3.0	800	800	100	18	300	15
45	400	13	1.2	1.0	2.0	3.0	800	800	100	18	300	15
45	400	12	1.1	1.0	2.0	3.0	800	800	80	10	300	15
60	800	+2	+0.3	+0.3	2.5	4.0	1,200	1,200	125	18+[h]	450	20
80	600	+4	+0.5	+0.3	2.5	4.0	1,200	1,200	150	18	450	25

[e]Total vitamin E activity, estimated to be 80 percent as α-tocopherol and 20 percent other tocopherols. See text for variation in allowances.

[f]The folacin allowances refer to dietary sources as determined by *Lactobacillus casei* assay. Pure forms of folacin may be effective in doses less than one fourth of the recommended dietary allowance.

[g]Although allowances are expressed as niacin, it is recognized that on the average 1 mg of niacin is derived from each 60 mg of dietary tryptophan.

[h]This increased requirement cannot be met by ordinary diets; therefore, the use of supplemental iron is recommended.

Nutrition in Action

Holt, Rinehart, and Winston
New York   Chicago   San Francisco   Atlanta
Dallas   Montreal   Toronto   London   Sydney

Ethel Austin Martin
Ardath Anders Coolidge
Purdue University *Calumet Campus*
Hammond, Indiana

Nutrition in Action

fourth edition

Ethel Austin Martin was formerly on the nutrition staffs and in the home economics departments of the University of Illinois, the University of Chicago and Northwestern University. She served as director of Nutrition Service for the National Dairy Council. Mrs. Martin holds Bachelor of Science and Master of Science degrees from Teachers College, Columbia University and the degree of Doctor of Science (honorary) from South Dakota University. She carries the title of Registered Dietitian (R.D.) granted by the American Dietetic Association. Her publications include *Robert's Nutrition Work with Children* and *Nutrition Education in Action*. She holds professional memberships in the American Dietetic Association and the Society for Nutrition Education and is a life member of the American Home Economics Association. She belongs to the honor societies Sigma Xi, Kappa Mu Sigma and Sigma Delta Epsilon and is a national honorary member of Phi Upsilon Omicron.

Ardath Anders Coolidge is Associate Professor of Consumer and Family Sciences in the Department of Behavioral Sciences, Purdue University, Calumet Campus. Dr. Coolidge holds a Bachelor of Arts degree from Earlham College and the degree of Doctor of Philosophy from Iowa State University, Ames, in human nutrition. Her professional memberships include the American Home Economics Association, the American Dietetic Association and the Society for Nutrition Education. Dr. Coolidge has had practical experience in the field of sensory evaluation of food products in conducting taste panel tests for Armour and Company's food research division. In her present capacity as professor of nutrition at the university level, she encounters and deals regularly with current nutrition problems of concern to students.

Editor   Joan Handelsman Greene
Project Editor   Susan Adams
Project Assistant   Christine Smith
Production Manager   Robert de Villeneuve
Designer   Karen Salsgiver
Other acknowledgments appear on page 531.

Library of Congress Cataloging in Publication Data

Martin, Ethel Austin
Nutrition in Action

  Includes bibliographies and index.
  1. Nutrition   2. Diet.
  I. Coolidge, Ardath A., joint author.   II Title.
TX354.M38   1978   641.1   77-24031
ISBN 0-03-020336-8

Composition by Precision Typographers Inc., New York
Printing and binding by Von Hoffmann Press, Missouri
 9 0 1 2 3   032   9 8 7 6 5 4 3 2

Preface

Courses in nutrition are being offered to college and university students in all disciplines. Courses without prerequisites provide a background of fundamental nutrition knowledge that primarily prepares students to make intelligent decisions about their own nutrition programs. It is for such courses that *Nutrition in Action* was originally intended and has continued to serve. Experience with previous editions of the book, however, has proved its adaptability in many areas. For example, students who have used the book as a text find that it helps them to introduce sound nutrition concepts when they become teachers in preschool, elementary and secondary classrooms. Nutritionists in public health programs have found *Nutrition in Action* a helpful resource in conducting orientation programs for non-nutrition staff personnel. And finally, adults in search of scientifically reliable information on nutrition, for independent study, have turned to the book as a text and reference.

Nutrition in Action covers the principles of nutrition with respect to basic body needs; the scope of nutrients and foods in satisfying those needs; and the results that can be expected in terms of human health when nutrient intake is adequate, deficient, or excessive. Student involvement and self-instruction are encouraged by the inclusion of extensive reading references with each chapter and frequent suggestions throughout the text to consider practical nutrition problems of a personal or community nature. Terms that may be unfamiliar are defined in the margins. More detailed descriptions of certain key words appear in the adjacent text. Illustrations—including many photographs, tables and charts—contribute to the interest and understanding of readers.

The fourth edition is completely updated and virtually rewritten. The text is oriented toward current nutrition concerns of students in their immediate environments but it also encompasses information that applies to the nutritional needs of individuals throughout the life cycle. It incorporates current nutrition developments based on recent research; an extensive table of nutrient content of foods derived from new official government compilations; new emphasis on such subjects as food additives, vegetarianism, safety in foods and nutrition labeling; new foods and meal concepts, including the ever-expanding array of convenience foods, snacks and fast food services. The material on ethnic diets has been updated and expanded. Structural formulas for certain nutrients have been added to the fourth edition to give students increased appreciation of the composition of their foods. Also new is the treatment of sensory perception as a factor in acceptance of foods in developing eating habits. The nutritional implications of health problems such as alcoholism and drug abuse are considered in light of present nutrition knowledge. New survey data on the health and nutritional status of the people in the United States are interpreted throughout the text. The need for a national nutrition policy and for establishing national dietary goals is explored. Consideration is given to contemporary nutrition problems and programs in the United States and in the world. As a whole, the fourth edition presents sound, balanced information on nutrition in a modern context.

Ardath Anders Coolidge has joined as co-author of this edition. As professor of nutrition at the university level she brings current knowledge of student interests and abilities. She is an observer of food practices of students, and, as the mother of teens and post-teens, she is in daily touch with food concerns of many of our reading audience. Her perception of the present-day eating habits of young people has kept our subject in focus.

It is impossible to name all those who have contributed in some manner to this text. Those who prepared specific material are cited at appropriate points in the book. To all others—those who provided information, illustrations or services, and who criticized and advised or encouraged us when we needed it most—we must be content to say a grateful "Thank you. May you feel rewarded by the gratitude of all those who find this book useful."

Chicago   E. A. M.
February, 1978   A. A. C.

Contents

Part 1
Nutrition Begins with Food

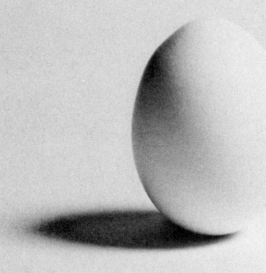

Good health, with its promise of vigor and achievement, is a coveted state. The term "health" is often confused with "nutrition," however. Health is a broad concept that includes nutrition as an essential factor. Total health cannot be attained without good nutrition, and good nutrition in turn depends upon adequate food intake. Thus nutrition does in fact begin with food, but it involves more than food alone. Nutrition implies all the things that happen to food from the time it is eaten until the time it finally nourishes the body. It is really a *process* in which food is digested and its nutrients are absorbed and transported to areas of the body where they are utilized. This process may be entirely successful, or faulty in varying degrees at different points— when reasonably successful, a person is considered well-nourished.

Faults in the nutrition process can result from too little, too much, or the wrong kinds of food, or there can be functional failure in any of its steps. Prolonged failure is characterized variously as *malnutrition, undernutrition, poor nutrition,* or *hunger.* As applied here, the first three terms suggest failure in some degree of one or more of the nutritional processes essential to the body's well-being. Hunger, on the other hand, is a physiological and psychological condition resulting from the deprivation of food. It can be relieved promptly by eating, but when hunger is prolonged, the outcome can be malnutrition.

The level of a person's nourishment is called his or her *nutritional status.* Food is obviously a critical element in determining whether nutritional status is good or poor. Food choices thus become a pivotal concern. Many psychological, cultural, and social factors influence individuals and groups in food selection. The ways these forces can modify eating habits offer a logical beginning for the study of nutrition.

Food Customs, Patterns, and Habits

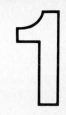

Personal Reactions to Food
Cultural Backgrounds
Eating Patterns in the United States
Educational Influences on Food Patterns

The foods people eat are crucial to their health and nutritional status. Both kinds and amounts of food make a difference in whether individuals will be well- or poorly nourished. If there is not enough food, they will go hungry and eventually become undernourished. On the other hand, when the food supply is plentiful, people may eat to excess or choose poorly. Abundance in itself does not guarantee an adequate diet or superior nutritional status.

People in every part of the world tend to develop patterns of eating, whether food is scarce or abundant. When they are long continued, such patterns characterize the food habits of groups living under similar conditions of food supplies. This is true for geographic areas such as small neighborhood units or subcontinents, as well as for ethnic groups or religious sects among whom special beliefs and customs are also involved. Under such circumstances, the food patterns—good or poor—ultimately provide presumptive evidence of the nutritional status of the group. Since eating practices of individuals closely resemble those of the group to which they belong, it is advantageous to explore some of the more obvious influences in personal food selection. Students can begin by identifying factors that have helped to shape their own current eating practices.

PERSONAL REACTIONS TO FOOD

Given a choice, people usually eat the foods they like—but what determines which foods these are? Individuals eat certain foods and refuse others for many different reasons, and often the reasons are related only indirectly to the foods themselves. Can you identify the reasons *you* particularly like or dislike certain foods?

As a means of focusing attention on your own food practices, keep a record of the food you eat for a period of 3 days. Choose days that are representative of your normal eating pattern. See Appendix A for the form and method of keeping your meal record. Since this record is to be the basis for other class activities, suggestions for keeping the record should be followed carefully.

When the record has been completed, classify the major items as follows: favorite foods; foods that you have learned to like and take some pleasure in eating now; and foods that you merely tolerate. Finally, note some common foods that do not appear on your meal record because you have an aversion to them. Make a serious effort to account for your attitudes toward the foods in each category.

A class discussion with comparisons of records can be helpful, and exchanging experiences will bring out similarities and differences. Students will mention foods they have always disliked, and why; foods they accepted from the first; and foods they have learned to like. Some will recall items their mothers insisted they eat as children, but which they rejected—perhaps carrots, beets, squash, grapefruit, spinach, or others. Did the urging prompt rejection, or the texture or flavor of the food itself? Other students may point out that many of these foods are their favorites, perhaps because of the special ways they were prepared at home, or because they planted, harvested, or cooked the foods themselves.

Many students will disclose that their attitudes toward some foods have been altered through the years, while other attitudes have remained unchanged. Some people have accepted certain foods because their peers ate them; they have taught themselves to like still other foods, such as shrimp, ripe olives, and avocados, because of their prestige value. Those who today enjoy eating most foods may recall home meals as enjoyable experiences with appetizing foods offered in a relaxed atmosphere, free of controversy and pressures. They may also be able to trace their present venturesome spirit with respect to eating new foods to enjoying ethnic meals with friends and neighbors in pleasant settings.

An exchange of experiences gives individuals added insight into the reasons for their own present food patterns. They may ask themselves, for example: Is my current choice of foods broad or limited? Do I give thought to the nutritional quality of my meals? Is food psychologically important to me? Answers to such questions lay the groundwork for exploring and understanding the many factors that enter into food preferences and acceptance.

Food Preferences

The food preferences of a considerable number of men, women, boys, and girls in the United States have been obtained by interview, observation, questionnaire, and food checklist. A few highlights of these many investigations are summarized here.

Attitudes of the majority of individuals studied were, on the whole, favorable to most of the food classes. Milk, meats, fruits, most cereals and breads, a few vegetables, and almost all desserts usually ranked high on the list of liked foods. There were, however, two chief drawbacks to this favorable picture. Investigators found a marked refusal of certain items *within* food groups, which had the effect of limiting selection. Beef and chicken, for example, were popular among meats, but organ meats were largely rejected. In one study of teenage food preferences, liver was found in more lists of "foods most disliked" than any other item (1). Cooked vegetables were the most unpopular food group, and green or yellow vegetables were disliked more consistently than others. Studies also discovered that nutritionally important foods were used sparingly. Most people professed a favorable attitude toward citrus fruits and milk, for instance, but used them in smaller-than-recommended amounts.

A recent nationwide study of consumers' preferences and uses of vegetables revealed that corn, white potatoes, and tomatoes—the vegetables best liked by adults—were also well liked by younger family members. Eggplant and turnips were disliked by both age groups. Children seemed to dislike more vegetables than adults did, and taste was the reason most frequently given for liking or disliking particular vegetables (2).

In another study, preschool children and their mothers were found to be in close agreement on preferences within the meat and bread-cereal groups. The children, all of whom were attending social intervention programs such as Head Start or day care centers, had a more diversified diet than their mothers. Yet, there was a high proportion overall of food items that were liked or disliked by both mother and child. (There was considerable variation in preferences for foods in the milk and fruit-vegetable groups, however.) Interestingly, many foods a mother had never tasted were also unfamiliar to her child. Most of the women felt that their own mothers or other relatives had exercised the greatest influence on their eating practices (3).

The generally negative attitude toward vegetables emphasizes the need for children to know and like items in this important food group at an early age. Teachers' and parents' attitudes toward all foods are major influences in creating children's preferences. Studies show that foods rejected by children—particularly vegetables—

are often those their parents dislike or do not serve at home. Tasting lessons at school and other experiences in classrooms and lunchrooms can help children to like many foods, including vegetables. But effort should be made to include parents in such projects as well.

Food Acceptance (4, 5)

Flavor is a major factor in food acceptance. This complex phenomenon involves the taste, aroma, texture, and temperature of food. Appearance, including color and form, also affects attitudes toward food. Thus, the physical characteristics of foods exert a profound influence on acceptance.

Acceptance of food has broad implications for nutrition. It can determine whether needy nations will adopt and use unfamiliar food products that provide the nutrients they require. It can also be the deciding factor in whether a new food product will be manufactured and marketed, perhaps on a worldwide scale. Food industries strive to capture in their processed foods the alluring flavors that the public associates with natural tastes, such as that of freshly baked homemade bread (Fig. 1.1).

In developing new products and in quality control, companies attempt to measure qualities that predict consumer acceptance. Instruments and tests have been devised for determining objectively some specific aspects of color, flavor, and texture. For example, a special apparatus measures relative shear resistance of meat that corresponds to human judgments of meat tenderness. Such laboratory tests supplement, but cannot replace, the evaluation of foods by human sense organs, since the ultimate success of a product depends on its acceptance by people. Results of sensory tests are used routinely and are highly regarded in new product development.

Sensory tests are of two general types: evaluations by small

Figure 1.1
Retention of fresh flavor characteristics and nutrient qualities are important goals of modern food processors. This rotary retort, shown in a pilot plant, reproduces commercial production conditions. (PFW/Hercules Food Technology Center)

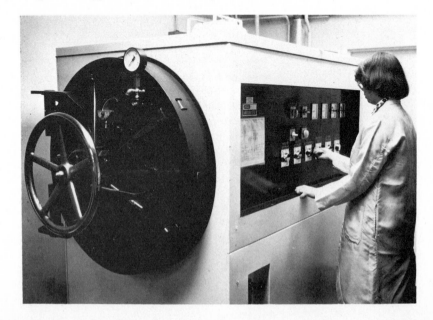

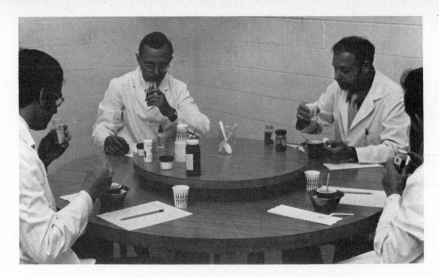

Figure 1.2
A specific type of sensory test is the flavor panel procedure carried out by a panel of judges highly trained in techniques of recognizing and describing separate flavor and aroma components of a particular kind of food. The panel as a group develops the flavor profile of the product under consideration. (Campbell Institute for Food Research)

groups of people who have been trained to make fine distinctions in flavor, aroma, and texture (Fig. 1.2); and preference tests in which large numbers of untrained subjects express their general likes and dislikes of products (Fig. 1.3). After careful pretesting to anticipate general consumer acceptance, food industries select for mass production only those items that give the greatest promise of consumer selection.

A look at the *physiological* mechanisms involved in each individual's judgment of food can shed some light on the complexity of food acceptance. Hunger and appetite are basic considerations.

physiological
Pertaining to functions of the body

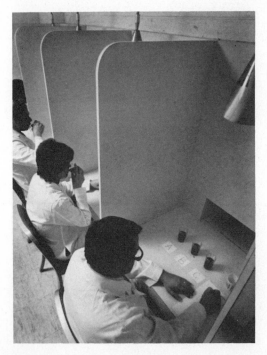

Figure 1.3
One type of sensory test involves a taste panel of experienced, but not necessarily trained, judges who make individual decisions regarding flavor, aroma and texture of foods. Many companies utilize data from such tests in the development and evaluation of products. (Campbell Institute for Food Research)

Hunger and Appetite (6)

Throughout life, every individual requires a continuous supply of energy and certain essential nutrients for survival. Hunger and appetite are sensations that serve as reminders of the need for food. People may say they are hungry at mealtime or that they have a good appetite. But hunger and appetite are not identical, and the difference between them is important in understanding food habits. *Hunger* is an unpleasant sensation resulting from deprivation of food. It is largely an unlearned, or instinctive, response. *Appetite*, a pleasant sensation to some degree, pertains to the desire to eat. It is largely a learned, or acquired, response.

Hunger   Hunger is a compelling drive with both a physiological and a psychological basis. People who are hungry are able to concentrate on little other than their physical need for food. Hunger is immediately relieved when food is eaten.

The sensation of hunger is perceived when a particular portion of the *hypothalamus* in the brain is stimulated (Fig. 1.4). There are many theories about conditions that constitute stimuli. Hunger pangs, or gastric contractions, are probably an important part of the sensory complex recognized as hunger. Numerous other sensations are recognized by various individuals as hunger signals. *Satiety*, the cessation of the urge to eat, is not linked with any particular sensation but frequently is associated with a change in mood. Sensations of gastric fullness may or may not accompany satiety. Research studies in animals and humans have resulted in many hypotheses, but as yet there is no well-substantiated theory to describe mechanisms controlling food intake.

hypothalamus
Concerned with control of appetite

Appetite   The desire to eat undoubtedly arises both from hunger and appetite; however, appetite may function long after the body's physiological need for food has been satisfied. An individual's appetite is affected by many factors relevant to both past and present experiences. These include cultural and meal-habit influences in childhood, as well as a multitude of stimuli operating in one's cur-

Figure 1.4
Hypothalamus

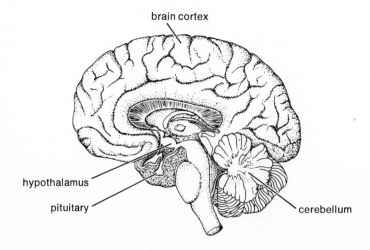

brain cortex

hypothalamus

pituitary

cerebellum

rent environment, such as the ready availability and palatability of food, the nature and atmosphere of the surroundings, and personal taste for individual foods.

Contrary to widely held opinion, human appetite is not guided by instinct. The high incidence of overweight in the United States bears witness to the fact that appetite is an unreliable guide to the *amount* of food needed. Nor is appetite a satisfactory indication of the *kinds* of nutrients required. Early research suggested the ability of experimental animals to select from their feed those elements that satisfied their nutrient needs. There is now evidence that such choices are not consistently reliable (7). The view that human cravings for certain foods signifies physiological need for specific nutrients has not been proved. Studies made half a century ago, purporting to demonstrate that infants can select from an array of foods those needed for an adequate diet, have since been discounted. Even casual observation shows that appetite is unreliable. Once children have eaten a variety of foods, they develop taste preferences based on factors entirely unrelated to nutritional values. Obviously, the same conclusion applies to adults. People accustomed to high-fat or high-sweet diets, for example, have a strong appetite for foods of this type, even though these may be the very foods they should avoid.

Certain perversions of appetite are well known, although not fully understood. A habit known as *pica* is observed chiefly in poorly fed pregnant women and preschool children in lower socioeconomic groups of the United States and in developing nations. It consists of eating certain foods such as cornstarch in large amounts, and the consumption of many nonfood items such as laundry starch, clay, and plaster.

Geophagia, an aspect of pica, is practiced in various parts of the world. There is some evidence that geophagia leads to iron deficiency, possibly because of the fact that it inhibits iron absorption (8, 9). Findings of the Ten-State Nutrition Survey (see p. 71) in low-income areas in the United States have shown pica to exist where *anemia* is also prevalent. The custom of pica is apparently passed on from one generation to another. It has been proposed that people experience this unusual craving due to nutrient lacks in their diets. In studies to determine its cause, however, vitamin and mineral supplements were found to be ineffective in dealing with pica. Current belief holds that pica may be a complicated cultural and psychological problem arising from unmet emotional needs.

Enjoyment of Food

The enjoyment of food has even wider implications for food habits than appetite does. It includes memory and experience, the atmosphere in which food is eaten, and the companionship enjoyed with it. Eating is a social rite among all cultures, and it is endowed with much symbolism for friendliness, sociability, and rapport. Eating alone is usually a dreary experience. Lone eaters are apt to eat a limited variety of foods, to undereat or overeat, and to hurry through their meals without enjoying them. Conversely, eating at-

geophagia
Earth-eating; a perversion of appetite

anemia
Deficiency in the oxygen-carrying capacity of the blood

tractive food in pleasant surroundings with congenial company is not only a satisfying social experience, but it also creates the most favorable conditions for the physiological utilization of food.

Enjoyment of food depends in part upon its stimulation of the sense organs. Impressions of food are usually general ones, with the various sensory perceptions coming in close succession. Sight and taste are well recognized as being important in stimulating and satisfying the appetite, but the senses of touch, hearing, and smell also add much to eating pleasure. The aroma of foods actually contributes more to our perception of flavor than does taste. Humans have several thousand taste-receptor cells but are endowed with millions of *olfactory* receptors. Thousands of odors are distinguishable, compared with only four basic tastes. Blending of tastes combined with numerous odors provide for countless interesting flavors. A brief examination of the sensory organs and the way they function can help in understanding and appreciating their roles in food selection and acceptance.

olfactory
Relating to the sense of smell

Sensory Perception of Food (10, 11, 12)

Appetite and the perception of food by the sense organs are closely related. Appearance, aroma, flavor, and texture are well-known and widely used as appetite stimulants. These attributes of food are very important in the acceptance of foods and in the establishment of food habits.

Vision   The first test foods must pass is the visual one, since a meal is often evaluated on the basis of its appearance on the plate. The colors, shapes, and forms of foods may have such eye appeal as to entice one to eat even when not hungry. On the other hand, an unattractive array of food may be rejected without even being tasted.

In addition to being appetite-stimulating, general appearance and color are useful indicators of quality, freshness, and ripeness. In the selection of fruits and vegetables, for example, one is guided by such visual aspects as size and degree of typical color development. The senses of touch and smell also participate in judgments of quality. Peaches that are small, green, and hard with no detectable aroma certainly have little appeal. On the other hand, long, straight, firm green beans with deep color pass the visual and touch tests, and a bright red, shiny slice of watermelon with its sweet aroma is hard to resist. Many food purchasing decisions are also made on the basis of color photography in advertisements.

Smell   Along with vision, the olfactory sense is utilized in evaluating food quality and detecting spoilage. The senses alone cannot be relied upon, however, as a means of protecting people from ingesting harmful substances.

Receptors for the sense of smell are the endings of olfactory nerve fibers, located in the upper part of the nose. The olfactory cells in the mucous membrane are surrounded by supporting cells and by glands (Fig. 1.5). Only volatile substances dissolved in the fluid of the mucous membrane stimulate these receptors of odor. In

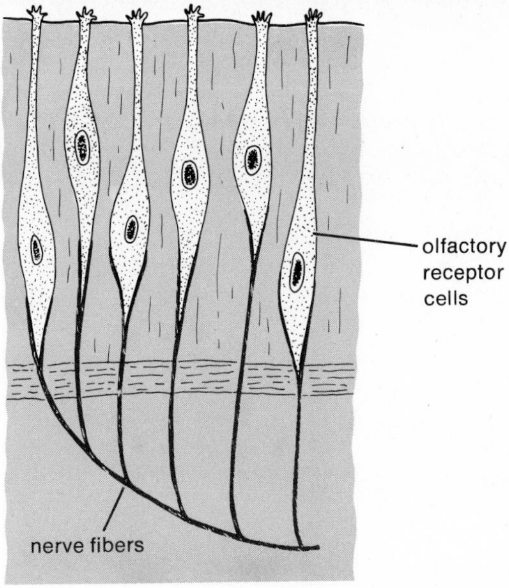

Figure 1.5
Olfactory Cells
(Dina Kazanowski, artist)

olfactory
receptor
cells

nerve fibers

normal breathing, very little air reaches the area where the olfactory receptors are located, but sniffing draws more air into the region. The olfactory system is extremely sensitive and can perceive very low concentrations of odorous substances. The aromas of foods such as fresh fruits, herbs, spices, and coffee are important factors in appetite stimulation and the consumption and enjoyment of food. The appeal of specific odors varies among cultures as well as between individuals.

papillae
Small projections on the upper surface of the tongue

Taste   Taste, often confused with smell, is a mixture of four sensations perceived in the mouth as sweet, bitter, salty, and sour. Taste buds, located chiefly in *papillae* on the tongue, are the receptors for the sense of taste. (Certain other regions of the mouth and throat are responsive to taste stimuli to a lesser degree.) Each taste bud is composed of ten to fifteen sensory cells. Solutions entering an opening or pore at the top of each taste bud stimulate taste receptors (Fig. 1.6). Only substances in solution can be tasted, and one of the functions of saliva is to dissolve foods that are dry when taken into the mouth. Particular areas of the tongue are more sensitive to certain tastes than to others. The tip of the tongue is especially sensitive to sweet, the back to bitter, the sides to sour, and both the tip and the sides to salt. A person who likes the taste of pretzels is responding positively to the salt stimulus.

Taste, as well as the other senses, is subject to adaptation. Continuous exposure to stimuli gradually results in reduced sensitivity, as in the case of overuse of salt or sugar. Sensitivity also varies with the temperature of the food and among individuals. When the same product is served both warm and cold, it will be perceived as saltier when cold.

Touch   The term *touch* includes a variety of sensations aroused in the skin. Pressure, pain, and temperature changes can be distin-

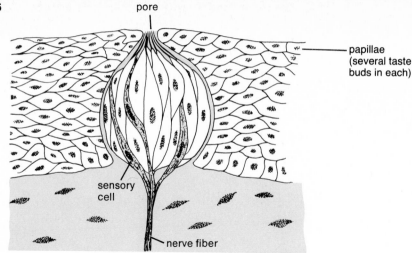

Figure 1.6
Taste Bud
(Dina Kazanowski, artist)

pore

papillae
(several taste
buds in each)

sensory
cell

nerve fiber

guished. Many more subdivisions of surface sensations are sometimes listed. Condiments such as pepper, curry, and other "hot" seasonings elicit a pain reaction. Some skin discriminations important in food selection and appreciation are stickiness, oiliness, hardness and softness, roughness and smoothness, wetness and dryness.

The *kinesthetic* sense is responsible for the appreciation of textures that offer some resistance to chewing. The receptors, located in the muscles of the jaw, are stimulated by chewing such foods as crisp raw vegetables or fruits, and crunchy dry cereals or crackers.

Temperature produces a direct hot or cold sensation, of course, but it also modifies odors and tastes and brings about physical and volatility changes in certain foods.

kinesthetic
Pertaining to the perception of muscular motion

Sound The *auditory* sense is of less significance with regard to food than the other senses described here, but it does play a role. Vibrations enter the external ear, reach the ear drum, and cause it to oscillate. The resulting vibrations are in turn transmitted through the middle ear by air conduction and then by bone conduction, until they reach the fluid of the inner ear in which the endings of the auditory nerve are immersed.

The spattering, sizzling sounds of meat cooking on the grill are appetite-stimulating to many people, especially when accompanied by the aroma. The clink of ice against glass when a cold drink is stirred, the crackle of eating potato chips, and the snapping sound made when a crisp apple or celery stalk is bitten are other familiar examples of auditory stimuli.

All normal, healthy human beings possess the same physiological mechanisms for sensory perception, although there are wide variations among individuals in sensitivity to stimuli. Understanding how the mechanisms function represents a challenge of considerable interest, but appreciating the various responses of individuals to sensory stimuli is even more fascinating. Why is it that the

auditory
Relating to the sense of hearing

very taste, odor, and textural characteristics that make some foods highly desirable to one cultural group make the same foods repugnant and intolerable to others?

Turn back to your food record and the lists you made of favorite foods, foods you tolerate, and foods you avoid. Can you explain why you like or dislike certain items in terms of your sensory reactions to them?

Have you attempted to distinguish between perception of taste and perception of aroma in considering why certain flavors appeal to you and others do not?

Are there any textural qualities of foods that you find particularly appealing? If so, why?

CULTURAL BACKGROUNDS

Just as sensory perception influences the foods people choose, so also does their cultural background determine their eating patterns. Culture consists of values, modes of thought, customs, and habits that are socially learned. Food habits of the people in any society develop within the framework of this broad concept. Eating practices of the society and its subgroups become those of individuals. They assume these habits as their own and—through the ideas associated with them—see and interpret all their experiences with food and eating.

Food habits of a group or an individual may be static, particularly when cultures are old and tradition rules the way of life. This is equally true when people live in closely integrated units and when food supplies have been limited for generations to a few staple items. Under such circumstances, people literally go hungry rather than defy tradition by eating foods not specifically prescribed by their cultural pattern.

History of Food Customs

Patterns of eating have been recognized since the beginning of history. Terrain, climate, and the life styles of peoples largely determined the nature of the food supply. The kinds of foods have also depended on whether the people were hunters or herdsmen, or were gatherers or growers of crops. For the herdsmen, meat and often milk were a major part of the diet; for the gatherers or growers, wild vegetables or grains were their chief foods. Even today, natural resources and traditions remain important determinants of dietary practice and habit formation.

Religions have also been linked with food habits of many peoples of the world, and cultural patterns often result from an intermingling of religious and other influences. Judaism probably traces its dietary practices more directly to biblical precept than does any other religion. Many of the present food habits of Orthodox Jews are based on Old Testament teachings, obeyed in greater or lesser degrees. Even among Jews who disregard routine directives, the ceremonial aspects of the diet code are often maintained, particularly during major religious festivals. This section simply points out some of the ways in which the code affects meal practices.

It is a well-known rule, for example, that meats and dairy foods cannot be served at the same meal, and that a specified amount of time must elapse after eating one before the other can be consumed. Meat selections are almost limitless, for the list of acceptable flesh food sources includes all cud-chewing quadrupeds with divided hooves. Pork is practically the only meat excluded. All animals must be selected and slaughtered under methods prescribed by Jewish law, and the meat must be drained of blood; that is, it must be *kosher*. All kinds of poultry and most kinds of fish (except shellfish) are allowed. Milk, cheese, cream, and butter may be used liberally, provided there is no conflict with the rule forbidding the use of meat and milk at the same meal.

Most of the diet regulations apply to the use of protein foods. Vegetables, fruits, cereal products, and breads can be eaten virtually without restriction. Thus the Jewish diet code allows for a varied eating pattern that can provide for nutritional adequacy. (For readers interested in the basis of the Jewish dietary code and details of its modern implementation, source material is available (13)).

Food Customs and Nutrition

The physiques and health of peoples living for generations on traditional diets reflect the nature of those diets. One of the earliest human nutrition experiments compared the diets of two neighboring tribes of East Indians—one tall, vigorous, and healthy; the other poorly developed and weak. The study was conducted by a British physician on assignment in India at the time (14). Traditionally, members of the more vigorous tribe were users of whole grains, meat, vegetables, and milk; the poorly developed tribe existed chiefly on polished rice, coffee with sugar, betel nuts, and little milk. To test his theory that diet was largely responsible for the physical differences between the tribes, the investigator fed the contrasting diets to two colonies of experimental animals. His findings convinced him that nutrition had made the difference.

Such a sharp contrast can rarely be seen except in a situation of the type cited. Differences are more clearcut and measurable among primitive peoples when there are few food items and even small variations in diet can make a significant impact on nutritional intake. This does not mean that it cannot happen in modern times nor to any nation or subgroup if certain of its food practices are altered. Chapter 3 cites the experiences of one nation—Japan—that has improved the physical growth pattern of its children in recent years by adopting certain new food practices in line with current nutrition knowledge. This was a dramatic nationwide development. It is more common to work for habit changes on a smaller scale and to expect somewhat less spectacular results in terms of improved nutritional status. The nutritional needs of small segments of populations are usually identified first, followed by specific efforts to improve dietary patterns. A problem encountered in older cultures is that long-standing taboos control eating practices and particularly decree which foods must be banned from diets.

Seemingly minor food customs that are contrary to good nutrition can have widespread consequences. This is true particularly when they represent deep-seated taboos that are all but impossible to eliminate, or when they apply through several generations to all members of the family. In many parts of the world customs and beliefs dictate the omission of certain foods, especially milk, eggs, meat, and fish. Unfortunately, the taboos usually affect the most vulnerable members of the family—infants, children, and pregnant and *lactating women* (15). Not only is the reasoning behind the taboos usually faulty, but these practices can result in undernourished peoples while valuable food goes to waste. For example, in many parts of the world where native fish are plentiful and needed as a source of protein, taboos prevent their consumption. Similarly, cattle abound in some areas where cultural customs rule against their use as food even though the population lacks meat and milk. Young children are undernourished in some countries where custom dictates that, at weaning, they be transferred immediately to an adult diet consisting chiefly of starchy foods lacking adequate nutrients for growth and development.

These examples could be multiplied many times, and they would not be confined to old cultures. Practices that distort eating patterns to the point at which they become detrimental to health exist in all industrial nations, including the United States. The following of food fads is one way in which desirable eating patterns may be seriously disrupted.

lactating women
Nursing mothers

> Obtain a typical day's menus of an individual or family whose eating habits are quite different from your own. Try to identify religious, national, racial, or other influences with these menus.
>
> Compile a list of beliefs, prejudices, and taboos about foods. Which of them do you think might stand in the way of obtaining an adequate diet?

As we have seen, food habits of the past are relevant in the present. Knowledge of past habits sheds light on ways to approach the study of current food patterns; many practices have come down through the centuries. But while food habits in ancient times were static, because the conditions that sustained them were fixed, now we are dealing with a fluid situation with many rapidly changing conditions. Even the oldest cultures are touched by change, including those that had been impervious for generations to inroads on their eating patterns. Aspects of such changes and conditions that create them are discussed elsewhere, notably in Chapters 3, 12, and 15.

Food patterns in the United States are unique in that they have been influenced by those of almost all sections of the world. A fascinating aspect of this development is the youth of the United States, and the fact that its recent—even current—cultural history is literally unfolding before our eyes. Our information about many events comes less from formal records than from participants at various stages in this evolution—our grandparents and parents—and from our own observations. The predominant eating patterns of the United States represent the contributions of foods and customs from many other cultures. The culmination is the varied patterns of eating that continue to change as the mix of the population shifts with continuing migrations and in-migrations.

FAMILY EATING PATTERNS IN THE UNITED STATES

The history of eating patterns in the United States covers nearly 400 years. This span of time has been divided by one student of the subject into three periods, each of which makes a distinctive contribution to its own time and to the periods that follow: the Colonial period (1600–1766); the period of westward exploration, development, and industrialization (1800–1900); and the period of the 20th century, which benefited from the influence of nutrition knowledge and technology (16, 17). Migrations have been a factor in all three periods.

Historical Origins

The early period of colonization saw a blending of the food habits brought by the colonists with those they adopted in the new land. Foods long grown in America by the Indians—such as corn, beans, and pumpkins—together with the abundant native fish, game, berries, and maple sugar, formed the basis of early meal patterns. Chickens, hogs, and cows, as well as apple trees and other fruit trees, were eventually brought from Europe to broaden the diet. In the first years, there were periods of near starvation. Later there was abundance and variety in some localities, particularly on the plantations of Virginia. Meals there were bountiful, with many foods served at one meal. Ham, beef, chicken, duck, and many lavish sweets were common items.

From the first, foods and meal patterns differed somewhat in the North and South, due in part to climatic conditions. Southern families enjoyed sweet potatoes, fruits, fowl, hot biscuits, corn products including fried mush, and puddings. Venison sometimes supplemented the meat supply. Sauces and condiments were used to make the meals more elaborate. Pies, including pumpkin and apple, were served frequently. In the North, breadstuffs from flour of home-grown wheat and rye were used to make pancakes, waffles, crullers, and doughnuts. Codfish was a staple item of diet. Boston brown bread, made from corn, wheat, or rye, was sweetened with native maple syrup (18).

The period of westward migration introduced different types of foods—those that could be carried easily across plains, such as salt pork, dry corn, and beans; those that could be obtained by hunting, including venison, bear meat, and game birds; and those that the settlers found plentiful in their new environments. In the Southwest and Far West, the pioneers encountered the Spanish influence in food, for example, the use of chili peppers. In the Midwest there were the contributions of European settlers—typical foods of Scandinavia, Holland, and England. The second half of the 19th century saw a great diversification of food supplies due to improved transportation, refrigeration, better facilities for cooking, new methods of preserving foods, and the tremendous influx of immigrants. In all newly settled areas there was active interchange of native dishes among the residents. Many foods were thus added to family meal patterns.

The 20th century brought a different influence on meal patterns—the new science of nutrition. For the first time people could choose certain foods because of their nutrient values. Food technology was also developing, and unprecedented strides were made in processing, manufacturing, and packaging foods. Many seasonal foods were made available year round. The boundaries of the American meal pattern became virtually limitless.

Eating Patterns Today

The United States today is regarded as a melting pot of ethnic groups, with no distinctive food-habit pattern of its own. The variety and abundance of its food supply, the different origins of the people who comprise its population, and its vast geographical area would seem to support this view. But the very size of the country gives rise to subcultures and regional food-habit patterns. Certain geographic regions have become known for their traditional foods. Boston baked beans, codfish cakes, and clam chowder are associated with New England; corn, beans, and peppers dominate the dishes of the Southwest; fried chicken, grits, turnip greens, and hot biscuits reflect traditional meal patterns of the Southeast. Household dietary surveys made periodically by the US Department of Agriculture substantiate the fact that some foods are eaten in greater quantities in one region of the country than another. For example, rural households in the southern region in 1965 were shown to be using ten times as much cornmeal and grits and sixteen times as much rice as rural households of comparable income in the north central region (19).

Ethnic and religious groups also have retained some of their food practices for generations. National and racial groups who migrate to the United States retain features of their original eating customs to some degree, depending on the length of their stay and the availability of their native foods. Thus some eating patterns persist. But influences for change are also at work; the melding process is never ending.

The Melding Process

Since Colonial times, families from all parts of the world have settled in the United States, bringing their food habits with them. Their customs have made, and continue to make, an impact on American eating patterns, as a few examples illustrate.

Europe   The so-called "historic core" of the traditional German diet is characterized by heavy soups, sausage, rye bread, and pork products such as pickled pigs' feet. These foods, once eaten only by German immigrants, are now relished by people of all origins (20). The Scots brought barley broth, oatmeal, oat cakes, and scones; the English, plum pudding, rabbit and chicken pie, turnip greens, and pecan turkey stuffing. With the arrival of the Irish, the white potato came back to its native American soil. The Dutch introduced the doughnut to America, along with cole slaw and head cheese (18). The Italians brought pastas, minestrone soup, olive oil, and Italian bread. In city centers where Italian families settle, neighborhood stores stock native foods that children of Italian parents learn to eat and enjoy. The dedication of Italian-Americans to their native foods has resulted in widespread acceptance of them throughout the United States. The influence continues; habits are perpetuated. As succeeding generations of Italians remain, their dietary patterns tend to diversify, but rarely do even second- or third-generation families relinquish their favorite native dishes. Meanwhile, many of these foods have become regular menu items in homes across the country.

Middle East (21)   Families coming from the Middle East have introduced not so much unfamiliar foods, as new ways of preparing those already known. Such dishes are distinctive in their use of spices and seasonings native to those areas of the world. Thus a different influence has been exerted on eating patterns in the United States. The Middle East embraces a vast area, from Morocco eastward to Pakistan, and from Greece and Turkey southward to the Sudan in Africa. Understandably, differences as well as similarities in eating patterns exist. Many dietary traditions and influences affect the habits in different areas. Religion, culture, and economics are modifying factors. Immigrants from such countries as Turkey, Armenia, and Syria enjoy certain foods in common, due to the similarities of climate and soil in that area. Their food habits have been shaped by the large assortment of agricultural products available to them in sections of their homelands where water is abundant. Many of their eating customs are continued when they come to the United States. Their dishes have interesting flavors, but generally speaking they are not highly seasoned. Combinations of spices are often used. Cardamom, fenugreek, and garlic are the individual seasonings that are frequently added, sometimes to the point of obscuring the natural flavors of the main foods. The United States annually imports many varieties of spices (such as cinnamon, marjoram, mint, and coriander) from the Middle East, as well as from other areas of the world. The demand is attributed in part to the needs of ethnic groups who use the spices in the preparation of their native dishes. Adventurous cooks of all ethnic backgrounds have learned to prepare such dishes, however, and many families have learned to enjoy them.

Lamb is a favorite meat in most Middle Eastern countries, although goat meat, chicken, duck, and goose are also well liked. A wide variety of vegetables and fruits grown in the Middle East—such as eggplant, artichoke, cucumbers, black olives, dates, raisins, figs, grapes, and melons—are being used in the United States in increasing quantities. Vegetables are traditionally prepared with native seasonings and often fried in olive oil. Pickled vegetables are also favorites. Fruits are usually eaten raw. Rice and wheat are the staple grains of the Middle East. Round, flat loaves of wheat bread are baked on griddles atop the stove. Cheeses and yogurt made of sour milk—often goat's milk—are preferred forms of dairy foods. People from the Middle East enjoy nuts, sugar, honey, molasses, and candied fruits in their rich desserts, and they drink large amounts of sweetened tea. Many of these preferences are evident in American eating patterns today.

East and Southeast Asia   Families coming to the United States from East and Southeast Asia have brought to the West new food combinations and unusual methods of preparing dishes. They have greatly widened our food selection, as evidenced by the popularity of Oriental restuarants and the demand for Oriental foods in convenient form for use in homes. Peoples of the Far East—Japan, China, Vietnam, and Thailand, as well as the Philippines, Indonesia, and the smaller islands—serve many of the same basic foods. Each major geographic division has certain of its own characteristic eating practices, however, traceable in part to the influence of various peoples who have occupied each territory at different periods in history. A major dietary similarity is the use of rice, which is preferred over other grains and takes the place of bread as it is used in the United States. Another important dietary item is fermented foods. Fermented grains, for example, are commonly used and thought to be superior in flavor and digestibility. These, too, have found favor in the United States. Milk—much of it in fermented form—is used sparingly throughout East and Southeast Asia. Seafoods are basic items of diet, and fish is often eaten raw. Soybeans provide an important source of protein, often in the form of soybean paste or soybean curd. Meats are generally eaten in small quantities, often cut into small pieces and cooked with vegetables. Bean sprouts and bamboo shoots, popular vegetables in most parts of the Far East, are being used in American households. With increased interest in Oriental foods and cookery, the *wok*, a frypan of Oriental origin, has become a familiar kitchen tool. It is designed particularly for stir-frying vegetables to the tender-crisp stage. Traditional foods and dishes of Japan and China, particularly, have become familiar items of eating patterns in the United States.

Latin America   In Latin America, Mexico stands out as the country having the most pronounced effect on food patterns of the United States. This would be expected, considering the proximity of the two countries, the frequent travel between them, and the constant migration north across the border. People in the United States have learned to know and like Mexican food, to enjoy it in many Mexican restaurants, and to prepare it regularly in their homes. The traditional diet of Mexico is a blend of Spanish and Indian foods. The core diet consists of dry beans, chili peppers, and corn. Mexican dishes have two outstanding characteristics: they

Figure 1.7
People of the United States adapt ethnic foods to their own tastes, using available ingredients, while retaining the unique characteristics of the dishes. Mexican tacos, for example, with their traditional beef, cheese and lettuce filling, lend themselves to a variety of additional fillings including peppers, tomatoes, onions and avocados. (United Dairy Industry Association)

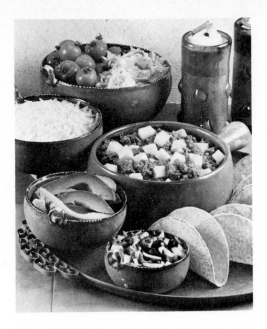

are most often mixtures of foods, and they are usually highly seasoned, due either to the seasonings added to the dishes themselves or to the hot chili sauces served over them. Probably the single food most appreciated and readily adopted in the United States is Mexico's pepper, in all of its sizes, shades, and varied degrees of hotness. These peppers are available in most supermarkets north of the border, and they not only provide the basis of many Mexican dishes but also add much to the general cuisine of the United States (22, 23).

Mexican dishes best known in the United States are tortillas, tacos, tamales, enchiladas, and pasolé. Their ingredients are increasingly available in large city markets, especially in Mexican communities. Convenience foods have made it possible to enjoy some Mexican dishes with little effort required for preparation. Tortillas and taco shells can be purchased ready for fillings. Some other foods or their essential ingredients are now available in canned or frozen form, and chili powders and sauces and chili con carne are available in various forms. With these opportunities to become familiar with Mexican foods, many non-Mexicans acquire a taste for them (Fig. 1.7). (See Appendix C for more detail on the Mexican diet.)

There is less migration to the United States from other countries of Central and South America than from Mexico. These countries have little direct impact on the United States eating pattern. Throughout the area there is great diversity in food supplies and eating practices due to differences in terrain, the vast territory some nations cover, and the range of soils and temperatures. The food habits of Brazil are covered in Chapter 15 in a discussion of daily food selection guides as a worldwide teaching tool.

Other Areas of the World   There are many other areas of the world that have contributed or are contributing in some degree to United States eating patterns. Africa is one example. Because of the developing nature of many nations, there is a minimum of migration. The greatest contact is probably through scholarship students to United States educational institutions, tourists, and official personnel of the United States stationed in these countries.

Puerto Rico (24, 25, 26)   The steady migration from the island of Puerto Rico to the mainland of the United States accounts for the spread of Puerto Rican food habit patterns in certain areas. The origin of the Puerto Rican diet, like that of Mexico, is strongly Spanish. The core of the traditional Puerto Rican diet is limited to a few basic foods—beans, rice, and *viandas* (starchy vegetables and unripe starchy fruits). Lard is commonly used for cooking, and café con leche (coffee with milk) is a regular accompaniment of the diet. The basic diet is typical for low-income rural families on the island, and it continues to serve as the nucleus for meals even in urban and industrialized areas where many other foods are increasingly available through supermarkets. Rice and beans are served together in a meal, and it is customary for many families to eat them twice daily. Puerto Ricans have a strong preference for their traditional diet and they do not accept substitutes easily. Migrants demand that supermarkets and neighborhood stores stock their favorite foods. The large numbers of migrants enhance their chances for success in obtaining these items. As these foods come into the market—beans of many kinds and descriptions, for example—non-Puerto Rican families try them and eventually incorporate the ones they like into their own eating patterns. (See Appendix B for more detail on the native Puerto Rican diet.)

In-Migrants   Still another potential for change in dietary patterns occurs when ethnic groups move from one geographic area to another within the boundaries of the United States. They often carry regional eating customs with them and to some degree stimulate change in the food patterns of those with whom they come in contact. Blacks and American Indians are two notable examples of current in-migrants.

Blacks often migrate from the rural south to urban areas, largely in the north (27). The basic pattern of the traditional southern diet consists of "greens," pork, and corn in various forms. The diet may be greatly improved, and even made nutritionally adequate, if there is opportunity to produce or gather additional foods. Fresh garden "greens" and the pot liquor in which the greens are cooked are important components of even an otherwise inferior southern diet. This dedication to "greens" remains strong even in new locations. If it has not stimulated the present enthusiasm for *fresh* vegetables now exhibited, especially among young vegetarians, at least it has reinforced a desirable trend. Rural southern blacks also bring to their new environments interest in and knowledge of soul foods (See Appendix D for more details on diets of blacks.)

American Indians migrate from some 300 reservations in various parts of the United States (26). Generally speaking, diets of reservation Indians reflect the traditional eating practices of the particular regions in which the reservations are located, as well as those of resident tribes. The diets of Indians from the *Southwest,* for example, reflect the Spanish influence of that section. They are high in chili peppers, corn and other grain products, fats, and sugar. Most tribes of the Southwest use large quantities of dry beans and eat meat regularly, the amount varying with income. Milk is used sparingly. Meals are normally limited to a relatively few food items. Diets of *Plains* Indians contain large quantities of meat, potatoes, and bread. Their meals are high in fats, cereals, and sugar, and low in vegetables, fruits, and milk. Diets of modern-day *Woodlands* Indians have a base of fish, beef, and some wild game. Potatoes, corn, and dry beans are staple items of diet, and in certain areas wild rice is available. With greater variety of foods obtainable through reservation stores and federal food programs, and with increasing contacts with residents outside reservations, it is becoming difficult to identify food patterns of Indians. Indians on reservations, especially those of the younger generation, are gradually adapting to a more general American diet while retaining a few of their favorite dishes.

These favorite dishes add to the ever expanding United States food pattern. Among the traditional dishes of the Plains Indians are *wasna* or *pemmican*, a pulverized meat combined with bone grease or suet and finely ground berries; *wajapi*, a puddinglike mixture made with boiled fruits, sugar, and suet, thickened with flour; and *jerky*, made by drying thin strips of various kinds of meat. All Indians eat "fry bread," a sweetened or unsweetened biscuit dough usually fried in deep fat. Many traditional dishes are nutritious mixtures of meat or cereals, combined with dried fruits. To preserve recipes of these traditional dishes, efforts have been made to compile them for the descendants of those who originated them and for all others who may wish to broaden the boundaries of their eating patterns. (See Appendix E for general locations of tribal groups mentioned and for details of their diets.)

Current Migrations and Food Habit Problems

When ethnic groups migrate in considerable numbers to new environments in the United States, the moves are usually motivated by the desire to improve their economic status. Migrants tend to settle in city neighborhoods near friends who have preceded them and close to places of prospective employment. This characterizes the situation of many current migrants, including Puerto Ricans, Mexicans, black Americans, and American Indians. We have briefly described some native food practices of these groups and what such practices may contribute to the United States eating pattern. But there is another angle to consider, and that is what health professionals can do to assist newcomers in adjusting to new foods and new conditions.

Federal, state, and local agencies dealing with health and nutrition problems provide professional advisory and educational services to these migrant groups. Appendixes B, C, D, and E are offered as a resource for agencies and staff who require current information on the native diets of the four ethnic groups, prior to their migrations. This is done in the plausible belief that the more the diet in the new environment is patterned on the old, the more contented the migrants will be, the better they will adjust to their altered eating pattern, and the better nourished they will be in the long run. Specialists with first-hand knowledge of the premigration diets have provided the dietary data for the first section in each of the four appendixes. Information for the second and third sections, which deal with postmigration nutrition problems, has been furnished by other professionals who know and understand the food and nutrition difficulties encountered by each of these migrant groups in their new environments.

Blending of Food Patterns in the United States

Food patterns in the United States are clearly in a state of constant change. There is a typical core of foods, but it is far from being a fixed entity. As the preceding pages suggest, many influences have pressed for change from Colonial times to the present. Ethnic eating customs are prominent among these. Nutrition research has also become an everpresent stimulus. As nutritional needs are discovered, various foods are recognized as important sources of nutrients. Citrus fruits, for example, have found an established place in breakfast patterns of the United States, largely as a result of the discovery that vitamin C is an essential nutrient for the human body and that citrus fruits are important sources of this vitamin. Technology has facilitated the use of citrus fruits by providing them year round, in a variety of forms to suit the different tastes and budgets of consumers. The overall effect of these and other changes has been the continual evolution of our eating pattern.

What generates and keeps alive these forces for change? The major factors are general scientific advancement, increased contact with the rest of the world and its people, and mass communications media. Our appreciation of foreign foods is traceable not only to the influence of migrant neighbors, but also to growing international travel, residence abroad as students and civil servants, and service in the armed forces overseas. This interest is constantly sharpened by illustrations of the foods of other countries, featured in national magazines and the food pages of metropolitan newspapers as well as by aggressive food advertising. A growing number of cookbooks feature recipes and meal plans of different ethnic groups. Flourishing cooking and gourmet clubs also acquaint interested persons with the food habits and cultures of other lands.

The result of all these factors is seen not only in the wider variety of most home-cooked meals, but also in the patronage enjoyed by ethnic restaurants featuring native dishes. There are many such restaurants representing major ethnic groups in all large cities of the United States. There are also numerous small neighborhood eating places that cater to migrants from their native lands. Both types of restaurants go far in acquainting people of the United States with unfamiliar foods. In addition, the scope of ethnic restaurants is widening. It is not uncommon to find establishments featuring the dishes of Turkey, Armenia, Korea, Indonesia, Vietnam, and Thailand, as well as the more familiar Greek, Chinese, Japanese, Mexican, and Italian restaurants.

Even school lunches serve to broaden the domestic meal pattern. In one high school, typical Italian dishes such as macaroni and spaghetti were as popular with the Oriental-Americans as with the Italian-Americans. The blending process is fostered in some schools by relating foods on the lunch menu to countries being studied in classrooms. Special authentic recipes native to the countries being studied are provided by families of the school. This lays the groundwork for students to taste and appreciate, if not to like, these new dishes. Many of them do become favorites and are served repeatedly. At commercial lunch counters and snack bars, such foods as pizza, chili con carne, and tacos—once available only in ethnic restaurants and native homes—are now enjoyed by all groups.

> What do you consider typical core foods in the diet of the United States? What do you regard as typical meal patterns in your section of the country? What effect do you think such types of food services as drive-ins, fast-food chains, and vending machines have had on food habit patterns? How have these influenced your own diet?

Eating patterns respond to intrinsic, natural forces such as sensory reactions to foods, cultural exchanges among ethnic groups, and the influence of migrating populations. These are interesting phenomena, but what are their implications for human nutrition? Are the resulting food patterns nutritionally adequate, and can they be depended upon to support good nutritional status in the populations where they are found? There is abundant evidence that significant segments of some populations are inadequately nourished on their characteristic eating patterns. People do not instinctively choose the foods they need in order to be well nourished. Each generation must learn the elements of good nutritional practice. Nutrition knowledge in itself does not guarantee the adoption of good eating habits, but it does provide the base for rational decisions crucial to the formation of desirable food patterns.

EDUCATIONAL INFLUENCES ON FOOD PATTERNS

Many educational influences—planned and unplanned—help to shape eating patterns throughout life. Attitudes toward food that develop during infancy may have permanent effects on later reactions to food. Infants respond favorably to surroundings that make them comfortable, unfavorably to those that make them uncomfortable. They have a receptive attitude toward food if they are fed when hungry, in a relaxed atmosphere, and with food that satisfies them. Food thus becomes a symbol for comfort, satisfaction, and security (28). The child who has this introduction to food has a foundation for good food habits. On the other hand, babies can develop a negative attitude toward food when feeding schedules are rigid, when they are given formulas that do not satisfy their hunger, or when they are fed in an atmosphere of tension. Under such circumstances food can come to symbolize dissatisfaction and conflict. This attitude may also persist into adulthood. As children grow older, they may come to reject certain foods, particularly those that were urged on them by oversolicitous adults. Parental guidance is important in encouraging a positive interest in food and eating. Some guidelines to follow in feeding young children are: attractive food, small servings, some freedom to choose their own foods and to eat in their own ways.

The School

Children acquire their first formal nutrition education when they enter school, whether it be nursery school, a day care center, or elementary school. They are introduced to simple facts about foods and nutrition and exposed to new foods and eating practices in meals and snacks they are served there (Fig. 1.8 and 1.9). Many current school nutrition programs leave much to be desired. They are often based chiefly on providing nutrition information, while little emphasis is placed on developing desirable attitudes and behavior with respect to food. Rarely is nutrition teaching coordinated effectively with the school lunch program in a way to encour-

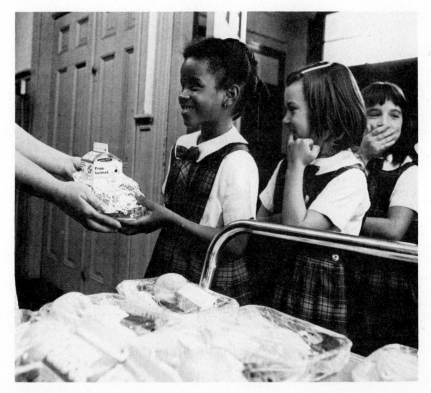

Figure 1.8
School meals may influence food patterns of children. Attractive, nutritious food offered in a friendly atmosphere and enjoyed with peers is an important aspect of nutrition education. (US Department of Agriculture)

Figure 1.9
A young Spanish-American is introduced to nutrition education through selection of a nourishing school meal. (US Department of Agriculture)

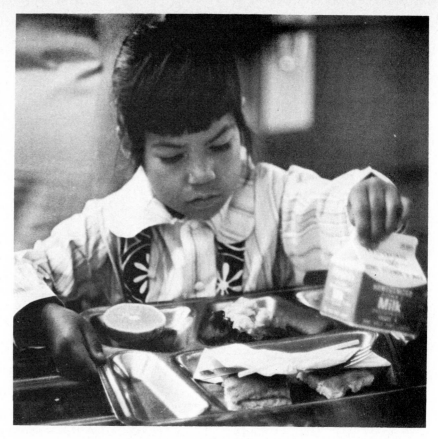

age desirable eating practices. At the elementary school level, the trend (though far from being realized) is toward planned, sequential curricula that relate nutrition to the living habits of the children. In high school, nutrition subject matter is usually coordinated with related subjects such as biology, health education, and home economics.

Community Resources

Community resources for nutrition education are extensive for people of all ages: organizations—official and private, community services—clinics and classes, mass media—including television and radio and the overwhelming supply of books, newspapers, magazines, and pamphlets. Much sound, helpful nutrition information emanates from these sources, but a great deal of it is superficial, misleading, or definitely erroneous. If good nutrition is to be served, there is the critical problem of sorting the sound from the unsound. Because fallacious statements and half-truths are often skilfully intermingled with accurate information, a knowledge of nutrition is required to identify them. Nutritionists serving health and nutrition agencies may themselves provide nutrition services that encourage desirable food practices or they may advise or direct individuals and groups to reliable sources of information. Many resources for nutrition education are referred to more specifically at appropriate points in the chapters that follow.

Food Advertising

Advertising that carries a nutrition message can constitute a type of nutrition education if it is factual and informative. But it can have a negative influence on food selection and eating patterns if it induces people to purchase foods they do not need, at unnecessary expense, by implying that these foods are essential to nutritional health. A case in point is the advertising of protein supplements and high-protein breads and cereals at premium prices. Food consumption surveys in the United States consistently show that protein intake at all income levels is adequate, and thus no supplementation is needed. Advertising does another disservice when it makes irresistable to consumers foods of little or no nutritional value, notably popular snacks. On the other hand, food advertising as a medium for announcing new forms of common foods, new processing methods, and new ways of serving familiar foods can be a positive influence in diversifying meal patterns and thus, in some measure, achieving desirable changes in food habits.

Modification of Eating Patterns

Resistance to Change   Eating patterns are subject to change as a result of the many influences we have discussed. Changes are made most easily in childhood; the younger the child, the more easily they are accomplished. Adult food practices are not easily altered, especially if they fall into a limited pattern. A person who has known no other way of eating is particularly inflexible. Adults complain of monotony and clamor for variety, particularly when meals planned by others are served to them in institutions. This attitude is universal, from college dormitories to retirement homes, and it occurs even when meals are well planned and reasonably varied. Left to themselves, these same persons often revert, day after day, to meals consisting of the core of foods to which they were accustomed. Many factors contribute to dissatisfaction with institutional meals. It seems likely, however, that the crux of the complaint is not monotony but the fact that the menus and the methods of preparing the foods are *different*. For some people, clinging to well known foods provides a feeling of security when they are experiencing other changes; for many it may simply offer a way of asserting their independence.

Approaches to Modification   Comprehensive food habit modification for groups should be attempted only after a careful study indicates that the present diet is nutritionally inadequate, and when the bases for present habits and the beliefs that support them are known. The same general principles govern the approach to food habit modification in individuals. The adequacy of the current diet should be judged on its known nutrient content and the nutritional status of the people who have been living on the diet. Customary diets usually form the best foundation on which to build in making the diet adequate.

Evidence of Changes in Patterns of Eating   Even deeply entrenched food habits can be altered. In the United States, Department of Agriculture data indicate a major shift in eating habits over the past 65 years (Fig. 1.10). There has been a steady decline in the use of flour and cereal grains, for example, and a sharp upward trend in the consumption of meat (29). This does not mean that everyone's eating practices have changed. These data represent foods available in the total food supply. Other studies show that some groups have made more change than others. The greatest adjustments have taken place in the diets of children and young adults; the diets of older people have undergone the least change. Young homemakers tend to adopt new meal patterns. As the planners and buyers for their households, they are in a position to create conditions for new eating patterns. When a group of homemakers was questioned about how they had learned to plan meals, many reported that they learned the basics in school (Fig. 1.11) (30). Thus

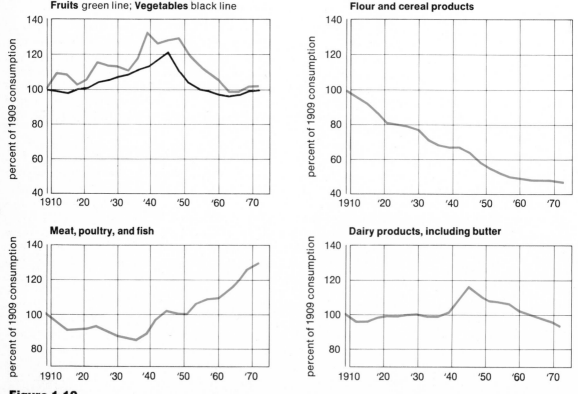

Figure 1.10
Food consumption trends per capita for selected categories from 1910 (1909=100%). Trends are expressed in 3-year intervals, based on a 5-year moving average. (Table 6, Agricultural Economic Report No. 138)

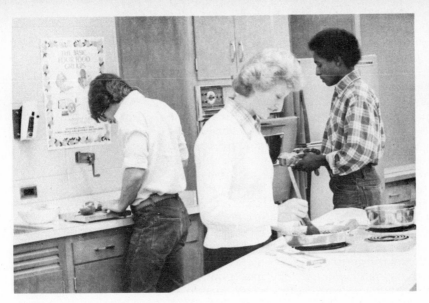

Figure 1.11
Homemakers' high school training in meal planning carries over to family meals. (Home economics class, Homewood-Flossmoor High School, Gregory Foster Bayles)

nutrition education of adults can begin in **elementary** school classrooms and lunchrooms.

Every time people are deprived of their accustomed ways of eating, they experience some change in their food patterns. If they are adaptable, they will accept the new diet or some part of it; but if their habits are rigid, they may merely endure the new until they can revert to the old. What happens when young men and women go away to college or join the armed services? In dormitories and mess halls, little can be done to cater to the preferences of individuals. Those who adapt to change make some lasting alteration in their way of eating and thus contribute to the gradual lessening of regional differences in food practices that is taking place in the United States today.

Food habits that differ from the conventional are not necessarily poor, nor do they indicate categorically a need for change. Nutrients can be obtained from many different food sources and from a multitude of food combinations. Meals that look and taste different from one's own or are served on a different time schedule can be entirely adequate nutritionally and suit perfectly the life styles of those who eat them. Even when food habits are poor, they are seldom all bad. Most people have relatively few things wrong with their diets, and many diets are deficient not because of the complete omission of important foods but because inadequate amounts of them are used. Adding only one food or one type of food or increasing the quantity of that food on a regular basis may accomplish the needed improvement. Satisfactory adjustments can usually best be made with gradual rather than radical changes in present eating patterns.

Personal Involvement in Habit Change

Personal involvement is a basic element of motivation, and motivation is the activating force in changing food habits. Motives are known by a variety of terms, such as *interests, problems,* and *needs.* The most compelling motive, of course, is *need.* People change when they *need* to change. But they must recognize that need and feel motivated by it. They must participate in the process of change. It is said that there are no unmotivated people, that individuals who appear to be unmotivated are those whose concerns, goals, and felt needs have not yet been discovered. An important challenge of nutrition education is to make those discoveries.

Felt needs are bases for action. If mature individuals analyze their own food habits objectively, identify their own needs, recognize the origin of their own problems, and face the advantages of making certain adjustments, dietary changes can be effected, provided people are convinced they need to change. Each individual must make the decision. Without doubt, the key to the outcome is the strength of the motivation to make the adjustment.

Specific Motivations   A driving urge to attain a concrete goal constitutes strong motivation for habit change. The goal may be to control an illness, such as diabetes or heart disease. The motive in this case is direct and compelling. Its intensity may be increased by fear of disability or even death. When an individual is so motivated, the diet change involved is often followed carefully, even though it may be a radical one. Also specific, but usually less demanding, are goals such as control of body weight. Motives to achieve weight loss may vary with sex and age, and they may range from the desire for a trim appearance to the need to lower blood pressure.

General Motivations   Motives are understandably weaker when the goal is more general and rewards are relatively remote. Everyone wants to enjoy the advantages of good general health. However, in the absence of specific objectives, people find it difficult to maintain a high level of motivation. They are interested in nutrition as it can be translated into specific benefits, and they want to see concrete evidence of those benefits. Often long-range goals can best be achieved through serious pursuit of a series of short-term goals.

REFERENCES

1. B. C. Schorr, D. Sanjur and E. C. Erickson, "Teen-age Food Habits," *J. Am. Dietet. Assoc.* 61 (Oct. 1972), pp. 415-20.

2. *Consumers' Preferences, Uses and Buying Practices for Selected Vegetables. A Nationwide Survey.* Marketing Res. Report No. 1019 (Washington, D.C.: Econ. Res. Serv. USDA, 1974).

3. D. Sanjur and A. D. Scoma, "Food Habits of Low-Income Children in Northern New York," *J. Nutr. Ed.* 2 (Winter 1971), pp. 85-95.

4. J. Sidel, A. Woolsey and H. Stone, "Sensory Analysis: Theory, Methodology and Evaluation," in E. G. Inglett, ed., *Fabricated Foods* (Westport, Conn.: Avi Publishing, 1975), Chap. 10.

5. M. C. Bourne, "Texture Properties and Evaluations of Fabricated Foods," in E. G. Inglett, ed., *Fabricated Foods* (Westport, Conn.: Avi Publishing, 1975), Chap. 11.

6. J. Mayer, "Physiology of Hunger and Satiety: Regulation of Food Intake," in R. S. Goodhart and M. E. Shils, eds., *Modern Nutrition in Health and Disease* (Philadelphia: Lea and Febiger, 1973), Chap. 14.

7. S. Lepkovsky, "Newer Concepts in the Regulation of Food Intake," *Am. J. Clin. Nutr.* 26 (Mar. 1973), pp. 271-84.

8. J. A. Halsted, "Geophagia (earth eating) in Man: Its Nature and Nutritional Effects," *Am. J. Clin. Nutr.* 21 (Dec. 1968), pp. 1384-93.

9. C. M. Bruhn and R. M. Pangborn, "Reported Incidence of Pica Among Migrant Families," *J. Am. Dietet. Assoc.* 58 (May 1971), pp. 417-20.

10. F. A. Geldard, *The Human Senses* (New York: John Wiley and Sons, 1972).

11. J. S. Wilentz, *The Senses of Man* (New York: Thomas Y. Crowell, 1968).

12. G. F. Stewart and M. A. Amerine, *Introduction to Food Science and Technology* (New York: Academic Press, 1973).

13. S. I. Korff, "The Jewish Dietary Code," *Food Tech.* 20 (July 1966), pp. 926-28.

14. R. McCarrison, "A Good Diet and a Bad One," *British Medical Journal* 2 (Oct. 23, 1926), pp. 730-32.

15. J. Cassel, "Social and Cultural Implications of Food and Habits," *Am. J. Public Health* 47 (June 1957), pp. 732-40.

16. E. N. Todhunter, *The History of Food Patterns in USA*, Proceedings of Third International Congress of Dietetics (London: Newman Books, 1961).

17. M. E. Lowenberg and B. L. Lucas, "Feeding Families and Children—1776-1976," *J. Am. Dietet. Assoc.* 68 (March 1976), pp. 207-15.

18. M. Bennion, "Food Preparation in Colonial America," *J. Am. Dietet. Assoc.* 69 (July 1976), pp. 16-23.

19. *Food Consumption of Households in the United States*, USDA, 1967. Household Food Consumption Survey, 1965-66, Reports No. 1, 3, 4.

20. National Research Council, Committee on Food Habits, *The Problem of Changing Food Habits,* Bull. 108 (Washington, D.C.: National Academy of Sciences, Oct. 1943, reprinted 1964).

21. L. E. Grivetti, "The Importance of Flavors in the Middle East," *Food Tech.* 29 (June, 1975), pp. 38-40.

22. V. M. Gladney, *Food Practices of the Mexican-American in Los Angeles County* (Los Angeles: Dept. of Health Services, Community Health Services, 1976).

23. H. B. Campbell, Texas Dept. of Health Resources—Personal communication, dietary and recipe material on Mexican-American food habits (Austin, Texas, 1976).

24. L. C. Reguero and S. R. Santiago, *Tabla de Composician de Alimentos de uso Corriente en Puerto Rico* (Rio Piedras, Puerto Rico: Editorial Universataria, 1976.)

25. R. L. Duyff, D. Sanjur and H. Y. Nelson, "Food Behavior and Related Factors of Puerto Rican Teenagers," *J. Nutr. Ed.* 7 (July-Sept. 1975), pp. 99-103.

26. The material relating to Puerto Rico was developed in consultation with nutritionists at the University of Puerto Rico; that concerned with the American Indian was acquired with the assistance of dietitians in US Public Health Service Hospitals on Indian reservations.

27. V. M. Gladney, *Food Practices of Some Black Americans in Los Angeles County* (Los Angeles: Dept. of Health Services, Community Health Services, 1976).

28. M. E. Lowenberg, "The Development of Food Patterns," *J. Am. Dietet. Assoc.* 65 (Sept. 1974), pp. 362-68.

29. S. J. Hiemstra, *Food Consumption, Prices and Expenditures,* Agric. Econ. Report No. 138 (Washington, D.C.: Econ. Res. Serv. USDA, July 1968; also Supplement for 1974, pub. Jan. 1976).

30. M. A. Walker, "Homemakers' Food and Nutrition Knowledge—Implications for Nutrition Education," *Nutrition Program News* (May-June 1975).

Booth, S. S., *A History of Eating in Colonial America*. (New York: Clarkson N. Potter, 1971).

Erhard, D., "The Vegetarians, Part One—Vegetarianism and its Medical Consequences," *Nutrition Today* 8 (Nov.-Dec. 1973), pp. 4-12.

Gaster, T. H., *Customs and Folkways of Jewish Life* (New York: William Sloane, 1955).

Gifft, H. H., M. B. Washbon and G. G. Harrison, *Nutrition, Behavior, and Change*. (Englewood Cliffs, N.J.: Prentice-Hall, 1972).

Grivetti, L. E. and R. M. Pangborn, "Origin of Selected Old Testament Dietary Prohibitions," *J. Am. Dietet. Assoc.* 65 (Dec. 1974), pp. 634-38.

Hofacker, R. and N. Brenner, "Vegetable Parade Persuades Children to Try New Foods," *J. Nutr. Ed.* 8 (Jan.-Mar. 1976), pp. 21-24.

Huenemann, R. L., L. R. Shapiro, M. C. Hampton and B. W. Mitchell, "Food and Eating Practices of Teen-Agers," *J. Am. Dietet. Assoc.* 53 (July 1968), pp. 17-24.

Jelliffe, D. B., "Parallel Food Classifications in Developing and Industrialized Countries," *Am. J. Clin. Nutr.* 20 (Mar. 1967), pp. 279-81.

Kight, M. A., *et al.*, "Nutritional Influences of Mexican-American Foods in Arizona," *J. Am. Dietet. Assoc.* 55 (Dec. 1969), pp. 557-61.

Lewis, C. E. and M. A. Lewis, "The Impact of Television Commercials on Health-Related Beliefs and Behaviors of Children," *Pediatrics* 53 (Mar. 1974), pp. 431-34.

Lowenberg, M. E., E. N. Todhunter, E. D. Wilson, J. R. Savage and J. L. Lubawski, *Food and Man*. (New York: John Wiley and Sons, 1974).

McBride, G., "Human Appetite, Eating Behavior Complexities Tantalize Scientists," *J. Am. Med. Assoc.* 236 (Sept. 27, 1976), pp. 1433-45.

McKenzie, J., "The Impact of Economic and Social Status on Food Choices," *Proc. Nutr. Soc.* 33 (May 1974).

Patwardhan, V. N. and W. J. Darby, *The State of Nutrition in the Arab Middle East* (Nashville, Tenn.: Vanderbilt University Press, 1972).

Present Knowledge in Nutrition (Washington, D.C.: The Nutrition Foundation, 1976).

Prideaux, J. S. and G. M. Shugart, "Students' Reactions to Residence Hall Food," *J. Am. Dietet. Assoc.* 49 (July 1966), pp. 38-41.

Robinson, L. G., A. Paulbitski, A. Jones and M. Roberts, "Nutrition Counseling and Children's Dental Health," *J. Nutr. Ed.* 8 (Jan.-Mar. 1976), pp. 33-34.

Senior, C. D. *The Puerto Ricans: Strangers—Then Neighbors* (Chicago: Quadrangle Books, 1965).

Nutritional Status

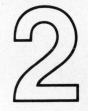

Methods of Assessing Nutritional Status
Diet and Nutritional Status
Standards of Dietary Adequacy
Standards for Nutrition Labeling
Application of Appraisal Techniques

Nutritional status, or one's level of nourishment, is an essential element in the total concept of health, as we have seen. This chapter is concerned with scientific methods of measuring the components of nutritional status.

To make a thorough assessment of nutritional status, it is necessary to see the task as a series of evaluations applied to the body as a whole or to body areas sensitive to nutritional measurements. Taken together—and reduced to the simplest terms—such evaluations are a measure of one's body structure and how one looks, feels, and functions. A person in an excellent state of nutrition from birth, for example, can be expected to have a well-developed skeleton with well-formed teeth and jaws, to exhibit a normal padding of fat over bones and muscles, and to have a blood supply that carries adequate amounts of oxygen and nutrients to the cells. Most people with these basic characteristics of good nutritional status will also be likely to display outward signs of vigor and health.

Judging nutritional status requires suitable measuring devices and appropriate standards for their use. Most of the measurement techniques are designed for use by specialists in various scientific fields. They are outlined here in lay terms, however, to suggest how each type of evaluation contributes to a comprehensive assessment of nutritional status.

METHODS OF ASSESSING NUTRITIONAL STATUS (1, 2)

The nutritional status of the body as a whole reflects the status of the various body parts and functions that relate in some manner to nutrition. In order to assess the body's state of nutrition, therefore, it is necessary to know what these parts and functions are and what each contributes. The methods of assessment fall into three general classes: physical appraisal, which includes measures of growth and development (*anthropometric* measurements) as well as clinical evaluations; biochemical analyses, which are made chiefly on blood and urine; and an accurate record of food intake over a specified period of time. Anthropometric and *biochemical* measurements provide objective data. Information on food habits and dietary intake helps to explain clinical and laboratory findings and to identify food practices that may be related to nutritional status. Certain facts about the community and the family are also important in interpreting a person's physical, biochemical, and dietary data, and in providing insight for recommending preventive measures, treatment, and follow-up.

anthropometric
Comparative human body measurements

biochemical
Relating to the chemical compounds and life processes of living organisms

Physical Appraisal

Growth and Development   Body measurements such as height and weight, have general implications with respect to nutritional status. A considerable variation from acceptable norms for weight may suggest either undernutrition or excessive intake of food in relation to energy use. Table 2.1 gives desirable weights for men and women 25 years of age and over. The weight of an adult can have greater nutritional significance at any given time if it coordinates with other evaluations, particularly the amount of body fat, the energy value of the diet, and the extent of usual physical activity.

For children, growth progress is one indication of the state of nutrition. Rate of growth provides a more accurate means of assessing nutritional status than a comparison of body measurements with average data at a given time. A child's growth pattern *over a period of time* can yield suggestive evidence of good or poor nutritional status.

Growth charts, based on measurements of thousands of children representative of the total child population of the United States, became available in 1976 for use as standards (3). Charts of stature-for-age and weight-for-age for boys 2 to 18 years old are reproduced in Figure 2.1. Charts are also available for girls of the same ages. The curved lines on each chart are numbered to show 5th, 10th, 25th, 50th, 90th, and 95th percentile values. As an example of how such charts may be used as longitudinal-type guidelines,

Table 2.1
Desirable weights for men and women
Weight in pounds according to frame (in indoor clothing)

Height with shoes on 1-in heels Feet	Inches	Small Frame	Medium Frame	Large Frame
5	2	112–120	118–129	126–141
5	3	115–123	121–133	129–144
5	4	118–126	124–136	132–148
5	5	121–129	127–139	135–152
5	6	124–133	130–143	138–156
5	7	128–137	134–147	142–161
5	8	132–141	138–152	147–166
5	9	136–145	142–156	151–170
5	10	140–150	146–160	155–174
5	11	144–154	150–165	159–179
6	0	148–158	154–170	164–184
6	1	152–162	158–175	168–189
6	2	156–167	162–180	173–194
6	3	160–171	167–185	178–199
6	4	164–175	172–190	182–204

desirable weights for men of ages 25 and over

Height with shoes on 2-in heels Feet	Inches	Small Frame	Medium Frame	Large Frame
4	10	92– 98	96–107	104–119
4	11	94–101	98–110	106–122
5	0	96–104	101–113	109–125
5	1	99–107	104–116	112–128
5	2	102–110	107–119	115–131
5	3	105–113	110–122	118–134
5	4	108–116	113–126	121–138
5	5	111–119	116–130	125–142
5	6	114–123	120–135	129–146
5	7	118–127	124–139	133–150
5	8	122–131	128–143	137–154
5	9	126–135	132–147	141–158
5	10	130–140	136–151	145–163
5	11	134–144	140–155	149–168
6	0	138–148	144–159	153–173

desirable weights for women of ages 25 and over

For women 18–25, subtract 1 lb for each year under 25.

Source: Metropolitan Life Insurance Company

the heights and weights of a hypothetical healthy boy are shown at yearly intervals. At 4 years of age, his height was 41 inches and his weight was 38 pounds. When plotted on the charts, the value of each measurement fell just above the 50th percentile line. This means that of every 100 boys in the large sample of 4-year-old boys on which the standard is based, more than fifty are shorter and weigh less than our subject. Each year as his height and weight were plotted on the charts, the marks continued to fall very close to the 50th percentile line, indicating that he was growing satisfactorily.

Figure 2.1
Growth charts with reference percentiles for boys 2 to 18 years of age (3).

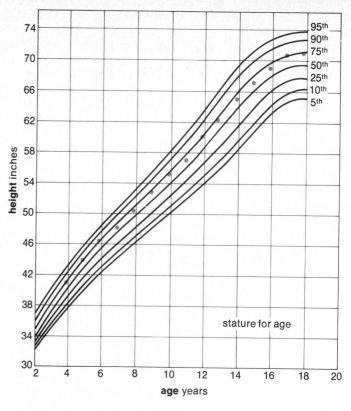

stature for age

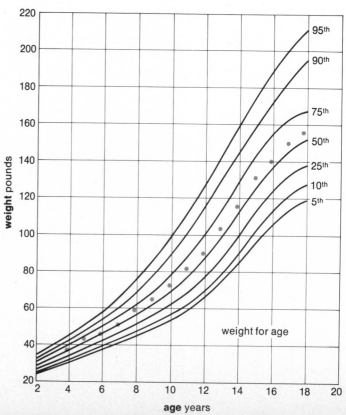

weight for age

The heights and weights of well-nourished children are likely to fall between the 25th and 75th percentiles and within corresponding ranks, as did those of the boy whose record is found in Figure 2.1. If a child's height and weight do *not* fall into corresponding percentile ranks, medical attention probably should be sought to determine whether the child is actually overweight (heavy and short) or underweight (thin and tall), or merely normally stocky or normally slender in build. Very low height and weight values (below the 5th percentile) indicate a child small for his or her age and suggest the possibility of chronic illness or nutritional deficiency. If a diet history reveals an inadequate nutrient intake, it might be assumed that the child's poor growth has a nutritional basis. However, some children who are consistently below the 5th percentile for height-for-age show steady growth and are found to be normal in all other respects.

Height and weight measurements have long been relied upon to evaluate growth and development of children, but the need for additional measures that relate more definitively to nutritional status has recently been recognized. The limitations of using gross body weight as an indicator of *obesity*, for example, led to studies of body composition and the development of methods for measuring various components of body mass. It was soon evident that higher-than-normal body weight may be due to heavy muscle mass, large bones, or obesity (a larger than normal amount of fat). There was an evident need to measure body fat itself. The quantity of total body fat varies greatly among individuals and has come to be another indicator of nutritional status.

obesity
Excessive amount of body fat

Body Fat   About 50 percent of the body's fat lies in a layer directly beneath the skin. The width of this *subcutaneous* fat layer can be estimated by measuring skinfold thickness with a pincer-like device called a *caliper* (Figs. 2.2 and 2.3). Skinfold thickness serves as an indicator of total body fat. The caliper is applied at specific sites that are considered to be representative of overall fat thickness. The triceps muscle along the back of the upper arm is one such area, and the *subscapular* region is another. Measurements of skinfold thickness have been generally accepted for use in evaluation of body fat in large population surveys.

subscapular
Lower back below the shoulder blade

Fat layer thickness varies with age and sex. There is a relatively steady increase with age in both males and females, but as early as the age of 2 there is a tendency for females to have a thicker layer of subcutaneous fat than males. Is it possible to determine what a reasonable skinfold thickness would be at any given age? Data on children aged 6 to 11 and 12 to 17 are available from the United States Health Examination Survey for use as norms in comparing survey findings on skinfold thickness (4, 5). An abnormally thick or thin layer of fat has significance in relation to good or poor nutritional status (6). Both are more meaningful when interpreted in the light of other body measures, especially body weight. If the value for an individual falls on the 50th percentile, half the population sample will have thicker fat layers and the other half thinner fat layers. When the value is greater than the 90th or less than the 5th percentile, medical supervision and coun-

Figure 2.2
Locating the midpoint between
specific positions at the
shoulder and elbow for
measurement of the triceps
skinfold.

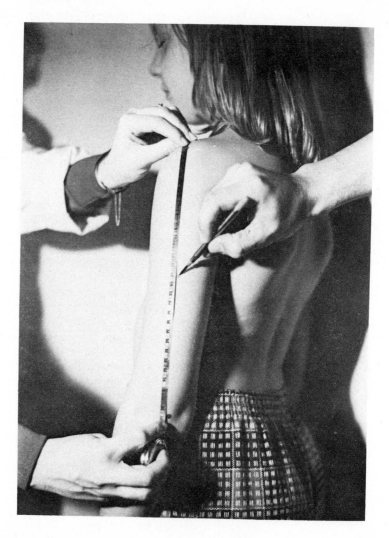

seling are recommended. A value exceeding the 95th percentile
suggests obesity, and the individual should be referred to an appropriate treatment facility.

An alternative way of judging fatness in children has been suggested. For children up to 9 years of age, the weight-for-height
chart is a reliable guide. Weight-for-height greater than the 95th
percentile can be considered presumptive evidence of obesity (7).
The correction of obesity at an early age is desirable, since this nutritional disorder tends to perpetuate itself and worsen over the
years, leading to many health problems later in life. (See Chap.
13.)

Figure 2.3
Applying the Lange caliper to
measure skinfold thickness at
the triceps muscle. (Samuel J.
Foman, MD. The University of
Iowa)

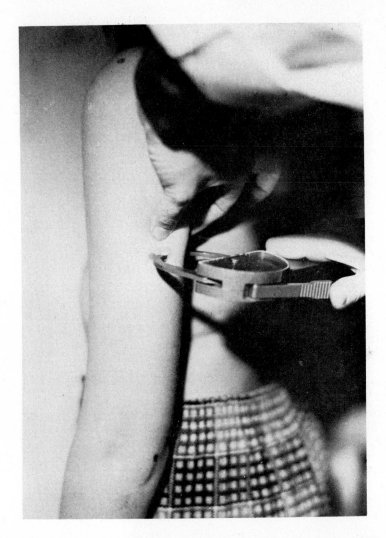

Skeletal Development (8)   Growth and development of the skeleton are also indicative of the state of nutrition, for nutrition influences the size and quality of bones. Periodic X-rays are used to
determine the age at which the different small bones of the wrists
of children first appear and how rapidly they develop (8). In well-
nourished children, the small bones become visible earlier and mature sooner than do those in poorly nourished children (Fig. 3.6).
There is also evidence to suggest that nutritional status may have
a bearing on the quality of bones in adults. People who have lived
for many years on poor diets—particularly diets low in bone-building nutrients—often have fragile and brittle bones.

Clinical Evaluation   In a clinical appraisal of nutritional status, the physician looks for signs and symptoms of nutritional deficiencies. These may be more or less pronounced, depending on the individual's age at the time of nutrient deprivation, as well as on the degree and duration of the nutrient lack. Certain parts of the body are particularly vulnerable to individual nutrient deficits. One example is the *thyroid gland*; when the food supply is deficient in iodine over a period of time, *goiter* may develop (see Chap. 8). The hair, skin, eyes, tongue, gums, and lips are also particularly sensitive to certain nutrient deficiencies. Descriptive lists of symptoms, photographs, and color slides depicting the actual lesions that result from such deficiencies are an aid to physicians in identifying nutritional disorders (9, 10). When there is a severe deficiency of any one of the nutrients, the results are usually apparent in well-marked, characteristic clinical signs. Such superficial signs as any of the following, which may be caused by a nutritional abnormality, should be considered a clue rather than a definitive diagnosis and should be pursued further: stiff and brittle hair; abnormally dry and rough skin; dry, dull, lusterless eyes with irritated lids; a deep red and fissured tongue; spongy and bleeding gums; lips that are swollen, chapped, and cracked at the corners. (Major deficiency diseases are described in later chapters, and the specific nutrients associated with each are identified.)

In mild nutrient deficiencies, there are problems of identification even for experienced physicians. The common clinical signs are less distinct than for severe deficiencies, and they are often similar to those arising from nonnutritional causes. Multiple nutrient deficiencies often exist simultaneously, thus causing a confusing variety of clinical signs to appear at the same time.

The assessment of dental health is usually included in the clinical appraisal. The relation of dentition to nutritional status is not a simple one. It is known, however, that the amount of fluoride in the water and the kind and frequency of consumption of dietary carbohydrate are important factors in controlling *dental caries*. When dental problems are severe, the kinds of foods that can be chewed may be limited. Thus, poor dental health may both be caused by, and contribute to, inadequate nutritional intake.

Certain nutritional deficiency diseases occur frequently in parts of the world where diets are grossly inadequate. Outright cases are not found routinely in the United States. But—as we will see later—recent evidence suggests that such diseases are perhaps more common, particularly among low-income groups, than was formerly suspected. Mild deficiency states without clinical manifestations may be fairly widespread among all income groups.

Biochemical Analysis

Two types of biochemical tests are employed for assessing nutritional status: those designed to measure levels in blood or urine of specific nutrients that reflect the adequacy of the diet; and functional tests that measure the effect of nutrient adequacy or deficiency on *enzymes*. These tests yield objective and precise data not influenced by human judgment. However, interpretation of the

thyroid gland
Situated at the base of the neck; secretes iodine-containing hormones

goiter
Enlargement of thyroid gland

dental caries
Tooth decay

enzymes
Proteins essential for stimulating reactions in the body

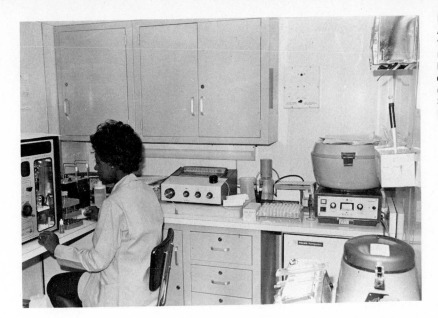

Figure 2.4
A laboratory technician using
the Coulter Counter that
measures the concentration of
hemoglobin and several other
constituents of blood samples.
(National Center for Health
Statistics, US Department of
Health, Education and Welfare)

hemoglobin
*Iron-containing protein pigment
in red blood cells*

**cholesterol and
triglycerides**
*Fatty substances; normal
constituents of blood*

glucose
Blood sugar

hormones
*Substances secreted by
glands and transported to
other parts of the body to
regulate specific processes*

findings may be difficult. Norms have been developed to serve as
guidelines in evaluating findings. A low concentration of certain
nutrients in the blood suggests that the body is malnourished with
respect to those nutrients. If the shortage is severe and continuous,
clinical evidence of the deficiency will eventually appear. Thus, unfavorable biochemical test results serve as early warnings of malnutrition. They are referred to as "risk signals." It is important to
realize that a deficiency in one nutrient is almost always accompanied by other nutrient inadequacies—a fact that calls for more
investigation.

Biochemical tests are applied to the blood in evaluating its content of protein and several vitamins. They also determine *hemoglobin* level, a possible indicator of anemia (Fig. 2.4). Biochemical tests
of the urine are used to evaluate body content of certain water-soluble vitamins (2). Determinations of blood levels of *cholesterol,
triglycerides, glucose,* and certain *hormones* provide important evidence regarding certain disease states as well as nutritional status.

DIET AND NUTRITIONAL STATUS

The nutritional status of individuals and groups is affected by the
amounts and kinds of foods that are consumed routinely. A record
of food intake, however, is not a valid measure of nutritional
status. A long-continued poor diet may be presumed to lead to a
malnourished condition, but the condition itself must be diagnosed
by measures discussed above. Thus, dietary analysis serves as one
phase of the total evaluation of nutritional status, along with physical and biochemical appraisals. The extent of agreement found in
the results of these three types of appraisals varies widely. Fairly
close agreement can be expected when the diet record reflects routine eating habits continued over a considerable period of time, and

when evaluations are made of groups, rather than of individuals. When groups have a limited and uniform diet, and when they are in a relatively poor state of nutrition, records of nutrient intake, physical examinations, and biochemical tests are most likely to be in good agreement.

Information about what and how much people eat is obtained in different ways. One method is to ask individuals to recall all the foods eaten in a recent time period—for example, during the preceding 24 hours; another is to ask them to recollect patterns of food intake over a period of years, called a diet history. A combination of the two methods may also be used (2). The quantities of foods consumed can be estimated, or they can be determined more precisely by weighing and measuring. The method chosen must fit the objective and type of each study. Dietary study methods will not be discussed here in detail. It is essential to emphasize, however, that diet records make a valid contribution to the total assessment of nutritional status only if they are accurate and represent typical, long-range eating habits (Fig. 2.5).

Dietary studies are made on individuals, on households, and on various segments of the population, as we will see in the following chapters. As a single device, they provide important background data about food choices and meal patterns, sources of nutrients, and food-preparation practices, all of which are indispensable to the realistic planning of dietary improvement programs. Thus, dietary findings often suggest approaches to the solutions of problems uncovered by clinical and biochemical evaluations.

Dietary information is more meaningful when physical and biochemical data are available on the same subjects at the same time. Studies that employ all three measures, such as the Health and Nutrition Examination Survey (HANES), are currently underway on a nationwide scale in the United States. In later chapters, findings from these studies will be examined in light of their purpose of determining the nutritional status of population samples.

Figure 2.5
When dietary surveys are made, people are asked to report kinds and amounts of foods consumed over a specified period of time. To ensure accuracy, food quantities are recorded in recognizable household measures such as cups and spoons. (National Center for Health Statistics; US Department of Health, Education and Welfare)

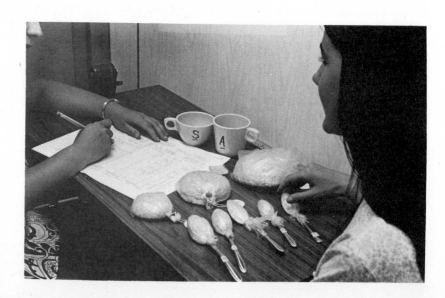

STANDARDS OF DIETARY ADEQUACY

More than fifty individual nutrients are known to be essential for human growth and health. Nutrients are the individual chemical substances contained in foods that are needed to nourish the body. Some of the nutrients provide energy, measured in *calories*. (See page 131 for the definition of a calorie and for guidelines for use of the term in this text.) Most nutrients are widely distributed in common foods, and for many of them there need be no concern about shortages. But some nutrients are less widely distributed, or the foods that contain them are eaten in insufficient quantities.

Guidelines are needed for use in assessing the adequacy of nutrients in diets. Dietary standards—amounts of certain nutrients recommended daily for different segments of the population—have been established to serve this purpose. Many countries have developed such guidelines with the needs of their own peoples in mind. Table 2.2 shows a sampling of these countries and the nutrient standards proposed for young men and women. (Standards have also been established for other age groups in these populations.) Each set of dietary standards represents a distinctive philosophy with respect to its purpose and use. The following brief discussion of the dietary standards developed jointly by two organizations of the United Nations, and the allowances developed for use in the United States represent different approaches.

FAO/WHO Dietary Requirements

Two United Nations organizations—the Food and Agriculture Organization (FAO) and the World Health Organization (WHO)—have developed a set of daily nutrient standards for adults and children in different age-sex categories (11). These groups have worked through joint committees and with many specialists throughout the world. FAO/WHO standards are intended primarily for the large number of nations without facilities and personnel for developing their own, and for population groups with limited food resources. They are aimed at the actual nutrient needs of different age and sex groups, rather than at providing a margin above physiological need. The FAO/WHO Expert Committee recently has begun to use "safe levels of intake" to describe its recommendations for protein. A close examination of Table 2.2 shows how FAO/WHO standards for adults differ from others on the list. For some nutrients there are minor variations; for protein the FAO/WHO standards are about one-fourth less; and for calcium the "suggested practical allowance" is lower than most countries' standards and scarcely more than half that of the United States.

Recommended Dietary Allowances (RDA)

The nutrient standards of the United States are known as the Recommended Dietary Allowances (RDA). Those for young men and women are shown in Table 2.2 for comparison with standards used in other parts of the world. The Recommended Dietary Allowances were first developed in 1943 by the Food and Nutrition Board of

Table 2.2
Comparative dietary standards of selected countries and United Nations agencies

Country	Sex	Age years	Weight kg	Kcal	Protein g	Calcium mg	Iron mg	Vit A activity IU	Thia-min mg	Ribo-flavin mg	Niacin equiv mg	Ascorbic acid mg
WHO/FAO	m	adults	65	3,000	37	400–500	7	2,500	1.2	1.8	19.8	30
	f	adults	55	2,200	29	400–500	21	2,500	0.9	1.3	14.5	30
USA	m	23–50	70	2,700	56	800	10	5,000	1.4	1.6	18.0	45
	f	23–50	58	2,000	46	800	18	4,000	1.0	1.2	13.0	45
Australia	m	18–35	70	2,800	70	400–800	10	2,500	1.1	1.4	18.0	30
	f	18–35	58	2,000	58	400–800	12	2,500	0.8	1.0	13.0	30
Canada	m	25–29	72	2,850	50	500	6	3,700	0.9	1.4	9.0	30
	f	25–29	57	2,400	39	500	10	3,700	0.7	1.2	7.0	30
Colombia	m	20–30	65	2,850	68	500	10	5,000	1.1	1.7	18.8	50
	f	20–30	55	1,900	60	500	15	5,000	0.8	1.1	12.5	50
Finland	m	20–44		2,400	60	700	8	2,500	0.8	1.2	8.0	30
	f	20–44		2,000	50	600	12	2,500	0.7	1.0	7.0	30
East Germany	m	19–35		2,700	85	800	10	3,000	1.6	1.6	18.0	70
	f	19–35		2,400	75	800	15	3,000	1.4	1.4	16.0	70
West Germany	m	25	72	2,550	72	800	10	5,000	1.7	1.8	18.0	75
	f	25	60	2,200	60	800	12	5,000	1.5	1.8	14.0	75
INCAP	m	adults		2,800	70	450	10	2,500	1.1	1.5	18.5	55
	f	adults		2,000	65	450	18	2,500	0.8	1.1	13.2	50
India	m	adults		2,400	55	400–500	20	2,500	1.2	1.3	16.0	50
	f	adults		1,900	45	400–500	30	2,500	1.0	1.0	13.0	50
Indonesia	m	20–40		2,600	65	500	10	4,000	1.0	1.4	17.0	60
	f	20–40		2,000	55	500	12	4,000	0.8	1.1	13.0	60
Japan	m	20–30	56	2,500	70	600	10	2,000	1.1	1.3	20.0	60
	f	20–30	49	2,000	60	600	15	2,000	0.9	1.0	16.0	50
Malaysia	m	18–35		2,500	55	450	10	7,500	1.0	1.4	16.5	30
	f	18–35		1,700	50	450	12	7,500	0.7	0.9	11.2	30
Netherlands	m	20–35		2,600	65	800	10	4,000	1.1	1.5	18.0	50
	f	20–35		2,000	55	800	12	4,000	0.8	1.3	13.0	50
Philippines	m	25	53	2,500	63	500	8	5,000	1.3	1.3	16.0	75
	f	25	46	1,900	55	500	18	5,000	1.0	1.0	13.0	70
Thailand	m	20–30		2,550	54	500	6	2,500	1.0	1.4	17.0	30
	f	20–30		1,800	47	400	16	2,500	0.7	1.0	12.0	30
Turkey	m	19–30		3,000	65	500	12	4,000	1.2	1.8	20.0	50
	f	19–30		2,300	55	500	22	4,000	1.0	1.2	14.0	50
United Kingdom	m	18–35		2,700	68	500	10	2,500	1.1	1.7	18.0	30
	f	18–55		2,200	55	500	12	2,500	0.9	1.3	15.0	30
WHO Western Pacific Region	m	adults		2,900	39	400	15	2,500	1.1	1.6	18.7	30
	f	adults		2,050	35	400	15	2,500	0.9	1.2	14.2	30

Adapted from "Report of the Committee on International Dietary Allowances of the International Union of Nutritional Sciences," *Nutr. Abst. Rev.* 45 (Feb. 1975) pp. 89–111. References to publications on standards are given in the report as well as footnotes interpreting the standards.

the National Academy of Sciences–National Research Council (NAS/NRC) (see Chap. 15). They were based on nutrition research applicable to quantitative human needs. Since 1943, adjustments have been made as new research has revealed the need for change, and revised editions have been published at about 5–year intervals. The 1974 table of Recommended Dietary Allowances includes amounts of energy, protein, ten vitamins, and six minerals for seventeen age-sex categories (see inside cover). Possible quantitative needs of a number of additional nutrients are considered in the text of the accompanying report (12).

Individuals are known to vary widely in their needs for nutrients. There is no way of determining a person's precise requirements except by expensive, time-consuming laboratory procedures. For this reason recommendations (except for energy) are for amounts of nutrients greater than those required by some, in order to provide an adequate supply for most individuals. "The Recommended Dietary Allowances are the levels of intake of essential nutrients considered, in the judgment of the Food and Nutrition Board on the basis of available scientific knowledge, to be adequate to meet the known nutritional needs of practically all healthy persons." (12) The RDA do not provide for the special nutritional needs resulting from abnormalities such as *metabolic* disorders or chronic diseases, nor for needs of premature infants. Long-term use of certain pharmaceutical preparations such as oral contraceptives may increase the requirement for specific nutrients to the extent that the RDA levels may not be sufficient (12).

metabolic
Concerned with body processes

Guidelines for the Use of RDA   It is important to understand the meaning and limitations of the RDA in order to recognize their proper uses. These allowances are intended to serve as a guide "for planning and procuring food supplies for population groups; for interpreting food consumption records; for establishing standards for public assistance programs; for evaluating the adequacy of food supplies in meeting national nutritional needs; for developing nutrition education programs; for the development of new products by industry; and for establishing guidelines for nutritional labeling of foods." (12)

The RDA are often employed in nutrition surveys as general guidelines for determining acceptable daily nutrient intakes. It is highly probable that a person's intake of a particular nutrient is adequate when it meets or exceeds the allowance. The lower the total intake, the greater the risk that nutrient needs are not being met. The RDA do not represent specific nutrient needs of individuals; therefore, an individual should not automatically be considered malnourished if the allowances are not met. As mentioned above, in assessment of nutritional status, records of nutrient intake are meaningful when considered along with physical and laboratory test findings.

Recommended allowances for energy are estimates of the average needs of population groups; they are not recommended intakes for individuals. Any margin over the requirement for energy usually is undesirable, for the surplus of energy is stored as fat and can lead to obesity.

The Food and Nutrition Board emphasizes the importance of obtaining the recommended amounts of nutrients through eating a wide variety of foods, to increase the likelihood of fulfilling possibly still unrecognized nutritional needs. In planning meals and

Table 2.3
United States Recommended Daily Allowances (US RDA)

Nutrient	Unit	Infants 0-12 mo.	Children under 4 yrs	Adults and children 4 or more yrs	Pregnant or lactating women
vitamin A	IU	1500.0	2500.0	5000.0	8000.0
vitamin D	IU	400.0	400.0	400.0	400.0
vitamin E	IU	5.0	10.0	30.0	30.0
vitamin C	mg	35.0	40.0	60.0	60.0
folic acid	mg	0.1	0.2	0.4	0.8
thiamine (B_1)	mg	0.5	0.7	1.5	1.7
riboflavin (B_2)	mg	0.6	0.8	1.7	2.0
niacin	mg	8.0	9.0	20.0	20.0
vitamin B_6	mg	0.4	0.7	2.0	2.5
vitamin B_{12}	mcg	2.0	3.0	6.0	8.0
biotin	mg	0.05	0.15	0.3	0.3
pantothenic acid	mg	3.0	5.0	10.0	10.0
calcium	g	0.6	0.8	1.0	1.3
phosphorus	g	0.5	0.8	1.0	1.3
iodine	mcg	45.0	70.0	150.0	150.0
iron	mg	15.0	10.0	18.0	18.0
magnesium	mg	70.0	200.0	400.0	450.0
copper	mg	0.6	1.0	2.0	2.0
zinc	mg	5.0	8.0	15.0	15.0

Source: US Department of Health, Education, and Welfare
Public Health Service, Food and Drug Administration, DHEW Publication No. (FDA) 74-2010

diets, the psychological and social values of foods must be taken into consideration; foods selected to meet nutritional needs must also be acceptable and palatable to ensure that they will be eaten and enjoyed.

United States Recommended Daily Allowances (US RDA)

The United States Food and Drug Administration (FDA) has adapted the Recommended Dietary Allowances in devising a standard to be used for food labeling. The modified, but very similar title of the FDA standard is United States Recommended Daily Allowances (US RDA) (13). The current standard is based on the 1968 NAS/NRC RDA, condensed to four categories: infants, children under 4 years, adults and children over 4 years, and pregnant and lactating women (Table 2.3). The highest values within each category on the RDA table were selected. The nutrition information on labels (except for infant foods or special dietary foods) is expressed as a percentage of the US RDA values for adults and children over 4 years, as shown in the third column of the table. The US RDA have replaced the Minimum Daily Requirements (MDR), formerly the legal standard for food labeling.

NUTRITION LABELING (14, 15)

Nutrition labeling is voluntary for most foods, but it is mandatory under certain conditions. Legislation that went into effect in 1975 requires that if a nutrient is added to any product, or if a nutritional claim is made on the label or in advertising, then food processors must provide complete nutrient composition information on the label. Products such as enriched bread or milk fortified with vitamin D thus require full nutrition labeling.

The label must follow a standard format, with the nutrition information panel to the right of the principal display panel. Serving size and the total number of servings in the container must be specified. A sample nutrition label is shown in Figure 10.5. Energy value (the number of calories) per serving and weights in grams of protein, carbohydrate, and fat per serving must be listed. The amounts of protein, vitamin A, vitamin C, thiamin, riboflavin, niacin, calcium, and iron present in each serving are given as a percentage of the US RDA. Certain additional information may be provided, such as the cholesterol content and the amounts of polyunsaturated fatty acids and saturated fatty acids per serving, and percentage of total calories from fat. The purpose of this information is stated on the label: "Information on fat (and/or cholesterol) content is provided for individuals who, on the advice of a physician, are modifying their total dietary intake of fat (and/or cholesterol)" (14). The sodium content of a serving of the food may also be listed for people who have been advised by a physician to limit the amount of sodium in their diets. Information about the twelve other vitamins and minerals for which standards have been established may be given if the processor wishes to include it.

APPLICATION OF APPRAISAL TECHNIQUES

In any branch of science, measurement techniques play an important role. As is evident, nutrition is no exception. Some of the tools and procedures described here, notably the Recommended Dietary Allowances and the United States Recommended Daily Allowances, will be used in the course of classwork. Other tools have been described chiefly to establish the function of each, in relation both to other measurements and to the concept of the total evaluation of nutritional status. As a whole, these procedures represent a major effort on the part of the worldwide scientific community to establish high—but attainable—nutritional goals for all peoples. This chapter should particularly prepare students to analyze and interpret the studies cited in Chapter 3 in answering the question dealt with next: Does nutrition make a difference?

REFERENCES

1. H. H. Sandstead and W. N. Pearson, "Clinical Evaluation of Nutrition Status," in R. S. Goodhart and M. E. Shils, eds., *Modern Nutrition in Health and Disease* (Philadelphia: Lea and Febiger, 1973), Chap. 19.

2. G. Christakis, ed., "Nutritional Assessment in Health Programs," *Am. J. Public Health* 63 (Nov. 1973), Part Two.

3. P. V. V. Hamill, T. Drizd, C. Johnson, R. Reed, and A. Roach, *NCHS Growth Charts, 1976*, Monthly Vital Statistics Report, 25, No. 3 Supp. (HRA) 76-1120 (Rockville, MD: Health Resources Administration, June, 1976).

4. F. E. Johnston, P. V. V. Hamill, and S. Lemeshow, *Skinfold Thickness of Children 6–11 Years, United States*. National Center for Health Statistics, Vital and Health Statistics, Series 11, Nov. 120, DHEW Publ. No. (HSM) 73-1602 (Washington, D.C.: US Gov. Print. Office, 1972).

5. F. E. Johnston, P. V. V. Hamill and S. Lemeshow, *Skinfold Thickness of Youths 12–17 Years, United States*, National Center for Health Statistics, Vital and Health Statistics, Series 11, No. 132, DHEW Publ. No. (HRA) 74-1614 (Washington, D.C.: US Gov. Print. Office, 1974).

6. J. Mayer, "Obesity," in R. S. Goodhart and M. E. Shils, eds., *Modern Nutrition in Health and Disease* (Philadelphia: Lea and Febiger, 1973), Chap. 22.

7. S. J. Fomon, *Nutritional Disorders of Children: Screening, Follow-Up, Prevention*. Health Services Administration DHEW Publ. No. (HSA) 76-5612 (Washington, D.C.: U.S. Gov. Print. Office, 1976).

8. S. Dreizen, R. M. Snodgrasse, H. Webb-Peploe and T. D. Spies, "The Retarding Effect of Protracted Undernutrition on the Appearance of the Postnatal Ossification Centers in the Hand and Wrist," *Human Biology* 30 (Dec. 1958), pp. 253-63.

9. H. H. Sandstead, J. P. Carter and W. J. Darby, "How to Diagnose Nutritional Disorders in Daily Practice," *Nutrition Today* 4 (Summer 1969), pp. 20-26.

10. H. H. Sandstead, J. P. Carter and W. J. Darby, *Teaching Aid No. 5: Nutrition Diagnosis* (kodachrome slides) (Washington, D.C.: *Nutrition Today*, 1969).

11. Food and Agriculture Organization, Rome: *Handbook of Human Nutritional Requirements*, FAO Nutritional Studies No. 28, 1974.

12. Food and Nutrition Board, National Research Council, *Recommended Dietary Allowances*, 8th revision. (Washington, D.C.: National Academy of Sciences–National Research Council, 1974).

13. FDA Consumer Memo, *Nutrition Labeling: Terms you Should Know,* DHEW Publication No. (FDA) 74-2010 (Rockville, MD: Food and Drug Administration, 1974).

14. National Nutrition Consortium, Inc. with R. M. Deutsch, *Nu-*

trition Labeling: How It Can Work for You (Bethesda, MD: National Nutrition Consortium, 1975).

15. B. Peterkin, J. Nichols, and C. Cromwell, *Nutrition Labeling: Tools for its Use*, Agric. Inform. Bull. No. 382 (Washington, D.C.: Consumer and Food Economics Inst., Agric. Res. Service, USDA, April 1975).

READINGS

Campbell, J. A., "Approaches in Revising Dietary Standards—Canadian, U.S., and International Standards Compared," *J. Am. Dietet. Assoc.* 64 (Feb. 1974), pp. 175-78.

Harper, A. E., "Those Pesky RDAs," *Nutr. Today* 9 (Mar.-Apr. 1974), pp. 15, 16, 19-22, 27, 28.

Hegsted, D. M., "Dietary Standards," *J. Am. Dietet. Assoc.* 66 (Jan. 1975), pp. 13-21.

Martin, E. A. and V. A. Beal, *Roberts' Nutrition Work with Children*. (Chicago: University of Chicago Press, 1978).

Does Nutrition Make a Difference?

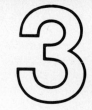

Body Size
Structure
Performance
Length of Life

Does nutrition really make a difference in the way people develop and function? In general, the answer is *yes*, but the breadth of the question calls for some explanation. Answers arise from research in the areas of physical, mental, and social development. The types of investigations conducted in these disciplines include laboratory research, population surveys, field studies, observations under known nutritional conditions, and statistical analyses of health data. Individual studies provide supporting information; collectively, they confirm the thesis that nutrition is a basic factor in shaping one's physical and mental being and in determining many patterns of performance.

Research cited here is confined for the most part to that on human beings. However, total accomplishments also depend on research with experimental animals that serves as a foundation for human studies. The short life spans of most animals, their brief growth periods, and the pure strains that can be utilized for study make animal research practical and advantageous. Feeding animals highly specialized diets can result in prompt and clear-cut bodily and functional changes. For obvious reasons, such experiments cannot be duplicated in humans. Often, however, they can point the way to modified studies with human subjects that yield evidence of the nutrition-health relationship.

All animals have much in common; they rely for health, strength, growth, biological performance, general appearance, and vigor on diets that are suitable and adequate for each species. Many people take the position that animal needs are different from those of humans and argue that research in one area does not apply to the other. It is true that the needs of various species differ; that physiological responses to individual nutrients can vary considerably; and that specific findings are not always transferable. Nevertheless, the broad results of animal feeding experiments reveal a strong cause-and-effect relationship between nutritional quality in diet and health and performance. This relationship is also seen in people.

The research findings reported here present evidence of the benefits of good nutrition and the disadvantages of poor nutrition, particularly as they relate to the basic form and functions of the human body at different ages. The findings are discussed in terms of *body size, body structure, body performance*, and *length of life*.

physiological
Pertaining to functions of the body

BODY SIZE AND NUTRITION

A person's eventual size and growth rate are determined by two chief factors, the inborn capacity to grow and various environmental conditions, important among which is nutrition. The two are interdependent, for while heredity limits the final size a person can reach, nutrition largely determines whether an individual achieves that limit. This concept has been aptly paraphrased: "The blueprint is in the chromosomes, but the bricks and mortar are in the market basket."

Body size in itself is not a prime concern. Size and growth are related, however, and the physical growth pattern of a child constitutes one of the most useful criteria for judging his or her nutritional status. When growth fails, malnutrition can be suspected. Physical growth is a complex process that involves not only increased size of the body as a whole but also the development of its different parts. Growth is now being studied as a cellular process marked by increases in both numbers and size of cells during development.

The availability of new and more sensitive instruments and techniques in recent years has made research at the cellular level possible. Significant gains in knowledge and understanding of *metabolic* processes have resulted. Research on animals suggests that energy restriction may tend to reduce cell multiplication, whereas the chief effect of protein restriction may be to reduce cell size. Apparently, the precise effect of malnutrition will be determined by the extent to which either or both of these deficiencies, and perhaps others, are present at the same time. Cells in various organs grow at different rates, as will be pointed out later in this chapter. There is also a difference between the sexes in the rate of cell

metabolic
Concerned with body processes

growth in muscles. Boys reach maturity with more muscle cells than do girls.

Cell Structure and Function (1)

Cell structures and functions are so complex that a full understanding of them requires a background in biochemistry and cell physiology. However, some appreciation of cell structure and function is possible for anyone who seeks merely to grasp the basic concept of body nourishment. The functioning of the body as a whole ultimately depends upon what happens in the cells. It is within the millions of individual cells that all growth and maintenance activity takes place. Only after food is digested to release nutrients and these are absorbed through the walls of the small intestine, carried by the blood to the cells, and have gained entry can the nutrients be of service to the body (see Chap. 5). Cells make up tissues, tissues make up organs, and groups of organs make up body systems. The living organism—you—consists of many systems working interdependently in an intricate and amazingly coordinated fashion to sustain and carry itself through the various stages of the life cycle.

Cells produce the substances required for their own functioning, such as enzymes, from nutrients made available to them. Some kinds of cells synthesize materials such as hormones, which are transported to other parts of the body where they perform specific functions. Obviously, cells of different tissues that perform different tasks vary somewhat in structure as well as in their nutrient requirements. The "typical" cell shown in Figure 3.1, therefore does not represent the precise structure of any *particular* cell but is a diagrammatic representation of cells in general. Figure 3.2 is a photograph of a cell.

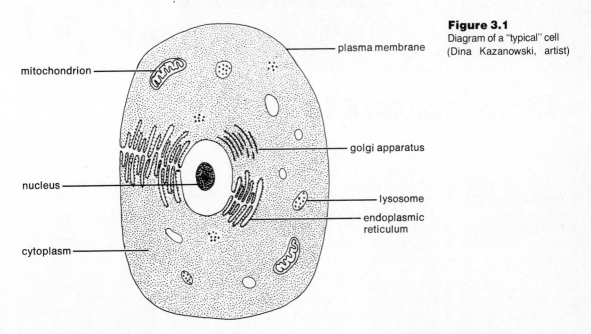

Figure 3.1
Diagram of a "typical" cell
(Dina Kazanowski, artist)

mitochondrion

plasma membrane

golgi apparatus

nucleus

lysosome

endoplasmic
reticulum

cytoplasm

Figure 3.2
Hampster suprarenal cortex
cell. Magnification 25,000 X.

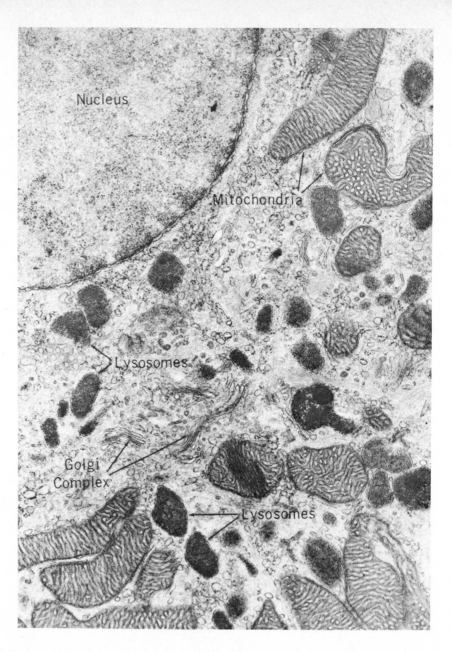

Every cell is bounded by a *plasma membrane* that separates its contents from the fluids and other cells surrounding it. The plasma membrane regulates the passage of substances into and out of the cell. Following is a brief description of certain other cell components that function in the nourishment process.

The *nucleus*, separated from the rest of the cell by a membrane, contains the genetic apparatus DNA (deoxyribonucleic acid) that ensures exact reproduction of the cell. This "data bank" also guides and controls the synthesis of all other materials produced in the cell by transcribing the specific information needed into RNA (ri-

plasma membrane
Semi-permeable film-like covering of the cell

bonucleic acid). Most of the several forms of RNA then move out of the nucleus into the *cytoplasm* of the cell.

The *cytoplasmic matrix* is the background substance that surrounds and supports all the organized, membrane-enclosed structures (*organelles*) within the cell. It contains water, all the soluble nutrients, enzymes, and other proteins of the cell.

The *mitochondria* are the sites of the complicated series of enzymatic changes known as Krebs' cycle, through which energy from the carbohydrates, fats, and proteins of food is transformed into *ATP* (adenosine triphosphate). The cell is totally dependent upon the availability of ATP for the energy needed to carry on all of its activities. The energy requirements of an individual are, after all, the sum total of the energy requirements of its constituent cells.

The *endoplasmic reticulum* is a system of channels in the cell that provides a passageway through the cytoplasm between the nucleus and the plasma membrane. Some of the endoplasmic reticulum appears to be rough, due to the presence of *ribosomes* composed of protein and RNA. Protein synthesis takes place on the ribosomes under the direction of RNA. The proteins formed then enter the endoplasmic reticulum to be transported to various parts of the cell or exported across the plasma membrane to be used elsewhere in the body.

The *Golgi apparatus* provides a packaging and storage facility for certain substances, such as hormones, that have been produced in the cell and are to be removed. The production of membranes is another important function of the Golgi apparatus.

Lysosomes contain a large assortment of powerful enzymes and act as the digestive organ of the cell. They also serve a protective function by destroying invading microorganisms and breaking down worn out cells and cell parts. The *catabolic* activities of this organelle are essential in maintaining the dynamic equilibrium that characterizes cell life.

The functioning of individual cells is clearly reflected in the nutritional status of the body as a whole. Body dimensions, for example, ultimately depend on cell nutrition. Of the many measures applied in assessing body size, standing height or length is among the most useful.

Increases in Body Size

Evidence of increased growth rates has been reported by many investigators. One study presents the increased size of boys and girls in the United States and Europe in the 60-year period from 1905 to 1965 at the ages of 5, 9, and 11 years (2). For example, 5-year-old boys and girls in comfortable economic circumstances were about 2 inches taller in 1965 than children of the same age and circumstances in 1905. In 1965, 9-year-olds were about 3 inches taller and 11-year-olds about 4 inches taller than their respective counterparts in 1905. These increases in height are represented in Figure 3.3. The investigator attributes the increased growth rates largely to improved nutrition and related environmental factors associated with health services for infants and children.

oganelles
Organized, membrane-enclosed structures in the cell

ATP
Compound in which energy is stored for use by the cell

catabolic
Destructive

Figure 3.3

Increased size of boys and girls in the United States and Europe over a sixty-year period, as represented at three age levels. Five-, 9-, and 11-year-old children averaged some 2, 3, and 4 inches taller respectively, in 1965 than their counterparts in 1905. [*Scientific American* 218 (Jan. 1968), p. 21]

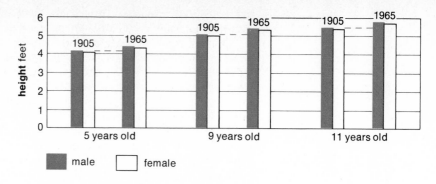

Higher economic status, which usually provides a favorable environment for nutritional development, apparently also fosters an increased rate of growth. This point has been emphasized in a study comparing body measurements of public school children with those of private school children at two different time periods—in the 1930s and in 1958–59 (3). Data show that acceleration in growth from one generation to the next had ended for private school children by the 1930s; their heights remained virtually unchanged in the period from the 1930s to 1958–59. The public school children, on the other hand, increased their stature appreciably during the same 30-year period. The inference is that the private school children were already fulfilling their growth potential by the 1930s, whereas the public school children had yet to reach that goal. Other studies that have explored this point confirm that gains become progressively smaller as more individuals in the population attain what appears to be their full growth potential set by heredity.

Adult Size (4)

Young men and women in the United States in the mid-20th century averaged about 2 inches taller than their counterparts 60 years earlier, and they reached that height at an earlier age. This conclusion was drawn from a compilation of studies made on the general population and on college students. The average heights of college men and women were slightly above the general average.

Freshmen students at two men's colleges advanced from a height of 67.5 inches in the early 1880s to over 70 inches in the 1950s; freshmen at two women's colleges advanced from about 63 inches in the late 1800s to slightly over 65 inches in the 1950s. Comparisons of college men and women with their fathers and mothers show the younger generation to be 1 inch taller on the average than their parents.

Another indication of the increased average height of the college population is the rising percentage of college men who are 6 feet tall. In 1883, only 4 percent of the young men entering two men's colleges measured 6 feet or more in height; by 1915 the percentage had risen to 10; and by 1965 more than 30 percent of the freshmen were at least 6 feet tall. Increases in stature in the United States are attributable to a combination of factors, including newer knowledge of nutritional needs and greater availability of nutritious foods to fulfill those needs.

Examination of height and weight data for varsity football players from 1899 to 1970 revealed that the teams from 1961 to 1970 averaged 2.6 inches taller and 35.3 pounds heavier than those from 1899 to 1910 (5). As might be expected, the football players were taller and heavier than their nonathlete age peers at any one time. Changes in recruiting practices, styles of play favoring larger players, and secular trends must be considered as factors in the observed size increases. Data on the sizes of participants in other sports are limited, but a tendency has been noted toward increases in the heights and weights of basketball players and participants in the Olympic Games.

Favored segments of the college group are experiencing a stabilization of these dramatic gains in height, however, as did the private school children in the study mentioned above. This trend was noted when the measurement records of Harvard University students who belong to old American families and whose male members habitually attend the university were singled out for special study (6). This study is unique in that its 85 subjects came from twelve four-generation families at Harvard, covering the years from 1870 to 1965. As "Old Americans," all the students had four grandparents born in the United States, a fact that minimized problems of genetic variation. Table 3.1 gives a summary of pertinent facts for each of the four generations: the number of men studied and mean birth dates for each generation; the mean ages when measurements were taken; and the average heights and weights for each generation.

There was a significant height increase from generation I to II (fathers to sons), a smaller rise in generation III (grandsons), and none at all in generation IV (great grandsons). The finding that height increases had tapered off and then ended for economically

Table 3.1
Secular trends in height and weight
Twelve four-generation families of old Americans at Harvard University

	Generations			
	I Fathers	II Sons	III Grandsons	IV Great grandsons
number	12	24	30	19
birth date mean	1858	1888	1918	1941*
age in years mean	21.9	19.0	18.9	18.8
height cm**	176.0	178.9	180.7	179.6
weight kg**	67.9	69.5	69.7	73.4

Adapted from Table 1, *Am. J. Phys. Anthropology* 29 (July 1968), p. 47.
*cutoff date 1965
**see Appendix F, Equivalents in Weights and Measures

favored men is in accord with observations of other investigators. Weight increases, however, continued simultaneously.

Unpublished data on more than six thousand men, members of more than two thousand two-, three-, and four-generation families at Harvard University, confirmed the findings on the 85 men represented in Table 3.1. Height increases stopped with men born in the decade preceding 1918; their sons were no taller than they (6). Environmental factors favoring growth in height can exert their influence only within the limits of genetic potential. Apparently the genetic potential of the Harvard men had been achieved by 1918. This point has not yet been reached in the general population, but there are indications that we are moving toward it. Relatively more men and women were found to be taller in the recent nationwide Health and Nutrition Examination Survey (*HANES, 1971–74*) than in a Health Examination Survey conducted in the United States about 10 years earlier (HES, 1960–62) (7). Mean heights of men and women grouped by age are shown in Figure 3.4. There is a small but consistent difference at all ages from 18 to 74, indicating that on the average adults in the United States were taller in 1971 to 1974 than in 1960 to 1962. They were also heavier. The HANES data on weights are consistently higher by an average of 6 pounds for men and by 3 pounds for women across the age range of 18 to 74 years. Body weight is not limited by genetic potential to the same extent that height is. The Harvard men were heavier than their fathers even when they were not taller.

HANES
Survey designed to measure the nutritional status of US population

Figure 3.4
Mean height in inches of US adults 18-74 years in HES (1960-62) and HANES (1971-74).

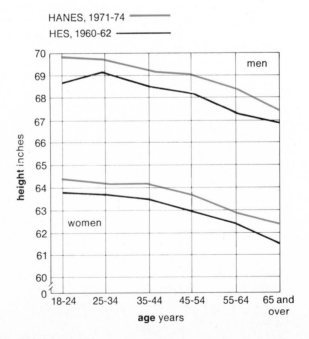

HANES, 1971-74 ————
HES, 1960-62 ————

Sizes of Racial Groups

The short stature of certain peoples has been popularly considered a racial characteristic based on heredity. In reality, this characteristic may result from poor environmental conditions continued through successive generations. The soundness of this theory has been demonstrated in a study of Japanese children, which offered a rare opportunity to isolate hereditary and environmental influences.

Japanese Children   The relative growth progress of Japanese children born and reared in their homeland and those born and reared in the United States has been compared (8). Measurement data were collected on nearly nine hundred American-born Japanese boys and girls between 6 and 19 years of age living in the San Francisco Bay area of California. These records were compared with those of children of the same sex and age in Japan, past and present. At every age considered in the study, the stature of the American-born Japanese boys exceeded that of native-born Japanese boys living in Japan by 4 to 13 centimeters, an amount greater than the increase that had taken place in the stature of boys in Japan during the preceding 53 years (3 to 5 centimeters). A similar superiority of stature was shown by American-born Japanese girls up to 14 years of age.

Figure 3.5 shows the height curves for the boys born in California (the highest line), those born and reared in Japan in fairly recent times (intermediate) and those born in Japan about 70 years ago (lowest). It reveals that considerable progress has been made in raising average height levels in Japan in the past three-quarters of a century. Despite these increases, the heights and weights of Japanese boys born and reared in the United States were strikingly greater. Thus heredity seems to be ruled out as a major limiting factor in the heights of Japanese people. The investigator believed the difference was due "rather to a more limited diet and to

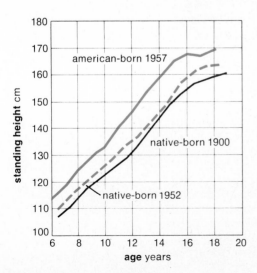

Figure 3.5
Average standing height of American-born Japanese boys compared with that of boys in Japan in 1900 and 1952. [Adapted from W.W. Greulich, "Growth of Children of the Same Race under Different Environmental Conditions," Science 127 (March 7, 1958), Fig. 1].

Does Nutrition Make a Difference?   **61**

other less favorable environmental conditions (then) existing in Japan" (8)

A more recent series of studies made by official agencies in Japan shows that native-born Japanese children have continued their accelerated gains in height in their homeland (9). In general, the increase has been attributed to a higher standard of living and a more varied and abundant diet than was previously available. Efforts have been made to identify the specific factors responsible for these gains. One investigator has explored possible diet relationships through two avenues of approach: by examining records of average food consumption in Japan for the period 1948 to 1962, when heights of children were increasing rapidly; and by comparing the diets of orphanage children with those of the notably taller public school children living in their own homes. Both approaches suggested that increased quantity and better quality of protein were distinguishing characteristics of the diets consumed by the taller children (10).

BODY STRUCTURE AND NUTRITION

Can good nutrition make a difference in the structure of the body itself? Is the body a sturdier, better developed, and more effective mechanism as a result of good nutrition? The answers to these questions, supplied by research, apply both to the skeleton and to the soft tissues which together compose the body's foundation.

The Bony Framework

The linear dimensions of the skeleton largely determine the body's stature. This relationship is implied in the preceding discussion of body size. Upward growth of the skeleton is in turn influenced by the development of the long bones of the legs, a feature with unmistakable nutrition connotations (10, 11). Nutrition also affects the quality of bone structure and the ability of bones to mature properly. (The growth of bones and the relationship between nutrition and bone size is discussed further in Chapter 8).

Periodic X-rays can be used to trace the progress of a child's developing bones. In making these measurements, the status of the wrist and hand bones is regarded as typical for the entire skeleton. To gauge a child's development at any one time, comparisons are made with a radiographic atlas showing representative X-ray pictures of the hands and wrists of children in the same age range (12). Minor variations from these norms may be meaningless, because there is considerable leeway within normal limits due to hereditary differences. However, wide divergence below the norm in skeletal development in children can indicate delays in the maturing process.

Do the bones of children in advanced countries such as the United States ever show delays in skeletal development? In one study, the retarding effect of prolonged undernutrition was shown dramatically in the bones of the hands and wrists of several hundred children (13). In every poorly nourished child of either sex, there was delay in the development of wrist bones when compared

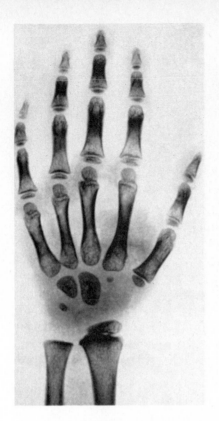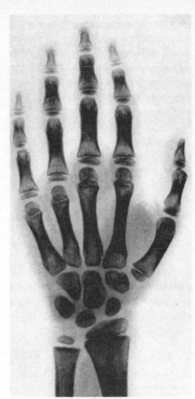

Figure 3.6
Effect of known undernutrition (left) and known adequate nutrition (right), as shown by X rays of hand skeletons of two 7-year-old girls. The X ray at left shows only four carpal centers (wrist bones); the one at right shows seven. The latter is regarded as normal for children of this age. [Human Biology 30 (Dec. 1958), p. 259, courtesy Samuel Dreizen, DDS, MD].

with those of well-nourished children of corresponding ages. Figure 3.6 demonstrates the characteristic differences in the wrists of two 7-year-old children in the study. The X-ray on the left shows a wrist typical for a poorly nourished child; that on the right, a wrist typical for a child with a history of good nutrition. At the age of these children, about seven carpal centers should be present. Only four are visible in the wrist of the undernourished child.

In severe malnutrition, retardation in skeletal development is readily detected, as exemplified in preschool children in Guatemalan villages (11). It is evident not only in the delayed appearance and development of the wrist bones, but also in the reduction in bone mineral in various parts of the skeleton. In extreme cases of malnutrition, bone thickness is notably diminished, and there is actual loss of volume.

Differences in bone quality extend into adult life. In the United States, many middle-aged and older people have fragile bones susceptible to easy breakage. Addition of bone-building nutrients to the diets of a group of elderly women resulted in significant increases in bone density (14).

dential caries
Tooth decay

Teeth (15, 16)   The teeth and jaws are part of the skeleton. Teeth merit serious attention, because dental caries is the most widespread of all chronic diseases. Almost 100 percent of the population of the United States is afflicted with this problem to some degree.

Despite many years of research on animals and humans, the cause or causes of dental decay have not been precisely defined. Nutrition is a basic factor in caries prevention and control and in the solution of the dental health problem. Studies with experimental animals indicate that malnutrition during tooth development may result in abnormal organic matrix formation and tooth structure. Such defective teeth are more susceptible to decay-promoting factors than are normal teeth.

The rising incidence of dental caries is closely associated with increasing replacement of dietary starch with sugar in many people's eating patterns. Certain microorganisms in *dental plaque* ferment the sugar, producing acid that penetrates the tooth enamel, thus causing tooth decay. Decay of susceptible teeth is directly related to the frequency of intake and the consistency of foods high in fermentable carbohydrate. Sweet foods that are sticky and adhere to the teeth are more destructive than sugar in liquid form. If such foods are eaten at very short intervals, the decay process can be practically continuous (17).

dental plaque
Sticky film of bacteria that clings to teeth

A well-balanced, nutritionally adequate, and satisfying diet is important for good nutrition under all circumstances. However, in caries control such a diet serves a special purpose. It would include adequate amounts of protein, calcium, and phosphate, plus moderate amounts of sugar, and its satisfying quality would tend to discourage excessive nibbling. A carefully controlled study with children has shown that, as their diets became more nearly adequate, the children tended to adjust voluntarily to lower sugar intake (18).

Dental caries is more prevalent in certain geographic areas than in others, regardless of the economic status of the people or the adequacy of their diet. Efforts to solve this puzzle eventually led investigators to the mineral fluoride as the critical factor. Fluoride is an essential trace element of proven value in producing decay-resistant teeth. Research has shown that a desirable amount of fluoride (approximately one part per million) occurring naturally in a community water supply, or a water supply adjusted properly in fluoride content, can provide a substantial degree of immunity to tooth decay (see Chap. 8).

Soft Tissues (19, 20)

The soft tissues of the body are muscle and fat. Muscles attached to the skeleton not only surround and support the body frame, but they are also essential in myriad ways to the functioning of the entire body. Fat in normal amounts serves protective functions. An estimate of the body's nutritional status can be obtained by determining the amounts of muscle and fat in the body (see Chap. 2).

Body Composition   Many methods and devices for assessing body composition have been developed during the past third of a century. Some of them are research procedures that must be carried out by skilled technicians in specially equipped laboratories. One such method estimates the amount of body fat by determining a person's *specific gravity*. Measuring specific gravity is a complicated process that involves weighing the body first in air and then under water. The principle involved is that lean body mass is relatively constant in composition, with a specific gravity of about 1.100. Fat has a lower specific gravity; therefore, the greater the proportion of fat in the body, the lower the specific gravity. The degree of reduction is an index of body fatness.

Other laboratory methods are employed, including X-rays, which make it possible to relate fat thickness to the size of the adjacent bones and muscles, and the "potassium 40" method, which gives a reasonably accurate estimate of a person's lean body mass.

Body Fat   A layer of subcutaneous fat of normal thickness is one indication of satisfactory nutritional status. The skinfold method for estimating body fat is described in Chapter 2.

A nutritionally adequate diet favors optimal body composition. The detrimental effects of a poor diet depend upon how inadequate the diet is and how long it has been continued. The results of prolonged malnutrition are often striking. It has been shown that the bodies of severely undernourished children characteristically have a much lower fat content and a much higher water content, for example, than those of well-nourished children of the same ages.

The amount of body fat is meaningful in relation to nutritional status at any age when it is considered in conjunction with other measurements, such as body weight. Multiple measurements make it possible to distinguish between overweight and obesity, for example (see Chap. 13). Obesity—a condition of excess body fat—is measured by determining body fat by the methods described. Overweight, on the other hand, may be ascribed to large bones or muscles rather than to excess fat. A person can be overweight without being obese. Measures of body weight and body fat supplement each other in providing some insights into body composition.

PERFORMANCE

Nutrition can make a significant difference in the physical development of peoples. This fact is important in itself, but there is also increasing scientific interest in potential benefits that may accompany physical gains and concern for the impairment that may result from prolonged undernutrition and subnormal growth. This solicitude has been focused on technically underdeveloped countries of the world. Infants and young children in lower socioeconomic groups characteristically grow at slower rates than do children of middle- and upper-income groups in their own countries and most children in North America and Europe. In the past, a major concern for these undersize children has been their high mortality rate—a rate ten to thirty times greater than that in industrial countries.

Major emphasis has shifted more recently to the fate of the children who do survive and to the significance of their malnourished condition in terms of effective living. Evidence has accumulated showing that the poor nutritional status of such children is one of several critical factors adversely affecting their ability to achieve growth potential and their capacity to perform as members of society.

The term "performance" here refers to the ways in which the body responds to contrasting conditions of good and poor nutrition. Differences in performance are considered in terms of mental capacity and learning behavior, ability to resist the inroads of infection, work capacity, and motor efficiency.

Mental Capacity and Learning Behavior (21, 22, 23, 24, 25)

Experiments with laboratory animals have demonstrated that gross *under*nutrition and serious growth failure in very early periods of development may permanently affect the development and functioning of the central nervous system. These findings led to the startling hypothesis that infants and young children might be similarly affected, and that severe undernutrition in late prenatal life and infancy may prevent children from achieving their full intellectual capacity.

Research with animals continues to explore basic aspects of the problem that cannot be pursued with human beings. At the same time, however, important studies are being conducted with severely undernourished children. Widely publicized early findings indicated that severe and prolonged nutritional deficiencies in prenatal life and infancy may have a permanently crippling effect on the intellectual potential and learning behavior of children.

Many newborn infants in lower economic groups of developing countries show a rapid decline in growth rate after the first few months of life, when breast milk becomes insufficient and supplementary foods are lacking in needed nutrients. If an unsatisfactory feeding regimen continues into the second year, the child's nutritional condition can worsen. The decline proceeds if the child then moves on to adult foods consisting predominately of carbohydrates, which fail to supply adequate nourishment. In extreme and prolonged undernutrition, especially when infection is involved, a child may lapse into a state of chronic starvation (*marasmus*) due to a generally poor, low-energy diet, or may develop *kwashiorkor*, a condition that results from a poor diet particularly inadequate in amount and kind of protein (see Chap. 7). While perhaps 20 percent of the children in poor, underdeveloped areas may suffer from such severe protein-calorie undernutrition, several times that number experience mild-to-moderate chronic malnutrition.

marasmus
Emaciation due to lack of food

What are the possible consequences of physical failure to a child's mental status? Some progress has been made in obtaining answers to this question. Various measures have been developed to assess mental capacity and learning ability, notably tests pertaining to structure and functioning of the central nervous system, growth rate and size of the brain, and level of intelligence.

Central Nervous System   The structure and functioning of the central nervous system have been studied primarily in experimental animals. Dietary restrictions imposed on animals to induce developmental changes are more severe than deficiencies generally found in human populations. Thus, direct application of animal experiments to human beings is unrealistic. However, procedures and findings in animal research do give direction to the study of physical-mental relationships in humans. Among the findings that have important implications for human conditions are factors affecting the reversibility of developmental changes in the central nervous system. Animal research shows that the earlier the onset of malnutrition, the more severe the growth failure. The more stringent the nutrient deficiencies and the longer these deficiencies persist, the more likely it is that changes in the central nervous system will be permanent.

These conclusions are compatible with the now generally accepted concept that nerve and brain cells are affected by good and poor nutrition, just as other cells of the body are. The degree to which brain and nerve tissues develop and function satisfactorily depends upon the adequacy of the nutrient supply. When extreme and prolonged deprivation of nutrients occurs during the period of greatest need, it is reasonable to assume that the consequences may be severe and perhaps permanent.

Brain Growth and Size   The brain of a child, as measured by head circumference, normally grows to approximately 90 percent of its ultimate size in the first 2 years of life. During this time, the child attains only about 20 percent of his or her adult body weight. If the period of most rapid brain growth—from the second half of pregnancy through the tenth month of infancy—is marred by severe undernutrition, the rate of brain growth may be diminished. The brains of children who died of marasmus during their first year of life had significantly fewer brain cells than those of normal children of corresponding age (23). The earlier the onset of malnutrition, the more marked were the effects. There is some evidence to suggest that retarded brain growth at this critical period cannot be reversed later, even if the child's nutritional condition improves. Reduced mental capacity appears to be a possible result of such circumstances.

Functioning of the Central Nervous System   Various tests have been devised in an effort to measure learning and behavior under conditions of good and extremely poor nutrition in children. In general, poor performance in such tests is positively related to both severe retardation in height-for-age and below-normal head circumference. Marasmic children who were so severely retarded in growth that their body weights were 50 percent below expectations for their age, and who were also retarded in height, were found to have behavioral deficits as much as 50 percent below normal (26).

Behavior deficits are of many types. They include sensory, perceptual, cognitive, motor, and social aspects. Because of the complex nature of behavior, no particular tests are yet generally accepted as best for measuring normal or subnormal behavior, nor is it known at what ages test results permit maximum predictability. One type of test has sought to measure mother-child interaction as it may be related to the child's state of nutrition. A malnourished child tends to be less active and less demanding, thereby eliciting

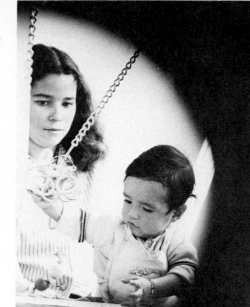

Figure 3.7
Researchers compare test results of poorly-nourished and well-nourished children to study the effects of malnutrition on mental development. Here an observer looks through a peephole to note a child's mental reactions as he is distracted by various objects. (UNICEF/Alastair Matheson)

less response from the mother. Decreased maternal attention may include failure to provide adequate nourishment for the child. Thus malnutrition can not only initiate, but also be perpetuated by, lack of mother-child interaction (27).

Research in this field is complicated by the diversity of factors that make up the environments of the subjects. Malnutrition almost universally exists under conditions of economic poverty with concomitant lack of social stimulation, due in part to low levels of education, motivation, and ability and interest in parenting. Animal studies and observations of humans have shown unquestionably that lack of stimulation is a major factor in subnormal mental development. It is very difficult, however, to distinguish nutritional factors from social-environmental factors as causative. Evaluating the effects of mild-to-moderate malnutrition on mental development and behavior is even more difficult than evaluating those of severe malnutrition. Attempts have been made to measure behavioral change resulting from hunger (due to the absence of breakfast and/or lunch) in school children in the United States. Reports suggest that hunger of this degree affects learning and behavior by interfering with the ability to concentrate, rather than by causing structural changes in the central nervous system. Some efforts at applying mental and behavioral tests in field studies are reported here (Figure 3.7).

Field Studies

Pioneering research in Mexico and Central America drew attention to the fact that poor intelligence-test scores of preschool and school-age children were consistently associated with subnormal body weight and height. Retardation in physical progress could be attributed primarily to poor dietary practices in the home and to the incidence of infectious disease. Genetic backgrounds of the children were similar, and general living conditions and social and economic status were essentially the same for all.

In a rural Mexican community a study was conducted to measure the physical and psychological effects of a nutritional supplement. Infants born in the community and living under the ordinary low socioeconomic conditions were compared with others whose diets had been supplemented continuously after weaning, and whose mothers had received a dietary supplement during pregnancy and *lactation*. The supplemented group was found to differ from the control group by several measures: there was an 8 percent increase in birth weight; physical activity was significantly greater; and psychological test scores were higher. The more rapidly growing, more active children in the supplemented group also had the additional advantage of receiving more attention and care from their fathers and other family members (28).

lactation
Period of milk secretion

Rural Guatemala (29)   A long-term field study is being conducted by the Institute of Nutrition of Central America and Panama (IN-CAP) in an area of Guatemala in which mild-to-moderate malnutrition is widespread and high infection and infant mortality rates are endemic. Basically its purpose is to clarify the relationship between malnutrition and intellectual development. Pregnant and lactating women and their children in two villages are offered a nutritional supplement that furnishes protein and energy. In two other villages, a supplement is offered that provides about one-third as much energy and no protein. The children and their mothers drink the supplements under supervision and the amount ingested by each person is recorded. A wide range of intake is observed since there are no restrictions on how much an individual may have. All participants receive vitamins, minerals and fluorides, and are provided free preventive and curative medical care. Participation in all phases of the project is voluntary. All the mothers and children are followed medically, nutritionally, and socially, and all children will also be followed psychologically until they are 5 years of age (Fig. 3.8).

Members of the interdisciplinary research team have developed new methodologies and refined older techniques to make them applicable to the special needs of this remote population group. Since the villages are matched in all respects except the dietary supplements, there is considerable hope for determining whether nutritional measures alone can prevent or alleviate intellectual and behavioral signs of malnutrition.

Preliminary analyses to date indicate that the effects of food supplementation are generally evident in the reduction of infant mortality, the significant gains in both height and weight of the children, and improved performance on some mental tests at particular ages from 6 months to 5 years. Statistical analysis of the data indicate that the results appear to be due to increased calories and not to proteins as previously thought. The dietary supplements

Figure 3.8
Dietary supplements provided
in rural Guatemala. (Institute of
Nutrition of Central America
and Panama)

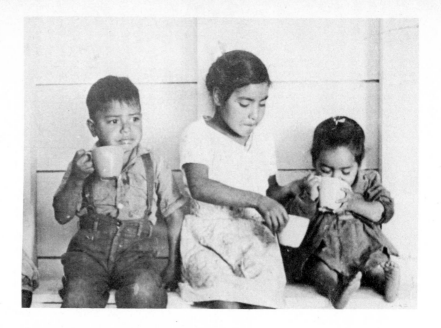

seem to have their greatest and most enduring effects when consumed by the pregnant mother or by the child from birth to 24
months (30). The findings strongly suggest that energy intake affects cognitive development as well as physical development and
general health.

Other field studies pertaining to nutritional status and mental
development have been reported, and most of them have contributed in some measure to our present body of knowledge. A fault
common to several studies, however, is their failure to pick for
comparison situations in which nutrition is the only major variant.
Cultural and social deprivations, which may have an impact equal
to or greater than that of nutritional deficiencies in depressing behavior, must be taken into consideration. Several studies have
been initiated to explore the effect of simultaneous nutritional improvement and social stimulation. In one such study underway in
Cali, Colombia, malnourished 3-year-old children were provided
with nutritional supplements. Some also participated in special
educational activities. After 1 year, and again after 2 years, the
nutritional supplement alone had not improved psychological test
results, while the supplement plus the special educational activities did bring about definite improvement (31).

Studies in the United States

For some time there has been concern that people in the United
States may not be as well nourished as the abundance of the food
supply would suggest. In 1967, Congress authorized the Nutrition
Program Division of the Public Health Service to conduct a National Nutrition Survey "to identify the incidence, magnitude, and
location of malnutrition and related health problems within the
United States" (32). Due to insufficient appropriation of funds to

carry out a study of that size, it became The Ten-State Nutrition Survey.

The Ten-State Nutrition Survey (32)   The Ten-State Survey was conducted in Washington, California, Texas, Louisiana, South Carolina, Kentucky, West Virginia, Michigan, Massachusetts, and New York, with a separate survey of New York City. The population sample within each state was drawn from the census districts with the lowest average income. Although some middle- and upper-income families live in these districts and were represented, the sample was composed largely of low-income people. The population studied was therefore not representative of the entire population within a state, nor of the entire United States. Thus the findings cannot be applied to the overall population, although they do have some application and importance.

The survey provides four types of information: general household socioeconomic data; physical examination findings; biochemical analyses; and dietary-intake data. Some major findings can be readily summarized. Evidence of malnutrition was found more commonly among blacks than among Spanish-Americans and least often among whites. In each ethnic group, nutritional deficiencies were more prevalent as the income level decreased. There was also an association seen between low hemoglobin levels and low dietary iron intakes. Poor dental health was found in many segments of the population. Certain nutrient deficits were more pronounced in vulnerable groups such as pregnant women and preschool children. A higher proportion of children in low income groups was found to be retarded in growth and development (Fig. 3.9). However, black children in general were taller and more advanced in skeletal and dental development than white children. The Ten-State Survey did not probe physical-mental relationships, but findings that show clear-cut evidence of retardation in growth suggest that this may be a productive area for other studies.

Nutritional Status of Preschool Children (33)   A nationwide study of the nutritional status of preschool children was conducted concur-

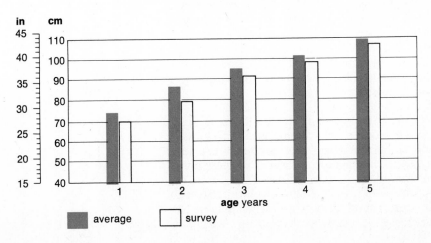

Figure 3.9
Ten-State Nutrition Survey (1968), Average heights of boys from 1 to 5 years of age in the survey, in relation to averages for children of the same ages in the United States (32).

rently with the Ten-State Nutrition Survey. All income groups were included. The sample was not truly representative of preschool children in the United States, but the findings do provide a general overview of the nutritional status of that age group. Growth achievement records and biochemical findings on the children lend support to dietary data and indicate that children of lower socioeconomic status are more "at risk" than are children from affluent homes. The nutritional *quality* of the diet was not highly correlated with socioeconomic status, however. Examination of dietary, clinical, anthropometric, and biochemical data together suggested that the basic nutritional problem of the children "nutritionally at risk" was insufficient *quantities* of food.

anthropometric
Comparative human body measurements

HANES (34, 35, 36)   A new type of program of greater dimensions than previous studies has recently been initiated in the United States to provide information for regional and national health care planning. The Division of Health Examination Statistics in the National Center for Health Statistics (Department of Health, Education, and Welfare) is responsible for planning and conducting the survey. The Health and Nutrition Examination Survey (HANES) will periodically measure the health and nutritional status of the United States population and monitor changes over time. The program was conceived as a surveillance system, implying continuous "watching over" and requiring the gathering of data on the same population at regular time intervals. This is the first time there has ever been a nutritional status study or surveillance of the United States population as a whole.

A sample of 28,000 people, ranging in age from 1 to 74 years, was carefully selected by standard procedures so as to be representative of the total population. On the basis of the findings obtained from examination of this sample, estimates can be made for the total population. The sample design also permits analysis of data pertaining to groups at high risk of malnutrition—the poor, preschool children, women of childbearing ages, and the elderly. Traveling teams of physicians, dentists, dietitians, interviewers, and technicians periodically visit 65 locations designated by the sampling design to collect the data. The first survey was completed in 1974; the second is now in progress.

The nutrition component of the survey consists of four parts: dietary intake data, based on a 24-hour recall and a food frequency questionnaire; biochemical levels of various nutrients, based on tests of blood and urine samples; clinical signs of possible nutritional deficiency disease as observed by a physician, a dermatologist, and a dentist; and anthropometric findings.

The data gathered in the Health and Nutrition Examination Survey bring to light problems related to malnutrition and also identify population groups in need of treatment, preventive services, and nutrition education. Preliminary findings show low intake levels of iron, correlated with evidence of iron deficiency anemia, to be particularly prevalent in young children aged 1 to 5, among blacks more than whites. Vitamin A deficiency, indicated by low *serum* levels, was also found in young children, with a greater percentage among blacks. There were signs of possible defi-

serum
Fluid portion of the blood that remains when blood clots

ciencies of the vitamin B complex, vitamins A, C, and D, calcium, and iron in other age groups as well, with blacks more affected than whites of the same age-sex-income group. Generally, however, black children were slightly taller than white children of the same age. Obese black women as a group are at greatest risk of *hypertension*, heart disease, and *diabetes*. (Specific findings of the surveys described above will be reported at appropriate points in the following chapters.)

hypertension
High blood pressure

diabetes
Disturbances of carbohydrate, fat and protein metabolism due to an inadequate supply of effective insulin

Smaller Surveys   Many surveys of more limited scope have been made on small segments of the population. For example, a nutritional assessment of seasonal farm workers in Florida identified about 20 percent of the individuals in these low-income families as having unsatisfactory nutritional status. Iron-deficiency anemia and *folacin* deficiency were the most common problems. Uncorrected dental defects were also widespread (37).

folacin
Vitamin of the B complex

A few studies in the United States have been designed to relate mental development of poorly nourished children to poor growth records. In one, the median values of height and weight of a group of deprived 4-year-old children were reported to be "below standard populations and closer to malnourished groups from underdeveloped countries." Of this group, 25 percent had "smaller head circumferences than the lowest 10 percent of the published standard population." (38)

In certain areas in the United States, unsatisfactory conditions exist for which malnutrition may be at least partially responsible. Among the clinic population of a municipal hospital in a black ghetto area of New York City, rates of low birth weight and infant mortality were much higher than in more affluent parts of the city. There is evidence that birth weight is affected by maternal nutrition, especially in poor populations. Low birth weight is closely associated with perinatal infant mortality and is also related to unsatisfactory development in later childhood. An investigation similar to the one in rural Guatemala described earlier has been undertaken in New York City (39). This study (the *Perinatal* Project) is an attempt to determine whether dietary improvement will make a difference in infant birth weights and mortality rates. Some of the pregnant women were given a nutritional supplement providing energy and protein. Comparisons of the physical and psychological measurements of their children with those of women who did not receive the supplement are underway. These will indicate whether malnutrition was a major cause of the poor health of infants born in this area of the city.

perinatal
At or about the time of birth

Additional studies are needed. Current data do not indicate whether the relatively mild level of malnutrition found in the United States is a threat to normal mental development. It *is* known that favorable social and public health environmental factors play a role in alleviating conditions surrounding malnutrition. For example, superior environmental sanitation (such as pure water, a safe food supply, and waste disposal systems) and the general availability of medical services in the United States may contribute to the generally better health of undernourished Americans when compared with the undernourished of developing countries.

A Classic Nutrition Study (40)

What are the consequences of malnutrition in maturity when previously well-nourished adults are subjected to severe dietary restrictions? This question was pertinent during World War II, when entire populations existed for long periods on substandard rations, and prisoners of war were grossly underfed in internment camps.

To answer the question, a classic experiment was implemented using as voluntary subjects conscientious objectors who served as noncombatants in the armed services. According to plan, the young men lived for 6 months on a diet providing about one-half the energy of the diet to which they were accustomed. During this time, various tests were administered to the men, and they were observed closely for behavioral changes. Their mental performance did not deteriorate to any degree as the period of undernutrition continued. Significantly, however, there was a sharp decline in spontaneous mental effort and in the capacity for sustained mental application and achievement, which returned to normal only gradually after the diet was restored to adequacy.

The men suffered periods of restlessness and irritability, alternating with periods of apathy and seeming loss of will power. Some of them became sullen and obstinate. They were moody, introspective, and uncooperative. When the men were tested on the Minnesota Multiphasic Personality Inventory, important deviations from the normal were observed. The investigators called the personality changes that occurred during the period of energy deficiency "semi-starvation neuroses."

In the refeeding period that followed, some of the manifestations disappeared in about 3 months' time; others—among them a feeling of depression—subsided less promptly. It seems clear, however, that the effects of the undernutrition were temporary. The condition simulated in this study may be comparable to that which exists when people in confinement are compelled to eat less than they need, or when individuals voluntarily curtail their intake, as in severely restricted reducing diets. It should be mentioned, however, that the diet used in this study was inadequate only in energy; nutrients were provided in adequate amounts. Under such circumstances, unfavorable results of a permanent nature would not be expected.

Resistance to Infection (41, 42, 43)

Nutritional deficiencies reduce the body's natural resistance to infection. Infection works by depressing the appetite, interfering with the absorption of nutrients, and increasing their loss from the body. Under these conditions it is impossible to maintain satisfactory dietary intake and thus overcome the nutritional deficiencies.

The interaction between infection and malnutrition is a *synergistic* one in which each condition makes the other more serious. The two frequently occur together and each perpetuates the other. Even mild infections significantly depress the appetite and thus lead to reduced food intake. A common practice among some groups of people is to offer only liquids to persons with fever or diarrhea; this further limits nutrient intake. When diarrhea is present or the intestinal tract is involved with the infection in some other way, nutrients are less efficiently absorbed than they normally are. Infections also cause metabolic changes, such as greater-than-normal loss of nitrogen and certain nutrients in the urine. This represents breakdown of muscle tissue, and there is loss of body weight. Another metabolic effect of infection occurs when iron loss associated with hookworm infection results in iron-deficiency anemia. Such parasitic intestinal infections as hookworm are very common in tropical and subtropical countries. Other types of anemia are known to be precipitated by different infectious diseases.

The consequences of inadequate child-feeding practices and poor sanitation and personal hygiene are frequent episodes of diarrhea, respiratory infections, and communicable diseases—major factors in the development of kwashiorkor, the protein deficiency disease. Among children treated for kwashiorkor in open hospital wards, there is a continuing high incidence of episodes of diarrhea and other infections. The *synergistic* relationship between infection and malnutrition makes for a long and hazardous recovery period. In many cases, protein-calorie malnutrition is more successfully treated with food alone in nutritional rehabilitation centers where chances of cross-infection are less.

Infection and malnutrition react with social and economic factors to inflict mental and physical injury on children (Fig. 3.10). The significance of an infectious episode on an individual depends on nutritional status, the duration and severity of the infection, and the diet during recovery. Diarrheal disease, upper respiratory tract infections, and the common communicable diseases of childhood are much more severe in grossly undernourished children than in well-nourished children. Among malnourished Guatemalan children, for example, the mortality rate for measles was 189 times that of the United States in 1959 (42). Even in the United States, however, malnutrition, to a degree at which it is as-

synergistic
Relating to the interaction of two or more influences whose total effect is greater than the effects of its parts

Figure 3.10
Schematic indication of relationships among environmental factors that may affect mental development. (*Saturday Review* March 16, 1968) *Central nervous system

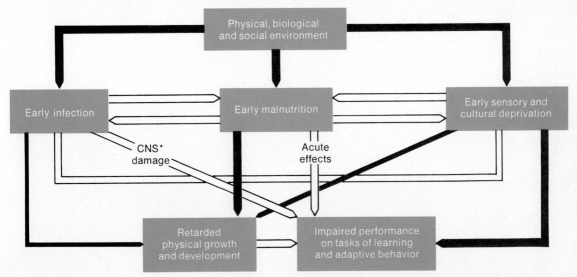

sociated with lowered immunity to infection, is seen in some large city hospitals (44).

The normal, healthy individual is protected against infection by an extremely complicated defense mechanism, some elements of which are not yet completely understood. Recent research findings indicate that while certain immune responses are drastically diminished by malnutrition, others seem not to be affected. This is of practical significance, for it emphasizes the importance of routine public health immunization programs against certain diseases, such as diphtheria, against which even malnourished children seem to develop a normal immune response.

Work Capacity (45)

Nutritional status is one of several factors that can affect work capacity, although its exact role is difficult to identify in real-life job situations. A complicating aspect is the part played by psychological factors, such as motivation, in increasing productivity, generally considered to be the prime measure of work capacity. There are few data that provide unquestionable, quantitative evidence of the effect of nutritional status alone on human work capacity. The studies cited here place major emphasis on the concept that a person's ability to work depends basically upon the supply of energy obtained from food.

The young conscientious objectors, in the experiment described earlier in this chapter were periodically subjected to a battery of motor tests while on their restricted diet. The tests included measures that would indicate energy loss, if such were the case, and suggest lowered productivity. Deterioration was evident in all of the test results, but the amounts varied considerably. By the end

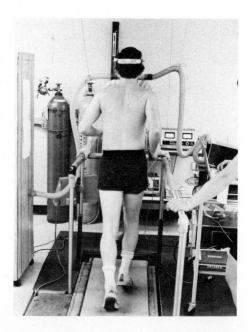

Figure 3.11
A subject runs on a treadmill while breathing into a respirometer that measures the volume of air inhaled and exhaled. The amount of energy required to run at a specific speed for a given period of time is determined by calculating the volume of oxygen consumed. (David L. Costill, PhD, Ball State University Photograph, courtesy National Dairy Council)

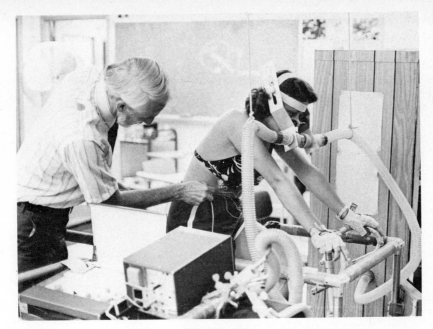

Figure 3.12
A bicycle ergometer is a stationary bicycle used to measure the work capacity of an individual. The energy cost of physical activity or work is usually expressed in terms of calories (units of heat produced). (David L. Costill, PhD, Ball State University Photograph, courtesy National Dairy Council)

ergometer
Apparatus for measuring amount of work done

of the experiment, about one third of the men's original strength—as measured by a grip test and a lifting test—was lost. The largest loss (80 percent) was shown in an endurance test that involved running to exhaustion on a treadmill (40) (Fig. 3.11).

Several studies of industrial workers have shown poor food habits to be associated with fatigue, physical inefficiency, and decreased work output. The productivity of men and women office and factory workers was measured on a bicycle *ergometer* (Fig. 3.12). All the subjects did significantly more work in the late morning hours when they started the day with a good breakfast than when they had omitted breakfast.

A dramatic example of the effects of lessened energy intake in a relatively short time, is that of troops stationed in the Canadian Arctic. Three companies were provided with rations on three different energy levels from high to low, and the behavior of the men was observed. By the end of a week, the companies on the two lower energy intakes began to show signs of deterioration. On returning to camp after a hard day in the field, each platoon cut down spruce trees for the night's shelter. There was a remarkable difference in response to this one operation among the three groups. The platoons on the best rations built proper shelters to protect themselves from the weather; those on the most energy-deficient diet merely spread the spruce branches on the ground and slept on them unprotected; the platoons on a diet with an energy level between the first two started to build shelters with the branches but were overtaken by inertia before they completed their tasks (46).

Several attempts are being made to measure the effect on productivity of two common types of nutritional problems: insufficient energy intake for sustained hard labor, and iron-deficiency ane-

Does Nutrition Make a Difference? **77**

mia, which might restrict work output by limiting the oxygen-carrying capacity of the blood. In rural Guatemala, where agricultural activities require considerable expenditures of human energy, two groups of workers were compared. One group consumed approximately 3500 calories per person per day; the other, approximately 2700 calories. The workers with the greater intake spent proportionately more energy in their daily activities, suggesting that productivity in energy-requiring tasks is limited by energy intake (47). Maximum capacity to consume oxygen was used as a measure of physical work capacity in a group of Colombian agricultural workers. The number of tons of sugarcane cut per day was established as a direct measure of the workers' productivity. Maximum oxygen-consumption capacity was consistently related to level of productivity—high producers had higher oxygen-consumption capacity. Highly productive workers were also somewhat taller and heavier, with more lean body mass, an indication of life-long better nutrition (48).

Among malnourished groups in developing countries, productivity potential can have a double relationship to nutrition: workers' daily work outputs may be extremely low, due primarily to the poor-quality, low-energy value of their diet; and their lifetime work output may be strikingly lower than that of their counterparts in industrial countries, due to fewer productive years. The life expectancy in developing nations is estimated to be 35 to 45 years, with 20 productive years. In industrial nations it is about 70 years, with almost 50 productive years.

Increasing realization of the importance that nutritional status holds for work capacity has revealed the need for including nutrition planning in the economic development of nations (49). A few countries—among them Chile, Colombia, Brazil, India, and Zambia—have already done this. The potential benefits of such planning were demonstrated with construction and plantation workers in Indonesia. There and in many other parts of the world iron-deficiency anemia is a nutrition-related impairment. The investigation in Indonesia studied the effect of the anemia on work capacity. Findings showed that when the anemia was corrected by iron therapy, work output increased measurably. An almost linear correlation was observed between hemoglobin levels and payments made to latex tappers on rubber plantations for output above the daily quota. It was estimated that the benefit-to-cost ratio for correcting the iron deficiency could be as high as 260-to-1. Such data provide planners with the evidence they need of the economic advantages of good nutritional status and the importance of programs to develop human resources. (45)

LENGTH OF LIFE AND NUTRITION

Statistics show that people in the United States are living longer now than at any time in history. A white male born in 1901 could expect to live about 48 years; by 1972, life expectancy for a male at birth had increased to more than 67 years. Comparable figures for females are even more favorable. In 1901, a white female at birth could expect to live about 51 years; by 1972, life expectancy

Table 3.2
Life expectation of white males and females in the United States in 1901 and 1972 (50)

Age	1901 Life expectation		1972 Life expectation		Gain by males 1901–1972	Gain by females 1901–1972
	Males	Females	Males	Females		
	years	years	years	years	years	years
0	48.2	50.7	67.4	75.1	19.2	24.4
1	54.6	56.1	67.8	75.3	13.2	19.2
10	50.6	51.9	59.2	66.6	8.6	14.7
20	42.2	43.6	49.7	56.9	7.5	13.3
30	34.9	36.3	40.7	47.3	5.8	11.0
40	27.7	29.1	31.6	37.9	3.9	8.8
50	20.8	21.8	23.3	29.0	2.5	7.2
60	14.4	15.2	16.1	20.8	1.7	5.6
70	9.0	9.6	10.4	13.5	1.4	3.9
80	5.1	5.5	6.4	7.9	1.3	2.4

for a female was 75 years—a gain of nearly a quarter-century. Table 3.2 bears out these facts, as well as providing additional information on the life expectancies of white men and women calculated at 10-year intervals from birth to 80 years of age (50).

Has nutrition entered into this picture of lengthened life in the United States? Does nutrition make a difference in how long life will last? A full answer to these questions calls for examining the data and exploring the possible causes for the present favorable picture.

Table 3.2 shows that while total gains in life expectancy have been spectacular, they have not been consistently good at all age levels. By far the greatest gains have been made in the early years of life. A major reason for this fact has been success in dealing with diseases of infectious origin, such as tuberculosis, dysentery, small-pox, and common childhood diseases. Contributing to this achievement are advances in medical knowledge, improvements in sanitation, better medical care, increased public health services, and greater knowledge of child-feeding requirements, as well as steady advancement in the newer area of nutrition knowledge. It is impossible to assess the exact proportionate role of nutrition in the life expectancy of children. Malnutrition is undoubtedly an important factor under all conditions—an overriding one when infection is involved. In countries where malnutrition and infectious disease continue to be severe, the average life span is as low as 35 to 45 years.

It is important that life-expectancy gains made in early childhood continue. A deterrent to this progress, however, is the relatively high infant mortality rate, particularly for the *neonatal period,* the first 28 days of life. Premature birth and low birth weight are clearly associated with neonatal mortality (51). In the United States prematurity and infant mortality are higher for infants of very young mothers and those with frequent pregnancies; inadequate prenatal care, poor nutrition, and low living standards are contributing factors. While there has been a steady overall downward trend in total infant mortality rate for the United States as a whole, there is a wide discrepancy between mortality rates for

neonatal period
First 28 days after birth

Table 3.3
Estimated average length of life in years
by color and sex in the United States 1900–1972 (50)

Year	White		Nonwhite		Differences in Favor of white	
	Male	Female	Male	Female	Male	Female
1900*	46.6	48.7	32.5	33.5	+14.1	+15.2
1910*	48.6	52.0	33.8	37.5	+14.8	+14.5
1920*	54.4	55.6	45.5	45.2	+8.9	+10.4
1930	59.7	63.5	47.3	49.2	+12.4	+14.3
1940	62.1	66.6	51.5	54.9	+10.6	+11.7
1950	66.5	72.2	59.1	62.9	+7.4	+9.3
1960	67.4	74.1	61.1	66.3	+6.3	+7.8
1970	68.0	75.6	61.3	69.4	+6.7	+6.2
1972	68.3	75.9	61.5	69.9	+6.7	+6.2

*Death Registration States

white and "all other" groups. In 1975, the rate for "all other" groups was still 58 percent higher than that for whites (51, 52, 53).

There is still room for gains in life expectancy, even in the early childhood years where most progress has already been made. In proportion to the effort expended, gains in the future will be relatively small in terms of years added to life. Gains will come not so much from medicine, which contributed so significantly to the original spurt early in the century, as from the social and cultural influences that impinge on health. Improved nutrition must be counted among the influences to be felt, and felt equally by all segments of the population, if life is to be enriched and lengthened for everyone. Merely narrowing the gap between the average length of life for white and nonwhite citizens of all ages will do much to continue the favorable trend toward greater life expectancy for all.

Table 3.3 shows estimated average lengths of life in the US by color and sex, at intervals from 1900 to 1972. The differences are striking. In 1900, the average white male could expect to live 14 years longer and the average white female 15 years longer than their nonwhite counterparts. In 1972, the corresponding advantage was less than 7 years. While the difference in average length of life between the races was cut in half in 70 years, the situation has changed little in the past 20 years (50). Studies show that in general the nutritional status of nonwhites in the United States is less favorable than that of whites.

Gains in Mature Years

Table 3.2 shows clearly the relatively small life-expectancy gains made in the ages beyond childhood between 1901 and 1972. By 10 years of age, the gains had begun to diminish noticeably. At 20 years of age, the average woman gained about 13 years in life expectancy; at 50 years of age she gained about 7 years; at 70 years she made a gain of about 4 years. The gains for men were smaller for the same periods. A major effort will be needed to extend life expectancy in these mature years.

The failure of the death rate to continue its sharp decline of early childhood into adult life is responsible for the contrast. This situation leads to a consideration of the chief causes of death in middle and later life. In the coming years, attention will be focused on the possibilities of conquering diseases common during these periods. Chronic degenerative diseases are major causes of death in adults, and heart diseases head the list (54). In most of these conditions the root of the disability lies in the arteries, which undergo deteriorative changes that impair their usefulness. There is evidence that artery changes of this character may be linked to diet (see Chap. 5). If research now in progress confirms such a relationship, it may also point to specific ways of preventing or reversing such changes. It is highly probable that new discoveries in nutrition can be the means of adding years to life.

Older people make up a steadily growing segment of the population. They are confronted with the problem of maintaining a level of health that will enable them to remain productive and enjoy living. Merely adding length to life is not enough, for added years can actually be a burden unless they bring with them vigor and independence. Forming good food habits at any age helps, but the person who has been well-nourished throughout life has the best propect of sustaining good nutritional status into later years.

REFERENCES

1. M. Mason, J. L. Mackin, G. G. Harrison and S. A. Seubert, *Nutrition and the Cell: The Inside Story* (Chicago: Year Book Medical Publishers, 1973).

2. J. M. Tanner, "Earlier Maturation in Man," *Scientific American* 218 (Jan. 1968), pp. 21-27.

3. H. Bakwin and S. M. McLaughlin, "Secular Increase in Height," *The Lancet* II (Dec. 5, 1964), pp. 1195-96.

4. M. L. Hathaway and E. D. Foard, *Heights and Weights in Adults in the United States,* Home Economics Res. Report (Washington, D.C.: USDA, 1960).

5. R. M. Malina, "Comparison of the Increase in Body Size between 1899 and 1970 in a Specially Selected Group with that in the General Population," *Am. J. Phys. Anthropology* 37 (Nov. 1971), pp. 135-42.

6. A. Damon, "Secular Trend in Height and Weight within Old American Families at Harvard, 1870-1965, I. Within Twelve Four-Generation Families," *Am. J. Phys. Anthropology* 29

(July 1968), pp. 45-50. (Certain additional information, as yet unpublished, has been supplied to the authors by this investigator.)

7. S. Abraham, C. L. Johnson and M. F. Najjar, "Height and Weight of Adults 18-74 Years of Age in the United States," Advance Data from Vital and Health Statistics of the National Center for Health Statistics, No. 3 (Rockville, Maryland: US Dept. of Health, Education and Welfare, Public Health Service, Nov. 19, 1976).

8. W. W. Greulich, "A Comparison of the Physical Growth and Development of American-born and Native Japanese Children," *Am. J. Phys. Anthropology* 15 (Dec. 1957), pp. 489-515.

9. W. Insull, T. Oiso, and K. Tsuchiya, "Diet and Nutritional Status of Japanese," *Am. J. Clin. Nutr.* 21 (July 1968), pp. 753-77.

10. H. S. Mitchell, "Protein Limitation and Growth," *J. Am. Dietet. Assoc.* 44 (March 1964), pp. 165-72.

11. S. M. Garn, "Malnutrition and Skeletal Development in the Preschool Child," *Preschool Child Malnutrition: Primary Deterrent to Progress* (Washington, D.C.: National Academy of Sciences—National Research Council, Pub. 1282, 1966), Chap. 5.

12. W. W. Greulich and S. I. Pyle, *Radiographic Atlas of Skeletal Development of the Hand and Wrist,* 2nd ed., (Stanford, Calif.: Stanford University Press, 1959).

13. S. Dreizen, R. M. Snodgrasse, H. Webb-Peploe and T. D. Spies, "The Retarding Effect of Protracted Undernutrition on the Appearance of the Postnatal Ossification Centers in the Hand and Wrist," *Human Biology* 30 (Dec. 1958), pp. 253-63.

14. A. A. Albanese, "Nutritional Aspects of Bone Loss," *Food and Nutrition News* 47 (Oct.-Nov. 1975 and Dec.-Jan. 1975-76), pp. 1, 4 in each.

15. A. E. Nizel, *Nutrition in Preventive Dentistry: Science and Practice,* (Philadelphia: W. B. Saunders 1972).

16. B. G. Bibby, "The Cariogenicity of Snack Foods and Confections," *J. Am. Dent. Assoc.* 90 (Jan. 1975), pp. 121-32.

17. L. E. Granath, *et al.,* "Variations in Caries Prevalence Related to Combinations of Dietary and Oral Hygiene Habits in 6-Year Old Children," *Caries Res.* 10 (April, 1976), pp. 308-17.

18. I. G. Macy, *Nutrition and Chemical Growth in Childhood,* Vol. I (Springfield, Ill.: Thomas Publishing, 1942).

19. J. Brozek, "Nutrition and Body Composition," *Review of Nutrition Research* 26:3 (July-Sept. 1965).

20. "Skinfold Thickness and Body Fat," *Nutr. Reviews* 26 (April 1968), pp. 104-7.

21. Subcommittee on Nutrition, Brain Development, and Behavior of the Committee on International Nutrition Programs, Food and Nutrition Board, *The Relationship of Nutrition to Brain Development and Behavior* (Washington, D.C.: National Academy of Sciences—National Research Council, 1973).

22. M. Winick, *Malnutrition and Brain Development* (New York: Oxford University Press, 1976).

23. M. S. Read, "Behavioral Correlates of Malnutrition," in M. A. B. Brazier, ed., *Growth and Development of the Brain* (New York: Raven Press, 1975), pp. 335-53.

24. J. Cravioto and E. R. DeLicardie, "Ecology of Malnutrition-Environmental Variables Associated with Clinical Severe Malnutrition," in C. A. Canosa, ed., *Nutrition, Growth and Development* (New York: S. Karger, 1975), pp. 157-66.

25. D. S. McLaren, U. S. Yaktin, A. A. Kanawati, S. Sabbagh, and Z. Kadi, "The Relationship of Severe Marasmic Protein-Energy Malnutrition and Rehabilitation in Infancy to Subsequent Mental Development," in R. E. Olson, ed., *Protein-Calorie Malnutrition* (New York: Academic Press, 1975), pp. 107-12.

26. E. Pollitt, "Behavioral Correlates of Severe Malnutrition in Man," in W. M. Moore, M. M. Silverberg and M. S. Read, eds., *Nutrition, Growth and Development of North American Indian Children,* DHEW Publication No. (NIH) 72-76, (Washington, D.C: US Gov. Print. Office, 1972), pp. 151-66.

27. P. L. Graves, "Nutrition, Infant Behavior and Maternal Characteristics: A Pilot Study in West Bengal, India," *Am. J. Clin. Nutr.* 29 (Mar. 1976), pp. 305-19.

28. A. Chavez, C. Martinez and T. Yaschine, "The Importance of Nutrition and Stimuli on Child Mental and Social Development," in J. Cravioto, L. Hambraeus and B. Vahlquist, eds., *Early Malnutrition and Mental Development* (Uppsala, Sweden: Almqvist and Wiksell, 1974), pp. 211-25.

29. A. Lechtig, H. Delgado, R. Lasky, C. Yarbrough, R. Martorell, J. P. Habicht and R. E. Klein, "Effect of Improved Nutrition

During Pregnancy and Lactation on Developmental Retardation and Infant Mortality," in P. L. White and N. Selvey, eds., *Proc. Western Hemisphere Nutrition Congress IV, 1974* (Acton, Mass.: Publishing Sciences Group, 1975), pp. 117-25.

30. J. Townsend, Psychologist, Division of Human Development, INCAP, Personal Communication, 1976.

31. H. E. McKay, A. McKay and L. Sinisterra, "Behavioral Intervention Studies with Malnourished Children: A Review of Experiences," in D. J. Kallen, ed., *Nutrition, Development and Social Behavior,* DHEW Publication No. (NIH) 73-242 (Washington, D.C.: US Gov. Print. Office, 1973).

32. "Highlights from the Ten-State Nutrition Survey," *Nutrition Today* 7 (July/Aug. 1972), pp. 4-11.

33. G. M. Owen, K. M. Kram, P. J. Garry, J. E. Lowe and A. H. Lubin, "A Study of Nutritional Status of Preschool Children in the United States, 1968-1970," *Pediatrics* 53 (April, 1974), pp. 597-646.

34. H. W. Miller, *Plan and Operation of the Health and Nutrition Examination Survey,* DHEW Publication No. (HRA) 76-1310 (Rockville, Maryland: US Dept. Health, Education and Welfare, Public Health Service, Health Resources Admin., 1973).

35. S. Abraham, F. W. Lowenstein, and C. L. Johnson, *Preliminary Findings of the First Health and Nutrition Examination Survey, United States, 1971-1972: Dietary Intake and Biochemical Findings,* DHEW Publication No. (HR) 76-1219-1 (Washington, D.C.: US Gov. Print. Office, 1974).

36. S. Abraham, F. W. Lowenstein, and D. E. O'Connell, *Preliminary Findings of the First Health and Nutrition Examination Survey, United States, 1971-1972: Anthropometric and Clinical Findings,* DHEW Publication No. (HRA) 75-1229 (Washington, D.C.: US Gov. Print. Office, 1975).

37. M. Kaufman, E. Lewis, A. V. Hardy, and J. Proulx, "Florida Seasonal Farm Workers: Follow-Up and Intervention Following a Nutrition Survey," *J. Am. Dietet. Assoc.* 66 (June 1975), pp. 605-9.

38. O. C. Stine, J. B. Saratsiotis and O. F. Furno, "Appraising the Health of Culturally Deprived Children," *Am. J. Clin. Nutr.* 20 (Oct. 1967), pp. 1084-95.

39. D. Rush, Z. Stein, G. Christakis and M. Susser, "The Prenatal Project: The First 20 months of Operation," in M. Winick, ed., *Nutrition and Fetal Development* (New York: John Wiley and Sons, 1974), pp. 95-125.

40. A. Keys, J. Brozek, A. Henschel, O. Michaelson and H. L. Taylor, *The Biology of Human Starvation* (Minneapolis: University of Minnesota Press, 1950).

41. N. S. Scrimshaw, "Interactions of Malnutrition and Infection: Advances in Understanding," in R. E. Olson, ed., *Protein-Calorie Malnutrition* (New York: Academic Press 1975), pp. 353-67.

42. C. G. Neumann, G. L. Lawlor, Jr., E. R. Stiehm, M. E. Swendseid, C. Newton, J. Herbert, A. J. Ammann and M. Jacob, "Immunologic Responses in Malnourished Children," *Am. J. Clin. Nutr.* 28 (Feb. 1975), pp. 89-104.

43. V. Reddy, V. Jagadeesan, N. Ragharamulu, C. Bhaskaram and S. G. Srikantia, "Functional Significance of Growth Retardation in Malnutrition," *Am. J. Clin. Nutr.* 29 (Jan. 1976), pp. 3-7.

44. B. R. Bistrian, G. L. Blackburn, N. S. Scrimshaw and J. P. Flatt, "Cellular Immunity in Semistarved States in Hospitalized Adults," *Am. J. Clin. Nutr.* 28 (Oct. 1975), pp. 1148-55.

45. M. S. Read, "Malnutrition and Human Performance," presented at Am. Assoc. Adv. Science meeting Boston, Feb. 1976. To be published.

46. R. M. Kark, "Food and Hunger in a World of Turmoil," in G. H. Bourne, *World Review of Nutrition and Dietetics* (New York: Hafner Publishing, 1966).

47. F. E. Viteri, B. Torun, J. C. Galicia, and E. Herrera, "Determining energy costs of agricultural activities by respirometer and energy balance techniques," *Am. J. Clin. Nutr.,* 24 (Dec. 1971), pp. 1418-30.

48. G. B. Spurr, M. Barac-Nieto, and M. D. Maksud, "Energy Expenditure Cutting Sugarcane," *J. Applied Physiol.,* 39 (Dec. 1975), pp. 990-96.

49. R. W. Longhurst and D. L. Call, "Scientific Consensus, Nutrition Programs and Economic Planning," *Am. J. Clin. Nutr.,* 28 (Oct. 1975), pp. 1177-82.

50. Vital Statistics of the United States, *Life Tables–1972, II, Section 5,* (Washington, D.C.: US Dept. Health, Education and Welfare, Public Health Service, 1975).

51. V. Vaughan and R. J. McKay, *Nelson Textbook of Pediatrics* (Philadelphia: W. B. Saunders Company, 1975).

52. G. Stickle and P. Ma, "Pregnancy in Adolescents: Scope of the Problem," *Contemporary Ob/Gyn* 5 (June 1975), pp. 85-91.

53. M. E. Wegman, "Annual Summary of Vital Statistics: 1975,"
    Pediatrics 58 (Dec. 1976), pp. 793-99.

54. Vital Statistics of the United States, Section 1, *General Mor-
    tality: 1972* (Washington, D.C.: US Dept. Health, Education
    and Welfare, Public Health Service, 1976).

READINGS

Cheek, D. B., *Fetal and Postnatal Cellular Growth*. (New York:
John Wiley and Sons, 1975).

Coursin, D. B. "Electrophysiological Studies in Malnutrition," in J.
Cravioto, L. Hambraeus and B. Vahlquist, eds., *Early Malnutri-
tion and Mental Development*. (Uppsala, Sweden: Almqvist and
Wiksell, 1974), pp. 72-84.

Faulk, W. P., E. M. Demaeyer, and A. J. S. Davies. "Some Effects of
Malnutrition on the Immune Response in Man." *Am. J. Clin.
Nutr.* 27 (June, 1974), pp. 638-46.

Freeman, H. E., R. E. Klein, J. Kagan and C. Yarbrough, "Relations
between Nutrition and Cognition in Rural Guatemala," *Am. J.
of Public Health* 67 (Mar. 1977), pp. 233-39.

"The Impact of Food and Nutrition on Oral Health." *Dairy Council
Digest* 44 (May-June, 1973), pp. 13-16.

Lowenstein, F. W., "Some Preliminary Findings from the First
Health and Nutrition Examination Survey," in P. L. White and
N. Selvey, eds., *Proc. Western Hemisphere Nutrition Congress
IV* (Acton, Mass.: Publishing Sciences Group, 1975).

Lowenstein, F. W. "The Health and Nutrition Examination Survey:
A Resume," *Am. J. Clin. Nutr.* 26 (Dec. 1973), pp. 1369-70.

Lowenstein, F. W. "Preliminary Clinical and Anthropometric Findings from the First Health and Nutrition Examination Survey,
U. S. A., 1971-1972," *Am. J. Clin. Nutr.* 29 (Aug. 1976), pp.
918-27.

Read, M. S., "Malnutrition, Hunger and Behavior I. Malnutrition
and Learning." *J. Am. Dietet. Assoc.* 63 (Oct. 1973), pp. 379-85.

Read, M. S. "Malnutrition, Hunger and Behavior II. Hunger, School
Feeding Programs, and Behavior." *J. Am. Dietet. Assoc.* 63
(Oct. 1973), pp. 386-91.

Sabry, Z. I., A. Campbell, M. E. Campbell and A. L. Forbes. "Nutrition Canada." *Nutrition Today* 9, (Jan.-Feb. 1974), pp. 5-13.

Scrimshaw, N. S. and V. R. Young, "The Requirements of Human
Nutrition." *Sci. American* 235, (Sept. 1976), pp. 50-64.

Shaw, J. H., "Diet Regulations for Caries Prevention." *Nutrition
News* 36 (Feb. 1973), pp. 1, 4.

Suskind, R., S. Sirishinka, V. Vithayasai, R. Edelman, D. Damrong-
sak, C. Charupatana and R. E. Olson. "Immunoglobulins and
Antibody Response in Children with Protein-Calorie Malnutrition." *Am. J. Clin. Nutr.* 29 (Aug. 1976), pp. 836-41.

Ten-State Nutrition Survey, 1968-1970, DHEW Publication No. (HSM) 72-8134, Volumes I-V (Atlanta, Georgia: Health Services and Mental Health Administration, 1972).

Weisberg, S. M., K. M. Reese and P. McDonald. *Nutrition and Productivity: Their Relationship in Developing Countries.* (Washington, D.C.: Office of Nutrition, Agency for International Development, 1972).

Part 2
The Science of Nutrition

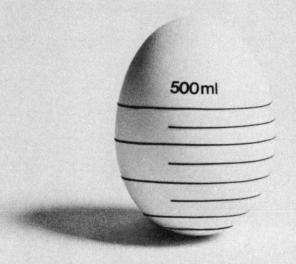

This Part introduces the fundamentals of the science of nutrition. It is intended to give students enough essential information to help them discover for themselves that nutrition is a living, growing science interrelated with biological and behavioral sciences, and that it has enormous significance in terms of their own well-being and that of all mankind. It should be evident that nutrition is a vast subject that cannot be encompassed in one college course. Nor can it be explored in depth without an extensive background in science. Nevertheless, there is much in store for those who seek a functional knowledge of nutrition, and the rewards are greatest for those who become actively involved in applying their learnings.

Involvement consists in becoming familiar with some of the tools of the science of nutrition and learning to evaluate their usefulness. For example, students should become acquainted with reliable reference materials in nutrition and related fields, and they should learn to distinguish the sound from the unsound in nutrition information. It would be useful for students to familiarize themselves with dietary criteria and how to apply them, to know the limitations as well as the strengths of such criteria. From exposure of this type comes an awareness of the practical benefits to be derived from applying the principles of the science of nutrition.

Lines of involvement are proposed throughout the text. It is urged that these be used as guides for class activities and discussion when possible. For classes too restricted by time limitations to develop their own materials, exhibits are provided in the chapters. These include food lists, specimen meal records, weight charts, and calculated diets.

Nutrients in Foods

Classification
Functions

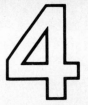

People are most familiar with the foods they eat for breakfast, lunch, dinner, and snacks. If you were to recall what you ate yesterday, the record might look something like the top half of Table 4.1. The food an individual eats in one day might include as many as twenty different items, each of which fits naturally into a grouping with other foods that are similar in composition and use. Thus, the separate food items can be classified into a small number of food groups, as shown in the lower half of Table 4.1.

A similar analysis of many menus would yield essentially the same results, with the food items classified under the same few headings. Such groupings are helpful in planning nutritionally adequate meals, as well as being a convenience in checking meals for variety in selection. Each food group contributes certain nutrients that your body needs. The complete assortment of the foods you choose determines the quality of your food intake, or the adequacy of your diet.

Table 4.1
Specimen meal record

Breakfast	Lunch	Snack	Dinner	Snack
doughnut	hamburger	cola type	pork chop	potato chips
coffee	bun	drink	mashed potato	
sugar	pickles		corn	
	catsup		cole slaw	
	mustard		rolls	
	onions		butter or	
	milk		margarine	
			ice cream	
			chocolate chip	
			cookies	

Food groups	Food items on the menu
milk group	milk, ice cream
meat group	hamburger, pork chop
vegetable group	potato, corn, cabbage
fruit group	—
bread-cereal group	doughnut, bun, rolls
fats group	butter or margarine
sweets group	sugar, cookies, soft drink

This specimen diet is not intended as a model in any sense; see footnote, p. 138.

Examine your 3-day food record (see Chap. 1, p. 4). How many different foods did you eat each day? Can you fit the individual food items into the food groups in Table 4.1?

Is the pattern of your meals and snacks similar to that in Table 4.1? If not, how does it vary?

To acquire a working knowledge of nutrition, foods are studied from two standpoints:

☐ as the foods themselves, including the ways they fit together to make good-tasting, satisfying, nutritionally adequate meals; and

☐ as those individual dietary substances, the nutrients, which in varying amounts and combinations constitute the foods.

Foods and eating practices are important to each of us for varied reasons, some of which were discussed in Chapter 1. Basically, however, food is important—regardless of one's age, culture, or socioeconomic status—because it is essential to sustain life. This physiological function is not dependent on individual food items, or even on the various food groups, but on the many separate nutrients of which all foods are composed. These nutrients are described below as background for an understanding of foods as they are considered in the remainder of the text.

CLASSES OF NUTRIENTS

The nutrients are grouped into six classes, on the basis of similarities in chemical structure and function. These classes are:

- ☐ carbohydrates
- ☐ fats
- ☐ proteins
- ☐ minerals
- ☐ vitamins
- ☐ water

Carbohydrates, fats, proteins, and water are by far the most abundant nutrients in foods. They account for almost the total weight of the nutrients in the diet. The minerals rank next in quantity, but they contribute only a fraction of an ounce to a total of some 4 pounds of food a person might eat in a day. The vitamins occur in even smaller quantities than that. In terms of total quantity, the amounts of minerals and vitamins in foods may seem negligible, but all of them are of critical importance to the normal growth and smooth functioning of the body. Each individual nutrient performs specific tasks, but no nutrient acts independently of others. Examples of the ways nutrients are interdependent and act together to achieve results will be cited throughout Part 2.

Most foods are composed of more than one type of nutrient, but it is customary to identify foods loosely according to their quantitative contributions of carbohydrates, fats, and proteins. For example, when a food contains more carbohydrate than protein or fat, it is referred to as a *carbohydrate food*; one with more fat than protein or carbohydrate is called a *fat food*; and a food with more protein than carbohydrate or fat is usually known as a *protein food*. This rule holds in spite of the fact that there are many exceptions, some of which are cited in the following discussion of these classes. There are obvious limitations to any plan that does not take into account all the nutrient classes in foods, or the fact that some foods supply significant amounts of all three kinds of nutrients—carbohydrates, fats, and proteins. Nevertheless, it is important to know and to understand the basis for a terminology that is widely applied in nutrition.

The bar graphs in Figure 4.1, showing the percentages of carbohydrate, fat, protein, mineral elements (total ash), and water in a few typical foods, illustrate the way in which the composition of a food qualifies it to be classified as a carbohydrate, a fat, or a protein food (1).

Carbohydrate Foods

Carbohydrates in foods are chiefly starches and sugars (Fig. 4.2). Some examples of starchy foods are grains, products made from grains, and starchy vegetables such as potatoes and root vegetables. Grain products include breads, other bakery items, pasta (noodles, spaghetti, and macaroni), and breakfast cereals. The sugars include granulated and brown sugar from sugarcane and sugar beets, syrups and sugars derived from corn, other syrups, honey, molasses, and the sugars occurring naturally in fruits, vegetables, and milk (2, 3). (Not included are the noncaloric sweeteners used as sugar substitutes.)

Figure 4.1

Composition of foods. Percent of carbohydrate, fat, protein, water, and ash. (Food values pertain to forms of foods as they are purchased.) [Data from Table 1, Agriculture Handbook No. 8, US Dept. of Agriculture]

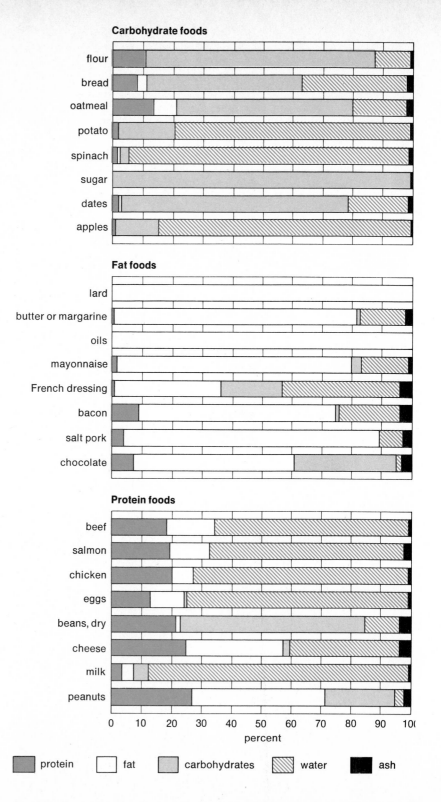

Carbohydrate foods in Figure 4.1 are composed of proportionately more carbohydrates than other nutrients except water. But sugar is the only food that is virtually 100 percent carbohydrate. Honey, jellies, jams, and candies are other sweets that rank as high-carbohydrate foods. Vegetables in general are higher in carbohydrates than in proteins or fats, but the proportion that is carbohydrate varies greatly among different kinds of vegetables. Although potatoes contain only about one-third as much carbohydrate as bread or oatmeal, they are concentrated sources of carbohydrate in comparison with leafy vegetables of high water content such as spinach. Essentially the same situation exists with respect to fruits. Dates, which are relatively concentrated sources of sugar, are carbohydrate-rich, while juicy fresh apples are a more dilute source.

Carbohydrates, particularly in the form of grains, are the most important sources of energy in the world. The types and amounts used and the proportion of the total diet they occupy differ widely. In some countries, for example, rice or corn is a major component of the food supply; in others, and in the higher income segments of some populations, the diet is more varied and includes a smaller proportion of carbohydrate foods. Because high-carbohydrate foods are relatively less expensive than protein-rich foods, they make up a large proportion of low-cost diets.

Patterns of Carbohydrate Consumption   One way to explore consumption patterns of foods and nutrients is to study estimates of the quantities of some major foods available to the population from the national food supply. Such estimates are referred to as "disappearance data," because they signify the quantity of food from all available sources that is moved into channels for civilian consumption in the United States. This quantity is assumed to have been

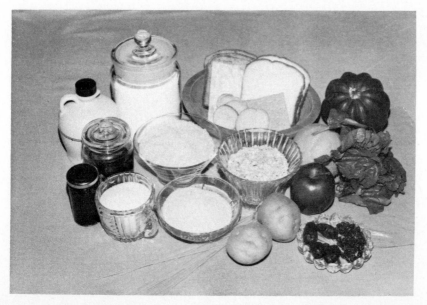

Figure 4.2
Common sources of carbohydrates: sugar, syrup, cereals, pasta, breadstuffs, fruits, vegetables. (Landon Gardiner)

Table 4.2
Per capita consumption of carbohydrate foods
in selected periods (disappearance data)

Time periods	Flour and cereal products lbs/year	Sugars and other sweeteners * lbs/year	 g/day
1909–13	291	89.1	111
1925–29	237	118.6	148
1935–39	204	110.5	137
1947–49	171	109.5	136
1957–59	148	106.5	132
1960	147	108.8	135
1961	147	109.2	135
1962	146	110.0	137
1963	144	110.5	137
1964	144	111.6	139
1965	144	111.7	139
1966	143	113.0	141
1967	144	112.6	140
1968	144	116.2	145
1969	145	116.9	145
1970	141	119.7	149
1971	142	120.0	149
1972	140	122.8	153
1973	140	125.1	156
1974	138	121.5	151
1975	139	114.5	142

*Does not include artificial sweeteners.
US Dept. of Agriculture (4)

consumed as food. Disappearance data are high estimates of the food actually consumed, since they include any food waste that occurs at or beyond the retail level. This is sometimes termed "economic consumption" as distinguished from true consumption data based on dietary studies. Information of this type is systematically assembled and made available by the US Department of Agriculture (4).

In the United States, carbohydrate from all sources currently yields somewhat less than half the calories available on the market. The percentage of energy obtained through carbohydrates has declined steadily from 56 percent to about 47 percent during the 1900s, but this decline does not apply to all carbohydrate foods. As shown in Table 4.2, the amount of flour and cereal products available, for example, has decreased significantly during this period from 291 pounds per person per year between 1909 and 1913 to 144 pounds in 1963, remaining steady at that level up to the present. The total amount of sugars marketed increased from 89 pounds per person in the earlier years to a high of 125 pounds in 1973. The decrease in 1974 clearly resulted from high prices. To facilitate relating the data on sugars to personal food habits, usage is also expressed in the table as grams per person per day. (One teaspoon of sugar weighs 4 grams.) It is hard to believe that sugar and sweetener consumption can indeed be as high as these data indicate. In many families very few pounds of sugar as such are purchased each year. But about two-thirds of the sugar consumed in the United States actually comes from commercial products such as candy, soft drinks, presweetened cereals, bakery goods and mixes, and other prepared foods.

Check the foods with the highest carbohydrate content on the table in appendix K. Group them by the amounts of carbohydrate per serving: 20 to 30 grams, 30 to 40, 40 to 50, and more than 50 grams, and note the types of foods that fall into these categories.

How much carbohydrate do you eat daily? Choose a representative day from the three you recorded earlier (see p. 4). Using Appendix K as the source, record the grams of carbohydrate in each food item you ate that day. What are your chief sources of carbohydrate?

How much sugar, as such, do you use? Which foods provide "unseen" sweetening? How much do you depend on sugar substitutes for sweetening?

Figure 4.3 illustrates trends in supplies of basic carbohydrate sources from 1909 through 1973 in the United States. As indicated above, total carbohydrate has dropped steadily; potatoes and flour and cereals have declined steeply through the years. In contrast, sugars and sweeteners have shown a strong upward trend.

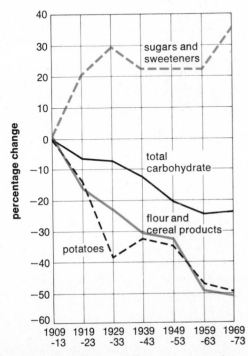

Figure 4.3
Percentage changes in supplies of carbohydrates from 1909-13 to 1969-73 (4).

One important result of the reversal in consumption patterns for cereals and sugars is a change of calorie and protein sources (4). Whereas in 1909 flour and cereal products provided 38 percent of the food energy in the United States, they now supply only one-half that amount (19 percent). In contrast, the percentage of calories obtained from sugars and sweeteners has increased from 12 percent in 1909 to 17 percent in 1974. Thus the sugar group has gained perceptibly on cereals as a source of calories in the diet of the United States. As for protein sources, in 1909 flour and cereals furnished a higher percentage of protein (36 percent) than did the total of meat, fish, and poultry (30 percent). By 1974 the cereals provided less than one-half (18 percent) of the amount supplied by meat, fish, and poultry combined (42 percent).

The change in carbohydrate use has been not only from starches (complex carbohydrates) to sugar (Fig. 4.3); within the sugar category there have been shifts in types of sweeteners used. In the base period 1910-13, 30 percent of sweeteners were from dietary (intrinsic) sugars. In other words, they were consumed as constituents of basic foods such as fruits, vegetables, and milk. By 1974, however, only 20 percent of sweeteners in the food supply were from basic foods. Use of refined sugar (sucrose) increased from 81 to 96 pounds per capita per year during that time. Because there was a substantial increase in use of corn sweeteners, however, the *percentage* of total sugars represented by sucrose actually dropped. By 1974 consumption of sugar substitutes (noncaloric sweeteners) had risen to be equivalent in sweetening power to 4 percent of the total sugars and sweeteners used in the United States.

Refined sugar produced from either sugarcane or sugar beets is the disaccharide sucrose. Corn sweeteners are produced by the hydrolysis of cornstarch—the breaking down of polysaccharide molecules into smaller molecules of dextrins, maltose, and glucose. Recently a process was developed to convert glucose to fructose; both are simple sugars (compare the similarity of their molecular structures, Fig. 5.2). This was a major breakthrough for the food industry, since fructose is sweeter per unit of weight than glucose, and cost is a major factor in the selection of ingredients for food processing. In 1974, production and use of the sweeter, high-fructose product amounted to more than a billion pounds.

Over two-thirds of all sweeteners consumed are delivered to processors and reach consumers as constituents of manufactured foods. In addition to fructose added to foods as such, much of the sucrose used as an ingredient in food manufacture is hydrolyzed in processing so that it is actually consumed as fructose and glucose. Taking this into account, dietary fructose consumption is estimated to be about 33 grams per person per day. Fructose is metabolized differently from glucose. In digestion sucrose is hydrolyzed to yield equal amounts of glucose and fructose. When fructose is made available gradually, the liver converts it to glucose. The effect on the body of relatively large quantities of fructose is now being studied (3).

Sweets have great appetite appeal, and much emphasis is placed on desserts in the United States. Many of us consider meals incomplete unless they conclude with something sweet. For children, dessert is often the reward for a clean plate. However, a concentrated sweet flavor tends to dull the appetite for bland foods. Routine overuse of sugar can thus result easily in unbalanced diets.

Sugars influence many qualities of foods. A relatively small amount of sugar can sometimes transform a tasteless dish into a palatable one. Kinds and amounts of sugars used also affect the physical properties of numerous common food products. Sugar contributes to the texture, tenderness, and crust color of baked products and influences the thickness of puddings and the firmness of jellies and custards. The size of sugar crystals critically affects the texture of candies, frostings, and frozen desserts (5).

diabetics
Persons unable to metabolize carbohydrate normally

Sugar Substitutes   Various substances other than natural sugars and sweeteners have been found to produce a sweet taste sensation. These substances are produced in several forms—liquid, granulated, and tablet. Because they are not carbohydrates and provide no calories, they have been widely used by *diabetics* and persons trying to reduce or control body weight. Saccharin, weight-for-weight three hundred times as sweet as sucrose, was commercially produced as early as 1900. It is the only artificial sweetener that has been in constant use in the United States. Its status as a safe additive is currently under review. Cyclamates, thirty times as sweet as sucrose, were used from 1950 until 1969 when they were banned by the Food and Drug Administration. Research is in progress on several other sweetening substances with desirable properties. One of these, Aspartame, is a molecule containing two *amino acids*. It is more than one hundred fifty times as sweet as sucrose.

amino acids
Structural units of proteins

Fat Foods

lipids
Fats and fat-like substances; soluble in organic solvents, insoluble in water

Fats are members of a larger group of compounds known as *lipids* (6). Fats appear in many forms—as butter, margarine, cream, salad and cooking oils, lard, bacon and other fat meats, and the visible fat on lean meats (Fig. 4.4). Fats are also present but invisible in such foods as nuts, avocados, chocolate, and—to a greater or lesser extent—in almost every food we eat. Finally, there are the fats and oils in pastries, salad dressings, luncheon meats, and gravies, and those that are absorbed when foods are fried. Fats are the most concentrated source of energy in the diet. They supply more than twice as many calories as equal weights of carbohydrates or proteins.

Fat foods shown in Figure 4.1 are composed of proportionately more fat than other nutrients. Cooking fats and salad and cooking oils are 100 percent fat. Butter and margarine contain more than 80 percent fat and negligible amounts of protein and carbohydrate. Bacon has proportionately more protein and carbohydrate, particularly protein. Crisp, drained bacon has lost a large part of its fat in preparation. Even so, the relatively small amount of protein in a serving of bacon prevents it from qualifying as a full alternate to lean meats as a protein source. Mayonnaise is predom-

Figure 4.4
Common sources of dietary fat: solid fats, oils, salad dressings, bacon, salt pork, avocado, chocolate, pastries and potato chips. (Landon Gardiner)

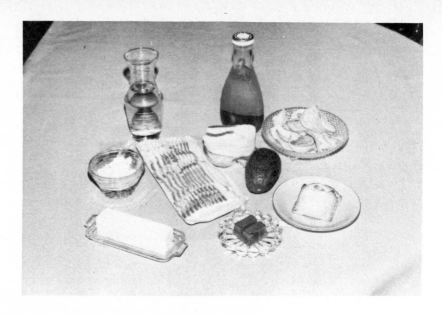

inantly fat, and French dressing is also sufficiently higher in fat than in the other nutrient classes to qualify for this grouping. (Other types of salad dressings are made from several ingredients and vary in fat content.) It may surprise you to learn that bitter chocolate is composed of more than 50 percent fat.

Patterns of Fat Consumption   Fats from all sources currently furnish about 43 percent of the total yield of energy from foods in the United States. This percentage has increased gradually from its 1909 level of 32 percent (Table 4.3). The major food sources of fat are meats, fish, poultry, dairy products, and fats and oils as such. Since 1909, fat consumption from the meat group has declined slightly; from dairy products, excluding butter, consumption has

Table 4.3
Calories per capita per day from available food supply disappearance data—Percent of calories from carbohydrate, fat, protein

Year	Food energy calories (kcal)	Approximate percent of calories from		
		Carbohydrate	Fat	Protein
1909	3530	56	32	12
1919	3440	55	34	11
1929	3460	54	35	11
1939	3340	52	37	11
1949	3200	49	39	12
1959	3170	47	41	12
1969	3270	46	42	12
1974	3290	46	42	12
1975	3210	46	43	12

US Dept. of Agriculture (4)

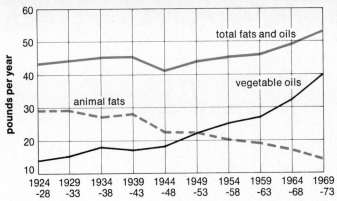

Figure 4.5
Trends in availability of fats and oils per capita (4).

also decreased. Consumer preferences within the fats and oils group have changed markedly. Figure 4.5 shows the spectacular rise since 1924 in the availability of vegetable oils (salad and cooking) per capita, in contrast to comparable figures for total fats and oils, which held relatively steady, and for animal fats (lard and butter), which declined (4, 7).

One way to obtain a practical knowledge of dietary fat sources is to examine food intake records for their fat content. The amount of fat in the specimen diet in Table 4.1 is shown in Appendix H. The grams of fat for each food are listed with the total fat consumption for the day coming to 96 grams. While there is no recommended dietary allowance for fat, 96 grams represents 45 percent of the total calories in the specimen diet. This is close to the average of about 43 percent in the United States food supply (Table 4.3). Most of the fat in the specimen diet comes from the same major sources chosen by the total population—the meat group, dairy products, and separated fats.

How much fat do you eat daily? Choose a typical day's meals from the three you recorded earlier (Chap. 1 see p. 4). Using Appendix K as the source, record the grams of fat yielded by each food serving on your meal record. What is the total for the day? What are your major sources of fat? Which meal of the day provided the most fat?

You may find that some of the foods with the highest percentage composition of fat, such as butter, margarine, or vegetable oils, appear on your diet record in very small quantities. On closer examination, however, they may prove to be present in significant amounts in prepared foods you use frequently.

A wider knowledge of fat sources can be obtained by studying the fat yield in grams per serving of a considerable number of common foods, such as those listed in Appendix K.

Check the foods with highest fat contents on the Appendix K table. (These could be the items that provide 10 grams or more of fat per serving.) Group the foods checked according to their fat content, and note the kinds of foods in each group. Of what significance are snack foods such as potato chips, chocolate candy bars, and milk shakes as sources of fat?

Fat helps to make foods palatable. A diet low in fat is dry and unappetizing and has little satiety value. Fat leaves the stomach more slowly than carbohydrate or protein, and thus it delays the feeling of hunger. Fat in itself is relatively tasteless, but it absorbs flavors and makes other foods more appetizing. Fat contributes desirable characteristic properties to many prepared foods, such as the smooth mouth-feel of salad dressings, the flakiness of pastries, and the tenderness of cakes and cookies. The popularity of fried foods—fried chicken, potato chips, French fries—is due largely to their crispness derived from contact with hot fat. It is not possible to measure the palatability of fat as easily or as accurately as it is to measure its calorie value. People become keenly aware of the importance of fat to palatability, however, when they must restrict their fat intake or are unable to obtain a favorite fat. Much of the characteristic flavor of meat products resides in the fat of the meat. The acceptability of many foods depends on the type of fat used in their preparation. Certain fats provide vitamins A, D, E, and K (see chap. 9).

Protein Foods

Lean meats, fish, poultry, and eggs are considered protein foods because they yield more proteins than they do fats or carbohydrates (Fig. 4.1). However, there are exceptions to this rule. Dry legumes (dry peas and beans) are included in the protein class, even though their carbohydrate content is higher than their protein content. Their protein contribution is a significant one—much higher than

Figure 4.6
Common sources of protein: lean meat, chicken, fish, eggs, legumes (split peas, black eye peas, kidney and lima beans), cheeses, milk, cottage cheese, peanuts and other nuts.
(Landon Gardiner)

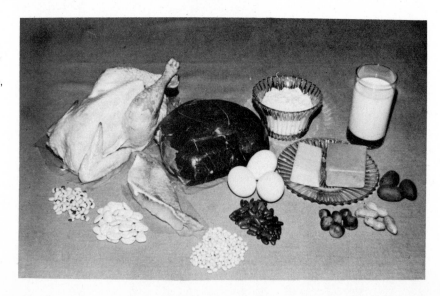

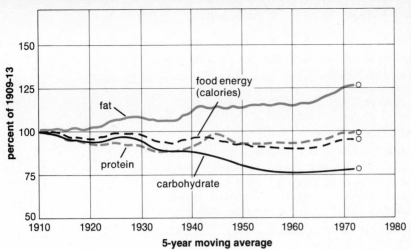

Figure 4.7
Food energy, protein, fat, and carbohydrate per capita civilian consumption. (US Department of Agriculture)

that of other vegetables—and dry legumes provide inexpensive alternates to meats and other protein foods. Nuts (particularly peanuts, which are legumes) are also classified as proteins for essentially the same reason, in spite of the fact that they contain more fat than protein.

Milk and most cheeses are classed as protein foods, even though whole milk has slightly more carbohydrate and fat than protein, and commonly used hard cheeses such as cheddar have more fat than protein. Both foods can provide a significant amount of protein in the daily diet. Children, for example, can obtain a considerable proportion of their daily protein intake from milk. When 2 or more ounces of cheese are eaten as the main dish of a meal, its protein yield is also significant.

Certain meats such as ham (not shown on the chart) may be higher in fat than in protein. In many cases the fat that is cooked out of them is not used, however, and edge fat is often cut off and discarded. The meats as eaten are then chiefly lean. Thus, they qualify as protein foods. (See Chap. 7 for additional information on protein foods.)

Trends in Nutrient Consumption

As we have seen, the consumption of carbohydrate foods has experienced a downward trend through the years; consumption of fats and oils has taken an upward trend. In both these groups the character of the foods has also changed. The amount of protein in the diet has held relatively constant, but there has been a sharp shift toward animal products and away from cereals as sources of protein. Average per capita calories available to the population have decreased by about 10 percent in the past 60 years. Table 4.3 summarizes data on daily food energy (calories) and percentage of calories from carbohydrate, fat, and protein by decades from 1909 to 1974. Figure 4.7 shows in chart form the trends in consumption of food energy in terms of carbohydrate, fat, and protein over essentially the same period (4, 8).

FUNCTIONS OF NUTRIENTS

Nutrients function in the body in three ways:

- ☐ *to sustain body structures and to provide for growth*: proteins, minerals, vitamins, water;
- ☐ *to control and coordinate its internal processes*: vitamins, minerals, proteins, water;
- ☐ *to provide energy for its activities and heat to maintain body temperature*: fats, carbohydrates, proteins.

All nutrient classes serve in one or more specific capacities, but there is great overlapping in function and there are many interrelationships between the actions of nutrients. Nutrients are therefore grouped under their main functions merely for convenience in discussion. It must be understood that each—alone and with other nutrients—contributes in many intricate ways to the nourishment of the body.

To Sustain Body Structure and to Provide for Growth

Proteins, minerals, vitamins, and water build and nourish the bones, muscles, organs, and blood that make up the body. There is no more dramatic demonstration of their contribution than the increase in body size from infancy to adulthood. This increase is evidence of the gradual enlargement of bones, organs, and muscles during the growth process and of the increased volume of blood. We have only to consider the inferior physiques of people who have been deprived of proper nourishment to appreciate the importance of adequate nutrient intakes throughout life (see Chaps. 3 and 14). When adult stature has been achieved, nutrients no longer serve to increase body size. All body structures require nutrients for their maintenance, however. Cells are continuously broken down and rebuilt throughout life.

The skeleton forms the rigid foundation of the body. The hardness and strength of bones and teeth are due to the depositing of certain mineral elements on a delicate framework that is composed largely of proteins. If bones grow normally, they acquire more and more of these mineral elements, chiefly calcium and phosphorus. Only to the extent that daily meals supply the kinds and amounts of mineral elements needed, however, do the bones grow to desirable size and become rigid and strong. Figure 4.8 illustrates the normal increases in the calcium content of bones that occur with increases in age and size. Average amounts of body calcium present at various ages are indicated for boys between infancy and 20 years of age. A normal young adult has acquired through the years some forty times the amount of calcium he or she had in infancy and has, indeed, grown in calcium.

Surrounding and covering the bones are the soft tissues—muscles, tendons, and skin. Bones are held in position and supported principally by the muscles, and the chief constituent of muscles is body protein. As a child grows, there must be an increasing deposit of protein in the muscles if he or she is to become steadily stronger.

The increasing need for muscle strength during growth is demonstrated when a baby advances from the crawling stage to an

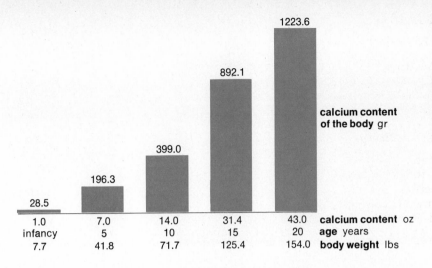

Figure 4.8
Body growth in calcium from
infancy to adulthood. [adapted
from I. Leitch and F. C. Aitken,
"The Estimation of Calcium
Requirement: A
Re-examination," Nutrition
Abstracts and Reviews 29
(April 1959), Table 3, pp.
393-411]

1223.6

892.1

**calcium content
of the body** gr

399.0

196.3

28.5

1.0	7.0	14.0	31.4	43.0	**calcium content** oz
infancy	5	10	15	20	**age** years
7.7	41.8	71.7	125.4	154.0	**body weight** lbs

epithelial tissue
*Cellular substance of the skin
and mucous membrane
covering or lining cavities and
passages in the body*

upright position. Good muscle development is required if the change is to be made without undue strain and posture is to remain good. As a child grows older, increasing demands are made on the muscles. Weak, sagging muscles can result from inadequate protein intake, and drooping posture and fatigue stance may be the outcome.

Vitamins have many functions in the building process. They are necessary for growth, and certain vitamins play important roles in the development of the teeth and in the building of healthy *epithelial tissues.* In conjunction with bone-building mineral elements and other nutrients, certain vitamins help to construct bone of good quality.

Water is necessary for all building functions in the body. It constitutes about two-thirds of the weight of the adult body and is present in greater or lesser amounts in every tissue. Even bone is composed of about one-third water. Body fluids are the most obvious carriers of water. Between 4 and 5 quarts of blood circulate constantly in the adult body, and digestive secretions probably make up an additional 5 to 10 quarts of fluid. Blood carries oxygen and all of the nutrients to the bones, muscles, and organs of the body for their use in maintaining their structures and for the synthesis of vital substances, as described in Chapter 1. Proteins, minerals, and other nutrients are required to build the blood itself.

To Control and Coordinate Internal Processes

The same nutrient classes that build the body—vitamins, mineral elements, proteins, and water—also regulate and control its internal processes. Practically all vitamins are related in some way to the successful functioning of the body when they are eaten in sufficient quantities; inadequate supplies contribute to poor functioning. In many cases, vitamins are associated with other nutrients in their coordinative activities. Certain mineral elements help to control such vital functions as the clotting of the blood and muscular contractions, including the beat of the heart (see Chap. 8).

Table 4.4
Body use of carbohydrates, fats, proteins

	Oxidized to yield energy	Other functions	Stored as	Excess changed to
carbo-hydrates	✓		glycogen	fat
fats	✓	formation of tissue fats	fat	carbohydrate (possibly some)
proteins	✓ (after removing nitrogen)	build, repair protein tissue; formation of enzymes and certain hormones	protein (in new tissue)	fat carbohydrate (when CHO intake is insufficient)

All enzymes produced in the body are proteins. Each has a highly specialized function. The enzymes in digestive juices, for example, prepare nutrients for use by the cells. Some of the hormones produced by the glands of internal secretion contain proteins. Thyroxine (secreted by the thyroid gland) is one of them. This hormone is a regulator of energy metabolism. Hemoglobin in the blood is largely protein. It serves the vital functions of carrying oxygen from the lungs to the tissues and some of the carbon dioxide from the tissues back to the lungs.

Water regulates body temperature. Heat is eliminated by means of evaporation of water from the lungs and from the surface of the skin. Probably as much as one-half of the water available to the body daily is disposed of from the skin surface. The amount of water loss through the skin is increased in hot weather through sweating. As water evaporates from the skin, there is a sense of cooling.

To Provide Energy for Activities and Heat to Maintain Body Temperature

Nutrients are needed to provide energy for involuntary, life-sustaining activities such as the beating of the heart, breathing, and the maintenance of muscle tone. In addition, all physical activities —sitting, standing, moving the body about in any manner—require energy. Carbohydrates, fats, and proteins (divested of their nitrogen) are the body's three sources of energy for all purposes. To create the body's capacity to work, these nutrients are *oxidized* in the cells. The three energy sources are interchangeable to a considerable extent; the body can use them in widely varying proportions. Table 4.4 lists the functions of carbohydrates, fats, and proteins in the body. Each is a source of energy to meet current needs; each is also a potential source of body fat.

enzymes
Proteins essential for stimulating reactions in the body

hormones
Substances secreted by glands and transported to other parts of the body to regulate specific processes

hemoglobin
Iron-containing protein pigment in red blood cells

oxidized
Combined with oxygen in a series of reactions resulting in energy release

REFERENCES

1. B. K. Watt and A. L. Merrill, *Composition of Foods: Raw, Processed, Prepared*, Agricultural Handbook No. 8 (Washington, D.C.: Consumer and Food Economics Research Division, USDA, Dec., 1963).

2. R. Levine, *Role of Carbohydrate in the Diet*, in R. S. Goodhart and M. E. Shils, eds., *Modern Nutrition in Health and Disease* (Philadelphia: Lea and Febiger, 1973), Chap. 3.

3. Academy Forum, *Sweeteners: Issues and Uncertainties* (Washington, D.C.: National Academy of Sciences, 1975).

4. S. J. Hiemstra, *Food Consumption, Prices and Expenditures*, Agric. Econ. Report No. 138 (Washington, D.C.: Econ. Res. Service, USDA, July 1968); also Supplement for 1975, pub. Jan. 1977.

5. M. Bennion and O. Hughes, *Introductory Foods* (New York: Macmillan Publishing, 1975).

6. Food and Nutrition Board, National Research Council, *Dietary Fat and Human Health*, Pub. 1147 (Washington, D.C.: National Academy of Sciences, 1966).

7. C. A. Chandler and R. M. Marston, *Fat in the US Diet* (Nutrition Program News, Washington, D.C.: Consumer and Food Economics Institute, Agric. Res. Service, USDA, May-Aug., 1976).

8. R. Marston and B. Friend, "Nutritional Review," *National Food Situation* (Washington, D.C.: Economic Research Service, USDA, Nov. 1976).

9. Food and Nutrition Board, National Research Council, *Recommended Dietary Allowances*, 8th revision. (Washington, D.C.: National Academy of Sciences—National Research Council, 1974).

READINGS

Food Fats and Oils (Washington, D.C.: Institute of Shortening and Edible Oils, 1974).

Guthrie, H. A., *Introductory Nutrition* (St. Louis: The C. V. Mosby Company, 1975).

White, P. L., D. C. Fletcher and M. Ellis, eds., *Nutrients in Processed Foods: Fats, Carbohydrates*. (Acton, Mass.: Publishing Sciences Group, 1975).

Wilson, E. D., K. H. Fisher, and M. E. Fuqua, *Principles of Nutrition* (New York: John Wiley and Sons, 1975).

Utilization of Nutrients

Carbohydrates
Lipids
Proteins
Minerals, Vitamins, and Water

Nutrients are taken into the body in complex assortments in the foods we eat. They are made useful to the body by the intricate processes of digestion, absorption, and assimilation. The total sequence of processes by which nutrients are utilized in the living body is referred to as *metabolism* (1). A thorough understanding of these processes requires a background in chemistry and physiology. The brief résumé that follows does not consider the subject in depth. It seeks chiefly to relate choice of kinds and amounts of foods consumed to the ultimate nourishment of the body.

DIGESTION AND ABSORPTION

In digestion, foods are broken down by mechanical means, and their nutrients are converted to simpler forms by chemical action. Proteins, fats, and carbohydrates (except monosaccharides) must be digested before they can be absorbed. *Monosaccharides*, water, vitamins, and minerals do not require digestion.

monosaccharides
Simple sugars

All chemical changes in the body are brought about by the action of enzymes, which are synthesized from amino acids. Enzymes function as *catalysts* and are essential for the thousands of chemical changes constantly taking place in the body. Each reaction requires a specific enzyme. Intricate chains of reactions, smoothly coordinated with each other, are essential to life.

Digestive enzymes are produced by glands embedded in the walls of the digestive organs and by glands adjacent to the digestive tract, with ducts leading into the tract. These enzymes are carried by digestive juices and thus are brought into contact with the food particles. Specific digestive enzymes are responsible for the chemical breakdown of proteins, fats, and carbohydrates to smaller molecules.

The digestive tract is composed of the mouth, esophagus, stomach, small intestine, and large intestine (Fig. 5.1). The process of digestion begins as soon as food is taken into the mouth; chewing is the important first step. This mechanical separation of large food particles into smaller ones and the mixing with saliva results in two changes: the food mass is liquified, making it easy to swallow; and the surface area of the food is greatly increased, exposing it to the digestive enzymes in the stomach and small intestine for efficient chemical breakdown. Strong contractions of the muscles in the walls of the digestive tract mechanically separate food into still smaller particles. At the same time, the food is mixed with a large

catalysts
Substances that participate in chemical reactions, undergoing change in the process and returning to their original state when reaction is completed

Figure 5.1
Diagram of the digestive tract.
[Johns, et al, Health for
Effective Living (New York:
McGraw Hill Book Co., 1966)]

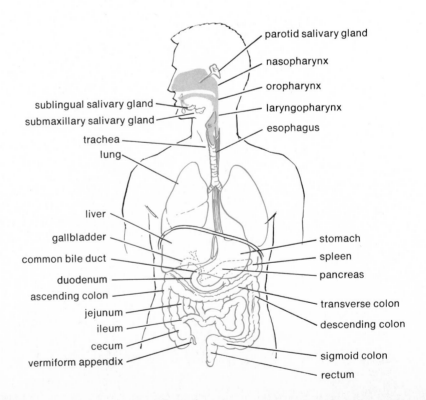

volume of digestive juices, so that when it passes from the stomach to the small intestine it is a thick, semifluid mass referred to as *chyme*.

Absorption and transportation of the simple liquid forms of the nutrients begin as digestion is completed. Absorption takes place largely through the walls of the small intestine. The *intestinal mucosa* is in large folds with *villi* projecting into the *lumen* of the small intestine. This structural arrangement provides an enormous surface area for the absorption of nutrients. Some absorption takes place by simple diffusion—movement of molecules in solution from the lumen of the small intestine, where they are highly concentrated, across the mucosa to the intercellular space on the other side, where they are less concentrated. For most nutrients, however, the assistance of special carriers and the expenditure of energy are required to facilitate their passage across the intestinal mucosa. From the intercellular space the nutrients then pass into the blood and lymph *capillaries* within the villi and are carried into larger vessels. With the bloodstream as the conveyer, nutrients are carried to every cell in every tissue of the body. Here chemical actions take place that prepare the nutrients to build tissue or release energy. It is at this point that the adequacy of the diet meets its real test. Does the diet provide all the nutrients in the amounts the body cells require? Or are there shortages that—if continued—will result in poorly nourished cells and eventually a poorly nourished person?

Carbohydrates, fats, and proteins all undergo the same general processes. They differ in the sections of the tract where they are digested, in the particular digestive enzymes that act on them, in the end products of digestion, and in the specific pathways they take to various organs and body parts. We will see later that having all the required nutrients present simultaneously at the point of need is an important consideration. Attention will be given now to individual nutrient classes to clarify the ways in which nutrients function in the body.

intestinal mucosa
Lining of the intestine

villi
Finger-like projections in the mucosa

lumen
Inner open space of the small intestine

capillaries
Minute vessels that conduct blood and lymph to and from the cells

CARBOHYDRATES

Carbohydrates are formed in nature by the remarkable process of photosynthesis, whereby light energy from the sun is transformed to chemical energy. Only green plants, with their *chlorophyll*, have the ability to utilize carbon dioxide from the air and water from the soil to capture the energy from the sun in the form of carbohydrate. Animals, including human beings, are thus ultimately dependent on plants for the nutrients necessary to sustain life.

chlorophyll
Substance in green leaves needed to produce carbohydrate

Structure

Almost all of the carbohydrates in foods fall into either of two general groupings—*starches* and *sugars* (see Chap. 4). These are similar in structure, and their breakdown in the body follows the same general pattern. Both are reduced in digestion to the same simple forms for absorption and use.

Carbohydrates are composed of just three elements: carbon (C), hydrogen (H), and oxygen (O). Combined according to a number of precise patterns, these elements form a variety of compounds classified according to structure as monosaccharides, disaccharides, or polysaccharides. The monosaccharides and disaccharides are sugars, characterized as being crystalline, sweet to the taste (in varying degrees) and soluble in water. The polysaccharides possess none of these qualities.

Monosaccharides (glucose, fructose, and galactose) are the simplest forms of carbohydrate in foods. Each molecule has six carbon atoms, to which twelve hydrogen and six oxygen atoms are attached. The structural formulae in Figure 5.2 illustrate how similar these compounds are, regardless of whether the simple sugar is glucose, fructose, or galactose. The slight differences in arrangement of the hydrogen and oxygen atoms on the carbon atoms account for the differences in properties of these three sugars, such as their degrees of sweetness and solubility. The monosaccharides also differ in chemical properties and how they are metabolized.

Glucose and fructose are present in fruits, vegetables, corn syrup, and honey. Galactose does not occur in the free state in foods. These three *hexoses* are the most significant ones in human nutrition.

hexoses
Six-carbon monosaccharides

Disaccharides (sucrose, lactose, and maltose) are composed of two molecules of monosaccharides linked together. Glucose joined to fructose produces a molecule of sucrose; glucose and galactose form lactose; and two molecules of glucose yield a molecule of maltose.

The structural formula for sucrose illustrates the way monosaccharides are attached to each other to form disaccharides (Fig. 5.3):

Sucrose is present in sugarcane and sugar beets. Through processes of extraction and crystallization, granulated sugar (practically 100 percent pure sucrose) and brown sugars are produced. Molasses, maple syrup, and maple sugars also are primarily sucrose.

Lactose is the sugar in milk and milk products. It is not found

Figure 5.2
Structural formulae of three common monosaccharides.

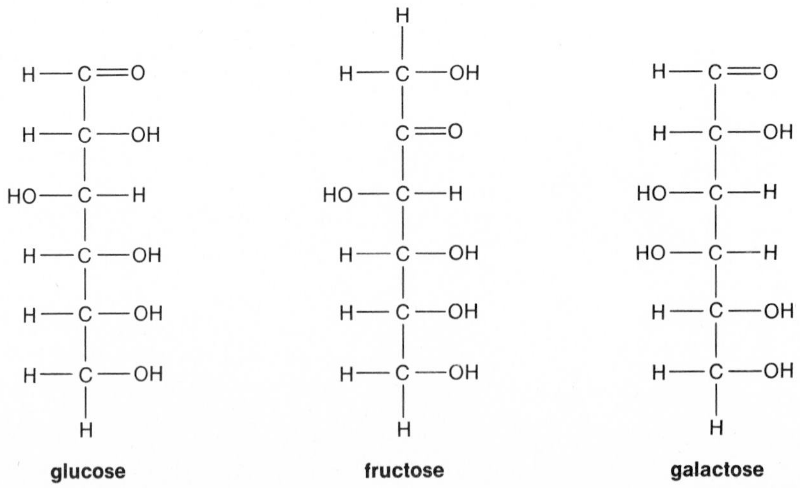

glucose   fructose   galactose

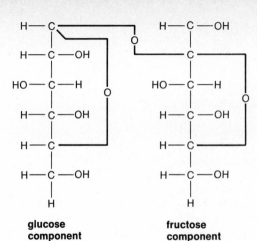

Figure 5.3
Structural formula of the most
common disaccharide,
sucrose.

**glucose
component**

**fructose
component**

in any other natural product. Maltose is present in sprouting
grains, in corn syrup and corn sugar, and in malted milk. (Malted
milk is a dried mixture of whole milk and the liquid obtained by
cooking barley malt and wheat in water.)

    Polysaccharides (dextrins, starch, glycogen, and cellulose) are
polymers of glucose molecules of varying lengths. Dextrins contain
relatively few glucose units, while starch molecules are made up of
hundreds or even thousands of them. Starches and dextrins are
found in grains and vegetables. Glycogen, the storage form of carbohydrate in animals, is also synthesized from glucose. It is present in liver and muscles and provides a limited quantity of readily
available glucose for the body. Cellulose is composed of glucose
units having a slightly different structure from those in starch
molecules. This polysaccharide is the main constituent of the cell
walls of all plants; thus it is present in grains, fruits, and vegetables. Cellulose, one type of *dietary fiber,* is not digested by
humans. Pectins, which occur in the pulp of certain fruits, are
compound carbohydrates that contain units other than monosaccharides.

    Noncaloric sweeteners are widely used as substitutes for the
sweet taste of sugar. They are not carbohydrates and, as components of food products, do not have the functional characteristics of
sugars (see Chap. 4).

Digestion

With an understanding of the structure of carbohydrates, it becomes obvious that starches are actually only complex forms of
sugar. Digestion of carbohydrate begins in the mouth. Saliva contains a digestive enzyme, ptyalin or salivary *amylase,* that acts on
starch and dextrins, breaking them down into shorter chains. This
step continues as the food is swallowed until the acidity of the gastric juice inactivates the enzyme. There is no amylase in gastric
juice. In the small intestine, digestive enzymes from the *pancreas*
resume the process. The final cleavage of disaccharides into monosaccharides takes place within the intestinal wall as the sugars are

polymers
Chains of one kind of molecule

dietary fiber
*Non-digestible components of
plant foods*

amylase
*Enzyme that acts on
carbohydrates in digestion*

pancreas
*Large gland below the
stomach; secretes the
hormone insulin and juice
containing digestive enzymes*

being absorbed. It is as monosaccharides, then, that carbohydrate enters the blood (Fig. 5.4).

When sugars are eaten, a minimum amount of digestion is required. If they are in the form of monosaccharides, they are ready for absorption with no digestive action whatsoever. Disaccharides must be split by digestive enzymes in the small intestine into their constituent monosaccharides.

Celluloses, the carbohydrates present in the cell walls of all plant materials, are not digested by humans. They are important in the mechanics of digestion, however, because they provide bulk and thus aid in discarding residues of digestion.

The monosaccharides, chiefly glucose, resulting from the complete digestion of carbohydrates are absorbed through the walls of the small intestine and pass into the blood capillaries in the villi. They reach the portal vein, which carries them to the liver where the fructose and galactose molecules are converted to glucose. The liver dispenses glucose to the blood, and it is thus made available to all the cells of the body.

Storage and Use

Carbohydrate as such is stored in the body as glycogen in very small quantities—less than 0.1 percent of total body weight. About

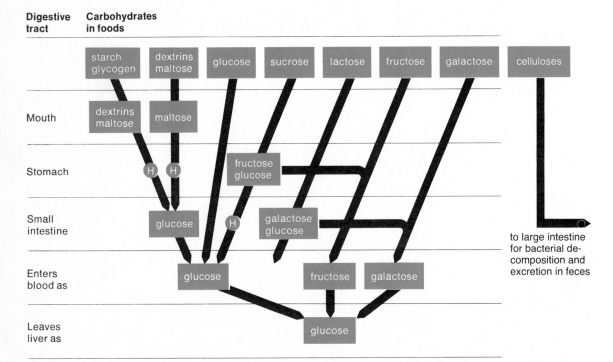

Ⓗ indicates that the same products as at the preceding level continue to appear

Figure 5.4
Products of carbohydrate digestion at various levels of the gastro-intestinal tract and the forms in which they are used in the body. [Adapted from R.S. Goodhart and M.E. Shils, eds., *Modern Nutrition in Health and Disease* (Philadelphia: Lea and Febiger, 1973), p. 103.]

two-thirds of this amount is stored in the muscles and about one-third in the liver. Glycogen is composed of glucose molecules joined together in chains. In muscles, it serves as an emergency reserve of fuel that can be rapidly converted back to glucose when needed for energy.

A small but essential amount of carbohydrate is present in the blood as glucose. The blood-sugar level normally remains stable, even though the cells of all tissues are continuously withdrawing glucose to replenish their supplies. The liver constantly adds sufficient amounts of glucose to the blood from dietary sources and from the breakdown of its store of glycogen to keep the blood glucose level normal.

Glucose is oxidized in the tissues. By a pattern of complex reactions involving many hormones, enzymes, and intermediate products it is converted to energy. Excess carbohydrate is converted to fat and stored.

Carbohydrate Intake and Health (1, 2)

The body has a specific need for carbohydrate, notably as a source of energy for the central nervous system. About 100 grams daily of digestible carbohydrate appears to be required. After this need has been met, the source of energy may be protein, fat, or carbohydrate, as shown in Table 4.4. However, dietary carbohydrate is most efficiently converted to energy.

There is no basis for a recommended dietary allowance for carbohydrate, according to the Food and Nutrition Board, because "diets compatible with good health may contain widely varying proportions of carbohydrates and fat" (2). There has been considerable discussion of desirable proportions of sugar and starch in the diet and the extent to which one can replace the other. Still, no specific dietary requirement for sugar has been demonstrated for normal individuals under ordinary circumstances. As pointed out in Chapter 4, sugar consumption in the United States has increased over the past half century; the use of starchy foods, such as flours and cereals, has declined over the same period.

Some investigators have linked high sugar consumption to increased incidence of *coronary heart disease*. There seems to be inadequate evidence at present that the current sugar consumption of most Americans has an adverse effect on their level of *blood lipids* (1). High sugar consumption has long been associated with high incidence of dental caries, however (see Chap. 3). There is evidence that caries-susceptible individuals may be able to reduce dental caries by restricting their intake of concentrated sweets.

Diabetes mellitus is a disease of metabolism in which there is an inadequate supply of effective insulin, causing disturbances of carbohydrate, fat, and protein metabolism. Factors projected as causes of diabetes include heredity, obesity, infection, and malfunction of the pituitary gland as well as diets high in sugar. Insulin, a hormone produced by the pancreas, is necessary for glucose to gain entry into the cells of certain tissues. Just how insulin functions to accomplish this is unknown. The importance of the efficient functioning of a system that facilitates the passage of glucose

coronary heart disease
Condition in which the flow of blood to heart muscle is impeded by deposits in the artery walls

blood lipids
Fats and fat-like substances, including cholesterol, circulating in the blood

dental caries
Tooth decay

into cells is obvious. Glucose is a very important source of energy, and the mechanism for releasing its energy is inside the cells.

Proper dietary management is the basic treatment of mild and moderately severe cases of diabetes. In some instances the disease can be controlled by diet alone; in others, administration of insulin is necessary. In all cases, the modified diet should provide optimum nutrition, as well as contribute to the maintenance of a normal blood-sugar level. Food exchange lists are widely used in prescribing and planning diets for diabetics (3, 4). Such diets usually furnish carbohydrate, fat, and protein in proportions generally used in well-balanced diets, but dietary sugar is restricted.

Lactose intolerance is a metabolic abnormality in which the digestive enzyme lactase is present in lower-than-normal quantities or is missing. Lactase is essential for the breakdown of lactose to its constituent monosaccharides, glucose and galactose. When lactose is not digested, its presence in the large intestine results in cramps and diarrhea. Eliminating or reducing the amounts of foods containing lactose provides relief (5).

Dietary fiber, sometimes referred to as "roughage" or "bulk," is present in variable quantities in all foods of vegetable origin and has long been recognized as important in normal bowel function. Attention has recently been focused on the decline of dietary fiber intake in industrialized countries and its possible relationship to a high incidence of a wide variety of diseases (6, 7, 8). The term "dietary fiber" is used to include a group of carbohydrate compounds: cellulose, hemicelluloses, mucilages, pectins, and gums, and the noncarbohydrate substance, lignin. These are all plant constituents that are resistant to digestion by secretions of the human gastrointestinal tract. They pass through the stomach and small intestine unchanged. In the colon, some are broken down into a number of by-products by the action of bacteria. Brief descriptions of some of the constituents of dietary fiber follow.

Cellulose is a high-molecular-weight polysaccharide consisting of glucose units. There is little decomposition of cellulose in the intestinal tract; most cellulose consumed is eliminated in the feces. Lignin, not a carbohydrate, makes up the principal part of the woody structure of plants along with cellulose. Lignin has the ability to combine with *bile acids* to form complexes that are not absorbed by the body. In some animal research studies, blood cholesterol levels have been reduced by the inclusion of dietary fiber. The availability of smaller quantities of bile acids for the synthesis of *cholesterol* apparently accounts for this finding. Hemicelluloses differ chemically from cellulose in that their unit of structure is not glucose. They are not *hydrolyzed* by enzymes in digestive juices but are broken down to some extent by bacteria in the colon. Some of the resulting compounds are absorbed and *metabolized* to yield energy. Pectin, familiar as the substance responsible for gelling fruit juices to make jelly, is closely associated with hemicelluloses in plant cell walls.

Whole grain products are good sources of dietary fiber, due to their bran content. Legumes, nuts, fruits, and vegetables are other contributors. Most of the fiber has been removed from white flour and refined cereals (Fig. 5.5). Animal products do not contain fiber.

bile acids
Compounds synthesized in the liver from cholesterol

cholesterol
Fatty substance; normal constituent of blood

hydrolyzed
Chemically broken down to simpler substances

metabolized
Changed by body processes

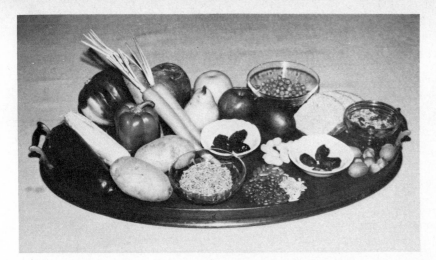

Figure 5.5
Food sources of dietary fiber:
Vegetables—carrots, potatoes,
cucumbers, peas, squash,
peppers, rutabagas, corn;
Fruits—oranges, apples,
avocados, prunes; Wholegrain
Cereals; Dry Legumes; Nuts.
(Landon Gardiner)

Data on the amount of dietary fiber in foods are limited, due to the complexity and expense of procedures for its estimation. Values for *crude fiber*, listed in some tables of food composition, are used as an index of dietary fiber content. (Crude fiber is the insoluble material remaining after severe acid and base hydrolysis.) Dietary fiber may be from two to seven times higher than the crude fiber value of a food.

Widespread coverage in the popular media concerning the importance of fiber in the diet suggests that fiber will prevent or cure many serious degenerative diseases, as well as some frustrating, less life-threatening health problems. Such publicity stems from epidemiological data associating fiber with certain diseases of the gastrointestinal tract, circulation-related conditions, and some metabolic diseases.

A well-documented function of dietary fiber is its action in promoting normal bowel function. The use of fiber to prevent constipation and possibly prevent *diverticular disease* and colon cancer is based on the observation that fiber absorbs water and softens and increases the size of feces. This results in faster passage of the contents through the gastrointestinal tract and greater distention of the colon. Under certain conditions, dietary fiber may reduce serum cholesterol levels, possibly by increasing the excretion of bile acids. This would not necessarily reduce the incidence of *cardiovascular disease*. It has been hypothesized that increased intake of dietary fiber may help to control *obesity* by diluting the concentration of energy-yielding nutrients. A larger quantity of fiber-containing food may be eaten to provide the same amount of energy as highly refined and concentrated foods. In addition, more chewing is required when the diet is high in fiber, providing time for recognition of the sensation of satiety.

The *epidemiological* evidence suggests that many people might benefit from the inclusion of foods providing moderate amounts of fiber. It is also most likely that high-fiber diets may have some negative effects. It has been reported that other constituents in the diet are less well digested and minerals particularly may be poorly

diverticular disease
Presence of small "blow-out" type protrusions of the wall of the large intestine

cardiovascular disease
Condition in which the flow of blood to heart muscle is impeded by deposits in the artery walls

obesity
Excessive amount of body fat

epidemiological
Concerned with the occurrence, distribution and control of a disease within a population

absorbed when dietary fiber is increased. Much remains to be learned from clinical and experimental studies to clarify the role of fiber in the diet. At present, large increases in dietary fiber are not recommended.

LIPIDS

Fats are synthesized in both plants and animals. The proportion of fat in different species of plants varies widely. In animals the

A Triglyceride, composed of a molecule of glycerol combined with three fatty acid molecules

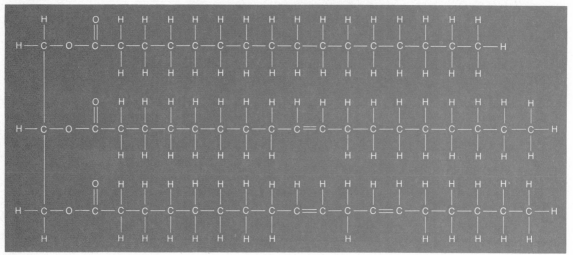

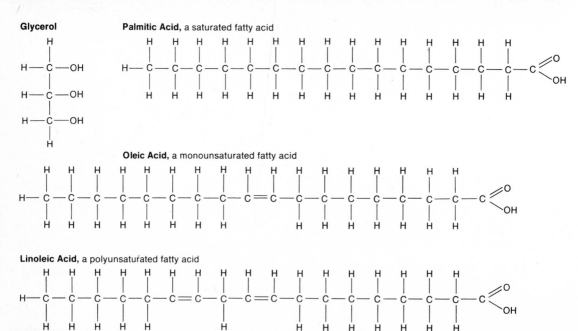

Glycerol

Palmitic Acid, a saturated fatty acid

Oleic Acid, a monounsaturated fatty acid

Linoleic Acid, a polyunsaturated fatty acid

Figure 5.6
Structural formulae of a triglyceride molecule and its components.

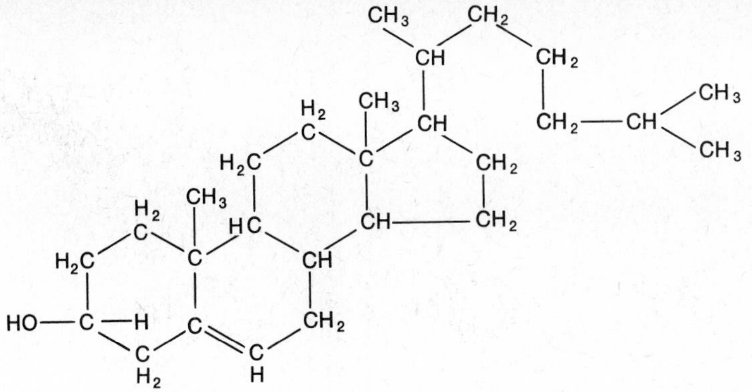

Figure 5.7
Structural formula of cholesterol.

amount of body fat varies not only among species, but also among individuals within the same species. Fat is an important component of the diet. It has been established that the body needs a regular source of dietary fat to carry the fat-soluble vitamins and to provide essential fatty acid. As we saw earlier, fats are our most concentrated source of energy, providing 9 calories per gram.

Structure of Fats

Fats are composed of the same three elements as carbohydrates—carbon, hydrogen, and oxygen—but in different proportions and in different arrangements. (Compare the structural formula for triglyceride in Figure 5.6 with that for sucrose in Figure 5.3). The terms "fat" and "lipid" are often used interchangeably. Lipid is the broader term, however, and it includes a variety of compounds related to the fatty acids. Triglycerides are *esters*, consisting of one molecule of glycerol (a three-carbon alcohol) attached to three molecules of fatty acids. Structural formulae for glycerol, several common fatty acids, and a triglyceride molecule are shown in Figure 5.6. About 98 percent of body and food fats are composed of these fat components. Monoglycerides and diglycerides are molecules of glycerol with either one or two molecules of fatty acids attached. Phospholipids are esters of fatty acids that include phosphoric acid and other constituents. Steroids are complex molecules often found in association with fat. Cholesterol (Fig. 5.7) is the most popularly known steroid because of its implication with fat metabolism. Ergosterol and a form of cholesterol have importance in nutrition also as precursors of vitamin D (see Chap. 9).

esters
Compounds formed from an alcohol and an acid by the removal of water

Fatty Acids   Fatty acids make up more than 90 percent of the fat molecule. The nature of a fat or oil is therefore largely determined by the types of fatty acids that predominate in its structure. These acids are chains of carbon atoms that vary in length, and they fall into two groups—saturated and unsaturated—with the latter consisting of mono- and polyunsaturated fatty acids.

Saturated fatty acids predominate in fats that are usually solid at room temperature. Their name is derived from the fact that they contain as much hydrogen as their carbon atoms will hold; they are

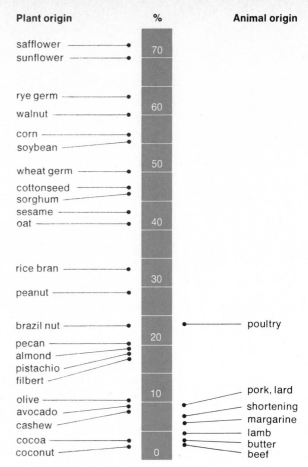

Figure 5.8
Percentage of linoleic acid in fats and oils of plant and animal origin. |C.M. Coons, "Fatty Acids in Foods," J. Am. Dietet. Assoc. 34:3 (March 1958), p. 242|

Plant origin

%

Animal origin

- safflower — 70
- sunflower

- rye germ — 60
- walnut

- corn
- soybean

- 50
- wheat germ
- cottonseed
- sorghum
- sesame
- oat — 40

- rice bran — 30
- peanut

- brazil nut — 20 ————— poultry
- pecan
- almond
- pistachio
- filbert

- 10
- olive
- avocado ————— pork, lard
- cashew ————— shortening
————— margarine
- cocoa ————— lamb
- coconut — 0 ————— butter
————— beef

"satisfied," or saturated. The structural formula of palmitic acid is shown in Figure 5.6 as an example of a saturated fatty acid. It is one of the most common saturated fatty acids in our food supply. Between 10 and 20 percent of the fatty acids in most fats are palmitic acid.

Unsaturated fatty acids predominate in fats that are liquid at room temperature. They are "unsatisfied," or unsaturated, because two or more hydrogen atoms are missing. *Monounsaturated* fatty acids have one double bond between two adjacent carbon atoms. Oleic acid, shown in Figure 5.6, is the most common monounsaturated fatty acid, constituting 30 percent or more of the total fatty acids in most fats. *Polyunsaturated* fatty acids have two or more double bonds in each molecule. Linoleic acid (Fig. 5.6), for example, has eighteen carbon atoms and two double bonds. Most seed oils have high proportions of linoleic acid. Commercially, oils are *hydrogenated* to produce fats that are solid at room temperature. This process lessens the degree of polyunsaturation of the fatty acids in the original oils and confers on them characteristics more like those of saturated fatty acids.

The terms "vegetable fat" and "animal fat" are not definitive with respect to the degree of saturation of their fatty acids (Fig.

hydrogenated
Hydrogen added to unsaturated fatty acids

5.6). It is necessary to be more specific. Beef and pork fats, for example, are relatively low in polyunsaturated fatty acids; poultry fat is relatively high. Most vegetable oils, on the other hand, are high in unsaturated fatty acids, but coconut oil and palm oil are low.

Linoleic acid, a polyunsaturated fatty acid, is virtually the only "essential" fatty acid. It is classed as essential because it must be provided from dietary sources; it cannot be synthesized by the body. Linoleic acid is present in high concentrations in such vegetable oils as safflower, corn, cottonseed, peanut, and soybean (Fig. 5.8). The body's requirement of this fatty acid is met when linoleic acid provides from 1 to 2 percent of the total caloric intake. A diet containing only 15 to 25 grams of appropriate food fats (less than 10 percent of the total caloric intake) can thus meet the specific requirement for fat, that is, it can furnish the essential fatty acid and all the fat-soluble vitamins required. Figure 5.8 shows the approximate percentage of linoleic acid in a wide variety of fats of plant and animal origin, suggesting the comparative importance of the different kinds of fats and oils as sources of essential fatty acid. Most fats are combinations of unsaturated and saturated fatty acids. Corn oil, for example, has 55 percent polyunsaturated linoleic acid. It also has 26 percent monounsaturated oleic acid and 13 percent of saturated fatty acids.

Table 5.1
Cholesterol content of common measures of selected foods
in ascending order

Food	Amount	Cholesterol mg
milk, skim, fluid or reconstituted dry	1 cup	5
cottage cheese, uncreamed	$1/2$ cup	7
lard	1 tbsp	12
cream, light table	1 fl oz	20
cottage cheese, creamed	$1/2$ cup	24
cream, half and half	$1/4$ cup	26
ice cream, regular, approximately 10% fat	$1/2$ cup	27
cheese, cheddar	1 oz	28
milk, whole	1 cup	34
butter	1 tbsp	35
oysters, salmon	3 oz, cooked	40
clams, halibut, tuna	3 oz, cooked	55
chicken, turkey, light meat	3 oz, cooked	67
beef, pork, lobster, chicken, turkey, dark meat	3 oz, cooked	75
lamb, veal, crab	3 oz, cooked	85
shrimp	3 oz, cooked	130
heart, beef	3 oz, cooked	230
egg	1 yolk or 1 egg	250
liver, beef, calf, hog, lamb	3 oz, cooked	370
kidney	3 oz, cooked	680
brains	3 oz, raw	more than 1700

Source: "Cholesterol Content of Foods," R. M. Feeley, P. E. Criner and B. K. Watt. *J. Am. Dietet. Assoc.* 61:134, 1972.

Cholesterol

The major sterol in the body, cholesterol has a large molecular size and complex structure (Fig. 5.7). It is synthesized in the body and is an essential constituent of cell membranes and *plasma lipoproteins*. It is also important as the substance from which bile acids and the steroid sex hormones (both male and female) are produced. Vitamin D is synthesized in the body from a derivative of cholesterol. Dietary cholesterol, as well as that produced *endogenously* (in the cells), is present in blood serum. Only foods of animal origin contain cholesterol. The cholesterol content of some common foods is shown in Table 5.1.

plasma lipoproteins
Compounds consisting of protein and lipid, circulating in the blood

Digestion of Fats

Fats from all sources are digested easily and almost completely if they are eaten in moderation. Most of the digestion and absorption of fats takes place in the small intestine (Fig. 5.9). Although there are no *lipases* in saliva and probably none in gastric juice, the action of chewing and the partial digestion of carbohydrates and proteins in the upper part of the digestive tract serve to separate fat from other nutrients, thus helping to prepare it for digestive action. As the fat enters the duodenum in small portions it is mixed with *bile* and pancreatic lipase, the principal enzyme concerned with fat digestion. About half of the triglyceride molecules are completely hydrolyzed to glycerol and fatty acids before absorption. Another major portion is partially broken down to monoglycerides, and about 10 percent remain as triglycerides or diglycerides. Some further hydrolysis may take place within the cells of the mucosa as absorption occurs.

lipases
Enzymes that act on fats in digestion

bile
Alkaline substance secreted by the liver; aids in digestion of fats

Figure 5.9
Products of fat digestion at various points in the digestive tract.

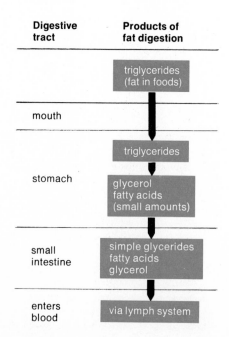

Digestive tract	Products of fat digestion
	triglycerides (fat in foods)
mouth	
	triglycerides
stomach	glycerol fatty acids (small amounts)
small intestine	simple glycerides fatty acids glycerol
enters blood	via lymph system

During absorption, some of the fatty acids are reunited with glycerol to form triglycerides again. These are combined with phospholipid, cholesterol, and protein into complex molecules called *chylomicrons*. The products of fat digestion pass into the *lacteals* of the villi and are carried to the *thoracic duct*. From here they pass into the blood system to be transported to all body cells. Short- and medium-chain fatty acids, present in food in very small quantities, are absorbed intact and pass directly into the blood capillaries. Droplets of fat in the blood are not in true solution but in suspension, much like the fat of homogenized milk. In the cells of the body, energy is released as the fatty acids are oxidized by an involved step-wise mechanism. All the tissues of the body except those of the central nervous system use fatty acids as a source of energy (1).

Storage and Use

Fat that is not needed immediately is stored as body fat. When needed it is moved into the bloodstream again, where it becomes available to the cells for energy. Since carbohydrates and proteins also can be converted into fat in the body, all foods are potential sources of body fat. The amount of stored fat therefore reflects the total amount of food that has been eaten in excess of immediate energy needs. About one-half of the body fat is stored directly under the skin; other stored fat serves as a protective covering for internal organs.

Fat Intake and Health

A deficiency of linoleic acid has long been recognized as a cause of growth failure and certain types of skin disorders in infants. It was believed until recently that linoleic acid might not be an essential dietary nutrient for adults. Under conditions of long-term parenteral nourishment, however, adults have been reported to develop symptoms of linoleic acid deficiency (9).

Wide use of the terms "cholesterol" and "polyunsaturated" in advertising has made the words familiar, often leaving the impression that cholesterol is a foreign substance to be disposed of. It is important to keep in mind that cholesterol is an essential component of the blood and of almost all body tissues. *Hypercholesterolemia* appears to be undesirable, and a high intake of saturated fatty acids has been associated with abnormally high levels of serum cholesterol. The amount of cholesterol in the diet may also affect the level of cholesterol in the blood. Hypercholesterolemia is in turn associated with an increase in the formation of fatty deposits in the linings of arteries. This condition is referred to as *atherosclerosis*. With the build-up of atheroma in the arteries that furnish blood for the nourishment of the heart muscles, coronary heart disease develops (10).

The association between types of fat in the diet and the incidence of coronary heart disease does not prove that a cause-and-effect relationship exists. Research findings indicate that *many* fac-

lacteals
Small lymph capillaries in intestinal villi

thoracic duct
Main vessel of the lymphatic system lying along the spinal column

hypercholesterolemia
Abnormally high amounts of cholesterol in the blood

atheroma
Fatty deposits in linings of arteries

tors are involved in the development of this disease. Hypertension and cigarette smoking, as well as hypercholesterolemia, have been identified as major risk factors. Reduction of these risk factors theoretically should result in reduced mortality from coronary heart disease, and this approach has been used repeatedly in research. For example, studies on animals and humans show that diets rich in polyunsaturated fatty acids can often lower blood cholesterol levels, although the mechanisms by which this takes place are not well understood. Limiting the intake of dietary cholesterol also tends to reduce high blood cholesterol levels. However, it has not yet been demonstrated conclusively that reduction of the major risk factors results in any substantial decrease in mortality from coronary heart disease (2).

Other factors positively associated with increased risk of developing coronary heart disease are obesity, diabetes, sedentary living, use of soft water for drinking, psychosocial tensions or stress, and a family history of premature atherosclerotic heart disease. The results of numerous investigations suggest that these factors may act singly or together in various ways to help create conditions that foster coronary heart disease. The possible role of high levels of dietary sucrose has also received attention. Currently additional dietary substances are being investigated, including dietary fiber, certain trace elements, the enzyme *xanthine oxidase*, and *trans-fatty* acids. Thus the possible relationship between diet and coronary heart disease continues to be explored in many laboratories, using different animal species as experimental subjects. Large-scale studies of free-living human subjects are also in progress (11).

In view of the difficulty of interpreting the findings of research completed to date, no quantitative recommendations for fat intake by the general population have been made by the Food and Nutrition Board (2). Likewise, no recommendation has been made with respect to a desirable ratio of unsaturated fatty acids in the diet. Until more definitive information is available, the Board recommends that American consumers eat a varied, balanced, and not overly rich diet and maintain a normal body weight by control of energy intake and by daily exercise (12). Moderation is the watchword of these recommendations.

The American Heart Association recommends that the proportion of energy derived from fat should not exceed 35 percent (see Chap 14: dietary goals for the United States). It is advised that foods containing complex carbohydrates be used to substitute for reduced dietary fat (2).

PROTEINS

Proteins are large molecules made up of many amino acids attached to each other. Proteins differ in chemical make-up from carbohydrates and fats in that they contain nitrogen in addition to carbon, hydrogen, and oxygen. Nitrogen is essential for the development, maintenance, and sustenance of every cell in the body—and thus of life itself.

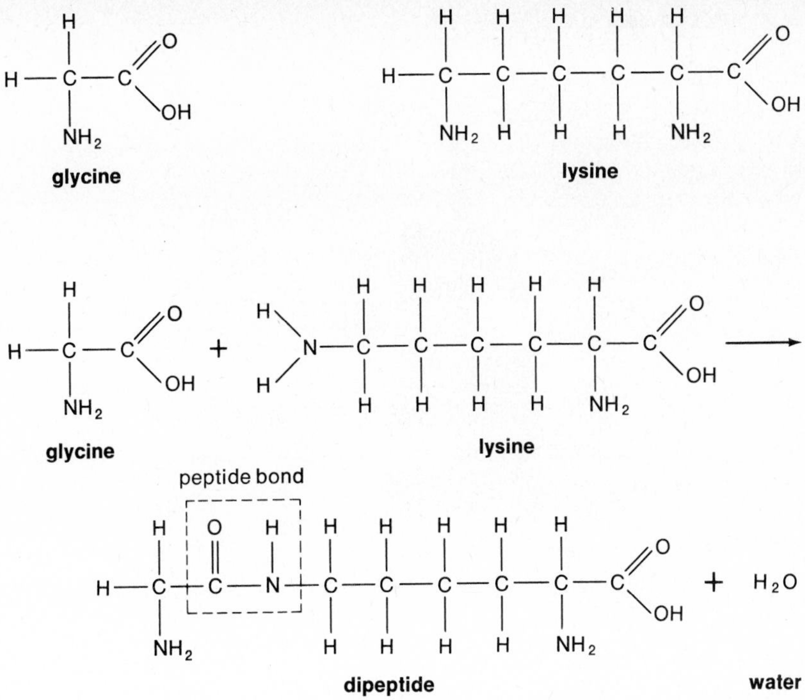

Figure 5.10
Structural formulae of certain
amino acids and a dipeptide.

glycine

lysine

glycine   +   lysine $\longrightarrow$

peptide bond

dipeptide $+$ H_2O

water

Structure

The structure of the individual amino acids that comprise proteins
varies, but all have in common at least one amino group (NH_2) and
one carboxyl group (COOH). The examples shown in Figure 5.10
are the structures for glycine, the simplest amino acid, and lysine,
an essential amino acid (see Chap. 7). Molecules of amino acids are
linked together by peptide bonds, involving an amino group of one
amino acid and a carboxyl group of the next amino acid in the
chain. When two amino acids are linked together (as in Figure
5.10), the new molecule is a *dipeptide*. Relatively short chains of
amino acids (up to about seventy units) are referred to as *polypep-
tides*. Still larger molecules are proteins. Proteins differ widely
from each other in size, shape, and molecular weight.

Digestion and Absorption

Digestion of proteins begins in the stomach, where they are acted
upon by the hydrochloric acid and digestive enzymes in the gastric
juice. In the small intestine digestion continues, with *proteolytic*
enzymes in the intestinal and pancreatic juices completing the process (Fig. 5.11). Amino acids are the final products of protein digestion. They are absorbed in watery solution through the walls of the
small intestine and into the bloodstream, to be carried (via the portal vein) to the liver and thence to all the cells.

Amino acids are regrouped in the cells into appropriate combinations required to rebuild tissues, form new ones, and synthesize

proteolytic
*Reducing proteins to simpler
products*

Figure 5.11
Products of protein digestion at various points in the digestive tract.

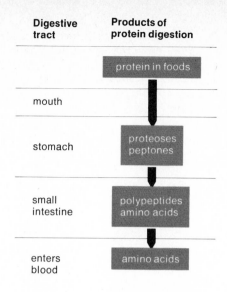

Digestive tract	Products of protein digestion
	protein in foods
mouth	
stomach	proteoses peptones
small intestine	polypeptides amino acids
enters blood	amino acids

certain active compounds such as hormones and enzymes. A nutritionally adequate diet provides proteins that yield the amounts and kinds of amino acids required for these functions. Amino acids also contribute to the energy needs of the body. When amino acids are not needed for the synthesis of body proteins, they are returned to the liver. There the nitrogen is removed and incorporated into *urea,* the form in which it can be excreted via the kidneys. The carbon, hydrogen, and oxygen that remain can be used for energy, just as they are when supplied by carbohydrates and fats. If the energy is not needed at once, body fat is formed and stored for future use (Table 4.4).

urea
Important end product of protein metabolism

OTHER CLASSES OF NUTRIENTS

Minerals, vitamins, and water are not sources of energy; neither are they acted upon by digestive juices as are proteins, fats, and carbohydrates. They are absorbed practically as they occur after being freed from foods during the digestive process.

Minerals

Minerals are absorbed through the walls of the small intestine into the bloodstream, and are carried to the tissues where they are used as needed. Unlike most other nutrients, mineral elements are not "used up" in the body, nor do they provide energy for body work. For the most part, when they have discharged their building and regulatory functions in the tissues, they are discarded. (This is not true of iron, which is retained by the body and reused.) A regular supply of mineral elements in the diet is essential in order to replace losses (see Chap. 8).

Vitamins

There is little exact information about the absorption of vitamins from the digestive tract. It is believed that the water-soluble vitamins enter the blood along with other water-soluble nutrients, such as amino acids and glucose. Fat-soluble vitamins probably accompany the fats. As chemical methods for detecting vitamins become increasingly reliable, more will undoubtedly be learned about the pathways for their absorption and utilization in the body. Vitamins are believed to reach the tissues in the same form in which they enter the body and to be used by the tissues as needed. Excesses of some vitamins are stored, while excesses of others are discarded from the body. Like minerals, vitamins are not sources of energy for work, but they serve in multiple ways in the development and functioning of the body (see Chap. 9).

Water

Water is the chief solvent in the body. Nutrients are reduced to a liquid state in digestion, in preparation for absorption. Water brings the digestive enzymes into the digestive tract and carries the products of digestion through the intestinal wall into the blood, which is largely composed of water. The blood distributes nutrients to all the cells of the body, which are bathed in water. Finally, some of the waste products from the cells are removed from the body in the urine, which is also largely water. Water is literally an indispensable nutrient (13).

REFERENCES

1. R. S. Goodhart and M. E. Shils, eds., *Modern Nutrition in Health and Disease* (Philadelphia: Lea and Febiger, 1973).

2. Food and Nutrition Board, National Research Council, *Recommended Dietary Allowances*, 8th revision. (Washington, D.C.: National Academy of Sciences—National Research Council, 1974).

3. *Exchange Lists for Meal Planning* (New York: American Diabetic Association, Inc. and Chicago: American Dietetic Association, 1976).

4. "What is an Exchange?" *J. Am. Dietet. Assoc.* 69 (Dec. 1976), p. 609.

5. R. L. Pike and M. L. Brown, *Nutrition: An Integrated Approach* (New York: John Wiley and Sons, 1975).

6. "The Role of Fiber in the Diet." *Dairy Council Digest* 46 (Jan-Feb. 1975), pp. 1-4.

7. D. L. Downing, ed., *The Role of Fiber in the Diet*, New York State Agric. Exp. Station Special Report 21, 1976.

8. G. A. Leveille, "Dietary Fiber," *Food and Nutrition News* 47 (Feb. 1976), pp. 1, 4.

9. "Essential Fatty Acid Deficiency in Continuous-drip Alimentation," *Nutr. Reviews,* 33 (Oct. 1975), p. 329.

10. C. Sirtori, G. Ricci, and S. Gorini, eds., *Diet and Atherosclerosis* (New York: Plenum Press, 1975).

11. "The Multiple Risk Factor Intervention Trial (MRFIT), A National Study of Primary Prevention of Coronary Heart Disease," *J. Am. Med. Assoc.* 235 (Feb. 23, 1976), pp. 825-27.

12. Food and Nutrition Board, National Research Council, *Dietary Fat and Human Health*, Pub. 1147 (Washington, D.C.: National Academy of Sciences, 1966).

13. J. R. Robinson, "Water—the Indispensable Nutrient," *Nutrition Today* 5 (Spring 1970), pp. 16-23, 28-29.

READINGS

Bing, F. C., "Dietary Fibers in Historical Perspective," *J. Am. Dietet. Assoc.* 69 (Nov. 1976), pp. 498-505.

Chaffee, E. E. and E. M. Greisheimer, *Basic Physiology and Anatomy* (Philadelphia: J.B. Lippincott Co., 1974).

Diabetes Mellitus (Indianapolis: Lilly Research Laboratories, 1973).

Fischer, A. D. and D. L. Horstman, *A Handbook for the Young Diabetic* (New York: Intercontinental Medical Book Corp., 1972).

Food and Fibre, Fifth Annual Marabou Symposium, *Nutrition Reviews,* 35 (March 1977), entire issue.

Garza, C. W. and N. S. Scrimshaw, "Relationship of Lactose Intolerance to Milk Intolerance in Young Children," *Am. J. Clin. Nutr.* 29 (Feb. 1976), pp. 192-96.

Gormican, A., *Controlling Diabetes With Diet* (Springfield: Charles C. Thomas 1976).

Hardinge, M. G., J. B. Swarmer, and H. Crooks, "Carbohydrates in Foods," *J. Am. Dietet. Assoc.* 46 (Feb. 1965) pp. 197-204.

Harper, H. A., *Review of Physiological Chemistry* (Los Altos, California: Lange Medical Publications, 1973).

Kagan, A. et al., "Epidemiologic Studies of Coronary Heart Disease and Stroke in Japanese Men Living in Japan, Hawaii and California: Demographic, Physical, Dietary and Biochemical Characteristics," *J. Chronic Dis.* 27 (Sept. 1974), pp. 345-64.

Kummerow, F. A., Y. Kim, M. D. Hull, J. Pollard, P. Ilinov, D. L. Dorossiev and J. Valek, "The Influence of Egg Consumption on the Serum Cholesterol Level in Human Subjects," *Am. J. Clin. Nutr.* 30 (May 1977), pp. 664-773.

Leverton, R. M., *Fats in Food and Diet,* Agricultural Information Bulletin No. 361 (Washington, D.C.: Gov. Print. Office, revised 1976).

Nichols, A. B., C. Ravenscroft, D. E. Lamphiear, and L. D. Ostrander, "Independence of Serum Lipid Levels and Dietary Habits," *J. Am. Med. Assoc.,* 236 (Oct. 25, 1976), pp. 1948-53.

Rosenweig, N. S., *A Review of Dietary Lactose and its Varied Utilization by Man* (Chicago: Whey Products Institute, 1974).

"Sucrose, Starch and Hyperlipidemia," *Nutr. Reviews* 33 (Feb. 1975), pp. 44-45.

"The Biological Effects of Polyunsaturated Fatty Acids," *Dairy Council Digest* 46 (Nov.-Dec. 1975), pp. 31-35.

"The Role of Lactose in the Diet," *Dairy Council Digest* 45 (Sept.-Oct. 1974), pp. 25-28.

Foods: Sources of Energy

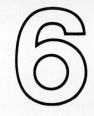

Calories—A Measurement of Energy
Calorie Values of Common Foods
Energy Needs of the Body
How the Body Uses Energy

oxidized
Combined with oxygen in a series of reactions resulting in energy release

Energy is the capacity to do work, and food is the fuel that serves as the source of energy. When nutrients are oxidized in the cells, energy is released. Heat is a by-product of that energy. Energy is measured in terms of *calories*, which are units of heat. Calorie is a familiar term that is used freely by everyone and with many interpretations, so that it is well to know its precise meaning. One calorie is the amount of heat required to raise the temperature of 1 kilogram (2.2 lbs or about 1 qt) of water 1 degree centigrade (1, 2). It is sometimes referred to as a kilocalorie or "kcal." Thus a calorie is not itself a nutrient but a convenient measure of the energy value of nutrients. The word "calorie," as used in this text, refers to the kilogram calorie. An equivalent measure of energy in the metric system is 4.184 kilojoules. Metric units of weight, volume and length have always been used in scientific work. Energy values, however, have been expressed in calories rather than the metric joules. With the gradual conversion to the metric system now underway in the United States and Canada, it is important to become familiar with metric equivalents. (See the conversion table in Appendix G.)

The sources of energy for the body are: foods supplying carbohydrates, fats, and proteins; the stored nutrients of the body, particularly body fat; and alcohol. Fat provides more than twice as many calories for a given weight as carbohydrate or protein. Alcohol, when completely metabolized, supplies nearly twice as many calories as carbohydrate or protein, or about 7 calories per gram. Food-supply statistics do not include alcoholic beverages, and long-term trend data on their use are not available.

metabolized
Changed by body processes

MEASUREMENT OF CALORIES

The energy values of separate nutrients and of many foods and food mixtures are determined by measuring the calories of heat given off when each is ignited and burned in equipment especially designed for the purpose. The objective of such efforts is to determine the relative calorie values of various foods that are potential sources of energy for the body. Two methods of measuring calories are used, one direct and one indirect.

Direct Measurement of Heat in a Bomb Calorimeter

In the direct method of calorie measurement, a weighed sample of food is placed in a capsule or bomb filled with pure oxygen. The bomb is immersed in a container holding a known amount of water (Fig. 6.1). The food in the bomb is burned completely when an electric spark ignites a fuse. As the food burns, sensitive thermometers

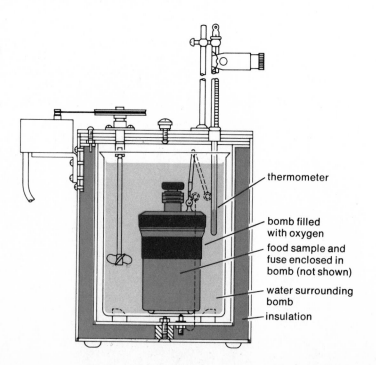

Figure 6.1
Parr oxygen bomb calorimeter (cross-section). Food contained in the bomb is burned, thereby releasing heat, which raises the temperature of the water surrounding the bomb. The number of calories of heat released by a given weight of food sample is computed from the rise in temperature of the water and the heat capacity of the apparatus. (Parr Instrument)

thermometer

bomb filled with oxygen

food sample and fuse enclosed in bomb (not shown)

water surrounding bomb

insulation

register the rise in temperature of the surrounding water. This rise indicates the amount of heat generated by burning the specified amount of the food. From the temperature reading the calorie yield is calculated.

Indirect Measurement of Heat in an Oxycalorimeter

In the indirect method, the amount of oxygen required to burn a weighed sample of food is measured. The energy yield of the food is then obtained by using standard factors established with the bomb calorimeter to convert the known volume of oxygen into calories. The dried sample—a single food or a mixture of foods—is ignited and burned in a stream of nearly pure oxygen in a closed circuit.

The original work of establishing calorie values was done with the bomb calorimeter, using weighed amounts of pure fat, pure carbohydrate, and pure protein. From those data it was possible to arrive at average energy values for a specified weight of each. Certain corrections are necessary when calculating energy values for human diets, because the body handles foods somewhat less efficiently than does the calorimeter. Extensive experimentation showed that the following rounded figures are suitable for practical use in calculating the calorie values of the usual mixed diets eaten in the United States:

1 gram of pure carbohydrate yields 4 calories.
1 gram of pure fat yields 9 calories.
1 gram of pure protein yields 4 calories.

Calculating Calorie Values

Once such calorie values were established, it was possible to calculate the energy yield of a given weight of any food if its percentage composition of protein, fat, and carbohydrate was known. This process is demonstrated in the calculation of the energy value of one egg (Table 6.1). The calculation can be carried a step further by combining a series of single foods in a recipe, such as that for cus-

Table 6.1
Calorie value of one egg

	Protein	Fat	Carbohydrate
composition of egg	12.9%	11.5%	0.9%
in 1 g of egg	0.129 g	0.115 g	0.009 g
energy factors	× 4	× 9	× 4
calories in 1 g of egg	0.516	1.035	0.036

0.516
1.035
0.036

1.587   total calorie value of 1 g of egg
  44   weight of 1 egg in grams (minus shell)

69.83   calories, the energy value of 1 egg
        (see Appendix K)

Table 6.2
Approximate calorie value of ½c serving of custard

½ egg	35 cal (from calculated value)
½ cup whole milk	80 cal (from Appendix K)
¾ tbsp sugar	35 cal (from Appendix K)
	150 cal

tard (Table 6.2), or can be elaborated to apply to custard pie or to any other food combination for which the ingredients and their calorie values are known. When an entire recipe is calculated—as for a pie—the calorie value of one portion is determined by dividing the total calories for the item by the number of servings. Obviously, servings of food combinations can vary widely in calorie value depending on the ingredients and their proportions. It is only by knowing the precise components of a recipe and the amount of each that the calorie value can be calculated with certainty. The size of servings is also a very important factor in determining the calorie value of portions, as we will see later in this chapter.

In studying calorie values of foods, one soon learns that fat-rich foods are concentrated sources of energy, and that small servings of such foods have the same calorie value as much larger servings of foods low in fat and/or high in water content and bulk. As already indicated, 1 gram of fat yields more than twice as much energy as 1 gram of either carbohydrate or protein. The comparison in Table 6.3 illustrates this point.

Table 6.3
Amounts of foods that yield approximately 100 calories each

1 tbsp mayonnaise	high fat
⅔ cup whole milk	low fat, high water
5 cups raw cabbage	low fat, high water, high bulk

The removal of fat from a food reduces its calorie content dramatically. A glass of skim milk, for example, from which much of the fat (cream) has been removed furnishes about 90 calories, while a glass of whole milk provides almost twice that amount. Two-percent milk falls between these in energy value (Table 6.4). The difference between pork chops with fat and those with the fat

Table 6.4
Comparison of calories from milks of different fat content

Milk	Protein percent	Fat percent	Carbohydrate percent	Approximate Calories per cup
skim	3.6	0.1	5.1	90
low fat (2%)	4.2	2.0	6.0	145
whole	3.5	3.7	4.9	160

Table 6.5
Comparison of calories from fat and lean pork

Cooked pork chop	Protein percent	Fat percent	Carbohydrate percent	Calories per chop
lean only (56 g)	31	16	—	150
lean and fat (78 g)	26	32	—	305

trimmed off is equally striking (Table 6.5). One cooked pork chop, with both lean meat and fat, yields 305 calories; the same chop with the fat removed yields about one-half that amount.

Thus calorie values of a food may vary greatly, particularly when there are differences in fat content. But calories themselves do not vary in value; one calorie of heat represents exactly the same amount of energy as every other calorie. Therefore no food can be said to be more "fattening" than any other food. Calories merely add up faster in a food that is high in fat (Fig. 6.2).

CALORIE VALUES OF COMMON FOODS

The calorie values of hundreds of foods are available today. Most of these data are issued by the US Department of Agriculture, which has derived and published them periodically since 1896 (3). They represent average calorie values based on the composition of individual foods as determined in many scientific laboratories. Calorie values of mixtures of foods (those found in "made" dishes) are usually calculated from the known content of carbohydrate, fat, and protein in each of the separate food ingredients (such as egg and milk in custard). The same information can be derived by direct or indirect *calorimetry*. The calorie values of food mixtures (beef stew, for example) can vary widely unless they are based on standard recipes.

Appendix K gives the calorie values of some four hundred single foods and prepared combinations of foods, such as main dishes,

calorimetry
Measurement of energy value of foods and energy needs of animals or people

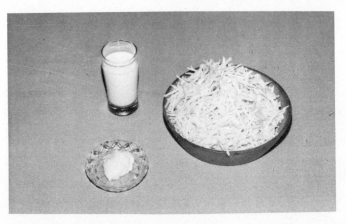

Figure 6.2
Three foods (milk, cabbage and mayonnaise) in different quantities provide the same amount of energy: 100 calories. (See Table 6.3 for amounts of foods and bases for differences.) (Landon Gardiner)

soups, beverages, and desserts.* They are presented in the familiar measures of cups, tablespoons, and teaspoons and, as far as possible, in practical serving sizes. A "serving", of course, may have a different connotation for each person who uses the term. The serving sizes indicated in the table are those used rather generally, such as 3 ounces of cooked meats, ½ cup of cooked vegetables, 1 slice of bread, and individual units of fruits. When necessary, the amounts can be either divided conveniently into smaller units or multiplied to take into account larger servings.

It is important to learn to visualize servings of common foods as they ordinarily appear at the table. There are various ways to do this. You can measure foods at home—½-cup servings of cooked vegetables, for example—and then form a mental image of how that amount looks on a plate or individual serving dish. If it is practical to do so, members of the class can also bring a few measured foods to make a collection for everyone to view and discuss. Food models, when they represent exact measures of foods, can be substituted for part or all of the foods to be studied (4). If an accurate small scale is available, certain foods such as meats and units of fruits can be weighed. In this way you can learn to recognize such standard serving sizes as 3 ounces of cooked meat, a large banana, or a small apple.

How to Use the Food Table in Appendix K

You can use a food composition table as a source of information to be drawn upon as needed, but you can also make it a valuable tool in the study of nutrition. One way of doing this is to concentrate on the relatively few foods that you eat most frequently.

Concentrate on Representative Foods   The average family uses about fifty different food items in a week's time. Your 3-day meal record (see Chap. 1) will reveal to some extent your own food range. The list of fifty foods in Table 6.6 was compiled from 3-day food records of one hundred university students and represents the foods of which their meals were usually composed. Thus, while each student ate meals that looked and tasted different from those of the others, they all drew upon this relatively small number of basic foods for the nucleus of their meals. There are fifty different food items in Table 6.6. They are divided among the food groups as follows: milk—5, meat—12, vegetables—13, fruits—8, bread-cereals—7, fats—3, and sweets—2.

> Make your own representative food list, beginning with the foods on your 3-day meal record. Enlarge it as necessary, but for practicality confine it, if possible, to thirty or forty foods. If the food lists of individual class members are quite similar they might be pooled to make a representative food list for the class.

* Appendix K also presents nutrient values for the same foods. The discussion of origin of data, determination of servings, and visualization of given quantities of foods applies to nutrients as well as to food energy.

Table 6.6
Specimen representative food list classified by food group
Calorie values in single servings

Food*	Weight or approximate measure**	Kilo-calories	Food*	Weight or approximate measure**	Kilo-calories
Milk group			**Fruit group**		
cheese, cheddar	1 oz	113	apple, raw	1 medium	80
cheese, cottage, creamed	¼ cup	65	banana, raw	1 medium	101
cream, half & half	1 tbsp	20	grapefruit, white	½ medium	46
milk, fluid, skim or buttermilk	1 cup	88	orange juice	½ cup	61
milk, fluid, whole	1 cup	159	peaches, canned	½ cup	100
			pineapple juice, canned	½ cup	69
Meat and Alternates group			raisins	¼ cup	105
			strawberries, raw	½ cup	28
beans, dry, canned	¾ cup	233			
beef, lean chuck	3 oz	212	**Bread-Cereal group**		
beef, hamburger	3 oz	186			
chicken, fried	½ breast	160	bread, white, enriched	1 slice	76
egg	1 medium	72	bread, whole wheat	1 slice	67
frankfurter	1 medium	139	bun or roll, enriched	1 bun	119
haddock, fried	1 fillet	182	cornflakes, fortified	1 cup	97
liver, beef	2 oz	130	macaroni, enriched, cooked	¾ cup	116
peanut butter	2 tbsp	188	oatmeal, cooked	⅔ cup	87
pork chop	1 chop	305	rice, enriched, cooked	¾ cup	167
tunafish, canned	½ cup	158			
sausage, bologna	2 oz	172	**Fat group**		
			butter or margarine	1 tbsp	102
Vegetable group			oils, salad or cooking	1 tbsp	120
			mayonnaise	1 tbsp	101
beans, green	½ cup	16			
broccoli	½ cup	20	**Sweets group**		
cabbage, chopped, raw	½ cup	11			
carrots, diced	½ cup	23	beverages, cola type	12 oz	144
corn, canned	½ cup	87	sugar, granulated	1 tbsp	46
lettuce, head	1 cup	10			
onions	½ cup	31			
peas, green, frozen	½ cup	55			
peppers, sweet, green, raw	½ medium	8			
potato, white	1 medium	88			
spinach	½ cup	24			
sweet potato	1 medium	172			
tomato juice, canned	½ cup	23			

*Foods on this list are in forms ready to eat. All meats and vegetables are cooked unless otherwise indicated.

**See Appendix K for further identification of these foods. All foods are described more fully there and both weights and measures are included. See Appendix F for equivalents in weights and measures.

With repeated use of a limited number of foods such as this, you will gradually become familiar with the calorie values of a sizable core of common foods. This is not to suggest that a limited selection of foods is desirable. Rather, it is simply a point of departure serving somewhat the same purpose as learning a few common words and phrases in beginning the study of a new language.

The items in Table 6.6 are confined largely to individual foods. The exceptions are items commonly bought as mixtures, such as breads and luncheon meats. The only feasible way of keeping the list short is to follow such a plan. Once the values of individual foods have been established, they can be combined as needed: milk on cereal, butter on bread, sugar on fruit, and so on. For the relatively few intricate recipes used in daily meals, Appendix K offers a source of information. If you eat certain food mixtures frequently, they should be included on your representative food list. The advantages in students' making their own representative lists is now evident: it offers the opportunity to include ethnic and regional foods as well as personal favorites. If it is not practical for you to make your own list, the list in Table 6.6 can serve the purpose. In either case, the following suggestion for putting to practical use the individual food items is offered as a time-saving step.

Enter the representative foods (your own or those in Table 6.6) on index cards or half sheets of paper, one food to a sheet. For each food add description, measure, weight, calorie value, and nutrient values from Appendix K, as follows:

hamburger, beef, broiled
1 patty: 3 in dia
weight: 3 oz (85 g)

calorie value	protein g	fat g	calcium mg	iron mg
186	23	10	10	3.0

vitamin A IU	thiamin mg	riboflavin mg	niacin mg	ascorbic acid mg
20	.08	.20	5.1	—

Sort the cards or sheets in the order of their concentration as sources of calories per serving.

Choose a typical day's meals from the three you recorded earlier. Enter the meals on the diet record form used in Appendix H*. Add the calorie value of each food and the totals as called for on the form. (Disregard all but calorie values for the present. The purpose of the activity is to coordinate study and discussion with actual dietary situations. It is therefore preferable that the various nutrients be entered on the meal record later as each is considered in the text.)

ENERGY NEEDS OF THE BODY

In the oxidation process in the body, oxygen unites slowly with the end products of digestion. This reaction takes place for the most part in the muscle cells. It consists of the chemical union of oxygen,

---

* The specimen diet, Appendix H, provides calorie and nutritive values for the sample meals given in Chapter 4. This diet purposely does not meet accepted dietary standards in all respects; it is not intended as a model. It is referred to throughout the text to suggest how nutritive requirements are met, or fail to be met, because of the food choices that are made.

breathed in and carried to the cells by the blood, with the carbon and hydrogen yielded by the assimilated food nutrients. Carbohydrates, fats, and proteins all yield carbon dioxide and water when oxidized. The chemical action releases energy, which makes it possible to do work, and heat, which helps to maintain a constant body temperature.

That the body's source of heat is internal is shown by the fact that body temperature does not normally fluctuate, irrespective of the temperature of the environment. Wearing heavier clothing in cold weather helps to hold in the heat already there; it does not actually warm the body. Wearing lightweight clothing in a warm environment facilitates the release of heat that the body has generated.

Measurement of Body Energy Needs

Scientific proof that oxidation in the body produces energy and heat has been provided by experiments with two types of equipment, one called a respiration calorimeter, the other a respiration apparatus.

The *respiration calorimeter* measures heat output directly. It consists, in essence, of an airtight chamber that can house an experimental subject. Body heat given off by the subject is measured as fast as it is produced by recording the rise in temperature of a current of cold water piped through the chamber. The amount of heat given off is then computed in terms of calories.

The *respiration apparatus* measures heat output indirectly. This apparatus consists of a closed circuit from which a subject breathes oxygen-enriched air through the mouth (Fig. 6.3). A nose

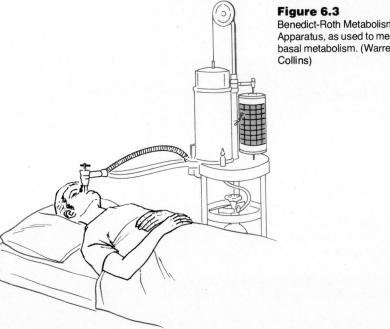

Figure 6.3
Benedict-Roth Metabolism Apparatus, as used to measure basal metabolism. (Warren E. Collins)

clip prevents inhalation of air through the nostrils. The oxygen consumed in a specified length of time is a measure of the amount of oxidation going on in the body during that period. By a series of calculations based on the number of calories represented by a given amount of oxygen consumed, oxygen consumption is translated into calories of heat.

Data obtained from both the direct and the indirect methods have demonstrated the relationship of the body's energy expenditure to its heat output. This has been accomplished by testing subjects when they are completely at rest as well as when they are performing many different types of activities. Such data make it possible to estimate the daily calorie needs of people engaged in various physical endeavors.

Keep in mind that the word "energy" as used here applies to the ability to perform work as a result of an adequate supply of body fuel. The same word is often used to refer to a feeling of fitness or animation. Energy in the true sense refers to food energy that precedes and makes possible physical activity. On the other hand, a feeling of vigor, often largely psychological, frequently follows and can be the result of physical activity.

HOW THE BODY USES ENERGY

The body uses energy in three ways:

☐ *for internal activities:* basic, involuntary processes such as heartbeat, breathing, circulation of blood, and metabolism of nutrients;

☐ *for external activities:* all physical activity or body motion that requires the slightest muscular effort or the most extreme exertion;

☐ *for storage of energy-yielding materials*, particularly when the body is producing new tissues, as in pregnancy and in growth during childhood.

Energy for Internal Body Activities

The energy level required to keep the internal mechanisms of the body functioning is called *basal metabolism*. This means the relatively constant, internal energy needs for sustaining life at its lowest ebb. (The term *basal* implies the minimum.) Obviously there is never even a brief letup in the need for activities such as breathing or heartbeat, over which the individual has no control. Never—day or night, awake or asleep—do those behind-the-scenes activities cease to function that are concerned with chemical changes in the cells and with processes involved in the oxidation of nutrients that serve as body fuels.

Basal Metabolism   One's basal energy requirement is determined with a respiration apparatus (Fig. 6.3). The findings can be translated into calories of heat that represent the amount of energy needed for internal activities for a period of 1 day. The basal metabolism is measured when a person is resting quietly, awake, in a comfortably warm room, 12 to 15 hours after eating.

Basal metabolic rate is related to the level of cellular activity, which varies in different types of cells, being high in muscle cells and low in fat cells. In general, males have a higher proportion of muscle tissue than females and younger individuals have a higher proportion of muscle than do older people. Norms have been developed for males and females of different ages and sizes from data accumulated on healthy individuals. An adult's basal energy rate is relatively constant from day to day but gradually decreases by a few calories a year, beginning at about the age of 20. At 75 years of age, the rate may be as much as 10 to 15 percent below that at 35 years. The basal metabolism of children fluctuates somewhat as the growth rate varies. It is highest during infancy and adolescence, the periods of accelerated growth. A number of conditions cause variations from the normal in basal metabolism, notably high or low levels of thyroxine, the hormone secreted by the thyroid gland. An overproduction of thyroxine causes a rise in the energy rate; an underproduction causes a fall. (Medical tests measuring protein-bound iodine in the blood are used to detect overproduction or underproduction of thyroxine.)

Data on the basal energy metabolism of large numbers of normal people have helped to identify some of the physical factors that determine basal metabolic rate, and this information has made it possible to devise ways of *estimating* basal metabolism. One simple procedure for making a rough estimate is based on the energy need per unit of body weight. The findings are reasonably satisfactory, assuming there are no upsetting factors such as an abnormal secretion of thyroxine. It has been found, for example, that normal young adults expend basal energy at the rate of about 1 calorie every hour for each 2.2 pounds (1 kg) of body weight. For an adult weighing 125 pounds (57 kg), therefore, the basal energy expenditure in 24 hours would be 1368 calories ($1 \times 24 \times 57$). A saving of about 10 percent of basal energy during sleep reduces the final figure slightly. For example, a person who sleeps 8 hours a day can deduct 46 calories ($0.1 \times 57 \times 8$), thus bringing his or her basal metabolic rate for the 24 hours down to 1322 calories ($1368 - 46$). The person is now ready to consider the additional factors that determine total daily energy needs.

Energy for External Activities

Muscular efforts of every type qualify as external activities. An activity can consist of such slight exertion as sitting up or standing, or it can involve the increasingly strenuous operations of walking, ironing, or playing tennis. Considerable data have been assembled on the energy required to carry on many different activities. This type of information has been classified by activities and occupations and is available for reference in various texts (5) (6). One author has presented the energy equivalents of a number of common foods by using the average energy expenditure for walking, bicycle riding, swimming, running, and reclining (7) (see Chap. 13). Such data can be used in calculating daily energy expenditures.

thyroid gland
Situated at the base of the neck; secretes iodine-containing hormones

Table 6.7
Estimation of calories for activities for various types of days

Type of activity	Calories * per lb per hr
a. **at rest most of day** sitting, reading, etc., very little walking and standing	0.23
b. **very light exercise** sitting most of the day, studying, with about 2 hr of walking and standing	0.27
c. **light exercise** sitting, typing, standing, laboratory work, walking, etc.	0.36
d. **moderate exercise** standing, walking, housework, gardening, carpentry, etc., little sitting	0.50
e. **severe exercise** standing, walking, skating, outdoor games, dancing, etc., little sitting	0.77
f. **very severe exercise** sports—tennis, swimming, basketball, football, running—heavy work, etc., little sitting	1.09

Adapted from C. M. Taylor and O. F. Pye, *Foundations of Nutrition* (New York: The Macmillan Company, 1966), p. 48.
*Exclusive of basal metabolism and the influence of food.

Calculation of daily energy expenditures involves a careful, hour-by-hour recording of all activities—work and play—and matching these activities to similar activities for which there are energy data. Simpler methods have been devised for use when an estimated figure is sufficiently accurate. One such method has been devised by Taylor and Pye (6). They have characterized six types of days on the basis of human activity levels, ranging from almost no activity to very strenuous exercise. Using this plan (Table 6.7), you can simply select the type of day most like your own. If, for example, you engage chiefly in light exercise, you would choose category "C" (0.36 cal per lb per hr). If moderate exercise characterizes your day, category "D" would be your choice. And if your level of activity seems to coincide with neither C nor D but is somewhere between the two, you can choose an intermediate figure (such as 0.43 cal per lb per hr). To estimate your total energy expenditure for external activities, merely multiply one of these calorie factors by your weight (for example, 125 lbs), and then multiply this result by the number of active hours (usually 16) in your day, giving in this case a total of 720 calories (0.36 × 125 × 16). This amount represents the energy expenditure for external activity alone.

Influence of Food   One additional item must be considered in estimating total daily energy need: increased energy expenditure, called *specific dynamic action*, due to the influence of food in the body. This increase has been referred to as a "tax" that is applied to the total calorie intake for handling the metabolic processes as the food nutrients are made available to the body. If the diet were

Table 6.8
To estimate your own daily calorie need
A short-cut method

a. weigh yourself; using your body weight as a basis, estimate your basal calorie need for 24 hours.
b. keep a diary of your activities for a typical day. Decide from Table 6.7 in which category your day falls—a, b, c, d, e, or f. Calculate the calorie need for your activities, for one day.
c. total your calorie needs, taking into consideration the 10 percent "tax" for influence of food.

Sample of calculation
Assume: an adult weighing 125 lbs (57 kg)
          a day with 16 hr of activity; 8 hr of sleep
Category of activity: c, light exercise

1. calories for basal metabolism (corrected for saving in sleep)	1322
basal metabolism for 24 hr: 1368 cal $(1 \times 57 \times 24)$	
saving in sleep, 8 hr: 46 cal $(0.1 \times 57 \times 8)$	
1322	
2. calories for activity $(0.36 \times 125 \times 16)$	+ 720
	2042
3. calories for the influence of food (10 percent of 2042)	+ 204
4. estimated total calories needed for the day	2246

almost exclusively carbohydrate, the tax would be about 6 percent; if it were almost exclusively fat, the tax could be as high as 14 percent; and if the diet were almost exclusively protein, the tax would be 30 percent or more. Because most people in the United States eat a mixed diet of the three nutrients, the average energy increase has been judged to be no more than 10 percent. This increase is accounted for in estimating the total calorie need for the day by adding 10 percent of the sum of the calories for basal energy metabolism and for external physical activities (in our example, $1322 + 720 = 2042 \times 0.10 = 204$).

Thus we have considered the separate components of the total energy metabolism of the adult—basal energy need, the energy required for physical activity, and the amount to be added to account for the influence of food (Table 6.8). For persons who are relatively inactive physically, the energy used by the body to maintain the vital functions is usually considerably greater than that used for physical activity.

Estimate your own daily energy requirements by the simple method suggested in Table 6.8.

How does your estimated daily calorie need compare with the total calorie intake recorded on your personal meal record? If they differ widely, how do you explain the discrepancy?

What is the difference in calories between your energy requirement for basal metabolism and your total caloric intake for one day? Is this sufficient to cover your energy needs for physical activity?

> If you did not record your own meals, compare your own estimated daily energy requirement with the grand total for calories on the specimen diet, Appendix H.

Desirable Goals for Energy Intake   Is it necessary to keep records of activities and perform the calculations shown in Table 6.8, or is there a convenient gauge of desirable energy intake? Are there recommended calorie-intake levels for various sex-age groups? The *Recommended Dietary Allowances* can be used in the United States as such a gauge, providing there is full understanding of the purpose of the allowances, and if conclusions from comparisons are drawn with caution. (Before proceeding, review the relevant material in Chapter 2.)

RDA
Nutrient standards for the United States

Recommended Dietary Allowances (RDA)   If you refer to the RDA for calories, identify yourself by sex and age. The column of the table labeled "kcal" presents the daily calorie allowances for categories of people of different ages, sexes, and conditions. Read from the table the recommended calorie level for the group into which you fall. The values are based on the knowledge that people similar in physical characteristics and activity often have similar energy needs (see inside cover) (8).

The calorie allowances apply to groups of people usually engaged in moderate physical activity. For those who take very little exercise, the allowances are excessive. People who lead sedentary lives probably will find that the allowances are above their daily calorie intakes or estimated energy needs. This is particularly true for individuals who are shorter and lighter than the height and weight given for the appropriate age group in the RDA table. The reverse can apply to those who are very active or taller and heavier than the height and weight indicated on the table.

The Food and Agriculture Organization (FAO) has proposed its own system of assessing energy requirements on an international scale. The FAO requirements are designed to be applied to populations of varied body size and age, living in different environments throughout the world (9). The system is subject to essentially the same limitations in use and interpretation as the RDA.

> Recognizing the need for caution in interpreting findings, make the following comparisons: RDA calorie allowance for your age-sex group *vs.* your estimated energy need; and RDA calorie allowance *vs.* your daily calorie intake, as shown on your personal meal record. Do the comparisons suggest problems in trying to estimate individual energy needs? What conclusions do you reach with regard to the use of the RDA as a guide for energy intake for individuals? How would you use your experience to guide others?

Body Weight and Energy Requirement   For practical purposes, an adult individual's daily energy need is one that assures a body weight that is best for that person. Therefore, no matter what the

RDA table or your own meal records indicate, the scales pass final judgment on desirable calorie intake. It is well then to know how much you weigh, how your weight compares with the desirable range for your age and height, and how steadily your weight holds from week to week. To obtain this information:

1. *Take your height and weight.* Observe the following rules in taking these and all future measurements. Measure your height against a flat wall or door, with heels, buttocks, and head touching the surface, eyes looking directly ahead. Have someone place a flat object such as a book atop your head; press the book straight back against the flat surface and mark the lower side to indicate your height. Measure the distance to the floor (Fig. 6.4).

   Weigh yourself on a balance (platform) scale, if possible. Use the same scale each week, and weigh yourself at the same time of day to minimize variations in weight resulting from bowel movements and food intake. Note suggestions for clothing in Chapter 2.

2. *Refer to Table 2.1 for desirable weights for men and women.* Classify yourself as of small, medium, or large frame. Select the weight range that corresponds to your height. For example, if you are a woman of medium frame, 5 feet 4 inches tall, your desirable weight is in the range of 113 to 126 pounds. Desirable weights are considerably below *average* weights. The latter are based on data obtained from a large number of individuals, many of whom are overweight (10, 11).

3. *Draw up a form for your own weight chart*, showing your desirable weight range as a "zone." (See the sample chart in Appendix I.) Allow sufficient space above and below the zone to indicate your actual weight if it falls above or below the desirable range and to permit the showing of gains or losses in the coming weeks. Keep the chart on a weekly basis as long as it has value as a guide to daily calorie intake.

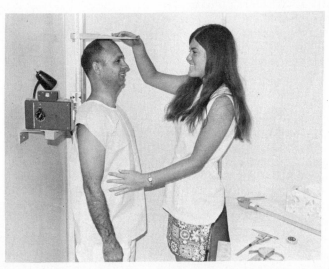

Figure 6.4
Measuring height in a laboratory setting with special measuring equipment. The same results are obtainable by method described in text. Proper stance of the subject is a critical factor in accuracy. (National Center for Health Statistics; US Department of Health, Education and Welfare)

Does your energy intake as shown on your personal meal record shed any light on your actual weight in relation to your desirable weight? On your estimated daily energy expenditure? On your energy allowance as taken from the RDA? How do you account for discrepancies if they exist?

Storage of Energy-Yielding Material during Growth

During childhood, total energy needs include not only the three components (basal metabolism, muscular activity, and specific dynamic action of food) considered thus far but also the energy requirements for growth. Unless there is enough energy-yielding material to permit reserves for growth during childhood, that growth is curtailed. There is no way of knowing exactly what proportion of energy-yielding nutrients is used for the needed reserve and what is used for muscular exercise. It *is* known that the need for reserve energy increases with a child's accelerated growth rate, and that the toll for activity is taken first. If a child does not have enough energy for both, growth suffers. Thus, a child with inadequate energy intake may be active at the expense of growth.

Energy allowances for age-sex groups of children are presented in the "kcal" column of the RDA table. Growth rate, size, and activity have all been considered in arriving at these values. Energy needs of individual children will not necessarily coincide with those of the corresponding group age ranges in the table. In general, large, rapidly growing, active children require more energy; smaller, slower growing, inactive children need less than the average. The energy intake of any child can be considered satisfactory if the child is growing at what appears to be a normal rate for that child.

Pregnancy and lactation also represent forms of growth. Additional amounts of energy at these periods are recommended in the RDA. Women's higher energy needs during pregnancy are due to a higher metabolic rate, which begins about the fourth month. The higher energy allowance for lactation is needed for milk production; the amount of additional energy corresponds with the actual amount of milk produced. (See Chap. 11 for more precise information on the increased needs of pregnancy and lactation.)

BUDGETING CALORIES

In this chapter we have considered the energy needs of the normal person and the energy values of foods that must satisfy these needs. Problems of achieving a balance between them, as related to weight control, are discussed in Chapter 13. Currently there is a tendency to regard calories as a necessary evil (12). However, the body's energy need is basic to all others. We cannot live and work without adequate sources of energy.

Rather than discount the importance of energy for good nutrition, we should conceive of it as an indispensable partner of the nutrients. This thought was forcefully expressed by M. S. Rose in the first edition of *Foundations of Nutrition* in 1927, and it is as true and important now as it was then: "Our first task is to learn how many calories we need and then to see how, by intelligent choice of foods which yield them, we may make them the carriers of every other dietary essential". Thus, we cannot do without calories, but we can make them serve us well.

This concept—that calories can be *good* or *poor* nutrient carriers—has led to the use of the term "empty calories" when a food yields little or no nutrient value. When the nutrient yield is good, calories can be said to pay a bonus. Variation in the nutrient yield among foods accounts for the fact that foods of the same calorie value often differ widely in nutritive value. Trading one food for another on the basis of calorie value alone is obviously a dangerous practice.

A consideration of calories, therefore, merely lays the groundwork for an appreciation of the various nutrients that are available in the foods we eat daily. The succeeding chapters point up the importance of these nutrients to good nutrition and show how intelligent choice of common foods can assure an adequate nutrient intake.

REFERENCES

1. R. S. Goodhart and M. E. Shils, eds., *Modern Nutrition in Health and Disease* (Philadelphia: Lea and Febiger, 1973).

2. R. L. Pike and M. L. Brown, *Nutrition: An Integrated Approach* (New York: John Wiley and Sons, 1975).

3. E. N. Todhunter, "Food Composition Tables in U.S.A., A History of, Bulletin 28," *J. Am. Dietet. Assoc.* 37 (Sept. 1960), pp. 209-14.

4. Food models can be purchased from the following sources: Nasco Company, Food Replicas (vinyl plastic models), Fort Atkinson, Wisc. 53538; National Dairy Council (pasteboard models, color), 6300 N. River Road, Rosemont, Ill. 60018.

5. E. D. Wilson, K. H. Fisher and M. E. Fuqua, *Principles of Nutrition* (New York: John Wiley and Sons, 1975).

6. C. M. Taylor and O. F. Pye, *Foundations of Nutrition* (New York: Macmillan, 1966).

7. F. Konishi, *Exercise Equivalents of Foods* (Carbondale, Ill.: Southern Illinois University Press, 1974).

8. Food and Nutrition Board, National Research Council, *Recommended Dietary Allowances*, 8th revision (Washington, D.C.: National Academy of Sciences—National Research Council, 1974).

9. Food and Agriculture Organization of the United Nations, *Handbook on Human Nutritional Requirements*, FAO Nutritional Studies, No. 28 (Rome: FAO, 1974).

10. National Center for Health Statistics, *Height and Weight Measurements of Adults 18–74 years: United States, 1971–74* (Washington, D.C.: Vital and Health Statistics, US Public Health Service, Series 11. To be published).

11. G. A. Bray, ed., *Obesity in Perspective*, DHEW Pub. No. (NIH) 75-708 (Washington, D.C.: US Gov. Print. Office, 1975).

12. L. E. Lamb, *Metabolics* (New York: Harper and Row, 1974).

Proteins

Functions
Needs and Allowances
Amino Acids
Food Sources of Protein
Unconventional Sources
Protein in the National Diet

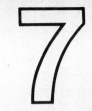

amino acids
Structural units of proteins

Certain aspects of proteins have already been considered: that proteins collectively, represent one of the six nutrient classes, that certain types of foods are more important than others as sources of dietary protein, and that proteins must be broken down into amino acids by the process of digestion before they can be absorbed and used by the body. Some of the ways in which the body uses protein have also been discussed. We are now ready to consider such matters as how much protein is needed daily, what is meant by protein quality, the relative importance of different food sources of protein, and what difference it makes whether or not we get the protein we need.

HOW PROTEINS ORIGINATE

Plants are the original source of all foods, including all food proteins. Only plants can use raw materials—nitrogen from soil, carbon dioxide from air, and water—to make their own proteins.

Energy for the task is furnished by the sun. Animals utilize mainly plant proteins in making their own body proteins. People, other than strict vegetarians, obtain their protein supply from both plant and animal sources. Food proteins are not utilized as such, but their constituent amino acids are rebuilt into the specific kinds of proteins required for body structures and processes (1).

The amino acids released by digestion and absorbed through the intestinal wall enter the bloodstream and are carried to all the cells. Within each cell nucleus, the *DNA* molecules hold the instructions that provide the means for lining up amino acids in proper sequence to produce a specific kind of protein. The message is transcribed when *messenger ribonucleic acid* (mRNA), daughter molecules of DNA, is formed. Other smaller *RNA* molecules, *transfer RNA* (a specific kind for each kind of amino acid), bring the amino acids to the *ribosomes* in the cell as the code in the RNA "calls" for them. As the amino acids are placed in appropriate order, enzymes link them into long chains that form protein (see Chap. 5).

If even one of the essential amino acids needed to make a specific protein is in short supply, utilization of all others is reduced proportionately. Figure 7.1 illustrates what happens when one essential amino acid is available in less than the required amount. The first bar in each group of three represents the relative amount of the designated amino acid required to build a specific protein. The second bar (green) indicates the amount of each amino acid available. Note that one of the essential amino acids, lysine, is present in just half the quantity required. As indicated by the third bar in each group, only half of all other essential amino acids can then be utilized, thus limiting protein synthesis to one half of its potential. The leftover amino acids will be metabolized for energy.

The body's specific need for protein is based on its building and

DNA
Genetic material in the nucleus of every cell

RNA
Substance that aids in synthesizing protein materials

ribosomes
Containing RNA; site of protein synthesis

enzymes
Proteins essential for stimulating reactions in the body

Figure 7.1
Limitation of protein synthesis when one essential amino acid (lysine) is in relatively short supply.

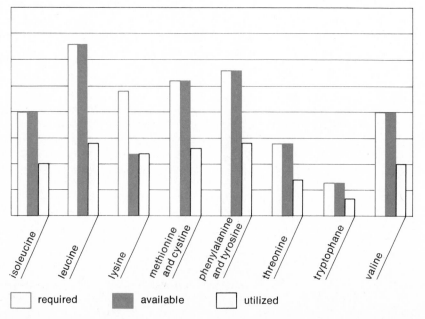

required   available   utilized

upkeep functions. Food protein can be used also for energy, but it is not specifically required for that purpose; carbohydrates and fats can perform just as satisfactorily in this regard and are more economical physiologically as well as in terms of the food budget.

FUNCTIONS OF PROTEIN (1, 2)

Formation of New Body Tissue   Growth during infancy and childhood, as well as the formation of new tissues during the course of pregnancy, depend upon an adequate supply of protein to provide amino acids in sufficient amounts and variety. Other situations in which new tissue must be built include wound healing and recovery from surgery, burns, and *febrile* and other wasting diseases. New tissue formation also takes place as muscle mass increases in response to certain types of athletic training.

febrile
Relating to fever

Maintenance of Body Structure   Body proteins are continuously undergoing a breaking-down and building-up process. Thus they are said to be in a *dynamic state* in the body. As proteins are broken down, some of the nitrogen from amino groups is excreted from the body, and new sources are continuously needed from the food supply.

Production of Compounds Essential for Normal Body Functions   All the thousands of kinds of enzymes that are produced in the body and that function in metabolism are protein in nature. Each has a specific structure and is responsible for catalyzing a specific reaction. Many of the hormones, which perform vital regulatory processes, are also proteins. Hemoglobin, essential for carrying oxygen to the cells and carbon dioxide to the lungs, is composed principally of protein, with a small amount of iron. Certain nonprotein but nitrogen-containing tissue constituents also use amino acids as a source of nitrogen.

hemoglobin
Iron-containing protein pigment in red blood cells

Regulation of Water Balance   Protein is one of many factors involved in regulating the exchange of fluids across the semipermeable membranes between the intracellular and intercellular compartments, and between the intercellular and *intravascular* compartments.

intravascular
Within the blood vessels

Maintenance of Blood Neutrality   Proteins normally present in blood *plasma* function as buffers—that is, they can react with either acids or bases. By this action they help to keep body fluids neutral, a condition essential for normal functioning of the cells.

plasma
Fluid part of circulating blood

Supply of Energy   After the amino group containing the nitrogen has been removed from an amino acid molecule, the remainder of the molecule can be metabolized to furnish energy.

PROTEIN QUALITY

It is not only the *quantity* of protein that counts but also the *quality*. The quality of proteins in the foods you eat determines to some

Table 7.1
Approximate percentage of essential amino acids in several proteins
(in grams per 100 grams of protein)

Essential amino acids	Egg whole	Cow's milk whole, skim	Beef	Fish	Gelatin	Soybeans and flour
lysine	6.4	7.9	8.7	8.8	4.4	6.3
tryptophan	1.6	1.4	1.2	1.0	—	1.4
phenylalanine	5.8	4.9	4.1	3.7	2.1	4.9
methionine	3.1	2.5	2.5	2.9	0.8	1.3
threonine	5.0	4.7	4.4	4.3	2.0	3.9
leucine	8.8	10.0	8.2	7.6	3.0	7.7
isoleucine	6.6	6.5	5.2	5.1	1.4	5.4
valine	7.4	7.0	5.6	5.3	2.5	5.2

Values calculated from *Amino Acid Content of Foods*, Table 1, Home Economics Research Report #4 (16% nitrogen). US Dept. Agriculture, 1966.

degree the quantity you need. In other words, if the quality is excellent, less protein suffices than if it is poor. Quality of food proteins is determined largely by the kinds and proportions of the amino acids they contain (1, 3).

Essential Amino Acids

There are some 22 amino acids, each a separate chemical entity having certain characteristics in common with all the others. Eight of them are known as "essential" amino acids for adult human beings. Because these eight cannot be synthesized from foods at the rate needed, they must be supplied readymade in foods. They are:

☐ lysine
☐ tryptophan
☐ phenylalanine
☐ methionine
☐ threonine
☐ leucine
☐ isoleucine
☐ valine

An additional one, histidine, is essential for infants. Some recent research has indicated that histidine may also be essential for adults (4). Practically all of the 22 amino acids are present in most proteins in greater or lesser amounts, but the amounts and proportions of the eight essential ones determine whether proteins are of high or low quality. The essential amino acid composition of a few representative proteins is shown in Table 7.1.

Progress has been made in determining human needs for the essential amino acids (5, 6), and allowances have thus far been proposed for young men, young women, and infants. Moreover, the amino acid content of a number of foods has been determined. Thus it is now possible to examine the diets of young adults for their yield of these amino acids and to compare intakes with proposed allowances. Such comparisons are interesting, and they indicate whether the diet is satisfactory with respect to the quality of protein. But a more revealing comparison is that of the *pattern* of es-

Table 7.1
continued

Chick-peas (garbanzos)	Beans navy, red, other	Peanuts, peanut butter	Cottonseed flour, meal	Corn, corn-meal	Rice, white, brown	Wheat, whole-grain, flour
6.9	7.4	3.6	4.3	2.9	3.8	2.6
0.8	0.9	1.1	1.2	0.6	1.0	1.2
4.9	5.5	5.1	5.2	4.5	4.8	4.6
1.3	1.0	0.9	1.4	1.9	1.7	1.4
3.6	4.3	2.7	3.5	4.0	3.7	2.7
7.4	8.6	6.1	5.9	13.0	8.2	6.3
5.7	5.7	4.1	3.8	4.6	4.5	4.0
4.9	6.1	5.0	4.9	5.1	6.7	4.3

sential amino acids, provided by individual foods or groups of foods, with body needs, as reflected by the amino acid composition of human tissue.

Nonessential Amino Acids

All proteins are made up of essential and nonessential amino acids. The so-called "nonessential" or "dispensable" amino acids are as important in metabolism as the essential amino acids. They are nonessential only in the sense that they need not be furnished preformed in food. The body can synthesize them, provided that sufficient nitrogen-containing substances are available. Thus the amounts and proportions of individual nonessential amino acids present in dietary protein are not of critical importance. What is important is their availability as a group, because they spare essential amino acids from being used to synthesize them (7).

Patterns of Essential Amino Acids

The amino acid pattern of a protein refers to the quantitative relationship or ratios between the essential amino acids it contains. Egg protein is often used as a reference standard for comparison of amino acid patterns of protein from other foods. The amino acid composition of proteins in animal foods—meats, poultry, fish, milk, cheese, and eggs—resembles the amino acid content of human tissues. Thus animal proteins provide amino acids in the approximate proportions needed by the body. This gives them a superior nutritional rating and helps to classify them as high-quality proteins. The nutritive value of proteins from most plant sources—vegetables, fruits, and grains—is lower, partly because their patterns of essential amino acids are less satisfactory. A poor pattern can be due to an incomplete assortment of essential amino acids, to their presence in too small quantities, or to unfavorable ratios among them. The amounts and proportions of essential amino acids in soybean proteins and in proteins of certain other legumes are similar to those in proteins of animal origin.

Table 7.1 shows the approximate percentage of essential amino acids in representative animal and vegetable proteins that are used throughout the world. The animal food proteins—eggs, milk, beef, and fish—appear first on the table. They represent desirable patterns of essential amino acids for human protein nutrition. Gelatin is an animal protein with a poor essential amino acid pattern. The remaining columns are devoted to vegetable proteins—those of legumes, seeds, and cereals. There is some variation in the content of essential amino acids between groups of vegetable proteins, as well as within the groups. Table 7.1 shows, for example, that legumes tend to be particularly low in methionine and cereals in lysine. It also shows considerable difference in essential amino acid content between individual legume proteins and between individual cereal proteins. This information gives some insight into the importance of combining proteins for effective supplementation of essential amino acids and also indicates where such supplementation is most needed. Although they are not of high quality individually, all proteins of vegetable sources make important contributions to the proteins in a mixed diet.

Other Factors

Protein quality cannot be determined solely on the basis of patterns of essential amino acids. Other factors that must be considered are the digestibility of proteins and the physiological availability of amino acids for absorption in the body (8). In the main, animal proteins are digested well. As a result, their satisfactory essential amino acid composition generally corresponds with efficient body use. Vegetable proteins are usually less well digested, and their amino acids are less efficiently released for body use. Their overall protein quality cannot be predicted accurately from the amino acid composition; it must be assessed by biological tests. Determination of biological value (BV), net protein utilization (NPU), and protein efficiency ratio (PER) provide measures of overall protein quality. These tests of protein quality are described in reference 1. Proteins from soybeans, for example, apparently furnish essential amino acids in good proportions. In animal feeding tests, however, raw soybeans do not promote growth as efficiently as would be expected from their amino acid composition. This is because raw soybeans contain a substance that inhibits the functioning of trypsin, an enzyme necessary for digesting the protein. Heating increases the overall utilization of the protein, but severe heat treatment reduces the protein quality. When properly processed, the proteins of soybeans and certain other legumes with good amino acid patterns are of higher quality than those of most vegetable sources and are nearly as useful as those in animal foods.

Processing of foods results in both favorable and adverse effects on their nutritional quality. Changes in the molecular structure of proteins during processing or storage can make them less useful to the body. Commercial processing of conventional food products, however, does not cause significant damage to biological values.

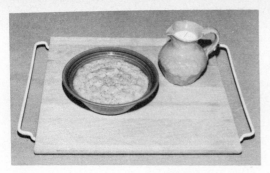

Figure 7.2
Cereal grain and milk combinations are examples of ways foods may supplement each other to improve the protein quality of meals. Milk supplies the essential amino acid lysine which is generally low in cereals. (Landon Gardiner)

Proteins in unconventional products, especially those made from isolated proteins, are more susceptible to adverse changes (9).

Supplementary Value of Proteins   When several foods containing protein are eaten together, the amino acids supplement each other naturally in behalf of good protein nutrition. When the day's meals provide proteins in sufficient quantity from a variety of sources (both animal and vegetable), as well as an adequate supply of energy from carbohydrates and fats, good protein nutrition is practically assured. Fortunately, foods that complement each other with respect to essential amino acids are often eaten together. Cereals and milk are an example of this type of combination. Milk furnishes extra lysine, which is the amino acid most deficient in the cereal protein (Fig. 7.2). A peanut butter sandwich and milk, or rice with fish or meat are other examples of common food combinations. The idea of providing essential amino acids through combinations of foods that can be produced locally is being pursued in parts of the world where animal sources of protein are scarce.

Such combinations represent the most practical means of amino acid supplementation. The addition of certain synthetic amino acids to diets is another possible method of improving protein quality. However, greater benefits result from use of complementary protein foods: protein quantity and energy value of the diet as well as protein quality are improved. It is the considered opinion of the Food and Nutrition Board and other professional groups that there is no need for supplementing the food supply of the United States with special protein or amino acid products. Furthermore, an imbalance of amino acids may result when an individual amino acid is added to the diet (10). There are some research data indicating that an excess of one amino acid may create a deficiency of another by reducing its potential for utilization.

PROTEIN REQUIREMENTS

We commonly speak of the body's protein need or protein requirement, even though we know it is the amino acids that are needed and not the proteins as such. Amino acids do not occur free in nature, but are available in the form of proteins in both animal and vegetable products. With this understanding, the term "protein need" is still a reasonable one.

There are several methods used for determining an individual's dietary protein requirement. One is the so-called *balance study*, in which nitrogen intake and output are measured, and the data obtained are converted mathematically into amounts of protein. If the amount of nitrogen consumed in food balances (or is approximately the same as) the amount excreted from the body on a daily basis, one is said to be in *nitrogen equilibrium*. When this condition exists in an adult, the individual's protein intake is believed to be adequate. However, the amount of protein consumed does not necessarily represent the amount required to meet actual needs; one will be in nitrogen equilibrium when dietary intake of protein meets or *exceeds* one's needs. The lowest protein intake on which an adult can maintain nitrogen equilibrium is considered to be the amount of protein required. The body has the ability to adapt to a less-than-adequate intake, since body tissues can compensate for a time by supplying the nitrogen needed to achieve equilibrium.

When a person is building new body tissue, less nitrogen is excreted than is taken in. The individual is said to be in *positive nitrogen balance*. This situation exists during the growth period (infancy, childhood, and adolescence), and during pregnancy. When more nitrogen is excreted than is taken in, a person is said to be in negative nitrogen balance. This happens when the diet is so deficient in protein that the body's needs for amino acids are not met. Body protein may be breaking down at the usual rate, but insufficient new amino acids from food proteins are available to replace it. Negative nitrogen balance also can result when body proteins break down at an excessive rate, as happens in surgery, in severe burns, during febrile illnesses, in the presence of infection, and during long periods of immobility.

Another method for estimating protein requirement involves maintaining individuals on a protein-free diet. After an adjustment period, the amount of protein that will compensate for the nitrogen lost in urine, feces, and sweat is determined, and the amounts required for increase in body mass during normal growth or pregnancy or for milk production during lactation are added.

There is considerable variation, even among normal, healthy individuals, in the amount of protein required to meet body needs. Several factors must be taken into consideration in determining the quantity required, one of which is the relationship between dietary protein and energy intake. The amount of protein required to maintain nitrogen equilibrium in adults varies directly with dietary energy intake. In studies to determine protein needs, care has been taken to avoid an energy deficit, but the opposite situation—provision of excess energy—has received less attention. Recent research findings have suggested that the current FAO Recommended Intakes for dietary protein may not be satisfactory, because they provide sufficient protein only when energy intake is so high as to result in gain of body weight. Reduction of energy intake to maintenance levels increases the need for protein to levels above those recommended (11).

The quality of dietary protein is another factor that must be taken into consideration in determining the quantity required.

Proteins of milk, meat, and eggs are of high nutritional quality; they furnish at least the minimum required quantity of each essential amino acid when the amount of protein consumed satisfies the requirement for nitrogen. Most people in the United States who use foods of animal origin in their diets also consume proteins of lower nutritional quality as well. For many population groups, dietary proteins consist almost entirely of vegetable proteins that fail to furnish one or more of the essential amino acids in sufficient amounts. In establishing the RDA for protein, the Food and Nutrition Board included a quality-correction factor as a safety measure. This is based on the assumption that efficiency of utilization of the mixed proteins in the United States diet is 75 percent of the ideal protein. The daily allowance also varies among individuals depending on size. Adults who are larger (that is, those who have a greater mass of living tissue) than the "average" person will obviously have higher daily protein allowances; those who are smaller will have correspondingly lower allowances. Note that the RDA for protein for men and women varies in proportion to their average weights (see inside cover).

Pregnancy and lactation call for more protein (see RDA table). During the second and third *trimesters* of pregnancy, the fetus has gained considerable size and is growing rapidly, thus increasing the mother's need for protein. Also more protein is needed during lactation to provide sufficient breast milk for the baby.

> What is the protein RDA for your sex-age group? Calculate the grams of protein needed per kilogram (2.2 lb) of body weight. Using this figure, determine your protein allowance based on your own body weight.

Protein Allowances for Children   Children need protein not only for upkeep but also for growth. They must be in positive nitrogen balance if their tissues are to grow and be nourished adequately. A child's protein requirement at any age depends on his or her size and rate of growth at that time. The RDA show a progression in protein allowances for children as they increase in age. Increases in height and weight, which normally accompany increases in age, indicate a growing mass of active body tissue. A steadily increasing protein intake is needed not only to support the growth of this tissue but also to nourish and sustain it.

Protein cannot be used for growth until after its maintenance function has been fulfilled. When there is not enough protein for both maintenance and growth, growth is the loser. Because of their growth needs, children have proportionately higher protein allowances in relation to their body weight than do adults. During the first 6 months of life, when growth is most rapid, the amount of protein recommended per kilogram of body weight is higher than at any other time. If you calculate the ratios of protein to body weight using the data in the RDA table, you will find that the ratio gradually decreases during the remainder of the growth period.

Figure 7.3
Protein: servings of representative foods in order of their protein content. (Each bar represents the approximate protein value for the foods listed below it.)

Food*	Weight or ** approximate measure	Protein grams
		24 g
chicken, fried	½ breast	26
beef, lean chuck	3 oz	25
beef, hamburger	3 oz	23
tunafish, canned	½ cup	23
haddock, fried	1 fillet (4 oz)	22
		15 g
pork chop	1 chop	19
liver, beef	2 oz	15
beans, dry, canned	¾ cup	12
		8 g
milk, fluid skim or buttermilk	1 cup	9
milk, fluid whole	1 cup	9
cheese, cottage creamed	¼ cup	8
peanut butter	2 tbsp	8
cheese, cheddar	1 oz	7
sausage, bologna	2 oz	7
egg	1 medium	6
frankfurter	1 medium	6
		3 g
macaroni, enriched, cooked	¾ cup	4
peas, green	½ cup	4
bread, whole wheat	1 slice	3
bun or roll, enriched	1 bun	3
corn, canned	½ cup	3
oatmeal, cooked	⅔ cup	3
potato, white	1 medium	3
rice, enriched, cooked	¾ cup	3
spinach	½ cup	3
sweet potato	1 medium	3
bread, white, enriched	1 slice	2
broccoli	½ cup	2
cornflakes, fortified	1 cup	2
		1 g or less
banana, raw	1 medium	1
beans, green	½ cup	1
cabbage, raw, chopped	½ cup	1
carrots, diced	½ cup	1
cream, half and half	1 tbsp	1
grapefruit, white	½ medium	1
lettuce, head, raw	1 cup	1
onions	½ cup	1
orange juice	½ cup	1
peaches, canned	½ cup	1
pineapple juice, canned	½ cup	1
raisins	¼ cup	1
strawberries, raw	½ cup	1
tomato juice, canned	½ cup	1
apple, raw	1 medium	tr
butter or margarine	1 tbsp	tr
mayonnaise	1 tbsp	tr
peppers, sweet, green, raw	½ medium	tr
beverages, cola type	12 oz	(0)†
oil, salad or cooking	1 tbsp	0†
sugar	1 tbsp	0†

*   Foods are in forms ready to eat. All meats and vegetables are cooked unless otherwise indicated.
** See Appendix K for further identification of these foods. All foods are described there more fully, and both weights and measures are indicated.
†   See Appendix J.

FOOD SOURCES OF PROTEIN

A glance at Figure 4.1 will refresh your memory about some of the types of foods regarded as important protein sources. On that figure, the protein content of the foods is represented on a percentage basis. This does not tell you how much protein you can obtain from eating a serving of any of the foods listed, but you can calculate the protein content of a serving of food from the percentage composition if you know its weight. For example, cooked lean beef yields about 26 percent protein, which means that every gram of cooked lean beef contains 0.26 gram of protein. It follows that a 3-ounce serving (85) grams) of beef furnishes about 22 grams of protein (85 × 0.26). Protein values can thus be determined by simple multiplication. However, making such calculations for foods would be tedious and time consuming. The protein contents of average servings of many foods have therefore been provided in Appendix K.

Comparative Protein Content of Foods

One way to become familiar with the amounts of protein in common foods in the portions in which they are usually served is to study the protein content of your own representative foods or of those on the specimen list. Note that the foods in Figure 7.3 are the identical fifty items that compose the specimen representative food list in Table 6.6. These fifty foods, in average servings, appear in Figure 7.3 in order of their quantitative importance as sources of protein. This is to help you associate levels of protein content with common food sources. Quantity, not quality, of protein is the basis for comparison.

Figure 7.3 provides the following assistance: the bars show by their length the comparative protein content of the foods, so that the more concentrated sources of protein are immediately evident by their top position. Foods with about the same protein content per serving can thus be associated. One approximate protein value is indicated on each bar for the foods listed below it. The figure also shows the types of foods that are not good sources of protein—those that contain only negligible amounts of protein in a serving and appear at the end. Much can be learned from a closer look at the figure.

Concentrated Sources   It is evident from Figure 7.3 that chicken, beef, and fish provide the most protein per portion when eaten in the amounts indicated. The values per serving in this assortment are very similar, ranging from 22 to 26 grams of protein, with a value of 24 grams fairly representative of all. Kinds of poultry, cuts of beef, and varieties of fish differ somewhat in protein content, but those listed here are reasonably typical.

All of the foods in the second section—pork chop, beef liver, and dry beans—as well as those above, belong to the meat group. The protein content of canned beans is representative of the different kinds of dry beans that are prepared as pork and beans and in various other ways. Taking 15 grams of protein as the amount representative of these foods, one serving of any of them furnishes roughly one-third of the protein needed each day.

Less Concentrated Sources Next in order on Figure 7.3 are several foods often called "meat alternates," because they can substitute for meat as protein sources in meals. These foods include cheese, eggs, milk, peanut butter, and sausages. Peanuts, which are legumes, are nearly twice as high in protein, weight for weight, as most other nuts, and peanut butter is similar to peanuts in protein content. A serving of any one of these foods yields about 8 grams of protein, one-fourth to one-third as much as the meats at the top of the list. Even though they are not concentrated sources of protein, they make a significant contribution to the day's total protein intake.

Serving size is a critical factor in determining the relative position of the foods in Figure 7.3. This is particularly true of the food groups we have been discussing. For example, many teenagers consider a pint of milk, rather than a cup, to be a serving. A 1-pint serving with its 18 grams of protein, would thus place milk higher on the list. In the same way, doubling the portion of cottage cheese from ¼ cup to ½ cup would elevate it to a higher category. On the other hand, reducing the size of a serving of baked beans from ¾ cup to ½ cup would move beans down on the list. In ranking foods on your own representative food list, be sure to adjust the sizes of servings to your own food habits.

Good and Fair Sources Still lower concentrations of protein are found in macaroni, green peas, cereals, bread, potatoes, and certain vegetables. These items range in protein value from 2 to 4 grams per serving, averaging about 3 grams. A check with Appendix K will show that the protein content of plain cooked macaroni is representative of the same amount of such similar foods as spaghetti and noodles, and that green peas yield about the same amount of protein as green lima beans. Fresh green legumes such as peas and lima beans are much higher in protein than other fresh vegetables. Both pastas and green legumes yield approximately 4 grams of protein per serving.

Cereals, bread, potatoes, and certain vegetables contribute 2 to 3 grams of protein per serving. In the main, 3 grams of protein per serving of oatmeal applies to other whole-grain cereals as well, such as rolled wheat and shredded wheat; commercially baked breads average about 2 grams of protein per slice; dry flaked or puffed cereals yield 2 to 3 grams per 1-ounce serving. Milled cooked cereals such as farina and grits yield about 2 grams of protein per serving. Although cereals and breads have relatively low yields of protein per serving, their total contribution to meals is considerable for individuals who eat large amounts of such foods. In the specimen diet given in Appendix H, there are no cereals and only three servings of bread; about 13 percent of the total day's protein comes from grains in various forms.

The vegetables that rank with cereals as protein sources are, for the most part, the starchy type: potatoes, corn, winter squash, and the dark green vegetables such as spinach and broccoli. Spin-

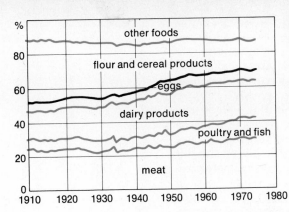

Figure 7.4
Sources of protein in the United
States (USDA)

ach runs somewhat higher in protein per serving than other
"greens" except collards and dandelion greens. Although none of
these can be considered a protein-rich source, they furnish two to
three times as much protein as vegetables appearing lower on the
list.

Almost half of the foods listed in Figure 7.3 yield less than 2
grams of protein per serving. The fruits and vegetables in this
category yield about 1 gram of protein per serving, while the fats
and sweets provide little or none.

> Arrange your own list of representative foods (see p. 136) by
> sorting your index cards or half sheets in order of their
> quantitative importance as sources of protein.

Meeting Protein Needs

In planning meals, both animal and vegetable sources of protein
are usually included. The RDA for protein were established on the
assumption that protein foods would be chosen from a variety of
sources yielding essential and other amino acids. One-half of the
total protein intake from animal sources is undoubtedly above actual needs; however, such a proportion is not out of line with eating practices in the United States (Fig. 7.4).

When animal protein food is eaten, all the essential amino
acids arrive in the cells at the same time. If animal protein is absent, however, the essential amino acids may not be available in
the amounts and proportions necessary to build body proteins. Now
that you understand how amino acids are put together to form proteins, you can appreciate the importance of providing the necessary
assortment and quantities of amino acids.

Experiments have suggested the wisdom of distributing animal
proteins throughout all the meals of the day as well. When college
women had animal protein with every meal, it helped to keep them
in nitrogen balance. For example, nitrogen was better utilized
when the students had one glass of milk with each of their three
meals than when they had none at breakfast (and no other source
of animal protein), one glass with lunch, and two glasses with din-

ner, along with other animal protein. Except for the variation in breakfast—with and without milk—the day's meals were identical and nutritionally adequate (12). Thus, timing of protein intake appeared to be a critical factor in the efficient use of amino acids. All essential amino acids, as well as adequate amounts of other amino acids, must be available *at the same time* to make body proteins. When an incomplete assortment of the essential amino acids is provided at a meal, there seems to be considerable wastage of those that are present, because they cannot be held over until others are provided at later meals (see Figure 7.1). This fact explains the difficulty of maintaining nitrogen balance under such circumstances.

Another investigation yielded different results. The effects of meal composition and pattern on efficiency of dietary nitrogen utilization was studied in college men. Protein was fed at relatively low levels—0.4 or 0.5 grams per kilogram of body weight per day with total protein intake ranging from 24 to 41 grams per day for the various subjects. Skim milk was the sole source of protein in the diet. The energy value of the diet was adjusted to maintain weight for each subject or to provide 80 percent of the amount required for weight maintenance. With different combinations of amounts of protein and energy, the efficiency of nitrogen utilization appeared not to be affected by the distribution throughout the day of energy and protein. The protein was as well utilized when consumed only at lunch and dinner as when it was included in the breakfast as well (13).

It is interesting to speculate on why the findings with regard to efficiency of nitrogen utilization were different in these two studies. It has been suggested that variations in the results might be related to such factors as the differences in sex of the subjects, the amounts of dietary protein, and the food sources of the protein (13).

The specimen diet in Appendix H shows how relatively simple it is for an adult to obtain a diet adequate in total protein, over three-fourths of which is derived from animal sources. The total protein intake for the day is 69 grams, which represents a substantial margin above the RDA. The animal sources of protein in this case are hamburger, milk, pork chop, and ice cream, with a total of 54 grams or 78 percent of the protein intake for the day.

Enter protein values from Appendix K on your personal meal record.

Compare your daily protein intake as shown on your personal meal record with the daily protein allowance you calculated on the basis of your own body weight.

Account for the effect of your food choices on your total protein intake.

What proportion of the total protein on your personal meal record came from animal sources? Did you have a source of animal protein at each meal?

In the United States, proteins commonly provide 10 to 15 percent of the total calorie intake in daily meals. The specimen diet in Appendix H shows a total calorie intake of 1927, of which 276 calories (69×4) are derived from protein. Protein in this case supplies about 14 percent of the calories ($276 \div 1927$).

> Determine what percent of the total calories on your personal meal record was provided by protein. Does it fall within the acceptable range?

Meeting Protein Needs with Vegetarian Diets

For most people in the United States who include meat and other animal products in their diets, protein intake meets or exceeds the RDA for their sex-age group. More and more people are adopting vegetarian diets, however. Are these diets adequate in quantity and quality of protein?

It is evident that the relative concentration of essential amino acids is the most important factor determining the biological value of a protein. This has led to recognition that the source of the protein, whether animal or plant, is not the critical consideration. The body cannot distinguish between amino acids from animal sources and those from plant sources. Diets composed entirely of foods from a variety of plant sources and furnishing sufficient energy for body maintenance from basic foods provide adequately for protein needs. Tests for adequacy have included nitrogen balance studies as well as comparison of total *serum protein*, and *albumin and globulin* values of subjects on vegetarian and nonvegetarian diets (14, 15).

A careful study of people eating different types of diets revealed that the *vegans* as well as the *lacto-ovo vegetarians* were actually eating more protein than proposed by the RDA. In addition to furnishing fully adequate amounts of protein, the diets of the vegans and the *lacto-ovo vegetarians* also supplied essential amino acids in greater than minimum quantities (16).

The proteins from milk and eggs in lacto-ovo vegetarian diets furnish a complete assortment of essential amino acids in good proportions. Proteins from plant sources in such diets supply important additional quantities of all amino acids. Strict vegetarian diets must be planned with greater concern for including a variety of sources of protein. These diets do not have the "safeguard" provided by milk and eggs in the lacto-ovo vegetarian diets. The essential amino acids in vegetable proteins are not as well balanced as in proteins from animal sources and therefore need to supplement each other to make a satisfactory amino acid pattern. Wheat, for example, is not satisfactory as the sole source of protein in the diet because it is relatively lacking in lysine, one of the essential amino acids. A deficiency of lysine limits the usefulness of other amino acids (see Figure 7.1). Legumes and nuts contain relatively greater amounts of lysine; including them in the diet compensates for the short supply in the grain. Total vegetarian diets should be supplemented with vitamin B_{12} (see Chap. 9), since this vitamin occurs only in foods of animal origin.

serum protein
Protein circulating in fluid portion of blood

albumin and globulin
Specific proteins in blood serum

vegans
Strict or total vegetarians who eat no animal products

lacto-ovo-vegetarians
Vegetarians who consume milk and eggs but no meat

Malnutrition among population groups subsisting mainly on foods of plant origin commonly has been ascribed to lack of sufficient dietary protein. Now it is recognized that in many instances such diets are adequate in protein in proportion to energy value; the problem results from an insufficient *amount* of food (17). Care must be taken, however, to avoid using large quantities of refined sugars and separated fats (such as salad oil), which provide energy but do not furnish a fair share of other nutrients. Attention is given to planning adequate vegetarian diets in Chapter 10.

Nutritionally adequate vegetarian diets are not to be confused with the severely restricted vegetarian diets such as the Zen macrobiotic type based solely on cereals. Such diets limit the kinds and amounts of foods and fluids that may be taken. They are dangerously inadequate. Dietary-deficiency diseases may develop and, with continued use, they may be life-threatening, particularly for children.

Protein in the National Diet

You have seen that many common foods are good sources of proteins, and that it is not difficult to obtain enough high-quality proteins if a free choice of foods is available. But is there sufficient protein to satisfy all individual needs? US Department of Agriculture data show that the total food supply in the United States is rich in protein. On the basis of proteins available for consumption, the intake would be about 102 grams per person per day if it were divided equally among all people. This amount is considerably above all RDA proposals for protein. Of the 102 grams, over two-thirds is from animal sources, a proportion in line with the substantial increase in proteins derived from animal products and the decreasing use of flour and cereal products (18). The change in protein sources and related facts are evident in Figure 7.4, which presents, on a percentage basis, the sources of protein in the U.S. food supply from 1910 to the present.

Nationwide dietary studies also suggest that there is a sufficiency of protein in the United States. A survey in 1965 showed that average intakes of protein for all age groups were over 100 percent of the RDA (19). In a nationwide survey of preschool children, the investigators concluded that the major nutritional problem of those children identified as "nutritionally at risk" was insufficient total food intake. Dietary levels of protein were so high, even among the lowest income groups, that it seemed protein had been given undue emphasis (20). Preliminary findings of the HANES also showed median intake of protein for all age groups to be above the RDA. No high-risk signs of protein deficiency were found, and the prevalence of moderate risk signs was low (21).

HANES
Survey designed to measure the nutritional status of US population

This evidence of high protein intakes brings up the possibility of getting too much protein. Is there harm in routinely eating more protein than is called for by the RDA? From observations on Arctic explorers existing for long periods almost exclusively on meat, it appears that normal adults can tolerate a protein intake far above their requirements. Infants and children, however, do not thrive as well on high-protein diets. When protein intake is to be increased, as in rehabilitation after malnutrition, it is recommended that it be done gradually. It is believed that excessive protein intake can result in fluid imbalances due to increased water requirements in the metabolism of protein.

High protein intakes can also pose a problem in weight control. Persons who need to limit their energy intake to maintain desirable body weight should be aware of the presence of fat, and therefore of high energy values, in many protein-rich foods. This factor will be apparent if you reexamine Figure 4.1 and look at the fat and energy values of high-protein foods listed in Appendix K.

Recent studies show that high-protein diets may adversely affect calcium balance in the body. Urinary calcium excretion was found to be directly correlated with the level of protein intake. Although there was a wide variation in urinary calcium excretion among individuals on the same diet, all subjects excreted more calcium in the urine whenever protein intake was increased (22).

hypertension
High blood pressure

The belief that hazards such as hypertension and damage to the kidneys or liver are associated with high protein intake has largely been proved erroneous. Nevertheless, excessive intakes of protein over prolonged periods of time are not advised. There has been no evidence that healthy human beings benefit from eating excessive amounts of protein (1, 23). The Food and Nutrition Board points out: "In healthy individuals, there is little evidence of nutritional benefit from intakes of protein that exceed requirements, nor is there evidence that intakes double or triple the recommended allowances are harmful (2)."

Despite the fact that most people in the United States eat proteins unsparingly, individuals do not share them equally or in accordance with need. Groups with special needs are infants, young children, and pregnant and lactating women. The elderly, often existing on limited amounts of food, are likely to have diets low in protein. For all people with low incomes and/or poor food habits, obtaining sufficient protein can be a problem.

PROTEIN AND FOOD PROBLEMS

In all countries there are undoubtedly individuals and groups who for various reasons do not consume sufficient protein. In many cases this is not entirely a matter of low protein intake, but of low total food intake. It is generally in the countries where protein supplies are low that energy values of diets are also low. Under such circumstances, emphasis should be placed on increasing the total food supply, rather than on increasing protein alone. There are exceptions, however. In some areas people subsist mainly on root crops such as manioc root, cassava, or bananas, which are so low in protein that even when the energy value of the diet is adequate, protein intake is still inadequate (24). In most developing countries grains form the basis for the diet. When these are supplemented with legumes or small amounts of animal products and eaten in quantities large enough to meet energy needs, protein requirements are also met.

Lack of sufficient food for all people is a problem that cannot be dealt with in isolation. It is the result of a complex of socioeconomic problems (see Chap. 15). Populations of some countries consume much more food per person than others. In the United States, for example, the per capita consumption of grain amounts to over 2,000 pounds per year, 150 pounds of which is eaten directly as grain products (bread, breakfast cereals, pasta, and such). The remaining 1,850 pounds are fed to animals that are used for human food. By contrast, it is estimated that in China the population is adequately nourished on 450 pounds of grain per person per year—350 pounds consumed directly as cereal and cereal products, and 100 pounds fed to animals (24).

Efficiency of conversion of plant food into animal food is variable, with the highest level, about 25 percent, attained in milk and egg production. Beef cattle convert feed nutrients into meat at a level of about 4 percent efficiency. From data such as these, the conclusion is often drawn that animals should not be used for food. It is true that to some extent animals and humans are competing for the same food—grains. However, *ruminants* (such as cows and sheep) need not be fed grain. They can utilize roughage such as crop residues (corn cobs and stalks), industrial byproducts, and forages from which humans could not otherwise benefit. Ruminants can also convert nonprotein nitrogen from sources such as urea into high-quality milk protein which is useful to humans (25). It is important to realize, too, that grains not fed to animals in developed countries do not necessarily reach hungry people in other parts of the world; economic considerations may serve as deterrents (26).

Also to be considered is the potential for increasing food production in developing countries by raising ruminants for food. Less fertilizer and energy are required to produce animals than to grow cereal grains. Much land that is unsuitable for crop production can support livestock and thus furnish high-quality proteins for human consumption. Ruminants are obviously an important link in the food chain (26).

ruminants
Cud-chewing animals with 3- or 4-chambered stomachs

urea
Important end product of protein metabolism; also synthesized commercially

The Food Gap

Organizations of the United Nations and other international and regional agencies concerned with the world's nutrition problems are engaged in programs designed to close the gap between food needs and food supplies in developing countries. Long-range plans deal with such basic considerations as increasing the production of animal, fish, and plant sources of protein, including grains genetically improved in protein content (27); improving the distribution and marketing of foods; and establishing research and personnel-training facilities. Such conventional methods of increasing food supplies are expected to meet present demands only for the next few years, and investigations into unconventional sources of protein for human consumption are in progress. Efforts to increase protein sources by conventional means are dealt with in Chapter 15. Following is a brief look at steps being taken to provide unconventional sources of protein.

UNCONVENTIONAL SOURCES OF PROTEIN

Goals

The aims of current research programs are to develop simple processes adaptable to the facilities of developing countries and to help those countries become self-sufficient in obtaining an adequate protein supply. Emphasis is placed upon the utilization of local resources and labor. Vast amounts of protein that are not now used for human food are available in the developing countries. Some unconventional sources of protein have been in experimental use for several years, and most of them are dependent on the application of modern technology rather than on the use of additional land.

Protein Concentrates from Oilseeds   About 40 to 50 percent of good-quality protein suited to human consumption is present in the meal remaining after the oil has been removed from such oilseeds as soya, peanut, cotton, sesame, and sunflower. Oilseed proteins can contribute importantly to the human diet. Research and development programs in the United States have already led to the production and use of a number of soy protein products (Figs. 7.5-7.9). Soybean meal requires processing to remove certain undesirable fractions. The defatted material can then be heated and ground to make grits or flour having a protein content of 40-50 percent. Products of higher protein content are prepared by removing more of the nonprotein constituents. Soy protein *concentrates* contain at least 70 percent protein. With further processing soy protein *isolates* containing 92 to 97 percent protein are obtained. The isolates —the most expensive of these products—cost about 5 to 6 times as

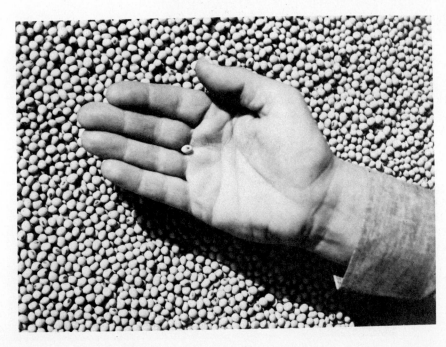

Figure 7.5
Mature soybeans ready for processing. (Central Soya)

Figure 7.6
Soybean products: soybean
meal, soy flour, soybean oil.
(General Mills)

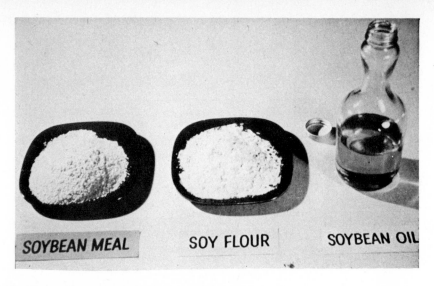

much as the least processed grits or flours and about twice as much
as the concentrates. Soy protein products are used in baked goods,
meat products, beverages, cereals, and pasta. Simulated meat products are made from soy protein by *extrusion* or spun-fiber techniques (28). Soy proteins have gained acceptance in institutional
feeding programs such as those of hospitals, nursing homes, and
schools.

    In the United States and other industrialized countries, protein
product development has been stimulated by economic and technical considerations as much as by nutritional and health objectives.
Some of these factors have been the high cost of meat, consumer
demand for protein products of low fat and cholesterol content, and
the search for materials that contribute functionally to new prod-

extrusion
*Process of shaping material by
forcing it through holes in a
metal block*

Figure 7.7
Schematic diagram of steps in
manufacturing soybeans into
meat analogs. (General Mills)

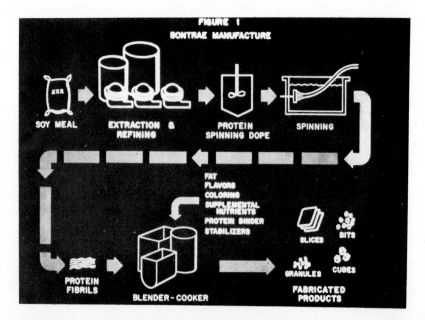

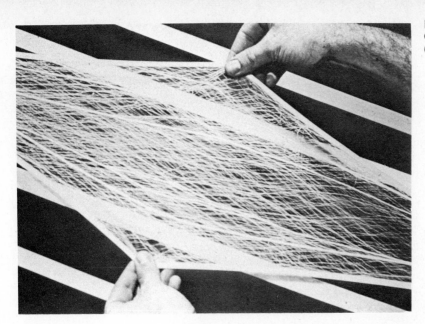

Figure 7.8
Close up of spun soy fibers.
(General Mills)

uct formulations. In developing countries, the use of oilseed meals is based more on their nutrient composition than on their functional qualities in manufactured products. Many traditional Asian soy recipes using whole soybeans or grits or flour would be more practical and effective in promoting good nutrition than the use of the more highly processed and expensive soy concentrates and isolates (28).

Whey

A watery byproduct of the manufacture of cheese, whey has often been disposed of as waste, although it has been used to some extent in animal feeds. Whey is an excellent source of nutrients—high quality proteins, vitamins, minerals, and sugar. A whey-soy drink has been developed and distributed to infants and young children through relief agencies around the world. The dry mixture consists of 42 percent sweet whey solids, 37 percent full-fat soy flour, 12 percent soybean oil, and 9 percent corn syrup solids. It can be fortified with additional vitamins and minerals, and is at least equivalent in nutritional value to nonfat dry milk. Another whey product,

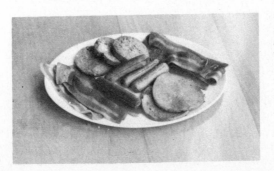

Figure 7.9
Samples of meat product analogs manufactured from textured vegetable proteins such as soy. (Landon Gardiner)

made from cottage cheese whey, consists of 80 to 90 percent protein and is suitable as an ingredient in breads and pastas. Various other whey blends are being used in the candy, bakery, and frozen dessert industries (29).

Single-Cell Protein

Techniques for producing single-cell protein (SCP) have been developed in many parts of the world, including Japan, Europe, and the United States. A variety of types of single-cell organisms—fungi, bacteria, and yeasts—are produced by fermentation, using many different materials as substrates. These include sugars, starches, and other substances from good-quality agricultural materials; hydrocarbons from petroleum or related sources; and cellulose and other industrial wastes. SCP has been proved to be safe and nutritious for animal feed; all types seem to be as dependable as traditional protein concentrates. Now being used for animal feed on an experimental basis in several countries, SCP will contribute to the food supply by freeing grains for human consumption (30). It cannot be approved for direct human use before further animal testing and clinical investigations with humans are carried out (31). Guidelines for human testing of supplementary food mixtures have been established by the Protein-Calorie Advisory Group of the United Nations System (32).

Leaf Protein Concentrates

The possibility of using concentrates prepared from green leaves such as alfalfa and tobacco has been investigated in a number of countries. In addition to protein, other constituents in the concentrate, particularly lipids, have potential nutritive value (30). Leaf protein was successful when used experimentally as a supplement in *kwashiorkor* cases in Nigeria, as well as when it was given to 9- to 12-year-old Indian boys on poor diets. Leaf protein extract is being tested in a large-scale comparative feeding trial with 2- to 5-year-old children in India (33).

lipids
Fats and fat-like substances
kwashiorkor
Severe protein deficiency disease

High-protein Products—Uses and Acceptance

Oilseed meals and other protein concentrates have essentially the same potential uses; that is, combination with other local foods to increase the quantity and quality of protein in the diet. For weaning foods, the meal or concentrate is usually mixed with nonfat dry milk solids; for school children essentially the same combination is used for supplementary snacks; for general household consumption the concentrate is combined with the staple cereal of the country.

The degree of acceptance of protein supplements in developing countries depends on the extent to which such foods fit into local eating patterns (34). In introducing them, there is need for knowledge of local food supplies, for understanding food tastes and customs of the area, and for acquaintance with channels of distribution. Nutrition education through existing agencies should also help to establish the new foods. But as these supplementary sources of protein gain some foothold, the fundamental problem of raising adequate yields of conventional food crops remains.

Table 7.2
Proteins a few highlights

What proteins do for you	Proteins build and maintain all body tissues: muscles, tendons, blood, skin, bone, nails, hair They help form hormones, digestive and other enzymes They help form antibodies to build resistance to disease They contribute to maintenance of normal water balance and acid-base balance They provide food energy
Some of the best food sources	lean meats, poultry, fish dry legumes cheese, milk, eggs cereals and breads (See Fig. 7.3)
The importance of proteins to good nutritional status	An adequate intake of proteins favors a well-developed body of desirable size and muscle texture; an inadequate protein intake is often associated with an undersized, poorly developed body with poor muscle tone. A diet providing an adequate supply of high-quality proteins contributes to a feeling of fitness and well-being; one providing an inadequate supply is a factor in low vigor and stamina Protein intake level is important in resistance to certain infections, recovery from disease, healing of wounds, and convalescence from surgery.

REFERENCES

1. A. A. Albanese and L. A. Orto, "The Proteins and Amino Acids," Chap. 2A in R. S. Goodhart and M. E. Shils, eds., *Modern Nutrition in Health and Disease* (5th edition), (Philadelphia: Lea and Febiger, 1973).

2. Food and Nutrition Board, National Research Council, *Recommended Dietary Allowances* (8th edition), (Washington, D.C.: National Academy of Sciences, 1974).

3. Food and Nutrition Board, *Evaluation of Protein Nutrition*, Pub. 711 (Washington, D.C.: National Academy of Sciences-National Research Council). Second edition in press.

4. M. E. Swendseid and J. D. Kopple, "Nitrogen Balance, Plasma Amino Acid Levels and Amino Acid Requirements," *Trans. New York Acad. Science* 35 (1973), 471-79.

5. W. C. Rose, "The Amino Acid Requirements of Adult Man," *Nutrition Abstracts and Reviews* 27 (July 1957), pp. 631-47.

6. M. S. Reynolds, "Amino Acid Requirements of Adults," *J. Am. Dietet. Assoc.* 33 (Oct. 1957), pp. 1015-18.

7. A. E. Harper, " 'Nonessential' Amino Acids," *J. Nutrition* 104 (1974), pp. 965-67.

8. J. B. Longenecker and G. S. Lo, "Protein Digestibility and Amino Acid Availability—Assessed by Concentration in Changes of Plasma Amino Acids," Chap. 15 in P. L. White and D. C. Fletcher, eds., *Nutrients in Processed Foods: Proteins* (Acton, Mass.: Publishing Sciences Group, 1974).

9. S. Tannenbaum, "Industrial Processing," Chap. 14 in P. L. White and D. C. Fletcher, eds., *Nutrients in Processed Foods: Proteins* (Acton, Mass.: Publishing Sciences Group, 1974).

10. A. E. Harper, "Amino Acid Excess," Chap. 5 in P. L. White and D. C. Fletcher, eds., *Nutrients in Processed Foods: Proteins* (Acton, Mass.: Publishing Sciences Group, 1974).

11. C. Garza, N. S. Scrimshaw and V. R. Young, "Human Protein Requirements: the Effect of Variations in Energy Intake within the Maintenance Range," *Am. J. Clin. Nutr.* 29 (March 1976), pp. 280-87.

12. R. M. Leverton and M. R. Gram, "Nitrogen Excretion of Women Related to the Distribution of Animal Protein in Daily Meals," *J. Nutrition* 39 (Sept. 1949), pp. 57-65.

13. Y. S. M. Taylor, V. R. Young, E. Murray, P. B. Pencharz and N. S. Scrimshaw, "Daily Protein and Meal Patterns Affecting Young Men Fed Adequate and Restricted Energy Intakes," *Am. J. Clin. Nutr.* 26 (Nov. 1973), pp. 1216-21.

14. M. G. Hardinge and F. J. Stare, "Nutritional Studies of Vegetarians: I. Nutritional, Physical and Laboratory Findings," *Am. J. Clin. Nutr.* 2 (Jan. 1954), pp. 73-82.

15. C. H. Edwards, L. K. Booker., C. H. Rumph, W. G. Wright and S. N. Ganapathy, "Utilization of Wheat by Adult Man: Nitrogen Metabolism, Plasma Amino Acids and Lipids," *Am. J. Clin. Nutr.* 24 (Feb. 1971), pp. 181-93.

16. M. G. Hardinge, H. Crooks and F. J. Stare, "Nutritional Studies of Vegetarians: V. Proteins and Essential Amino Acids," *J. Am. Dietet. Assoc.* 48 (Jan. 1966), pp. 25-28.

17. U. S. Register and L. M. Sonnenberg, "The Vegetarian Diet," *J. Am. Dietet. Assoc.* 62 (Mar. 1973), pp. 253-61.

18. S. J. Hiemstra, *Food Consumption, Prices and Expenditures*, Agric. Econ. Report No. 138 (Washington, D.C.: Economic Re-

search Service, USDA July, 1968). Supplement for 1974 published Jan. 1976.

19. *Food Intake and Nutritive Value of Diets of Men, Women and Children in the United States, Spring 1965* (Washington, D.C.: USDA, March 1969), ARS 62-78.

20. G. M. Owen, K. M. Kram, P. J. Garry, J. E. Lowe and A. H. Lubin, "A Study of Nutritional Status of Preschool Children in the United States, 1968-1970," *Pediatrics* 53 (April 1974), pp. 597-646.

21. S. Abraham, F. W. Lowenstein and C. L. Johnson, *Preliminary Findings of the First Health and Nutrition Examination Survey, United States, 1971-1972: Dietary Intake and Biochemical Findings*, DHEW Publication No. (HRA) 76-1219-1 (Washington, D.C.: US Gov. Print. Office, 1974).

22. S. Margen, J. Y. Chu, N. A. Kaufmann and D. H. Calloway, "Studies in Calcium Metabolism I. The Calciuretic Effect of Dietary Protein," *Am. J. Clin. Nutr.* 27 (June 1974), pp. 584-89.

23. R. A. Nelson, "Implications of Excessive Protein" in P. L. White and N. Selvey, eds., *Proc. Western Hemisphere Congress IV* (Acton, Mass.: Publishing Sciences Group, 1975).

24. J. Mayer, "The Dimensions of Human Hunger," *Sci. American* 235 (Sept. 1976), pp. 40-49.

25. Council for Agricultural Science and Technology, "Ruminants as Food Producers Now and for the Future," Special Publication No. 4 (March 1975).

26. "Role of the Dairy Cow in Providing Food," *Dairy Council Digest* 47 (Jan.-Feb. 1976).

27. H. E. Clark, "Meeting Protein Requirements of Man," *J. Am. Dietet. Assoc.* 52 (June 1968), pp. 475-79.

28. W. J. Wolf and J. C. Cowan, *Soybeans as a Food Source* (Cleveland: CRC Press, 1975).

29. N. E. Roberts, "Nutrition-Related Research at USDA's Eastern Regional Research Center," *J. Am. Dietet. Assoc.* 69 (July 1976), pp. 56-60.

30. F. Aylward, "Development of Regulations Pertaining to Novel Foods," *Food and Nutrition* 1 (No. 3, 1975), pp. 24-29.

31. "PAG *ad hoc* Working Group Meeting on Clinical Evaluation and Acceptable Nucleic Acid Levels of SCP for Human Consumption," *PAG Bulletin* 5 (Sept. 1975), pp. 17-26.

32. "Guideline No. 7 for Human Testing of Supplementary Food Mixtures, 1972" in *Documents on Single Cell Protein Issued by PAG* (New York: Protein-Calorie Advisory Group of the United Nations System, 1976).

33. C. Martin, "Leaf Protein Child Feeding Trial," League for International Food Educ. Newsletter (March 1975).

34. S. Veil, "Food and Health," *Food and Nutrition* 1 (no. 4, 1975).

Brown, P. T. and J. G. Bergan, "The Dietary Status of the 'New' Vegetarians," *J. Am. Dietet. Assoc.* 67 (Nov. 1975), pp. 455-59.

Cravioto, J. and E. R. DeLicardie, "Mother-Infant Relationship Prior to the Development of Clinically Severe Malnutrition in the Child," in P. L. White and N. Selvey, eds., *Proc. Western Hemisphere Nutrition Congress IV* (Acton, Mass.: Publishing Sciences Group, 1975).

Erhard, D., "The New Vegetarians: Vegetarianism and its Medical Consequences," *Nutrition Today* 8 (Nov.-Dec. 1973), pp. 4-12.

Erhard, D., "The New Vegetarians: The Zen Macrobiotic Movement and Other Cults Based on Vegetarianism," *Nutrition Today*, 9 (Jan.-Feb., 1974), pp. 20-27.

Hegsted, D. M., "Protein Needs and Possible Modifications of the American Diet," *J. Am. Dietet. Assoc.* 68 (April 1976) pp. 317-20.

MacLean, W. C., Jr. and G. G. Graham, "Growth and Nitrogen Retention of Children Consuming all of the Day's Protein Intake in One Meal," *Am. J. Clin. Nutr.* 29 (Jan. 1976), pp. 78-86.

Scrimshaw, N. S. and V. R. Young, "The Requirements of Human Nutrition," *Sci. American* 235 (Sept. 1976), pp. 50-64.

Vemury, M. K. D., C. Kies and H. M. Fox, "Comparative Protein Value of Several Vegetable Protein Products Fed at Equal Nitrogen Levels to Human Adults," *J. Food Science* 41 (Sept.-Oct. 1976), 1086–9.

Vegetarian Diets, Statement of the Food and Nutrition Board, National Res. Council-National Acad. Sciences (May 1974).

Wortman, S., "Food and Agriculture," *Sci. American* 235 (Sept. 1976), pp. 30-39.

Minerals

Calcium, Phosphorus, Magnesium
Potassium, Sodium, Chlorine, Sulfur
Iron, Copper, Iodine, Fluoride, Zinc

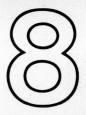

Certain facts about minerals have been established in previous chapters. You know, for example, that minerals collectively represent one of the six nutrient classes; that the presence of particular kinds of mineral elements is more important than the total quantity in foods; that they are not broken down in digestive processes in preparation for performing their specific functions in the body but, if soluble, are absorbed and used essentially as they occur in foods; and that, in broad terms, minerals help build the body structure and coordinate its processes.

You are now ready to consider: certain individual mineral elements that require particular attention in food selection, their more specific functions, and their food sources; how much you need of these mineral elements; and what you can expect in terms of nutritional well-being when your diet contains enough, or is deficient in, certain of them. Some general considerations will give a background for this chapter.

ORIGIN OF MINERAL ELEMENTS

Mineral elements originate in the soil—soil fed by rocks that have disintegrated through the ages. Plants require only inorganic materials for subsistence. They take from the soil the elements they need to form their roots, stems, and leaves. Animals eat the plants and in turn utilize the minerals they require for their own body development and functioning. You obtain your mineral elements by eating not only plants but also animal tissue and such products of animals as milk and eggs. Thus, indirectly, the minerals of the soil become the minerals of your body (1).

Soils differ in mineral content as well as in many other respects. Although the composition of plants is determined principally by their genetic makeup, it is affected by the kind of soil in which the plants are grown and the type and quantity of fertilizer used. Climate, seasonal conditions, and the state of maturity of the plant when harvested are other factors that influence the mineral content. In general, soil improvement increases the yield and size of crops but does not affect their major nutritional characteristics (2). There are certain exceptions. The concentration of a few minerals such as fluoride in the soil is reflected in crops grown in that soil. Soils deficient in iodine, zinc, or cobalt have caused nutritional diseases in grazing animals. An excess of selenium in some soils has led to *toxicity* in animals. But diseases caused by soil characteristics have been much less frequent in humans. The relationship between iodine in soils and plants and the incidence of goiter was discovered when long-distance shipments of foods were uncommon. When the food supply was limited to crops grown locally, the effect of deficiency in the soil was reflected in the inadequacy of iodine in the food supply. With modern food distribution methods, our food supply includes components from a variety of geographic areas, thus minimizing the effects of a mineral deficiency in any soil (3). Furthermore, commercial fertilizers are now balanced to provide minerals lacking in the soil.

toxicity
Related to or caused by a poison

The above information is relevant to the subject of "organic" foods. No legal definition has been established for the term, but generally speaking "organic" refers to foods grown without the use of pesticides or chemical fertilizers. Since all living things are organic, the designation "organically-grown" is more correct. Plants have specific nutrient requirements just as animals do. They use inorganic elements in the soil for growth. When organic fertilizers are used, the inorganic constituents—such as potassium, phosphorous and nitrogen—must be released from the organic components by the action of microorganisms in the soil before the plant can use them. Claims that organically-grown foods are nutritionally superior to those grown with the use of chemical fertilizers have not been substantiated. Studies have failed to show that organically-grown crops are higher in nutrients than those grown under standard agricultural conditions (2).

In a way, minerals are merely on loan from the soil to the body. They are released from the complexes in which they occur in food by the process of digestion, then are absorbed and dispensed to the parts of the body that need them. When they have performed the functions for which they are responsible, the minerals are excreted in most cases and eventually returned to the soil.

Minerals Required by the Body

For convenience in discussing them, mineral elements usually are separated into two groups: those that occur in the body and in foods in relatively large amounts, and those called *trace elements*, which occur in traces only and are needed in minute amounts. Calcium, phosphorus, magnesium, potassium, sodium, chlorine, and sulfur belong to the first group. The second category includes iron, copper, iodine, fluoride, cobalt, manganese, and zinc—trace elements that are known to be useful in nutrition. Recent evidence shows that the trace elements nickel, tin, vanadium, and silicon are also essential for animals. The Food and Nutrition Board has tabulated daily dietary allowances for calcium, phosphorus, magnesium, iron, iodine, and zinc (see inside cover). If allowances for these and other nutrients on the recommended dietary allowance table are met by basic foods, the remaining minerals probably will be present in adequate amounts.

Mineral elements are identified separately, but they act together and render service in many different combinations. Thus, while certain minerals perform specific functions in the body, they probably never act alone.

CALCIUM AND PHOSPHORUS

A notable example of collaboration between minerals is that of calcium and phosphorus. These two minerals occur together in different parts of the body and jointly meet many body needs. Both are present in relatively large amounts. The body of an adult contains from 1½ to 2 percent of its weight as calcium and about 1 percent as phosphorus, although the minerals are distributed unevenly. About 99 percent of the calcium and 80 percent of the phosphorus is in the bones and teeth; the small remainder of each element is in the soft tissues and body fluids (4).

How the Body Uses Calcium and Phosphorus

During digestion, calcium and phosphorus are separated from food and are eventually absorbed through the intestinal wall into the bloodstream, which carries them to the areas of the body where they are needed. These minerals are not absorbed completely; the extent of absorption varies widely with individuals and with certain physical conditions (4). Human adults are reported to absorb from 20 to 50 percent of calcium on a mixed diet. About 70 percent of phosphorus is absorbed. Calcium is excreted in feces and urine, while phosphorus is eliminated chiefly in the urine.

Factors Affecting Calcium Absorption

Nature of the Food   The nature of the food in which calcium is consumed can have a marked effect on the percent of the mineral that is absorbed. When a diet is high in cereal fiber, for example, the food mass moves along the intestinal tract at a rate that allows less time for calcium to be in contact with the intestinal wall, thus reducing the efficiency of calcium absorption (5).

Body's Need for Calcium   During child growth, pregnancy, and lactation, when the demands for calcium are greatest, the absorption is usually most efficient. Apparently, 40 percent or more absorption of dietary calcium can be assumed during the second and third trimesters of pregnancy. Breast-fed infants absorb 50 to 70 percent of the calcium ingested.

Amount of Calcium Provided by the Diet   The more calcium provided by food, the greater the total amount absorbed. However, the body uses calcium more economically (that is, it absorbs a larger proportion of the intake) when the intake is small. In countries with very low calcium supplies, people utilize this mineral more efficiently than do people in regions where sources are more abundant and intakes are higher. People adapt to different intake levels with time. Some adults can maintain equilibrium on intakes as low as 300 to 400 milligrams of calcium daily. It is not certain, however, that any particular individual can adapt to such relatively low calcium intakes (4).

Vitamin D   Vitamin D is a major facilitator in the absorption of calcium from the gastrointestinal tract. When inadequate amounts of vitamin D are present, calcium is poorly absorbed, and eventually evidence of calcium deficiency becomes apparent. Studies done with animals and believed to be applicable to humans indicate that the action of vitamin D in improving calcium absorption is dependent on the formation of a calcium-binding protein in the lining of the intestinal wall (6).

Fat   Evidence also suggests that the absorption of calcium requires the presence of fat in the diet, and that the absorption of fat requires the presence of calcium (6). Impairment in the absorption of one leads to impaired absorption of the other.

Oxalic Acid   Certain "greens," rhubarb, and cocoa contain oxalic acid, which combines with calcium. The oxalate that results is insoluble in intestinal fluids; thus, the calcium cannot be absorbed (it is unavailable) and is lost in the feces. The extent to which oxalic acid limits the absorption of calcium from various foods in which it occurs is not accurately known (7). Fortunately, foods containing oxalic acid are not highly concentrated sources of calcium. It has been shown, however, that the action of oxalic acid does not extend beyond the calcium of the food in which it is contained. The cocoa in chocolate milk, for example, does not depress the absorption of calcium from the milk.

Other Factors   Increased intestinal acidity favors calcium absorption. This condition exists when the stomach secretes excessive amounts of hydrochloric acid. The presence of lactose also enhances the absorption of calcium. On the other hand, phytic acid, present in the outer coats of grains, forms an insoluble salt with calcium and thus depresses calcium absorption. Emotional stress has also been observed to decrease the ability to absorb calcium (4).

Regulation of Calcium Level in Blood

Most of the calcium in the body is in the bones, but the very small remainder distributed in the soft tissues and blood is extremely important. This portion, less than 10 grams in adults, is responsible for a long list of body functions, all of which depend on the maintenance of a relatively constant level of blood calcium. The parathyroid hormone and vitamin D are involved in maintaining this level.

There is ample evidence that vitamin D increases the absorption of calcium from the small intestine. The parathyroid hormone acts with vitamin D in affecting the rate of calcium absorption and in mobilizing calcium from the bones to maintain the normal concentration in the blood. The bones are the source of supply of calcium for the blood. Two mechanisms move calcium from bone to blood: an exchange of blood calcium and bone calcium, which is dependent on chemical dynamics; and regulation by the secretion of hormones. A lower-than-normal level of calcium in the blood stimulates the parathyroid glands—four tiny bodies embedded in the thyroid gland in the neck—to increase their secretion of hormone, which, in turn, mobilizes bone calcium to bring the blood level up to normal. Elevation of the plasma calcium level stimulates the secretion of another hormone, *calcitonin*, formed by the thyroid gland. Calcitonin lowers plasma calcium level, apparently by diminishing bone resorption. When the blood calcium level is temporarily above normal, as when dietary calcium is being absorbed, there is some deposition of calcium in the bones and some excretion of calcium in the urine (4).

Functions of Calcium and Phosphorus (4, 8)

The very small, precisely regulated amount of calcium in the blood serves with sodium and potassium in promoting normal action of the heart muscle to maintain a rhythmic beat. It is essential for the clotting of blood, for helping to control the passage of fluids through cell walls, and for the actions of certain enzymes. These extremely important functions of calcium are rarely influenced by the level of intake. Phosphorus is an indispensable part of every cell of the body, for it is concerned with practically all metabolic processes. It plays a distinctive role in maintaining the neutrality of the blood and reacts chemically with the energy-yielding nutrients—proteins, fats, and carbohydrates—to release energy. The end products of carbohydrate digestion require phosphorus in many stages of their *metabolism*. Furthermore, phosphorus is a component of the high-energy compound ATP (adenosine triphosphate)—the form of energy that the body can use. Phosphorus is also an integral part of nucleoproteins that carry the genetic code. Thus we have the first examples of the regulatory and coordinative

metabolism
Process by which a nutrient is utilized by the body

ATP
Compound in which energy is stored for use by the cell

Figure 8.1
Long Bone
(Dina Kazanowski, artist)

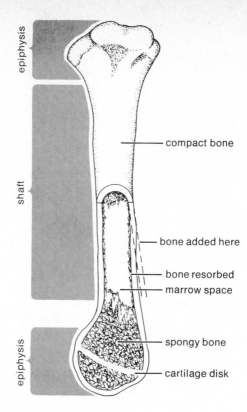

epiphysis

shaft

epiphysis

compact bone

bone added here

bone resorbed
marrow space

spongy bone

cartilage disk

functions of specific mineral elements. Calcium and phosphorus are equally important to body structure.

Bone Formation (4, 8)   In the developing embryo, the skeleton is originally constructed of cartilage. Bone formation is initiated when *osteoblasts* invade the cartilage. The osteoblasts secrete an organic substance around themselves that consists of fibers composed of proteins (*collagen* and *elastin*) embedded in a ground substance of *mucopolysaccharide* (a complex carbohydrate). This provides the framework into which minerals transported by the blood are deposited. Calcium and phosphorus are the principal minerals in bone and account for its characteristic strength and hardness. The mineral substance of young bone consists of a considerable amount of *amorphous* material that becomes more crystalline as bone matures. Osteoblasts and *osteoclasts* function throughout life, in the continuous formation of bone at certain parts of the structure and the removal of bone at others. The substances for bone repair are provided by the intercellular fluid.

Bones change in size and character with age (Fig. 8.1). Growth in length is provided for by a band of cartilage between the shaft and the epiphysis at each end of long bones. The cartilage grows, is invaded by osteoblasts, and becomes ossified. During childhood the cartilage disk remains a fairly constant thickness, but eventually its rate of growth slows down and finally it stops growing. *Ossification* of the remaining cartilage then fuses the shaft and epiphysis together and further growth in length is impossible.

osteoblasts
Bone-forming cells

amorphous
Without definite shape or form
osteoclasts
Cells that remove bone tissue

ossification
Mineralization of bone

Bones grow in width by a series of coordinated processes in which new bone is formed on the outer surface of the bone while resorption occurs at the inner surface, increasing the width of the marrow cavity. During the growth period when skeletal size is increasing, the rate of bone formation exceeds that of resorption. In the normal adult, formation and resorption are approximately equal, whereas in old age resorption may predominate.

As bones grow and are ossified, the amount of calcium in the body increases. The quantitative increase in body calcium with age is shown graphically in Figure 4.8. Normally the increase in calcium is in direct proportion to size as the individual grows into an adult. The proportion of body weight contributed by the skeleton varies with age, amounting to about 3 percent at birth, increasing to a maximum value of 5.5 percent in the female and 6.5 percent in the male, and declining to about 4 percent in the aged female (9).

Estimates of the weight of the skeleton have been converted mathematically into estimates of the amounts of calcium and phosphorus retained daily in the form of bone. Figure 8.2 presents data indicating that in the first few years of life approximately 100 milligrams of calcium per day is retained, increasing to 200 milligrams per day in the adolescent female and almost 300 milligrams per day in the adolescent male. Note that in adulthood (beginning earlier in females than in males), the amount of calcium retained as bone diminishes. After the age of 50 in both males and females there is a small daily loss of calcium from bone (9).

Bone building is probably affected by all or most of the factors involved in general body growth. In addition to calcium and phosphorus, magnesium and several other minerals are essential in the bone-building process; protein is required for building and main-

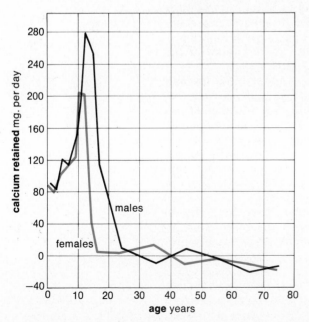

Figure 8.2
Calcium retained as bone (mg. per day). Adapted from Table 36, Reference 9.

taining the bone matrix; energy is essential, as it is for the growth of any tissue; and vitamins A, C, and D are needed for specialized functions (see Chap. 9). As would be expected, bones and teeth calcify more slowly when the diet is deficient in calcium, phosphorus, and the other nutrients. This fact was demonstrated in Figure 3.6, in which the retarding effect of undernutrition was shown in the poorly calcified wrist bones of a 7-year-old child.

Tooth Formation   In the first few weeks of fetal life, tooth buds begin to form; the first teeth start to calcify by the midpoint of pregnancy. Certain permanent tooth buds begin to calcify at birth, and most others start the process in the period between birth and 3 years of age. Wisdom teeth often begin to calcify as late as the tenth year of age. The enamel, dentin, and cementum of the teeth are all highly calcified tissues, with enamel containing only 2 to 3 percent organic matter. Unfortunately, calcified dental tissues do not have the capacity to repair themselves as bone tissues do.

Assessing Nutritional Status

A reserve of calcium and allied minerals, with adequate replenishment from daily food, serves the body in ways that have been discussed. The result to be expected is a well-functioning body with good bone growth and development. When the diet is deficient in calcium and phosphorus, these minerals are taken from reserves in the bone structure. If this situation continues, the bones become deficient in calcium content.

Difference in Growth   Growth imposes heavy demands for calcium, a fact that is taken into account by the dietary allowances recommended during childhood and adolescence. Thus it is advantageous to build body stores with generous intakes of calcium in the preadolescent years. The increase in height of the United States population above that of some other peoples may well imply a higher calcium requirement to provide for growth and maintenance of the larger skeleton.

Studies with young experimental animals indicate that low calcium intakes result in smaller, poorer bones. Because comparable experiments with children are not feasible, such a direct cause-and-effect relationship has not been demonstrated in human beings. Moreover, the mixed heritage of humans clouds the picture of growth possibilities. The sizes of people in various parts of the world do suggest a calcium-growth relationship. For example, populations who have lived for generations on low calcium intakes are of notably small frame and short stature. Children in these areas may be several years behind the children of other countries in terms of skeletal growth (10). In populations with low calcium intakes there are usually shortages of other nutrients (notably protein) contributing to slower growth rates.

Difference in Quality of Bone   It seems logical that a poorly calcified, weakened bone would break easily and heal slowly. Research and observations on animals show this to be the case. However, clear-cut experimental evidence on human beings has not been available. When a child or adult has bone-healing difficulties, many factors frequently complicate the picture. More and more, however, it seems evident that diet—and notably a prolonged calcium deficiency—is an important factor. Repeated cases of slow bone healing in patients with a history of allergy to milk since birth, for example, have strengthened the conviction that there is a relationship between low calcium reserves and the ability of the bones to mend promptly. Middle-aged and older persons who have routinely consumed calcium-poor diets can be expected to have brittle, demineralized bones that are susceptible to breakage and present problems in healing (11).

Abnormalities in Bone   Several abnormal conditions in bones are related directly or indirectly to diet. Rickets in children results when there is an imbalance of calcium, phosphorus, and vitamin D in the body. The period of greatest susceptibility is from prebirth through the preschool age. This condition was common in the United States until the discovery of vitamin D and recognition of its function in bone formation. Now that vitamin D has become part of the routine diet during pregnancy and early childhood—in the form of vitamin-D milk—rickets is not commonly seen in the United States (see Chap. 9).

Osteoporosis is the condition existing when bones become porous and fragile due to decreased density of total bone substance. The diagnosis implies a lessening of total bone, including the organic matrix as well as mineral substance, in the affected areas. Bones of the spine and pelvis are most often involved. The precise cause of this type of faulty bone structure is not known, and there is lack of agreement in research evidence on the role of dietary calcium. It appears certain that the *etiology* of osteoporosis is complex. Factors that may be involved include level of calcium intake, ability to absorb calcium adequately from the gastrointestinal tract, level of fluoride intake, sex hormones, and amount of dietary protein (4, 9, 12).

etiology
Cause or causes of a disease

Osteoporosis is not uncommon in the United States, usually occurring in older people, especially women. It has been estimated that 14 million women in the United States suffer from this disorder. The prevalence of osteoporosis was observed to be similar among different population groups in the United States and in six Central American countries. The pooled data indicated that more than 50 percent of all women from the sixth decade on had osteoporosis. In these studies, no systematic relationship was found between calcium intake and the rate of bone loss (9).

In a recent long-term study, a group of "normal healthy" elderly women (average age 80.2 yrs) were found to have histories of low intake of dairy products, as well as current low calcium intakes averaging 450 milligrams per day. A series of radiographic measurements showed that a reversal of bone losses occurred with the administration of supplements providing 750 milligrams of calcium and 375 units of vitamin D per day over periods of 12 to 48 months. In the control group, bone loss continued at the previous rate of 2 to 3 percent per year (13).

With the present incomplete understanding of osteoporosis, prevention is more realistic than cure. Calcium intake sufficient to produce maximum bone density during growing years and to prevent bone loss during adult years should be maintained. Adequate amounts of vitamin D and other nutrients are also indicated, along with an optimal amount of fluoride in the drinking water. Treatment often recommended includes at least 1 gram of calcium daily, vitamin D, adequate protein, fluoride, other nutrients, and physical activity. In some cases, estrogens may be beneficial for women (9, 12, 13).

Some concern has been expressed recently that people in the United States may be receiving too much calcium, rather than too little. Those who take this position cite cases of the calcification of soft tissues in the body, and particularly the formation of kidney stones. There appears to be no adequate evidence, however, that high calcium intakes are a primary causal factor in the formation of kidney stones, although low calcium intakes are often important in therapy. The underlying abnormality responsible for stone formation has not yet been identified.

There are some indications that the actual calcium intakes of certain groups in the United States population may be low. In the first HANES, some clinical evidence indicated "moderate risk" of calcium deficiency or calcium-phosphorus imbalance. The highest prevalence of such evidence, about 13 percent, was found among persons in the 12- to 17-year age group and among women aged 18 to 44 years (14).

HANES
Survey designed to measure the nutritional status of US population

Comparative Calcium Food Values

Your day-to-day intakes of calcium and phosphorus come from the foods you eat. How well you are nourished with respect to these two mineral elements depends on how well you choose your food. It is of first importance, therefore, to know reliable food sources of both minerals and some practical ways of applying this information to food selection. The task is somewhat simplified because diets that supply enough protein and calcium usually carry enough phosphorus as well. Important sources of phosphorus are lean meats, milk, cheeses, fish, dry legumes, whole grain cereals, and eggs. Our chief concern at this point, then, is the calcium values of familiar foods in portions commonly served.

One way to obtain a perspective on calcium values in foods is to study the comparative calcium yields of the different foods on your own representative food list. The specimen representative list (Fig. 8.3) serves as a basis for drawing general conclusions with respect to important food sources.

It is apparent from Figure 8.3 that calcium is present in many foods but that only milk and cheese are rich sources. Spinach is next on the list, but its high position is misleading; spinach has a relatively high concentration of oxalic acid that combines with calcium, making it unavailable to the body. The amount of calcium present in a food thus does not necessarily indicate its importance as a dietary source of the mineral. The amounts of such foods that are served and how often they are served, as well as whether the

Food*	Weight or ** approximate measure	Calcium milligrams	
			250 mg
milk, fluid skim or buttermilk	1 cup	296	
milk, fluid whole	1 cup	288	
cheese, cheddar	1 oz	213	
	100 mg		
spinach	½ cup	116 unavailable	
beans, dry, canned	¾ cup	104	
	55 mg		
broccoli	½ cup	68	
cheese, cottage, creamed	¼ cup	58	
sweet potato	1 medium	48	
haddock, fried	1 fillet (4 oz)	44	
	25 mg		
beans, green	½ cup	32	
bun or roll, enriched	1 bun	30	
onions	½ cup	25	
bread, white, enriched	1 slice	24	
bread, whole wheat	1 slice	24	
carrots, diced	½ cup	24	
egg	1 medium	24	
raisins	¼ cup	23	
cabbage, raw, chopped	½ cup	22	
	15 mg		
grapefruit, white	½ medium	19	
pineapple juice, canned	½ cup	19	
peanut butter	2 tbsp	18	
cream, half and half	1 tbsp	16	
rice, enriched, cooked	¾ cup	16	
strawberries, raw	½ cup	16	
lettuce, raw	1 cup	15	
oatmeal, cooked	⅔ cup	15	
peas, green	½ cup	15	
orange juice	½ cup	13	
	9 mg		
beef, lean chuck	3 oz	11	
apple, raw	1 medium	10	
banana, raw	1 medium	10	
beef, hamburger	3 oz	10	
chicken, fried	½ breast	9	
pork chop	1 chop	9	
tomato juice, canned	½ cup	9	
macaroni, enriched, cooked	¾ cup	8	
potato, white	1 medium	8	
tunafish, canned	½ cup	7	
liver, beef	2 oz	6	
	5 mg and less		
peaches, canned	½ cup	5	
peppers, sweet, green, raw	½ medium	4	
sausage, bologna	2 oz	4	
butter or margarine	1 tbsp	3	
corn, canned	½ cup	3	
frankfurter	1 medium	3	
mayonnaise	1 tbsp	3	
beverages, cola type	12 oz	— †	
cornflakes, fortified	1 cup	neg.	
oil, salad or cooking	1 tbsp	0	
sugar	1 tbsp	0	

Figure 8.3
Calcium: Servings of representative foods in order of their calcium content. (Each bar represents the approximate calcium value for the foods listed below it.)

* Foods are in forms ready to eat. All meats and vegetables are cooked unless otherwise indicated.
** See Appendix K for further identification of these foods. All foods are described there more fully, and both weights and measures are indicated.
† See Appendix J.

calcium present can be absorbed by the body, must be taken into consideration. Milk is in a particularly favorable position because it lends itself to frequent use. It is also consumed in different forms, such as cheese and ice cream. Routine inclusion of milk and foods made from milk in a day's meals makes it feasible to double or triple the calcium values of the individual milk items in Figure 8.3.

Certain "greens" that are not high in oxalic acid, such as collards and kale, may be significant sources of calcium if used daily in liberal amounts. For example, collards have 180 milligrams of calcium per ½-cup serving; mustard greens and kale each have about 100 milligrams. For many people in the United States, however, dry legumes and "greens" are not daily items of diet. Another rich source of calcium, not shown in Figure 8.3, is canned salmon when the bones are eaten. Consumption of canned salmon is so low, however, that its high concentration of calcium is not of practical importance. Therefore, regular use of milk and foods made with milk, along with *carefully chosen* secondary sources of calcium, give the greatest promise of an adequate calcium intake.

Secondary sources of calcium shown in Figure 8.3 are certain vegetables (broccoli and sweet potatoes), cottage cheese, and fish. The difference in values between primary and secondary sources is striking. It takes about four servings of a high secondary source (for example, broccoli, 68 mg per serving) to equal the calcium yield of one serving of a primary source (milk, 288 mg per 1-cup serving). The calcium values then drop off sharply, and only halfway down the list it takes about nineteen servings of a food such as lettuce to equal the calcium value of 1 cup of milk.

Foods that furnish less than 20 milligrams of calcium per serving include all meats, most fruits, and many cereals and vegetables. Meats, cereals (unless prepared with or served with milk, or fortified with calcium), and pure fats and sweets can therefore be eliminated from consideration as practical sources of dietary calcium.

Arrange your own list of representative foods by sorting your index cards or half sheets in order of their quantitative importance as sources of calcium. Analyze the list. Consider the groups of foods representing similar calcium values, and try to characterize them.

Enter calcium values on your personal meal record, and total your calcium intake for the day.

List the "greens" in Appendix K, with their calcium values per ½-cup serving. Which of them provide available sources of calcium? How much do you depend on "greens" as a source of calcium?

List the different kinds of dry legumes in Appendix K with their calcium values per serving. Which—if any—do you have on your personal meal record? Would it be practical for you to depend on legumes as a source of calcium?

Determining Calcium Need

Daily needs for calcium have been assessed with balance studies similar to those for protein. The term "balance" refers to the condition of equilibrium that exists in an adult body when the daily intake of calcium in foods approximately equals the amount in excreta. The smallest amount of calcium necessary to bring this about in an adult is proposed as the daily requirement. To establish the requirements for childhood, pregnancy, and lactation, essentially the same procedure is followed; the difference is that the proposed requirement ensures the maximum storage that can be achieved at these periods, rather than equilibrium.

There is some dissatisfaction with the balance method as a means of determining calcium requirements, but an acceptable alternative method has not been found. People who live on relatively low-calcium diets become "adapted"—their metabolism adjusts to achieve balance at the level they habitually consume. Thus, calcium balance data may not provide a satisfactory estimate of calcium need (4).

RDA
Nutrient standards for the United States

Recommended Dietary Allowances (RDA) for Calcium

In establishing allowances for calcium, the Food and Nutrition Board recognizes that people vary considerably in individual need, but the proposed allowance is believed to be sufficiently liberal to provide for wide differences (see the RDA table on inside cover).

Note that the daily allowance for calcium during pregnancy is higher than the amount recommended for nonpregnant women 18 years of age and older. Calcium and phosphorus are chiefly involved in the development of the bones and teeth of the fetus. About 65 percent of the total amount of these two minerals present in the infant's body at term are normally deposited in the last 2 months of pregnancy. The mother's diet therefore requires the largest amounts of calcium and phosphorus during that period. If she enters pregnancy with low calcium stores, she should increase her intake in early pregnancy and thus begin replenishing her stores before she reaches the period of greatest stress.

The mother's daily allowance for calcium during lactation is also greater than that of the nonpregnant woman. This increased allowance reflects the needs of the baby's rapidly growing skeleton. The mother's diet must supply the bone-building ingredients through her breast milk if the baby's growth is to proceed normally.

Children need calcium not only for upkeep but also for the growth of their bones. The RDA table shows the progression in daily calcium allowances from infancy to adolescence. The increased storage and use of calcium by the growing body is shown in Figure 4.8. Because of their growth need, children have a proportionately higher allowance in relation to their body weight than do adults, and some actual calcium allowances for children are higher than those for adults except in pregnancy and lactation.

Table 8.1
Food combinations that provide 800 milligrams of calcium

1		Calcium mg
milk, skim	1 pt (2 cups)	592
cheese, cheddar	1 oz	213
	total	**805**

2		Calcium mg
milk, skim	1 cup	296
cheese, cheddar	1 oz	213
broccoli	½ cup	68
oranges	2 medium	108
cheese, cottage	¼ cup	58
sweet potato	1 medium	48
egg	1 medium	24
	total	**815**

3		Calcium mg
cheese, cheddar	2 oz	426
cheese, cottage	½ cup	116
turnip greens	½ cup	134
oranges	2 medium	108
egg	1 medium	24
	total	**808**

4		Calcium mg
salmon, canned (with bones)	½ cup	215
beans, dry, canned	¾ cup	104
broccoli	½ cup	68
oranges	1 medium	54
sweet potato	1 medium	48
muskmelon	½ melon	38
egg	1 medium	24
apricots, stewed	½ cup	30
squash, winter	½ cup	29
cabbage, raw	½ cup	22
prunes	½ cup, with juice	23
bread, enriched	3 slices	72
carrots, cooked	½ cup	24
peas, green	½ cup	15
beets	½ cup	16
strawberries	½ cup	16
	total	**798**

Meeting Calcium Allowances

The specimen diet in Appendix H shows that milk and milk products stand out as sources of calcium in an ordinary mixed diet; breads and vegetables provide small but important amounts of calcium; meat makes a negligible contribution to the day's calcium; and sugar and soft drinks provide none.

The food combinations grouped in Table 8.1 show four ways in which calcium allowances can be met, with and without milk and dairy foods. No other nutrient allowance is as easily attained by discriminating food selection as that for calcium, and none is so difficult to attain or so easily missed if the few rich sources are omitted or used in inadequate quantities. Food combinations 1, 2, and 3 in Table 8.1 show ways to provide about 800 milligrams of calcium by using milk products exclusively or with other good sources of calcium. Combination 4 omits dairy foods but includes other good sources, and this demonstrates how difficult it is to obtain enough calcium when milk and milk-made dishes are omitted from the diet. Under such circumstances vegetables and fruits must be eaten in quantities scarcely practicable. In addition, main-dish foods must regularly include certain selected kinds of fish, such as salmon (with bones), eggs, and dry legumes, such as beans. This is not to minimize the nutritional importance of fruits and vegetables. Both groups make significant dietary contributions, as will be shown.

> What is the RDA for calcium for your sex-age group (see the RDA table)?
>
> How does your daily calcium intake as shown on your meal record compare with the calcium allowance figure? Account for the effect of your food choices on your total calcium intake, and on whether it is high or low in relation to the allowance.
>
> List some foods that would provide 800 milligrams of calcium for a person on a strict vegetarian diet.
>
> How would you reply to a person who said to you, "I don't use milk but I eat lots of salads. Will they give me the calcium I need?"

Sources of Calcium in the World

In many parts of the world, little milk is available. Some countries traditionally use cheeses and fermented milk products, such as yogurt, made from the small amount of milk obtained from their various domesticated animals. In other countries condensed forms of milk are imported. Even with such measures, milk and milk products still are negligible sources of calcium in parts of the Western Hemisphere and in much of the Eastern Hemisphere. Under these circumstances, babies are often breast-fed for a prolonged period, giving them the benefit of calcium from the mother's milk. After weaning, however, the calcium content of the diet is usually very low; this deficiency contributes to the small bones and short stature of the peoples on such diets. Sometimes dietary customs, such as eating tiny bones of fish and other animals, using them in pulverized form in food mixtures, drinking the liquid after boiling such bones in vinegar (which dissolves the calcium), soaking corn in lime before making certain native dishes such as tortillas, and eating very large amounts of green vegetables, are responsible for raising the calcium content of diets. In areas where the drinking water contains calcium, it makes a small contribution to the total supply.

When milk is available but for some reason a person cannot use it, a physician may recommend calcium and phosphorus as supplements. The body can utilize these elements in tablets and capsules as well as in food, but the user is deprived of the other essential nutrients in milk and must therefore make special plans to obtain them from other foods.

Large proportions of people in nonwhite population groups are reported to be lactose intolerant (see Chap. 5). The relationship between *lactose intolerance* and milk intolerance is now receiving attention. Research has indicated that persons diagnosed as lactose intolerant by the standard lactose tolerance test do not necessarily have to eliminate milk from their diets. In one study, 4- to 9-year-old lactose intolerant children were observed after being given graded amounts of milk. None of the children, black or white, developed symptoms of intolerance after drinking 1 cup of milk (15).

lactose intolerance
Resulting from insufficient lactase enzyme to digest lactose

Calcium in the National Diet

The question of whether people in the United States get enough calcium can be answered in different ways, depending on the basis for the reply. One basis is the average amount of calcium available per person per day from the total food supply (16). The figure is now about 930 milligrams. This amount is above the recommended dietary allowance for some groups but below the allowances for adolescence, pregnancy, and lactation. Like other nutrients, however, calcium is not distributed equally to all people, nor is it allocated on the basis of need. To determine whether we are actually getting enough calcium, therefore, we require information on the food habits of families and their individual members.

The comprehensive dietary study of households made by the US Department of Agriculture in 1965 showed that the calcium intake of one-fourth or more of the families in this sample failed to reach

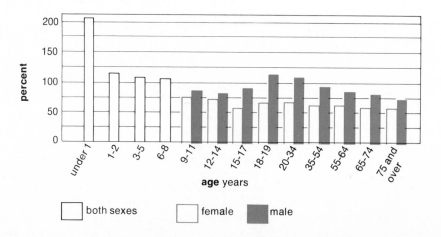

Figure 8.4

Calcium from one day's diet, as a percent of the then current Recommended Dietary Allowances (18).

Table 8.2
Standards for evaluation of daily dietary intake used in the
Health and Nutrition Examination Survey, United States, 1971-72 (19)

Age and sex		Calories per kg	Protein g per kg	Calcium mg	Iron mg	Vitamin A* I.U.	Vitamin C mg
1-5 years:							
12-23 months, male and female		90	1.9	450	15	2,000	40
24-47 months, male and female		86	1.7	450	15	2,000	40
48-71 months, male and female		82	1.5	450	10	2,000	40
6-7 years, male and female		82	1.3	450	10	2,500	40
8-9 years, male and female		82	1.3	450	10	2,500	40
10-12 years	male	68	1.2	650	10	2,500	40
	female	64	1.2	650	18	2,500	40
13-16 years	male	60	1.2	650	18	3,500	50
	female	48	1.2	650	18	3,500	50
17-19 years	male	44	1.1	550	18	3,500	55
	female	35	1.1	550	18	3,500	50
20-29 years	male	40	1.0	400	10	3,500	60
	female	35	1.0	600	18	3,500	55
30-39 years	male	38	1.0	400	10	3,500	60
	female	33	1.0	600	18	3,500	55
40-49 years	male	37	1.0	400	10	3,500	60
	female	31	1.0	600	18	3,500	55
50-54 years	male	36	1.0	400	10	3,500	60
	female	30	1.0	600	18	3,500	55
55-59 years	male	36	1.0	400	10	3,500	60
	female	30	1.0	600	10	3,500	55
60-69 years	male	34	1.0	400	10	3,500	60
	female	29	1.0	600	10	3,500	55
70 years and over	male	34	1.0	400	10	3,500	60
	female	29	1.0	600	10	3,500	55
Pregnancy (fifth month and beyond), add to basic standard		200	20	200		1,000	5**
Lactating, add to basic standard		1,000	25	500		1,000	5

*Assumed 70 percent carotene, 30 percent retinol.
**For all pregnant women.

their recommended dietary allowances for calcium at that time (17). Only 68 percent of urban families and 75 percent of rural families had diets that met the allowances for calcium.

Family consumption data still do not pinpoint the specific groups in which calcium intakes are lowest. To correct this shortcoming, dietary data for 1 day were obtained on more than fourteen thousand men, women, and children in the households just mentioned. On the basis of average quantities in the diets, calcium proved to be one of the nutrients most often consumed in amounts below the RDA at that time (18). Figure 8.4 shows the percent of RDA attained by various age-sex groups throughout the life cycle. The line representing one hundred percent at the center of the figure represents the RDA goals. The perpendicular bars show a tendency for both males and females to drop below the allowances after 8 years of age. Women and girls failed their goals by wider margins than did men and boys, particularly in the 15- to 17-year age span. This group, and several age groups of women 35 years of age and older, were more than 30 percent below the RDA for calcium at that time.

The preliminary findings of HANES, 1971–72 indicated that mean intakes of calcium for all age, income, and race groups—with the exception of black women aged 18 to 44—reached or exceeded the standard. (The standards shown in Table 8.2 are estimates of desirable intakes of nutrients that were developed particularly for the evaluation of the HANES dietary data.) Averages can be misleading, however. When data were examined in terms of percentage distribution of intake levels a large proportion of individuals were found to have intakes below the standards. More than half of all women, black and white, from 18 to 44 years of age, had calcium intakes below the standards. About one-third of the black children aged 1 to 5 years and black men from 18 to 44 years also had intakes below standards. Less than half as many white children and white men in those age groups had intakes below standards (19).

Because calcium is so closely identified with milk, consumption data on calcium usually reflect the status of milk consumption. Milk and milk products, other than butter, currently provide three-fourths of all the calcium available to consumers in the United States (16).

Figure 8.5 shows average daily quantities of milk and milk products consumed by the same age groups represented in Figure 8.4. In Figure 8.5 the milk and milk products are expressed in terms of their calcium equivalents. In general, the two figures support each other, as would be expected. Young children and boys use the most milk; men and boys use more nearly recommended amounts than do women and girls; and girls from adolescence through adulthood consistently use less milk than do all other groups.

Figure 8.5
Milk and milk products (calcium equivalent)—quantity per person per day (18).

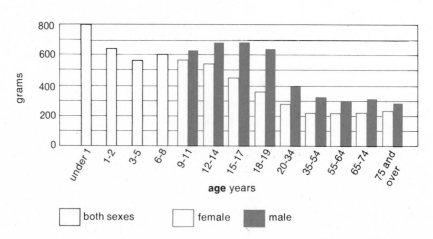

MAGNESIUM (12, 20, 21)

The average adult human body contains somewhat less than 1 ounce of magnesium. This is in sharp contrast to the nearly 3 pounds of calcium and 1½ pounds of phosphorus that are present. One-half to three-fourths of the magnesium is in the skeleton; the remainder is in the soft tissues and blood. Magnesium is an essential nutrient for plants and animals. Research on the metabolism of this mineral in animals and the identification of magnesium deficiency symptoms in human beings have generated considerable interest. Many nutrients are also known to be involved in magnesium metabolism, including protein, lactose, vitamin D, calcium, and phosphorus.

Functions of Magnesium

chlorophyll
Substance in green leaves needed to produce carbohydrate

Magnesium has basic functions in the metabolism of both plants and animals, thus exerting an influence on all the processes of life. As a constituent of the chlorophyll molecule, magnesium plays a significant role in photosynthesis, the process by which solar energy is used by green plants to convert carbon dioxide and water to carbohydrate. In animals, magnesium contributes to the structure of the body as one of the elements in bone and is necessary for the normal transmission of nerve impulses and for muscular contraction. It also is essential as an activator of many enzyme systems utilizing ATP. Magnesium is involved in the metabolism of carbohydrate, protein, and fat, as well as in the synthesis of many other substances.

Magnesium Deficiency

tetany
Muscular spasms

Magnesium deficiency has been observed in farm animals and induced in laboratory animals. A fall in serum magnesium levels usually occurs with the onset of deficiency, resulting in great sensitivity to noise or stimulation. *Tetany* and convulsions often follow. Magnesium-deficient animals deposit calcium phosphate in the soft tissues. In humans, the deficiency manifests itself in muscular tremors and convulsions. Its occurrence is most often the result of conditions other than, or in combination with, a dietary deficiency, rather than simply a lack of sufficient dietary magnesium. Magnesium deficiency is noted particularly in alcoholics and in persons with certain disorders of the parathyroid gland. Malabsorption, *diuretic* therapy, and post-surgical stress can also contribute to its development. Persons on prolonged restricted feedings (for example, children with the protein-calorie deficiency disease kwashiorkor) can become deficient in magnesium. Long-term magnesium deficiency in adults may contribute to *renal, neuromuscular,* and *cardiovascular* abnormalities.

diuretic
Drug to increase excretion of urine

renal
Pertaining to kidney

neuromuscular
Affecting nerves and muscles

cardiovascular
Relating to heart and blood vessels

The blood level of magnesium can decline sharply when dietary magnesium is reduced because the body has no mechanism for maintaining a constant level of magnesium in the blood, as it has for calcium. Excess magnesium in the blood can cause problems, as can too little. Massive doses of magnesium-containing drugs, usually antacids, can result in abnormally high blood levels of magnesium, particularly in individuals with renal insufficiency. Very high blood levels of magnesium are associated with paralysis of skeletal muscles and respiratory depression.

Magnesium Sources and RDA (12, 22)

Magnesium is widespread in nature. Dairy products furnish about a fifth of the magnesium in the United States food supply; another fifth comes from fruits and vegetables; and another from flour and grain products. Meats, poultry, and fish provide about 14 percent; dry legumes and nuts about 12 percent. Persons eating a varied diet can thus be reasonably certain of obtaining all the magnesium they need. In 1968 magnesium was included in the RDA table for the first time, with specified amounts recommended for people in different age-sex groups. The amount suggested for women is greater during pregnancy and lactation.

POTASSIUM, SODIUM, CHLORINE, AND SULFUR

Other minerals that occur in relatively large amounts in the body also play important roles in nutrition. Most of them are widely distributed in plant and animal foods, although none of this group, which includes potassium, sodium, chlorine, and sulfur, appears on the table of recommended daily dietary allowances. Exact information about needed amounts is generally lacking, but presumably dietary shortage is not common. In several cases the Food and Nutrition Board has suggested desirable daily intakes; in others it has indicated the use of certain foods to cover probable needs.

POTASSIUM, SODIUM, AND CHLORINE (12)

Potassium, sodium, and chlorine are found in relative abundance in the body. Only calcium and phosphorus occur in greater quantity. Sodium and chlorine, well known because they occur together in common salt, are found chiefly in the fluids that circulate *outside* body cells; potassium is present mostly in the fluids *inside* the cells. Sodium is involved primarily with the maintenance of *osmotic equilibrium* and keeps the concentrations of water and other substances passing back and forth between the cells and the surrounding fluids relatively constant. Potassium and chlorine, too, are necessary in keeping a normal balance of water between fluids and cells. A sharp increase or decrease in one of these minerals can create an imbalance. Nerve response to stimulation, the conduction of nerve impulses to the muscles, and muscle contractions (including the beat of the heart) are all dependent on the presence of sodium and potassium. Together with chlorine they help to keep a balance between the amounts of acid and of alkali in the blood. Chlorine is also essential for the formation of the hydrochloric acid in gastric juice.

There is usually no deficiency of these minerals, unless there are large losses from the body. Excessive losses of potassium may occur due to diarrhea, diabetic acidosis, or use of certain diuretic drugs or purgatives. Many common foods furnish potassium. Some

osmotic equilibrium
Constant concentration of water and other substances passing between cells and their surrounding fluids

of the richest sources include potatos, prunes, winter squash, bananas and oranges. Extreme heat that causes heavy perspiration can result in large losses of sodium. The Food and Nutrition Board suggests that when there is excessive sweating and when more than 4 quarts of water are consumed to satisfy thirst, approximately 2 grams of sodium chloride should be provided for each additional quart of water (12). Some other situations in which abnormal losses can occur include renal disorders, prolonged diarrhea, and vomiting.

Sodium in excess of needs can be handled well under ordinary circumstances; the excess is excreted in the urine. When the body's mechanism fails to rid itself of excess sodium, however—as in certain types of heart and kidney diseases—the patient suffers from *edema*. In such cases, professionally planned sodium-restricted diets are prescribed.

edema
Condition in which abnormally large amounts of water are retained in the tissues

Table salt is our most concentrated source of sodium (43 percent). Most foods contain some sodium naturally, and many have sodium or salt added to them in such preparation processes as curing meats or brining fish and vegetables. Many popular snack items such as various kinds of crackers, chips, and pretzels obviously are high in salt. With high consumption of these processed foods and liberal use of table salt, many people eat far more sodium than they need. Foods of animal origin are the richest natural sources of this mineral. Fruits and most vegetables are low in sodium, except when sodium products are added in preparing or preserving them. Cereal grains are also low in sodium unless it is used in processing. Drinking waters vary greatly in sodium content. Moderation in the use of table salt and salty processed foods is the simplest way to avoid excessive intake of sodium.

SULFUR (8)

Sulfur is closely identified with protein. As an integral part of sulfur-containing amino acids, it is found in every cell of the body as well as in several essential compounds and active *metabolites*. Sulfur functions in certain oxidation-reduction reactions and in some detoxification reactions. No dietary allowance for sulfur has been proposed. It seems safe to assume that the sulfur needs of the body will be met if the protein intake is adequate.

metabolites
Products formed as a result of normal physical and chemical body processes

TRACE MINERALS

Life depends on the maintenance of a delicate balance of numerous competing chemical and physiological processes. The trace elements are known to be of critical importance to those processes and to that balance although their precise functions are not yet completely understood. Certain trace elements are indispensable parts of the catalytic systems that speed up metabolic activities in the cells, and some of them are structural components of enzymes and other essential substances in the body. A large number of the vital processes of life depend upon the activities of enzyme systems.

IRON

The amount of iron in the body normally amounts to about 50 milligrams per kilogram of body weight in adult men, and about 35 milligrams per kilogram in adult women. This is a very small quantity when compared with calcium, about one three-hundredths as much. The total amount of iron in the body varies with the concentration of hemoglobin in the blood and with the size of iron stores, as well as with the weight and sex of individuals. Iron is distributed roughly as follows: about three-fourths as functional iron, chiefly in the red blood cells as hemoglobin; and about one-fourth in storage forms. Iron is closely related to other nutrients in its functions. Its relationship with vitamin B_{12} and folic acid in the prevention of anemias is well known, and its connection with copper will be discussed later. Iron is found in various combinations and associations with proteins. Before exploring iron's role as a nutrient in the body, it is necessary to understand its general mode of action and movement in the body and its storage and absorption patterns.

hemoglobin
Iron-containing protein pigment in red blood cells

How the Body Uses Iron (12, 23)

When iron is absorbed into the bloodstream from the small intestine, it becomes attached to *transferrin*, an iron-binding protein in plasma. A large part of the iron is transported immediately by transferrin to the bone marrow, where it is incorporated in new red blood cells. The changes necessary to produce red blood cells from precursor stem cells require about 7 days; the cells are then ready to circulate in the blood. After functioning for about 4 months the red blood cells are destroyed, but the iron in them is salvaged and returned to the bone marrow for reuse. This highly efficient process is carried on continuously with very little loss of iron. Its concept is fundamental to our consideration of the body's quantitative needs for iron.

Hemoglobin performs the basic function of carrying oxygen from the lungs to the tissues, where it is released for use. Hemoglobin then combines loosely with carbon dioxide (a waste product of cell metabolism), carries it to the lungs, and releases it there to be excreted from the body. The hemoglobin is now ready to pick up oxygen again in the start of a new cycle. This ability of hemoglobin to take up and release oxygen is a unique function that depends on the presence of iron within the assembled molecule. Without iron, this essential link in the tissue's oxygen-supply mechanism would be lacking.

Myoglobin, an iron-containing molecule similar in structure to hemoglobin, is present in muscle tissue, where it serves as a convenient source of oxygen for muscle metabolism. Iron is also an essential component of the enzyme system in cells, which converts energy from carbohydrate, fat, and protein to ATP, the form the body can use.

Absorption of Food Iron   A relatively small proportion of dietary iron is absorbed for use by the body. Many factors influence iron absorption, among them the chemical form in which the iron occurs, the character of the food of which it is a part, and the nature of other foods eaten at the same time. For example, iron in the form of ferrous sulfate or ascorbate is absorbed very efficiently, while compounds containing iron in the ferric state are not. *Heme iron*, the natural compound in animal meats, is absorbed much more efficiently than iron from other animal protein sources or from vegetables. Furthermore, research studies with human subjects have shown that meat in a meal enhances the absorption of nonheme iron from other foods eaten at the same time. Ascorbic acid, when present in the same meal as foods containing nonheme iron, also increases iron absorption. On the other hand, eating certain foods of animal origin that do not contain heme iron (such as cheese or eggs) with other nonheme iron-containing foods (such as vegetables) reduces the availability of iron from those foods. Phytic acid is also known to reduce iron absorption. Such evidence suggests the importance of considering the nutritive iron value of foods not only on the basis of their iron content, but also on iron availability and the influence on iron availability of other foods eaten at the same time (24).

Wide variations in efficiency of iron absorption are observed among normal healthy subjects on the same diets. In general, iron-deficient individuals absorb a higher percentage of iron than do those with adequate iron stores. The Food and Nutrition Board, after taking into consideration all the known factors influencing iron absorption, based the RDA for iron on the assumption that 10 percent of dietary iron is available to the body (12).

Storage of Iron   When iron is absorbed, that which is not used immediately is stored. The liver, spleen, and bone marrow are the chief storage sites. Stored iron exists with protein mainly as *ferritin*, in a combination that can be mobilized by the body when necessary for hemoglobin synthesis. When large amounts of iron accumulate, they are stored as *hemosiderin*, a more complex molecule than ferritin.

Losses of Iron   There is no mechanism for removing iron from the body once it has been absorbed. The limited passage of iron from food through the intestinal mucosa is the means of regulating the amount of iron in the body. A small amount is lost daily, however, despite the body's remarkable ability to conserve its iron content. This occurs almost entirely through the loss of iron-containing cells such as epithelial cells and blood cells. Iron balance experiments and tracer studies have been employed to establish these facts about iron. Such methods also provide a means of investigating special body needs for iron in different segments of the population.

Demands of the Body for Iron

The body's daily needs for iron are summarized for various age and sex groups and for certain stress conditions in Table 8.3. Column 1 on the table names the specific groups whose needs are considered. Columns 2 to 5 provide data on estimated daily iron needs for

heme
Iron-containing component of hemoglobin

ferritin
Iron-protein complex; chief storage form of iron in the body

hemosiderin
Iron-storing protein

Table 8.3
Estimated iron requirements mg per day

	Loss* in urine, sweat, feces	menses	Average requirement for pregnancy	growth	Total requirement absorbed iron	Daily food iron intake requirement **
1	2	3	4	5	6	7
normal men and non-menstruating women	0.7–1.3				0.7–1.3	7–13
menstruating women	0.6–0.9	0.1–1.4			0.7–2.3	7–23
pregnant women	0.7–1.0		1.0–2.5 or more		1.7–3.5 or more	17–35
adolescent girls	0.6–0.9	0.1–1.4		0.3–0.5	1.0–2.8	10–28
adolescent boys	0.7–1.3			0.4–0.7	1.1–2.0	10–20
children 2-12 yrs					0.4–1.0	4–10

Adapted from C. V. Moore, "Iron," in R. S. Goodhart and M. E. Shils, eds. *Modern Nutrition in Health and Disease* (Philadelphia: Lea and Febiger, 1973).
*0.013 mg/kg
**Assuming 10% absorption of iron

each of the groups, to cover all types of iron losses and to provide for growth in all of its forms. Column 6 gives the estimated total needs for absorbed iron for each group, and column 7 lists the amount of iron in food that must be ingested daily to cover the total needs. Thus Table 8.3 provides the factors that enter into the assessment of human iron requirements. The following discussion of the various demands of the human body for iron is based on these factors. The discussion will be more meaningful if you follow closely the references made to the table in the text. In interpreting the table, remember that losses as indicated in columns 2 and 3 are to be regarded as needs because they must be replaced, and that the requirements for dietary iron (column 7) assume 10 percent absorption of food iron. To compare the estimated requirements for iron with the RDA turn to the RDA table (see inside cover).

Iron Needs of Adults

The loss in excretion of 0.7 to 1.3 milligrams of iron daily (column 2) for normal men and nonmenstruating women represents a basic requirement. With no additional needs for growth, the RDA for iron should be met easily with a varied, well-balanced diet, provided that as much as 10 percent of the iron intake is absorbed. At all other periods of life there are stresses that call for additional amounts of iron.

Iron Needs of Women—Stresses in Menses and Childbearing (23)

Menses   The menstrual blood loss for any individual normal woman is fairly constant from month to month, but differences among women are great. A loss of about 45 milliliters of blood every 28 days can be considered average, with most normal women losing less than 80 milliliters. The resulting loss of iron amounts to something between 0.1 and 1.4 milligrams daily. Excessive menstrual flow, which occurs in about 5 percent of women, brings the loss to more than 1.4 milligrams per day (Table 8.3, column 3). The total loss, including that from routine excretion, (column 2), could thus reach between 0.7 and 2.3 milligrams daily. Even if menstruating women meet the RDA for food iron, they may still be in a marginal situation with respect to iron balance. With the recognized difficulties of attaining the RDA for food iron, together with the possibility that losses are greater than stated and absorption less than 10 percent, the probability of iron deficiency is real. It is very likely that many menstruating women are unable to accumulate adequate iron stores. Failure to store iron at this period can mean entering pregnancy in poor nutritional status with respect to iron.

Childbearing   Although there are no menstrual losses during pregnancy, the needs of the developing fetus and the supporting tissues of the mother's body require extra amounts of iron, estimated at 1.0 to 2.5 or more milligrams daily (Table 8.3, column 4), particularly in the latter part of pregnancy. This is a significantly greater amount than the loss during menstruation shown in column 3. The total iron loss in pregnancy, including routine excretion losses (column 2), may well reach considerably more than 2 milligrams (column 6) per day. Table 8.4 shows an estimated breakdown of the distribution of iron "cost" in pregnancy. Additional iron is required for the increase in red blood cell volume that occurs during the last half of pregnancy, although this is not part of the iron "cost" since most of it remains in the body when the red blood cell volume returns to normal after delivery (23). It is obvious that meeting iron needs with iron from food alone is almost impossible during pregnancy.

Iron transfer from the maternal organism to the fetus seems to be restricted to a one-way flow. Even when maternal requirements are not being met, the transfer of iron to the fetus continues (23). The extent to which the pregnant woman's iron nutrition affects the amount of iron in her infant at birth is unknown (25). A num-

Table 8.4
Iron "cost" of a normal pregnancy

iron contributed to fetus	200–370 mg*
in placenta and cord	30–170 mg
in blood loss at delivery	90–310 mg
in milk, lactation 6 months	100–180 mg
total	420–1030 mg
average per day (pregnancy 9 mo. lactation 6 mo):	**1.0–2.5 mg**

Source: C. V. Moore, "Iron" in R. S. Goodhart and M. E. Shils eds., *Modern Nutrition in Health and Disease* (Philadelphia: Lea and Febiger, 1973).
*These figures are in addition to the normal excretory loss of 0.5 to 1.0 mg/day.

Figure 8.6

Mean iron intake as a percent of standard by age, sex and race for income levels, United States, 1971-72 (19).

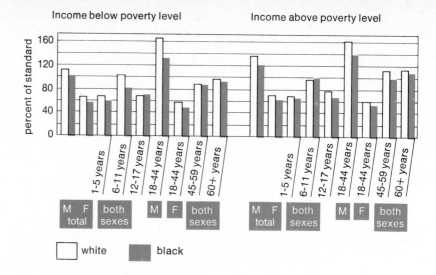

The y-axis is labeled "percent of standard" with values 0, 40, 80, 120, 160.

Two main groups: "Income below poverty level" and "Income above poverty level".

Age categories: 1-5 years, 6-11 years, 12-17 years, 18-44 years, 18-44 years, 45-59 years, 60+ years. Grouped by M and F total, and both sexes.

Legend: □ white ■ black

ber of studies have shown that girls and women have low iron intakes at the ages when stresses are greatest. Dietary data collected for the HANES, 1971–72 indicate that the mean iron intake of women of childbearing age (from 18 to 44 years), including blacks and whites with incomes above and below the poverty level, was about 58 percent below the standard (19). No other group had a mean intake that far below standard (Fig. 8.6).

The loss of iron during lactation is approximately 0.5 to 1.0 milligram per day (23). This amounts roughly to the menstrual loss, which may not be a factor in lactation.

Iron Needs of Childhood—Stresses in Growth

The requirement for iron for growth is closely related to the growth rate. Increases in hemoglobin mass during infancy and adolescence, the periods of most rapid growth, make heavy demands on iron. The iron endowment of normal, full-term infants at birth varies widely but in any case it cannot be depended upon to meet iron needs beyond 6 months of age. Infants of low birth weight often begin life with only one-half to two-thirds as much iron in their bodies as full-term infants. The body of an infant contains on the average about 0.5 gram of iron; the adult body, 3.0 to 5.0 grams. There must therefore be a steady gain in body content of iron over the period from infancy to adulthood. The total gain would be 2.5 to 4.5 grams, with a net increase of about 0.3 to 0.6 *milligram* per day over the entire period. Adequate amounts of iron, in some form, must be supplied regularly in infancy and early childhood in order to satisfy the extremely high needs during that period. If an infant receives 7 milligrams of dietary iron in a form that is efficiently absorbed every day beginning at 4 weeks of age, the iron requirement for the first year of life will be met. If dietary iron is not provided until the infant is several months old, a larger daily amount is required to meet the baby's needs (25).

Human milk and cow's milk are poor sources of iron. An iron

supplement must be provided for breast-fed infants and for those on cow's-milk formulas. Commercially prepared formulas supplemented with iron will provide a major portion of the iron needed daily during the early months of life. Iron-fortified dry cereals commercially prepared for infants are also rich sources of iron. Use of these cereals on a daily basis at least until the infant reaches 18 months of age should be encouraged. Few other foods commonly fed to infants provide such generous amounts of iron (25).

Assuming that a 7-year-old child has a daily iron intake of 10 milligrams (see Table 8.3, Column 7) and absorbs 10 percent of it (1.0 milligram), he or she may utilize 0.5 milligram (Column 5) for growth and have a small surplus. How much of this surplus contributes to a positive balance depends on how much iron is excreted, a subject about which little is known for the childhood years. There is certain to be some iron excretion, however. A small positive balance can be eliminated easily by a diet poor in iron, by usually poor absorption of iron, or even by a mild infection.

Table 8.3 shows that adolescents have a substantial iron requirement based on growth (column 5), as well as routine excretion losses. In addition, an adolescent girl has a menstrual loss of iron (column 3). Her total requirement of absorbed iron could be close to 3 milligrams to compensate for excretion, menses, and growth. Thus, even a girl who has a daily iron intake of 18 milligrams could be in negative iron balance. Data on iron intake suggest that it commonly falls below the standard in adolescent years (Fig. 8.6). If a girl is pregnant during adolescence, the stress becomes intensified. Evidence suggests, however, that a higher percentage of food iron is absorbed during the latter half of pregnancy and whenever red blood cell formation is stimulated than at other times (23).

Blood Donations

Donations of blood for transfusions result in a considerable loss of iron and therefore constitute a type of stress. When a pint of blood is given, the donor may lose as much as 250 milligrams of iron. Spread over a period of a year, this means a loss of about 0.6 to 0.7 milligram per day. A blood donor can replace the loss as hemoglobin within a few days if he or she has adequate stores. If stores are inadequate, however, and the iron replacement must come from iron in the diet, the blood regeneration may require 2 to 3 months or longer.

Assessing Nutritional Status

Data from a number of recent studies conducted in various parts of the United States reveal that anemia is prevalent in infants and children. Anemia in children aged 6 months to 6 years is arbitrarily defined as a concentration of hemoglobin in the blood of less than 11.0 grams per 100 milliliters. Between 14 and 48 percent of infants less than 1 year of age were anemic by this standard, with as many as 53 percent of low-birth-weight infants so classified. Among children aged 1 to 5, the prevalence of anemia ranged from 3 to 58 percent. Incidence was highest among the younger children,

Table 8.5
Guidelines for classification of biochemical determinations used in the Health and Nutrition Examination Survey, United States, 1971–72 (19)

Biochemical determination age and sex	Classification category		
	Low	Acceptable	High
hemoglobin g/100 ml			
1–5 years	<10.0	10.0–11.0	>11.0
6–11 years	<11.5	11.5–12.5	>12.5
12–17 years, male	<13.0	13.0–14.0	>14.0
12–17 years, female	<11.5	11.5–12.5	>12.5
18 years and over, male	<14.0	14.0–16.5	>16.5
18 years and over, female	<12.0	12.0–14.5	>14.5
hematocrit percent			
1–5 years	<31	31–34	>34
6–11 years	<35	35–39	>39
12–17 years, male	<40	40–44	>44
12–17 years, female	<36	36–38	>38
18 years and over, male	<44	44–52	>52
18 years and over, female	<38	38–48	>48
serum iron µg/100 ml			
1–5 years	<40	40– 49	> 49
6–11 years	<50	50– 59	> 59
12 years and over, male	<60	60–149	>149
12 years and over, female	<40	40–119	>119
transferrin saturation percent			
1–5 years	<15	15–29	>30
6–11 years	<20	20–29	>30
12 years and over, male	<20	20–29	>30
12 years and over, female	<15	15–29	>30
serum protein g/100 ml			
1–5 years	<5.0	5.0–6.0	>6.0
6–17 years	<6.0	6.0–8.0	>8.0
adult	<6.5	6.5–8.5	>8.5
serum albumin g/100 ml			
1–5 years	<2.5	2.5–3.5	>3.5
6–17 years	<3.0	3.0–4.0	>4.0
adult	<3.5	3.5–5.5	>5.5
serum vitamin A µg/100 ml			
all ages	<20	20–80	>80

< = less tnan; > = greater than

those of low birth weight, and those from families with the lowest incomes (25).

Preliminary findings from the HANES, 1971–72, provide information with regard to the prevalence of unsatisfactory iron nutrition among various groups in the United States population (19). Measurements of concentration of hemoglobin and *hematocrit* are used to assess iron deficiency anemia. Both are general rather than specific indicators of the cause of anemia. Guidelines for the classification of biochemical determinations used in the HANES are shown in Table 8.5. The table lists the biochemical determinations made with acceptable ranges for different age and sex groups as well as what are considered high and low values for each.

hematocrit
Percentage of red cells in the blood by volume

Blacks had a higher incidence of low hemoglobin values than did whites for all age groups regardless of income level, as can be seen in Figure 8.7. Blacks aged 60 years and over had the highest prevalence of low hemoglobin values for any age group regardless of income level—about 30 percent in the low income group and 23 percent in the income group above poverty. In the 18- to 44-year age group, females had a higher percentage of low hemoglobin values than did males for all race and income groups, while males had a much higher percentage than females in the 12- to 17-year age group—7.4 and 1.9 percent respectively. The reader is referred to the report of the findings (19) for values of the hematocrit measurements as well as those of serum iron and transferrin saturation.

Hemoglobin Concentration   The determination of hemoglobin concentration in the blood is a time-honored method for indicating the level of iron nutrition. Findings are evaluated in comparison with so-called standard values, based on averages for many hemoglobin determinations at different ages (see Table 8.5). Variations below the norms have been considered indicative of poor iron nutrition. At a specified low level for each age group, the person is said to be anemic. This is sometimes called presumptive evidence of iron deficiency. Iron-deficiency anemia usually develops over an extended period of time, because excretion of iron from the body is limited, except as blood loss. When the iron absorbed from dietary sources is insufficient to meet current needs, iron stored as ferritin and hemosiderin is withdrawn and used. At the same time, there is an increase in the iron-binding capacity of plasma, and the levels of iron in the plasma are decreased. As body stores of iron are exhausted, the rate of red blood cell production slows down, and the new cells that are formed contain less-than-normal amounts of iron. This sequence of changes may take months or years. The time required for anemia to develop depends on the size of iron stores and the relative deficiency of dietary iron absorbed (23).

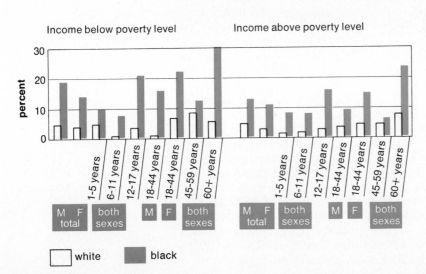

Figure 8.7
Percent of persons with low hemoglobin values by age, sex and race for income levels, United States, 1971-72 (19). (HANES Preliminary)

Continuous shortages of iron in the diet, poor absorption, and types of stresses, already discussed, that increase the need for iron are believed to be among the chief causes of iron-deficiency anemia, the commonest type of nutritional anemia. However, shortages of certain other nutrients, notably vitamin B_{12}, folic acid, and protein are also involved. They presumably act with iron in the development of red blood cells in the bone marrow. Shortages of these nutrients contribute to lowered amounts of hemoglobin per red cell, and lowered hemoglobin results in decreased ability of the cells to carry oxygen to the tissues. When cardiorespiratory functions are thus affected, a decrease in capacity for physical work occurs. With less oxygen and more carbon dioxide in the cells, body processes can become sluggish. In this situation, a person may be pale in appearance because the color-bearing (red) hemoglobin of the blood has been reduced.

Iron Stores   Hemoglobin values do not give a complete picture of nutritional status with respect to iron. One may be in a state of poor iron nutrition without exhibiting low hemoglobin levels. Moderately decreased hemoglobin levels appear to have no clinical significance, and there may be no subjective indications of a problem. If the hemoglobin level is corrected so that iron balance is restored, the person may live with nearly depleted iron stores for years without suffering any apparent health problems. This situation has been found to exist in many otherwise healthy girls and women. Even though their hemoglobin levels are within the normal range, they are at risk of developing anemia very quickly if there is an increased need for iron due to pregnancy or increased blood loss. It is now apparent that an appraisal of iron stores is necessary for a total evaluation of nutritional status with respect to iron. Several methods of determining iron stores have been tried, and one that measures bone marrow iron appears to be the most reliable. With this method, it has been possible to demonstrate that the body may show a deficiency of iron even when the hemoglobin values are well above anemia levels. Unfortunately, the bone-marrow method of measurement is a *biopsy* technique and not suited to mass survey studies. A simpler method for measuring iron stores is needed.

biopsy
Examination of tissue removed from a living subject

Dietary iron   At the present time it is not known whether meeting the RDA for iron will ensure adequate iron stores in women and girls. We can assume, however, that routinely high intakes of iron will tend to build iron stores or at least to prevent their depletion. Various types of dietary studies shed some light on whether population groups in the United States are consuming iron in amounts that approach the RDA for iron. Preliminary findings of the HANES, 1971–72 showed that the diets for three age groups among blacks and whites both above and below the poverty level were below the standards for iron intake—children aged 1 to 5 years, adolescents aged 12 to 17, and females aged 18 to 44 years (Fig. 8.7). Mean intakes of iron failed to meet the standard for all blacks in the lowest income group except males aged 18 to 44 years. About 95 percent of all children aged 1 to 5 years and all women aged 18 to 44 in both race and income groups had iron in-

Food*	Weight or ** approximate measure	Iron milligrams	

Figure 8.8

Iron: Servings of representative foods in order of their iron content. (Each bar represents an approximate iron value for the group of foods listed below it.)

███████████████████████████████████ 5 mg

liver, beef	2 oz	5.0

███████████████ 3 mg

beans, dry, canned	¾ cup	3.5
beef, lean, chuck	3 oz	3.1
beef, hamburger	3 oz	3.6
pork chop	1 chop	2.7

███████ 1.5 mg

spinach	½ cup	2.2
peas, green	½ cup	1.5
tunafish, canned	½ cup	1.5
rice, enriched, cooked	¾ cup	1.4
chicken, fried	½ breast	1.3
haddock, fried	1 fillet (4 oz)	1.3
raisins	¼ cup	1.3

█████ 0.8 mg

sweet potato	1 medium	1.1
tomato juice, canned	½ cup	1.1
egg	1 medium	1.0
macaroni, enriched, cooked	¾ cup	1.0
sausage, bologna	2 oz	1.0
frankfurter	1 medium	0.9
oatmeal, cooked	⅔ cup	0.9
banana, raw	1 medium	0.8
bread, whole wheat	1 slice	0.8
bun or roll, enriched	1 bun	0.8
strawberries, raw	½ cup	0.8
bread, white, enriched	1 slice	0.7
potato, white	1 medium	0.7

███ 0.5 mg

broccoli	½ cup	0.6
corn, canned	½ cup	0.6
cornflakes, fortified	1 cup	0.6
peanut butter	2 tbsp	0.6
grapefruit, white	½ medium	0.5
carrots, diced	½ cup	0.5
apple, raw	1 medium	0.4
beans, green	½ cup	0.4
lettuce, head	1 cup	0.4
peaches, canned	½ cup	0.4
onions	½ cup	0.4
pineapple juice, canned	½ cup	0.4

██ 0.2 mg and less

cheese, cheddar	1 oz	0.3
peppers, sweet, green, raw	½ medium	0.3
Cabbage, raw, chopped	½ cup	0.2
Cheese, cottage, creamed	¼ cup	0.2
mayonnaise	1 tbsp	0.1
milk, fluid skim or buttermilk	1 cup	0.1
milk, fluid, whole	1 cup	0.1
orange juice	½ cup	0.1
sugar	1 tbsp	tr
cream, half and half	1 tbsp	tr
butter or margarine	1 tbsp	0†
oil, salad or cooking	1 tbsp	0
beverages, cola type	12 oz	—

* Foods are in forms ready to eat. All meats and vegetables are cooked unless otherwise indicated.
** See Appendix K for further identification of these foods. All foods are described there more fully, and both weights and measures are indicated.
† See Appendix J.

takes below the standard. Women in the childbearing years were the group most consistently low in iron intake in relation to the HANES standard (19). A major problem for women is their relatively low energy intake. Although most women require considerably less food energy than men do, their iron allowances are much higher than those for men.

Comparative Iron Values in Foods

With iron widely distributed but not highly concentrated in commonly used foods, it is most important to evaluate food sources of this mineral with a view to making wise choices. The comparative iron yield of the items on your representative food list will indicate the range of values among common foods. The specimen representative list in Figure 8.8 can be used as a basis for discussion of comparative iron sources. Average servings of the foods are arranged in order of their concentration in iron, from the rich sources at the top to those with little or no iron at the end.

The importance of protein foods as concentrated sources of iron is apparent. Organ meats such as liver, lean muscle meats of all kinds and dry legumes head the list; 2 ounces of cooked beef liver furnishes more than one-and-one-half times as much iron as 3 ounces of cooked lean beef. The livers of different animals and some other organ meats are likewise higher in iron than similar amounts of lean muscle meats.

Dark green leafy vegetables (represented by spinach on this list), fish, enriched rice, dried fruits (represented by raisins), eggs (yolk) whole-grain and restored or enriched cereals and breads are all good sources of iron.

Foods that supply ½ milligram of iron or less per serving (most of the lower half of the list) and are thus negligible sources of iron include: fresh fruits; several vegetables of high water content other than the dark green leafy varieties; unenriched, highly milled cereals; fat meats such as bacon; milk and cheeses. These foods can be counted on to provide some iron, but the greater part of the allowance must be met by the more concentrated sources. Note that the positions of milk and meat on the calcium list have been practically reversed (Fig. 8.3).

The pure fats, sugar, and soft drinks provide no iron, although molasses, a less refined sweetener than sugar, does contain some. For individuals who prefer dark molasses and use it on a regular basis, it can provide significant amounts of iron. However, molasses cannot be considered an important source of iron in the food supply of the United States because of the relatively small amount that is consumed overall.

Iron in the National Diet

US Department of Agriculture data show that nearly one-third of the iron available to consumers in the United States comes from meat, poultry, and fish; almost as much from flour and cereal products, many of them enriched; about one-fifth from all kinds of vegetables, including dry legumes; and the remainder, in small

Table 8.6
Enrichment standards for certain conventional foods
mg per lb unless otherwise indicated

	Enriched flour	Enriched Bread Rolls Buns	Enriched Corn Meal		Enriched Rice		Enriched macaroni products		Enriched noodle products	
			Minimum	Maximum	Minimum	Maximum	Minimum	Maximum	Minimum	Maximum
thiamin	2.9	1.8	2.0	3.0	2.0	4.0	4.0	5.0	4.0	5.0
riboflavin	1.8	1.1	1.2	1.8	1.2	2.4	1.7	2.2	1.7	2.2
niacin	24.0	15.0	16.0	24.0	16.0	32.0	27.0	34.0	27.0	34.0
iron	not more than 16.5	not more than 12.5 not less than 8.0	13.0	26.0	13.0	26.0	13.0	16.5	13.0	16.5
calcium*	960.0**	600.0**	500.0	750.0	500.0	750.0	500.0	625.0	500.0	625.0
vitamin D*			250.0	1000.0	250.0	1000.0	250.0	1000.0	250.0	1000.0
USP units wheat germ or partly defatted wheat germ*	not more than 5% by weight	not more than 5% by weight of flour ingredient					not more than 5% by weight of finished food (partly defatted wheat germ)		not more than 5% by weight of finished food (partly defatted wheat germ)	

Source: Code of Federal Regulations. Food & Drug Administration 1976 (FDA)
Tryptophan not to be considered as source of Niacin
*Optional additions
**Enriched flour and bread may contain added calcium in such quantity that total calcium content, respectively, is 960 and 600 mg per lb.

amounts, from other food groups. This widespread distribution is in sharp contrast to the high concentration of calcium in a single food group—76 percent in milk and dairy foods. Because we must "shop around" for iron, it is important to be familiar with the types of foods where it is most likely to be found.

Enrichment of Foods   Whole-grain, restored, and enriched cereals and breads are important for iron intake, not only because they are relatively concentrated sources but also because cereals are eaten in some form at practically every meal. Whole-grain cereals are those that retain the germ and outer coats of the grain and the nutrients therein. Restored cereals are those in which certain nutrients lost in the milling process are returned to their natural levels or higher. Enriched cereals and breads are made from highly milled grains and flours to which specified amounts of iron and certain vitamins are added.

The practice of food enrichment emerged from World War II. Before the war, nutritionists became aware that the average diet in the United States was declining in its content of iron and those vitamins affected by lessened use of potatoes and whole-grain cereals. In 1940, therefore, the Food and Nutrition Board had developed suggested levels of enrichment for white flour and baker's bread. In 1943, War Food Order No. 1 was issued, requiring nationwide enrichment of white bread and rolls with iron, thiamin, riboflavin, and niacin, with calcium and vitamin D as optional ingredients. By the end of the war when the order was revoked (1946), nineteen states had made enrichment compulsory. Now most enrichment takes place at the mills, and almost all flour sold in the United States is enriched. Table 8.6 shows present Federal enrichment standards for flour, bread, cornmeal, rice, and macaroni and noodle products.

Breakfast cereals undoubtedly add a considerable amount of iron to the American diet. Most manufacturers voluntarily enrich cereal products when nutrients have been lost in processing. Cereals, including those for infants, are subject to the same nutritional labeling regulations as other products; if nutrients have been added or nutritional claims are made, the standard nutritional label must appear on the box or container.

Other Aspects of Iron Sources   Despite active programs for the enrichment and restoration of flour and cereal products, the amount of iron from such foods in the national food supply has not increased in recent years. This is due in part to the fact that the consumption of many cereal foods is decreasing. There is other evidence that the iron content of diets in the United States is not increasing. Household diet surveys made in 1955 and 1965 showed that iron intake from all food sources remained essentially the same in the two time periods. (17). It even appears possible that the amount of iron in foods has *decreased* over the years, due to changes in commercial processing and home cooking equipment. Canned foods, for example, are now carefully guarded against rust in cans, whereas they once were subject to harmless "contamination" with iron from this source. Iron pots, frypans, and skillets, undoubtedly a source of added iron at one time, are now little used (23).

Various plans have been proposed to raise iron intake automatically. One is to enrich heavily one staple food (as has been done with vitamin D in milk), which would ensure meeting the total daily iron requirement. The choice of a suitable food for this proposal has been much debated. Another plan proposes that current iron levels in flours and cereals be raised, and that enrichment be extended to other grain foods, such as rolls, crackers, and all pastas. Testing of various iron compounds is required to ensure that forms of iron used for enrichment are available for absorption.

An important consideration in any plan for heavy enrichment is that the food or foods selected should be those that the most vulnerable group—women and girls—now eat routinely or could be encouraged to eat in sufficient amounts to accomplish the purpose. The potential danger of iron overload for men who have lower requirements for iron has also been pointed out. Some active men would likely consume large quantities of one or several highly enriched foods, which might lead to a daily iron intake in excess of 30 milligrams. This should not have adverse consequences (12).

Further aspects of enrichment will be considered in connection with the B vitamins, the other enrichment factors, in Chapter 9.

Arrange your own list of representative foods (see p. 136) in order of their importance as sources of iron. Analyze the list. Suggest groups representing similar iron values. Characterize the foods in each group.

Enter iron values from Appendix K on your personal meal record. Total the iron intake for the day. How does the total compare with the RDA for iron for your sex-age group (see the RDA table)?

Problems in Selecting Foods for Iron

The specimen diet in Appendix H shows one way an adult can choose a day's meals furnishing about 1900 calories and about 10 milligrams of iron. Representatives of good, but not highly concentrated, sources of iron are evident in the diet—hamburger, pork chop, and enriched flour (in buns and rolls). This selection suggests that, with ordinary mixed diets, no trouble need be anticipated in meeting the iron allowance for men. The real challenge, however, lies in reaching the much higher level of iron that has been recommended for older girls and women throughout the childbearing period. In the United States, this means greatly increasing the average amount of iron now consumed by these groups (Fig. 8.6). The problem is augmented by the fact that the relatively low daily energy intake of these groups limits the amount of food that must carry the relatively large amount of iron. To attack this puzzling problem effectively, it is necessary to acquire a working knowledge of iron values in common foods and to find practical ways of adapt-

Figure 8.9
Five foods providing about 20
mg. of iron. (See Table 8.7,
columns 1 and 2 for names of
foods, their amounts and iron
content). (Landon Gardiner)

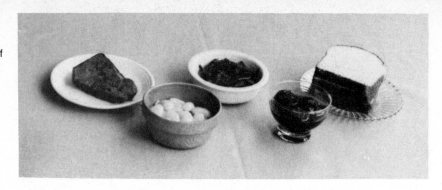

ing such information to personal and family meal planning (Figs. 8.9 and 8.10).

Meeting Iron Needs for Women and Older Girls

Table 8.7 demonstrates the practical problems of food choice that must be faced in planning a diet that will furnish a sufficient amount of iron to meet the needs of women and older girls. The table presents two lists of foods containing meats, meat alternates, vegetables, fruits, and grain foods that might serve as the core of a day's diet. List 1 on the left purposely consists of concentrated sources of iron; list 2 on the right consists of corresponding types of foods in similar amounts but representing less concentrated sources of iron. Iron values are given for average servings of foods on both lists. The Table makes it apparent that the iron content of meals can be varied greatly by merely substituting one type of food for another within the same classification of foods. This fact is emphasized by the differences in iron yields of corresponding food items and in the total amounts of iron provided by the two lists.

List 1 obviously does not offer a practical solution to the problem of meeting the RDA for iron for women even though the foods listed supply that amount. Liver and spinach generally are not popular items of diet, and they would not be served daily in most homes. Actually, in the case of liver, it is doubtful that there would

Table 8.7
Alternatives in choosing a diet high in iron

1	Amount	Iron mg	2	Amount	Iron mg
beef liver	4 oz	10.0	**beef pot roast**	4 oz	3.5
lima beans (dry, cooked)	¾ cup	4.4	**navy beans** (dry, cooked)	¾ cup	3.8
spinach	½ cup	2.2	**carrots**	½ cup	0.5
prunes	½ cup	1.8	**apple sauce**	½ cup	0.7
bread, white, enriched	3 slices	2.1	**bread**, white, unenriched	3 slices	0.6
	total	20.5		total	9.1

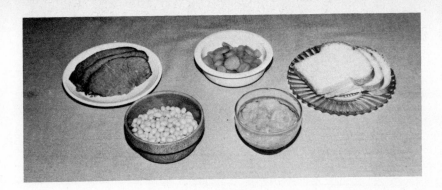

Figure 8.10
Five foods, matching in type to those in 8.9 but supplying less than half the amount of iron. (See Table 8.7, column 2.) (Landon Gardiner)

be enough available in the market to supply even the most vulnerable groups on a daily basis.

List 2 offers a more practical working base. Even though they are lower in iron than liver, muscle meats are more acceptable for regular use. Furthermore, there is a relatively wide choice among lean muscle meats of similar iron content, from various cuts and from different meat animals. Likewise, vegetables other than "greens" are more acceptable for daily use in most regions, and there is a considerable variety of such vegetables even though their iron yield is meager for the most part. The dry beans on the two lists are not significantly different in their yield of iron. Either kind would be acceptable for daily use in diets of certain ethnic groups. Apple sauce and many other cooked fruits of similarly low iron value are probably used more regularly than prunes in most family meals. Only the breads on lists 1 and 2 look and taste the same. Many considerations enter into choices of foods: personal preferences, family meal patterns, cost, and availability. A knowledge of the iron values of common foods can serve as a framework within which to exercise preferences that will provide maximum dietary iron.

The problem of meeting a child's dietary allowance for iron is similar to that of meeting an adult's. It is a matter of giving special consideration to good sources. The RDA is especially high for both boys and girls approaching and during adolescence. However, boys at these ages have a better chance of attaining the RDA than girls do, because their energy requirements are considerably higher. The same foods that can form the nucleus of an adult's diet can also serve for a child's. Children of different ages can meet their varying iron needs at the family table chiefly by adjusting the size of servings of certain foods in line with their total energy needs.

A Practical Approach

Is there a practical solution to obtaining a diet that will provide an adequate amount of iron daily, particularly if the quantity of food served must be limited to about 2000 calories or less? How much iron can a palatable, moderately low-calorie diet consistently provide from day to day?

Obviously, neither list 1 nor list 2 in Table 8.7 provides the complete answer. It is not feasible to "pack" the diet with highly concentrated sources of iron, as list 1 might suggest. It *is* practical, however, to apply information from list 1 in mapping a compromise dietary plan, based largely on the sources of iron found in list 2. For example:

1. *Use liver and other organ meats on a regular basis*, perhaps once a week. Choose liver from different meat animals; the liver of young animals (calves' liver) is higher in iron than the liver of mature animals. Pork liver is an even more concentrated source of iron than beef or calves' liver. Prices of livers vary widely. Some of them are moderate in cost compared with other meats.

> Make a list of livers from different animal sources in Appendix K with their iron values per serving. Compare the iron values of liver with those of other organ meats. How much do you depend upon liver as a source of iron?

2. *Form the habit of eating dry legumes often.* Beans are not only an excellent source of iron at moderate cost but they provide protein, calcium, and certain vitamins as well.

> Compare the iron yields of different kinds of dry beans (cooked and canned) per serving in Appendix K.

3. *Use "greens" frequently in place of other vegetables.* Try different varieties. Also select vegetables other than "greens" that are relatively good sources of iron. Take care to include some meat in the meal for the enhancing effect it has on the absorption of iron from vegetables and legumes. If meat is not part of the meal, select a food rich in ascorbic acid to increase the availability of iron from the vegetables, legumes, and grains.

> Compare servings of various "greens" in Appendix K with spinach as sources of iron. Choose six to ten vegetables other than "greens" that are the best vegetable sources of iron.

4. *Confine your selection of breads and cereals* to those that are whole grain, or that have been restored or enriched. Such foods can add a significant amount of iron to the diet.

> Study the breads and breakfast foods listed in Appendix K for information on the practice of enriching and restoring cereal foods. Read bread wrappers and box labels for the iron content of cereal foods.

5. *Make a habit of using dried fruits.*

> Compare the iron content of the various dried fruits listed in Appendix K. Look elsewhere for the iron content of servings of the same fruits in fresh and dried forms.

6. *Test the plan.*

> Plan a day's meals compatible with your usual eating pattern, incorporating iron-rich foods at levels that would be acceptable to you on a continuing basis. Estimate iron and energy values. (If certain foods are planned on a less-than-daily basis, indicate at what intervals you could accept them.)
>
> On the basis of your findings, how much iron can you expect to obtain daily at a calorie level that maintains your desirable body weight?

It is estimated that, on the basis of the total United States food supply, there are about 6 milligrams of iron in every 1000 calories. Diets providing 2000 calories a day might thus be expected to furnish 12 milligrams of iron if they consist primarily of a wide variety of basic foods. The inclusion of large amounts of refined sugars and fats would reduce the iron-to-calorie ratio. Requirements for iron vary widely even among individuals within any population group (see Table 8.3). It may be that the level of 12 milligrams a day meets the iron needs for many women and girls. More liberal intakes of iron, of course, provide greater assurance of desirable iron stores.

Supplementary Iron

If dietary measures are inadequate and iron intake is low, medicinal iron supplementation may be prescribed by a physician, especially if hemoglobin values are also below normal. An iron supplement is routinely prescribed during pregnancy.

COPPER, IODINE, AND FLUORIDE
COPPER (12, 26)

Copper is an essential nutrient for mammals. It is present in all body tissues, with the highest concentrations in liver, kidney, brain, and heart. A number of copper-containing proteins and enzymes have been identified. This mineral is also involved in many ways with the functioning of iron in the body. It appears to be necessary for the normal absorption of iron from the gastrointestinal tract, for its transport, and for its incorporation into certain iron-containing enzymes and hemoglobin. Normal use of iron in the body is therefore dependent on adequate intake and utilization of copper. The first proof of the existence of a copper deficiency in laboratory animals was furnished when an anemic condition was relieved by the administration of a copper salt. A copper-containing protein, *ceruloplasmin,* is necessary for the release of iron from storage in the body. Thus a copper deficiency may result in iron-deficiency anemia even when the body has adequate iron stores. Copper is also essential for the normal development of bone, the central nervous system, and connective tissue.

Deficiency of copper is rare in human beings. It has been seen in children with iron-deficiency anemia and with kwashiorkor. About 2 milligrams daily will apparently maintain copper balance in an adult; 0.05 to 0.10 milligram of copper per kilogram of body weight is probably sufficient during growth. Copper is contained in a variety of foods and can be transferred to food from copper cooking dishes if the food actually comes in contact with the copper. Ordinary diets in the United States provide about 2 milligrams of copper daily; there appears to be little danger of an insufficient intake. Copper occurs in many of the same foods as does iron. Meats, particularly liver and kidney, some shellfish, nuts, raisins, and dried legumes are excellent sources.

IODINE (12, 27, 28)

The only known function of iodine in the body is as an essential constituent of thyroid hormones. These hormones control reactions involving cellular energy, and—as we saw in Chapter 6—they are a vital factor in regulating basal energy metabolism. Thyroid hormones are also necessary for growth and development in the young and for successful pregnancy and lactation. When there is a deficiency in the secretion of these hormones, a child's physical development is retarded. With prolonged, severe deficiency, *cretinism,* which involves both physical and mental retardation, can result.

cretinism
Arrested physical and mental development due to severe deficiency of thyroid secretion

Dietary iodine is absorbed rapidly from the digestive tract, most of it from the small intestine. About three-fourths of the iodine in the body is concentrated in the thyroid gland. By a series of metabolic processes (largely regulated by a hormone secreted by the pituitary gland), dietary iodine is ultimately released from the thyroid gland into the blood as a constituent of the hormones *thyroxine* and *triiodothyronine.* The normal level of thyroid hormones in the blood is maintained by a sensitive feedback mechanism between the pituitary and thyroid glands. When insufficient amounts of iodine are available for normal functioning of this system, compensatory alterations in the thyroid gland result in considerable increase in its size. Simple *goiter* occurs chiefly in areas of the world where the soil is poor in iodine. Goiter is still endemic and a worldwide problem.

goiter
Enlargement of thyroid gland

Careful study of the varying incidence of goiter from one section to another in certain *endemic* areas has led some researchers to conclude that other factors besides iodine deficiency may contribute to the development of goiter. It has been suggested that the stress of iodine deficiency serves to uncover subtle biochemical defects in hormone synthesis in certain individuals (27). This would

endemic
Prevalent in a particular locality

help to explain why *all* people in a region where the soil is lacking in iodine do not develop goiter.

In the United States, the soil lacks iodine around the Great Lakes and in the Pacific Northwest; goiter was prevalent in these areas until about 60 years ago. Although goiter has been known for centuries, the importance of iodine as a preventive measure was not demonstrated until the 1900s. A study was begun in Akron, Ohio, in 1917 in which 2 grams of sodium iodide were fed semiannually for 2½ years to more than two thousand young girls. About the same number of girls served as controls, with no iodine added to their diets. Of the group receiving iodine, only five developed goiter; of those receiving no iodine, about *five hundred* developed goiter.

As a result of this and other studies, a movement was launched in 1922 to produce and sell iodized salt as a means of supplying iodine to goitrous regions. Follow-up studies through the mid-1950s showed that the incidence of goiter among children in Great Lakes regions had dropped dramatically in that 30-year period. This decline is attributed largely to the use of iodized salt, which is manufactured and distributed on a voluntary basis.

Another contributing factor to the decline in simple goiter is the present system of marketing foods far from their points of origin, thus increasing the possibility that people in goitrous regions will receive some of their foods from areas where the soil is iodine-rich.

Recommendations for daily intakes of iodine were first included in the RDA in 1968. They are based on indications from balance studies that adults require 50 to 75 micrograms daily. It is assumed that growing children and pregnant and lactating women need more. Intakes of 50 to 1000 micrograms of iodine a day have been estimated to be safe for adults; intakes between 100 and 300 micrograms a day are desirable (12).

There is a very small amount of iodine in the body. This mineral is also present in foods in minute quantities. Shellfish, salt-water fish, and fish that live a part of their lives in salt water are the best food sources of iodine. Foods grown on iodine-rich soils are good secondary sources. The same kind of food can vary widely in iodine content from sample to sample, depending on the iodine content of the soil in which it is grown. Iodized salt, if used routinely, is the most dependable source of iodine. At the current level of enrichment, iodized salt furnishes 75 micrograms of iodine per gram. The average use of table salt in the United States is estimated to be about 3.4 grams per person per day; slightly over half this salt is iodized. Salt used in commercial food processing and by schools and restaurant chains usually does not contain iodine. It has been suggested that all products designed to provide complete nutrient maintenance, such as infant formulas and meal replacers for adults, should contain sufficient iodine to provide their proportion of the RDA (12).

Recently there has been concern that excessive iodine intake may be a possibility for some people in the United States due to changes in agricultural practices, food manufacturing methods, medications, and other factors. The average consumption of iodine in the United States has actually increased in recent years and now may be five to ten times the RDA. Such rather large iodine intakes are harmless for most people; body mechanisms can adapt to differences of this magnitude. The few individuals who are predisposed to diet-induced *thyrotoxicosis*, causing an enlarged and hyperactive thyroid, should be under medical supervision. Grossly excessive intakes, however, cannot be accommodated even by normal individuals. For example, some inhabitants of Japan develop thyrotoxicosis as a result of consuming amounts of seaweed that contain on the average up to 20,000 micrograms of iodine per day (28).

thyrotoxicosis
Hyperthyroidism resulting in rapid heartbeat and tremors

Although intakes of iodine in the United States are high *on the average*, they are currently extremely variable. For this reason, it is still advisable that persons living in regions where goiter is endemic continue to use iodized salt to ensure an adequate intake of dietary iodine. Continued use of iodized salt by inhabitants of non-goitrous areas would probably not have adverse effects (28).

Data from the Ten-State Nutrition Survey showed no evidence of iodine deficiency in the United States population. In the first HANES, enlargement of the thyroid gland to the degree that it was classified as grade 1 goiter showed a prevalence of 10 percent or less in six of the eight survey groups. Blacks aged 12 to 17 years in the income group above poverty level (11.0 percent prevalance) and black women aged 18 to 44 years (10.1 percent prevalence) in the same income group were the exceptions (14).

FLUORIDE (8, 12, 25, 29)

Fluoride, an essential nutrient, is required for optimal dental health. This mineral is incorporated into the structure of teeth, providing maximum resistance to dental caries. The relationship of fluoride to dental caries was discovered through observations of the effects of excessive fluoride in drinking water in certain regions of the United States. Although the excess fluoride caused a mottled, unsightly condition in teeth, particularly in children who used the water from birth, these teeth did not decay readily. When the water naturally contained a small but definite amount of fluoride, the teeth were *not* mottled and they still resisted decay. This finding led in 1945 to the first experiments to test the effects of fluoride on the incidence of dental caries.

The studies were carried on in two cities on a control basis: the drinking water in one city was fortified with fluoride; that in a comparable second city was not fortified. The drinking water in Newburgh, New York, which was naturally low in fluoride content, was treated with 1 part fluoride per million parts water. The water in Kingston, New York, 30 miles distant, was not treated. Groups of children in both cities were given annual dental and medical examinations, in some cases for as long as 10 years. The findings were startling. At the end of the 10-year period, the children in Newburgh had an average of 60 percent fewer decayed teeth than the children in Kingston. The greatest benefits in Newburgh were observed in children who had used the fluoridated water since birth, and no unfavorable effects were found in any medical examinations. This type of experiment, which was repeated in many other locations in the United States and abroad, clearly demonstrated the safety and nutritional advantages of fluoride in the water supply.

Standardization of water supplies by the addition of enough fluoride to bring the concentration to 1 milligram per liter is an economical and efficient way to provide optimum intakes. Recognizing that people drink more water in hot weather, the Federal Environmental Protection Agency recommends a slight adjustment of the concentration of fluoride to allow for differences in consumption with seasonal temperature changes.

Fluoridation of community water supplies has been endorsed by the American Dental Association and leading medical and public health groups as desirable for dental health and harmless to general health. In spite of campaigns for fluoridation of public water supplies, it was estimated that probably less than one-half the United States population in 1972 received desirable intakes of fluoride from water. Attempts to provide fluoride by adding it to milk, salt, or flour for people who do not have access to water supplies containing fluoride have been partially successful in several European countries. A major advantage of fluoridated water, however, is that it provides a continuous source of fluoride automatically (see Chap. 3).

While fluoride is widely distributed in nature, few foods are rich sources. Milk, meat, fruits, and vegetables contain little fluoride. Fish and dry legumes are fair sources, tea is a good source. The daily intake in the diet, other than that from drinking water, is estimated to vary from 0.3 to 3.1 milligrams. Like other trace elements, fluoride is toxic when consumed in excessive amounts. Daily intakes of 20 to 80 milligrams or more, continued over long periods of time, produce symptoms of chronic toxicity.

Since the discovery that fluoride is a deterrent to dental caries, research has been directed to basic body functions of this mineral. Because fluoride is present in minute quantities in almost all soils, plants, and animals, it is difficult to produce a deficiency. Preparation of an experimental diet and control of conditions to ensure absolute lack of fluoride require special facilities and care. Only recently, therefore, has fluoride been demonstrated to be essential for normal growth in rats. A number of studies have suggested that fluoride plays a role in the maintenance of bone structure; its successful use in the treatment of osteoporosis seems to support this possibility.

ZINC (8, 12, 26)

Zinc is present in small or trace amounts in all living matter. In humans, a total of 2 to 3 grams of zinc is distributed throughout the body, with the highest concentrations found in tissues of the eye and in male sex organs. Zinc is an essential nutrient, functioning primarily as a constituent of numerous enzyme systems. Important in the formation of protein, zinc is necessary for growth and for normal sexual development in children. Zinc was included in the RDA table in 1974 for the first time.

Zinc deficiency syndromes have developed in farm animals in areas of the United States where soils were lacking in available zinc, necessitating addition of the mineral to animal feeds. Zinc deficiency in humans has resulted in *hypogonadism* and dwarfism in the Middle East. Marginal states of zinc deficiency have been recognized in the United States. In several studies, more rapid rates of wound healing and improved taste acuity were observed with increased zinc intake, suggesting that the subjects' needs for zinc had not been fully satisfied by their diets. Marginal zinc deficiency has also been observed in some apparently healthy children in the United States. Deficiency symptoms, including *hypogeusia*, lower-than-normal concentrations of zinc in hair, poor appetite, and suboptimal growth, were all improved by increasing the daily zinc intake.

Recently the effect of supplementing a commercial infant formula with zinc was investigated. The male infants, but not the females, in the supplemented group grew more in length and weight in the first 6 months of life than their counterparts in the control group. A lower incidence of disturbed gastrointestinal function also was associated with the addition of zinc to the infants' formula (30).

The average adult dietary intake of zinc is estimated to be 10 to 15 milligrams daily, of which about 5 milligrams are retained. Balance studies have shown that intakes in this range result in zinc equilibrium. The availability of dietary zinc for absorption is decreased by the presence of phytic acid, which forms an insoluble complex with zinc. The presence of calcium with phytate appears to further impair zinc absorption.

Foods of animal origin—meat, liver, eggs, seafood (especially oysters), cheese, and milk—are the best sources of available zinc. Legumes, nuts, and whole grains are also good sources. Fruits and parts of plants other than seeds (leaves, stems, roots, and blossoms) are very low in zinc. Milled grains, such as white flour, in which the bran and germ have been removed, furnish only about one-tenth to one-half as much zinc as the whole grain (Figure 8.11)

hypogonadism
Retardation of growth and sexual development due to decreased functional activity of testes and ovaries

hypogeusia
Impairment of the sense of taste

Figure 8.11
Excellent food sources of zinc.
(Landon Gardiner)

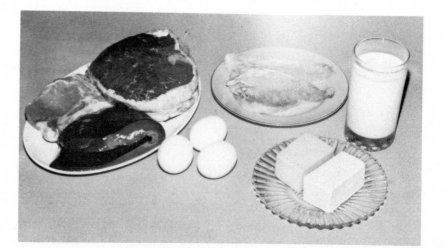

(31). (See Freeland and Cousins, 1976 and Murphy, Willis, and Watt, 1975 for zinc content of foods on page 227.)

> Do you feel somewhat overwhelmed by the large number of mineral elements important in nutrition? Organize the material pertaining to the functions and food sources of these nutrients. Try preparing a table similar to the one at the end of the chapter on proteins (Table 7.2, "Proteins—A Few Highlights").

OTHER TRACE MINERALS (12, 26, 32)

Research continues to reveal evidence of essential functions for other trace minerals in humans. Chromium, cobalt, manganese, molybdenum, and selenium are known to have relationships to human nutrition. No RDA have been established, and the amounts of these minerals found in most common foods are unknown. A balanced diet composed of basic foods would undoubtedly cover human needs for these minerals. It is conceivable that deficiencies might occur if highly refined foods and food product analogs comprise the major part of the diet. The brief comments that follow on the elements mentioned serve chiefly to indicate the functional interrelationships between these trace elements and other nutrients. This may be the key to an eventual clarification of their full nutritional importance to human beings.

COBALT

Cobalt is a component of the vitamin B_{12} molecule. This mineral is bound to protein in foods of animal origin. Cobalt is essential to the functioning of all cells—particularly those of the bone marrow, the nervous system, and the gastrointestinal tract. By its association with B_{12}, it plays a part in the prevention of pernicious anemia.

MANGANESE

Manganese is an essential element of normal bone structure and is found in highest concentration in bone. This mineral is part of certain human enzyme systems. In mammals, manganese deficiency is characterized by defective growth, bone abnormalities, and reproductive irregularities, as well as by disturbances in lipid metabolism. No human deficiency has been demonstrated. Nuts and whole grains are excellent sources of manganese; vegetables and fruits also provide important amounts. Meat, poultry, seafood, and fish are poor sources.

MOLYBDENUM

nucleic acids
Components of cell-nucleus proteins

Trace amounts of molybdenum and iron, along with riboflavin, function in an enzyme system involved in the digestion of certain *nucleic acids*. Molybdenum deficiencies have been produced in animals, but not in humans, indicating that amounts present in ordinary diets probably meet the human requirement for this mineral.

SELENIUM

Although several species of animals are known to require selenium, the biochemical function of this element is not yet clear. It is known to be capable of replacing vitamin E to a certain extent, particularly as an inhibitor of *lipid peroxidation*.

NICKEL, SILICON, TIN AND VANADIUM

Since 1970 nickel, silicon, tin, and vanadium have been found to be essential for normal growth and development of laboratory animals. It seems likely that they may also be essential for humans (32). A report of research findings related to these elements is beyond the scope of this book. You may wish to follow the scientific literature for the fascinating accounts of these little-understood elements as the stories of their development unfold.

lipid peroxidation
Formation from lipids of compounds unusually high in oxygen content believed to bring about disintegration of cell membranes

REFERENCES

1. J. Janick, C. H. Noller, and C. L. Rhykerd, "The Cycles of Plant and Animal Nutrition," *Scientific American* 235 (Sept. 1976), pp. 74-86.

2. W. H. Allaway, "The Effect of Soils and Fertilizers on Human and Animal Nutrition," USDA Agric. Inform. Bull. No. 378, 1975.

3. Committee on Nutritional Misinformation, *Soil Fertility and the Nutritive Value of Crops: a Statement of the Food and Nutrition Board* (Washington, D.C.: National Academy of Sciences, Sept. 1976).

4. D. M. Hegsted, "Calcium and Phosphorus," Chap. 6, Section A in R. S. Goodhart and M. E. Shils, eds., *Modern Nutrition in Health and Disease* (Philadelphia: Lea and Febiger, 1973).

5. J. H. Cummings, M. J. Hill, D. J. A. Jenkins, J. R. Pearson and H. S. Wiggins, "Changes in Fecal Composition and Colonic Function due to Cereal Fiber," *Am. J. Clin. Nutr.* 29 (Dec. 1976), pp. 1468-73.

6. L. D. McBean and E. W. Speckmann, "A Recognition of the Interrelationship of Calcium with Various Dietary Components," *Am. J. Clin. Nutr.* 27 (June 1974), pp. 603-09.

7. C. A. Adams, *Nutritive Value of American Foods in Common Units* (Washington, D.C.: USDA Agr. Res. Service, 1975).

8. R. L. Pike and M. L. Brown, *Nutrition: An Integrated Approach* (New York: John Wiley and Sons, Inc., 1975).

9. S. M. Garn, *The Earlier Gain and the Later Lo*
Bone in Nutritional Perspective (Springfield
Thomas, 1970).

10. S. M. Garn, "Malnutrition and Skeletal Deve
Preschool Child," Chap. 5 in *Preschool Child M.*
Primary Deterrent to Human Progress (Washington, D.C
tional Academy of Sciences—National Research Council, Pu
1282, 1966).

11. A. P. Iskrant, "The Etiology of Fractured Hips in Females,"
Am. J. Public Health 58 (March 1968), pp. 485-90.

12. Food and Nutrition Board, National Research Council, *Recommended Dietary Allowances*, 8th revision. (Washington, D.C.:
National Academy of Sciences, 1974).

13. A. A. Albanese, "Nutritional Aspects of Bone Loss," *Food and Nutrition News* 47 No. 1 and 2, pp. 1, 4 in each, 1975-1976.

14. S. Abraham, F. W. Lowenstein and D. E. O'Connell, *Preliminary Findings of the First Health and Nutrition Examination Survey, United States, 1971–72: Anthropometric and Clinical Findings*, DHEW Publication No. (HRA) 75-1229 (Washington, D.C.: US Gov. Print. Office, 1975).

15. C. Garza and N. S. Scrimshaw, "Relationship of lactose intolerance to milk intolerance in young children," *Am. J. Clin. Nutr.* 29 (Feb. 1976), pp. 192-96.

16. R. Marston and B. Friend, "Nutritional Review," *National Food Situation* 158, (Nov. 1976), pp. 25-32.

17. *Food Consumption of Households in the United States* (Washington, D.C.: USDA, 1967, Household Food Consumption Survey, 1965-66, Report Nos. 1, 2, 3, 4).

18. *Food Intake and Nutritive Value of Diets of Men, Women, and Children in the United States, Spring 1965* (Washington, D.C.: USDA, March 1969), ARS 62-18.

19. S. Abraham, F. W. Lowenstein, and C. L. Johnson, *Preliminary Findings of the First Health and Nutrition Examination Survey, United States, 1971-72: Dietary Intake and Biochemical Findings*, DHEW Publication No. (HRA) 76-1219-1 (Washington, D.C.: US Gov. Print. Office, 1974).

20. M. E. Shils, "Magnesium," Chap. 6, Section B in R. S. Goodhart and M. E. Shils, eds., *Modern Nutrition in Health and Disease* (Philadelphia: Lea and Febiger, 1973).

21. "Magnesium in Human Nutrition," *Dairy Council Digest* 42 (March-April 1971), pp. 7-10.

, J. Hiemstra, *Food Consumption, Prices and Expenditures*, Agric. Econ. Report No. 138 (Washington, D.C.: Econ. Res. Service, USDA, July 1968). (Also Supplement for 1975, published Jan. 1977.)

23. C. V. Moore, "Iron," Chap. 6, Section C in R. S. Goodhart and M. E. Shils, eds., *Modern Nutrition in Health and Disease* (Philadelphia: Lea and Febiger, 1973).

24. J. D. Cook and E. R. Monsen, "Food Iron Absorption in Human Subjects. III. Comparison of the Effect of Animal Proteins on Nonheme Iron Absorption," *Am. J. Clin. Nutr.* 29 (Aug. 1976), pp. 859-67.

25. S. J. Fomon, *Infant Nutrition* (Philadelphia: Saunders, 1974).

26. Ting-Kai Li and B. L. Vallee, "The Biochemical and Nutritional Role of Trace Elements" Chap. 8, Section B, in R. S. Goodhart and M. E. Shils, eds., *Modern Nutrition in Health and Disease* (Philadelphia: Lea and Febiger, 1973).

27. R. R. Cavalieri, "Trace Elements," Chap. 8, Section A, "Iodine" in R. S. Goodhart and M. E. Shils, eds., *Modern Nutrition in Health and Disease* (Philadelphia: Lea and Febiger, 1973).

28. R. W. Cullen and S. M. Oace, "Iodine: Current Status," *J. Nutr. Educ.* 6 (July-Sept. 1976), pp. 101-2.

29. J. H. Shaw and E. A. Sweeney, "Nutrition in Relation to Dental Medicine," Chap. 27 in R. S. Goodhart and M. E. Shils, eds., *Modern Nutrition in Health and Disease* (Philadelphia: Lea and Febiger, 1973).

30. P. A. Walravens and K. M. Hambidge, "Growth of Infants Fed a Zinc Supplemented Formula," *Am. J. Clin. Nutr.* 29 (Oct. 1976), pp. 1114-21.

31. B. W. Willis and A. P. Mangubat, "Zinc in Foods," *Family Econ. Rev.* (Spring 1975), pp. 16-17.

32. F. H. Nielsen, " 'Newer' Trace Elements in Human Nutrition," *Food Technology,* 28 (Jan. 1974), pp. 38-44.

READINGS

"Are Selenium Supplements Needed (By the General Public)?" *J. Am. Dietet. Assoc.* 70 (March 1977), pp. 249-50.

Baer, M. J., *Growth and Maturation* (Cambridge, Mass.: Howard A. Doyle Publishing, 1973).

Burch, R. E., H. K. J. Hahan and J. F. Sullivan, "Newer Aspects of the Roles of Zinc, Manganese, and Copper in Human Nutrition," *Clin. Chem.* 21 (April 1975), pp. 501-20.

Cook, J. D. and E. R. Monsen. "Vitamin C, the Common Cold, and Iron Absorption," *Am. J. Clin. Nutr.* 30 (Feb. 1977), pp. 235-41.

Fourman, P., P. Royer, M. J. Levell, and D. B. Morgan, *Calcium Metabolism and the Bone*, (Philadelphia: F. A. Davis, 1968).

Freeland, J. H. and R. J. Cousins, "Zinc Content of Selected Foods," *J. Am. Dietet. Assoc.* 68 (June 1976), pp. 526-29.

Kidd, P. S., F. L. Trowbridge, J. B. Goldsby, and M. A. Nichaman, "Sources of Dietary Iodine," *J. Am. Dietet. Assoc.* 65 (Oct. 1974), pp. 420-22.

Levander, O. A., "Selenium and Chromium in Human Nutrition," *J. Am. Dietet. Assoc.* 66 (April, 1975), pp. 338-44.

Murphy, E. W., B. W. Willis, and B. K. Watt, "Provisional Tables on the Zinc Content of Foods," *J. Am. Dietet. Assoc.* 66 (April, 1975), pp. 345-55.

Talbot, J. M., K. D. Fisher and C. J. Carr, *A Review of the Effects of Dietary Iodine on Certain Thyroid Disorders*, July 1976. Life Sciences Research Office, Federation of American Societies for Experimental Biology.

Vitamins

Fat-Soluble Vitamins:
A, D, E, and K
Water-Soluble Vitamins:
B-complex
Ascorbic Acid (Vitamin C)

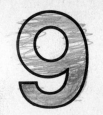

229 -231 - 242 -
245
248 - 49
250 - 57
67 - 70
70 - 71 - 79

In earlier chapters certain facts about vitamins were established: that vitamins, as a group, represent one of the six nutrient classes; that their importance in nutrition is out of all proportion to the minute quantities in which they are found in foods and are required by the body; that vitamins in foods are not broken down in the digestive processes but are absorbed essentially as they occur; and that vitamins, in broad terms, contribute to the building of the body structure and help regulate its processes.

You are now prepared to consider some of the individual vitamins in relation to nutrition and health; your need for those vitamins for which daily dietary allowances have been established; how you obtain the vitamins to which attention must be given in food selection; and the outcomes in nutritional status when there is enough, too much, or a deficiency of certain vitamins. Some general considerations will give a background for this chapter.

VITAMINS AS A GROUP

Vitamins make up the most recently discovered nutrient group. Scientists involved with animal feeding studies in the early part of this century realized that natural foods contained what they referred to as "accessory factors," which were necessary for the life and health of experimental animals. These substances were not present in pure proteins, fats, carbohydrates, and minerals—previously believed to be the sole components of an adequate diet. It was not until 1913, however, that the first of the vitamins was recognized as an individual nutrient. As more vitamins were discovered they were identified by letters of the alphabet. The term vitamin was derived from the Latin *vita*, meaning life. At first vitamins were thought to be chemically related to each other, but after several vitamins were identified and studied, it became apparent that they differed in chemical nature and in body functions and had little in common except the title "vitamin." Most of the vitamins have now been given scientific names that describe their individual characteristics. The discovery of vitamins introduced what came to be known as the newer knowledge of nutrition.

Vitamins are "essential" in the sense that they must be provided by foods; they cannot be synthesized by the body in sufficient quantities to satisfy its needs. More than a dozen vitamins occur naturally in foods and have been shown to contribute to human nutrition. They do not furnish energy, even though they are organic substances. The vitamins included by the Food and Nutrition Board on its dietary allowance table (see the RDA table) are the ones to which we must give special attention in selecting meals. When they and the other nutrients listed on the table are supplied through basic foods in amounts sufficient to meet the allowances, other vitamins required by the human body probably also will be provided adequately. Tentative allowances have been suggested for several of these other vitamins.

Vitamins act with each other and with other nutrients in coordinating body functions. This action is chiefly catalytic. Beyond that, their exact functions differ so greatly that it is impossible to generalize about them. Each vitamin has distinct and essential functions, and a severe shortage of any one vitamin leads eventually to a characteristic nutritional disorder. In some cases such disorders have been known for centuries, and frequently food "cures" (such as lemons for scurvy) were applied successfully long before vitamins were discovered. It was not until a deficiency of each major vitamin was linked by research to a specific nutritional disorder in humans that the cause-and-effect relationships were fully established.

Much present-day information about vitamins originated in studies with animals. Some of the basic research regarding the functions of vitamins in metabolic processes could be done only with animals, but suitable methods of working with human subjects are constantly being explored and developed. All research was strengthened when pure vitamins were made available. These made it possible to determine more precisely the characteristic responses of animals to specific vitamins. When comparable effects are identified in human beings, the functions of an individual vitamin in human nutrition are clarified. There is increasing interest in understanding how vitamins function in chemical reactions within the cells, and scientists of many disciplines have joined in a broad approach to vitamin research.

The vitamins on the RDA table and certain others are discussed here individually, with special emphasis on the positive contributions that adequate amounts of vitamins furnished by foods make to nutritional well-being. The conditions created by serious vitamin deficiencies are also described.

All vitamins fall into one of two classes with respect to their solubility: some are soluble in water; others are soluble in fat and in the solvents of fat, such as ether.

FAT-SOLUBLE VITAMINS

Solubility offers a practical basis for a discussion of vitamins because of its relation to the retention of vitamin values in foods. Vitamins A, D, E, and K—the fat-soluble vitamins—are generally more stable in ordinary handling and cooking processes than are the water-soluble vitamins. All fat-soluble vitamins are stored in the body to some extent. This fact has a bearing on the distribution of fat-soluble vitamins in the animal foods people eat and on the human body's ability to build up a reserve of them. Vitamins A and D were among the first to be discovered, and much is known about their functions, their food sources, and the body's need for them under different conditions. But more remains to be learned, and research continues to disclose more detailed information about them.

VITAMIN A

retinol
Chemical term for vitamin-A alcohol; form in which vitamin A functions in the body

provitamin
Compound chemically related to a vitamin; has vitamin value when converted to the biologically active form

Vitamin A occurs in nature in several slightly different forms. The related compounds that possess vitamin A value or activity may be classified under two headings: vitamin A as such (*retinol*), also referred to as *preformed vitamin A*, and certain carotenoid plant pigments, chiefly *beta-carotene* (β-carotene), which are called *provitamins A*. Both preformed vitamin A and provitamin A occur in the body and in foods. Vitamin A (retinol) is present only in foods of animal origin; carotene is found in both animal and vegetable foods (1, 2).

Carotene must be associated with dietary fat to be efficiently absorbed from the small intestine. Some of the carotenoids provided by foods are converted into retinol during or following absorption of the molecules through the intestinal wall. Their ability to undergo this conversion to vitamin A explains their classification as provitamin A.

Functions of Vitamin A

epithelial tissues
Skin and mucous membranes

Vitamin A is essential for maintaining *epithelial* tissues in normal condition. It also functions in the visual process. In this case the specific relationship of vitamin A to a bodily function is quite well established.

Vitamin A and Vision (1)   Vitamin A is known to be needed for vision. Vitamin-A deficiency results in *night blindness*, the first symptom of disability. In this condition one is unable to see well in dim light, particularly after exposure to a bright light. The blindness is explained by the fact that vitamin A, combined with a protein in the retina of the eye, forms a pigment called *visual purple* that is bleached in strong light. Some vitamin A is lost when this occurs. If the body has sufficient reserve vitamin A to draw upon, the regeneration of visual purple is rapid and the eyes adapt very quickly to subdued light. Vision returns almost at once. When there is a vitamin-A deficiency, however, the regeneration of visual purple is slow, and night blindness is a consequence. You may experience a mild degree of night blindness when you step from a brightly lighted lobby or from brilliant sunshine into a partially darkened theater, or when you face a dark road at night after being confronted with the glare of oncoming automobile headlights. Since night blindness can sometimes be due to a physical defect in the eye or some other cause, the vitamin-A-deficient condition is referred to as *functional* night blindness.

There is no sure way of knowing precisely how much functional night blindness there is in the United States or how severe it is. The condition is well known to people who are subjected routinely to strong light for long periods and then are plunged into darkness, such as those who fish or ski in the glare of sun on water or snow for hours and then try to make their way home after dark. Tragic stories are told of the fishermen of Newfoundland and Labrador, who in earlier days were lost at sea under these circumstances. Their basic diets were almost devoid of vitamin-A activity, and they did not realize that one of the richest sources was within their reach—the livers of the fish that filled their boats.

Vitamin A and Health of Epithelial Tissues   Vitamin A is needed for the maintenance and functioning of epithelial membranes: the skin and the linings of various body passages and cavities, such as the eyelids, eyes, nose, and mouth, and the respiratory, genitourinary, and digestive tracts. When a sufficient amount of vitamin A is available from the diet or from body stores, the membranes are moist, pliable, and intact; they provide a protective covering for the organs and resist bacterial invasion. When the diet is deficient in vitamin A and the stores are depleted, the membranes become thin, dry, horny, porous, and flaky. They are unable to perform their protective functions, and bacteria have ready access. A prolonged shortage of vitamin A therefore lowers barriers to certain infections.

Vitamin-A deficiency can also result in a dermatosis (*follicular hyperkeratosis*) that begins with a dry, rough, itching skin. Eruptive lesions appear at the sites of hair follicles on the surface of the skin. The lesions often appear on the back of the upper arm. This symptom is one that physicians participating in nutritional status surveys in the United States usually look for (3).

xerophthalmia
Dry, lusterless condition of the eye

Vitamin A and Eye Disease   The epithelial membranes of the eye are particularly susceptible to vitamin-A deficiency. In cases of extreme and prolonged shortages of vitamin A, *xerophthalmia* can result from changes in the epithelial tissue. Failure of the tear glands to function causes a dry eye and severe damage to the cornea. Unless vitamin A is introduced, further changes can develop, advancing to *keratomalacia*. The cornea softens, melting into a gelatinous mass, and blindness results due to damage of the lens (1).

A now-famous outbreak of xerophthalmia occurred in Denmark during World War I. Butter, the country's chief source of vitamin A, was being exported to England. The Danish children, drinking only skim milk, developed xerophthalmia, and many lost their eyesight. Danish physicians associated the condition with the recent discovery of fat-soluble vitamin A. When they restored whole milk to the children's diets, the eye disease was brought under control.

Xerophthalmia is almost never seen in the United States. The disease is prevalent in areas of the Far East and in certain regions of Africa and South America, where it is responsible for a high percentage of blindness, especially among children. Xerophthalmia occurs partly because many diets are low in fats that carry vitamin A, even when such fats are at hand. In Indonesia, for example, xerophthalmia was a serious menace at one time while a local product, red palm oil containing β-carotene, was being exported for the manufacture of soap. Xerophthalmia may also be due indirectly to inadequate fat intake. In certain areas of Central Africa, the consumption of carotene-containing green vegetables is sufficient to meet the vitamin-A requirements of most children, but because of the extremely low fat content of the diet, only a small percentage of the carotene is absorbed and made useful as vitamin A. In many cases xerophthalmia and *kwashiorkor* occur together in children (Fig. 9.1) (4).

kwashiorkor
Severe protein deficiency disease

Vitamin A and Growth   Vitamin A has some functions that are also attributed to other nutrients, such as growth, but this does not detract from the proved relationship of vitamin A to the growth process. In fact, the failure of laboratory animals to grow under certain feeding conditions led to the discovery of vitamin A, and the vitamin content of foods was first assessed by their ability to produce growth. The way in which vitamin A acts in growth is not clear, but apparently the skeleton is first to show growth retardation. Research with laboratory animals suggests that inadequate growth of the skull can lead to brain and nerve injury due to crowding. Vitamin A functions in tooth formation and calcification. In a severe, prolonged deficiency of vitamin A, the enamel-forming cells are affected resulting in abnormalities of the pulp, dentin and enamel (1, 5).

physiological
Pertaining to functions of the body

pathological
Pertaining to or caused by disease

lysosomal membranes
Tissue surrounding the lysosomes, which are structures in cells containing destructive enzymes

Other Functions of Vitamin A   Evidence shows that vitamin A affects many *physiological* functions, and a number of *pathological* lesions are seen in vitamin-A-deficient animals. It seems probable that vitamin A is involved in the regulation of membrane structure and function. Studies have demonstrated that normal concentrations of vitamin A ensure optimum stability of *lysosomal mem-*

branes (see Chap. 3), whereas in vitamin-A-deficiency *or* excess the membranes are destroyed (1).

Meeting Vitamin A Needs

As mentioned earlier, vitamin A in the human diet is derived from preformed vitamin A and from carotenoid "precursors" of the vitamin. Some foods of animal origin contain both vitamin A and various carotenes. Of the latter, β-carotene is most efficiently converted to vitamin A and is the most plentiful in human foods. The usual foods available to people in the United States are estimated to provide about half their total vitamin-A activity as retinol and half as provitamin A carotenoids (2).

In the past, the vitamin-A value of foods has been expressed as International Units (IU) of vitamin A. In arriving at a value for the total vitamin-A activity of a food, carotene was given only a fraction of the value of the preformed vitamin, because it is used less efficiently by the body. The expression of total vitamin-A activity as IU thus requires specifying the percentages of activity coming from retinol and from provitamins. In 1974, however, the Food and Nutrition Board gave the RDA for vitamin A both as IU and as *retinol equivalents* (see the RDA table). It is planned that vitamin-A activity eventually will be expressed only in terms of retinol equivalents. By definition, 1 retinol equivalent is equal to 1 microgram of retinol, 6 micrograms of β-carotene, or 12 micrograms of other provitamin A carotenoid. One retinol equivalent is equal to 3.33 IU of retinol or 10 IU of β-carotene (2). The expression of vitamin A needs only as retinol equivalents will be impractical, however, until tables of food composition provide vitamin-A activity in terms of retinol equivalents. The amount of carotene absorbed and the efficiency of its conversion to vitamin A varies with individuals. It depends also on such factors as the types of foods that provide the carotene, the way they are prepared, and the presence or absence of certain other nutrients. A high intake in terms of total vitamin-A activity, if obtained largely from vegetable sources, could present an overly optimistic picture of vitamin-A nutrition. A practical solution for meeting vitamin-A needs is to choose some foods daily that supply the preformed vitamin and to use an abundance of foods rich in the provitamin.

Certain losses can prevent an individual from meeting vitamin-A needs. For example, antibiotics and laxatives tend to decrease absorption of vitamin A from the intestinal tract. A common type of loss results from the indiscriminate use of mineral oil as a laxative. Vitamin A, as well as carotene, may be dissolved in the oil in the digestive tract. Since this oil is not absorbed, the vitamin is discarded from the body along with the oil. The loss can be minimized by taking the oil several hours after eating a meal.

Food Sources of Vitamin A and Carotene   The US Department of Agriculture reports that about 25 percent of all the available vitamin-A activity in the food supply of the United States comes from leafy green vegetables and orange-colored vegetables and fruits (6). Other vegetables and fruits can provide an additional 25 percent.

RDA
Nutrient standards for the United States

retinol equivalents
Measure of vitamin-A activity

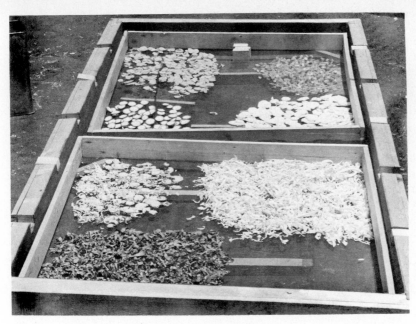

the remaining 50 percent of the vitamin-A activity comes chiefly
from four sources: 15 percent from dairy products, including butter;
6 percent each from other fats and from eggs; and 22 percent from
meats and poultry, largely from liver.

Color is a distinguishing feature of vitamin-A activity in foods.
Vitamin A itself is a very pale yellow. Carotene (so called because
it was first found in carrots) is a deep yellow-orange. Carotene is
present in both animal and vegetable foods, and it can be readily
identified in the yellow color of egg yolk, butter, fish-liver oils, and
the yellow cast of liver, as well as in the orange color of carrots,
sweet potatoes, winter squash, apricots, and cantaloupe. Carotene
is also present in green vegetables, although its color is obscured
by the green chlorophyll in these plants.

The specimen list of representative foods in Figure 9.2 is arranged in descending order of vitamin-A activity (total content of
β-carotene and vitamin A) per serving. The values are expressed in
IU rather than in grams or milligrams. One IU of vitamin-A activity equals the amount provided by 0.3 microgram of pure vitamin
A (retinol) or by 0.6 microgram of carotene. The USP (US Pharma-
copeia) unit is identical to the IU.

A 2-ounce serving of cooked beef liver stands at the top of Figure 9.2. It provides more than three times as much vitamin-A activity as does the average of 1 serving of each of the next three
sources: sweet potatoes, spinach, and carrots. Liver is the chief
storage organ for vitamin A in the animal body. The striking contrast between liver and muscle as storage points for vitamin A in
the meat animal is demonstrated by the difference between beef
liver and beef roast as sources of vitamin-A activity: 30,260 IU
compared to 20 IU. Livers of different animals vary in vitamin-A
activity, but all are concentrated sources. The richness of vitamin

Figure 9.2
Vitamin A: Servings of representative foods in order of their vitamin A content. (Each bar represents an approximate vitamin A value for the group of foods listed below it.)

Food*	Weight or ** approximate measure	Vitamin A activity International units
		30,000 IU
liver, beef	2 oz	30,260
		9,000 IU
sweet potato	1 medium	11,940
spinach	½ cup	8,100
carrots	½ cup	7,615
		1300 IU
broccoli	½ cup	1,940
cornflakes, fortified vit. A	1 cup	1,180
tomato juice	½ cup	970
		450 IU
peaches, canned, yellow flesh	½ cup	550
egg	1 medium	520
milk, skim, fortified	1 cup	510
peas, green	½ cup	480
butter or margarine	1 tbsp	470
corn, canned, yellow	½ cup	370
cheese, cheddar	1 oz	370
milk, whole	1 cup	350
beans, green	½ cup	340
		200 IU
orange juice	½ cup	270
lettuce, raw	1 cup	250
beans, dry, canned	¾ cup	248
banana, raw	1 medium	230
peppers, sweet, green, raw	½ medium	155
apple, raw	1 medium	120
cheese, cottage, creamed	¼ cup	105
		70 IU
chicken, fried	½ breast	70
cream, half and half	1 tbsp	70
pineapple juice	½ cup	65
tunafish	½ cup	65
cabbage, raw, chopped	½ cup	60
		35 IU
strawberries	½ cup	45
mayonnaise	1 tbsp	40
onions, yellow flesh	½ cup	40
beef, hamburger	3 oz	20
beef, lean chuck	3 oz	20
		10 IU and less
grapefruit, white	½ medium	10
buttermilk, no added vit. A	1 cup	10
raisins	¼ cup	8
bread, white, enriched	1 slice	tr
bread, whole wheat	1 slice	tr
bun or roll, enriched	1 bun	tr
potato, white	1 medium	tr
sugar	1 tbsp	0
beverages, cola type	12 oz	(0)†
macaroni, enriched, cooked	¾ cup	(0)
oatmeal, cooked	⅔ cup	(0)
pork chop	1 chop	(0)
rice, enriched, cooked	¾ cup	(0)
frankfurter	1 medium	—
haddock, fried	1 fillet (4 oz)	—
oil, salad or cooking	1 tbsp	—
peanut butter	2 tbsp	—
sausage, bologna	2 oz	—

* Foods are in forms ready to eat. All meats and vegetables are cooked unless otherwise indicated.
** See Appendix K for further identification of these foods. All foods are described there more fully, and both weights and measures are indicated.
† See Appendix J.

Table 9.1
Fortification standards for milks of different fat content

Milks	% Fat	Vitamin D	Vitamin A	Nonfat Milk Solids
		International Units	International Units	
fluid whole milk*	3.25, not less than	400 per qt (optional)	not less than 2000 per qt (optional)	no provision
fluid lowfat milk*	0.5, 1.0, 1.5, or 2	400 per qt (optional)	not less than 2000 per qt (mandatory)	optional
fluid skim milk*	0.5, less than	400 per qt (optional)	not less than 2000 per qt (mandatory)	optional
evaporated milk	7.5, not less than	25 per fluid oz (mandatory)	125 per fluid oz (optional)	no provision
nonfat dry milk fortified with vitamins A & D**	1.5, not more than by weight of milk fat	400 per reconstituted qt (mandatory)	2000 per reconstituted qt (mandatory)	no provision

Source: Code of Federal Regulations, Food & Drug Administration (FDA) 1976
*Must be pasteurized or sterilized
**There are also standards for a nonfortified dry milk, identified as nonfat dry milk.

A in liver and other organ meats is largely responsible for the fact that the meat group supplies about 20 percent of the vitamin A in the United States diet, despite the fact that the amount of liver in a meat animal represents a very small proportion of the total meat available.

In general, the vitamin-A value of foods decreases as the orange color diminishes in intensity. Sweet potatoes, for example, are richer in vitamin-A value than carrots; carrots much higher than peaches, and peaches more than twice as rich as bananas (Fig. 9.2).

Depth of color is not the sole gauge of vitamin-A activity in egg yolks and butterfat (whole milk, cream, and butter), which contain both carotene and preformed vitamin A. Different breeds of animals differ in their ability to convert carotene to vitamin A in their bodies. Therefore, deep yellow egg yolks or butterfat do not necessarily contain more vitamin-A activity than those of paler color. The deep yellow may merely indicate the presence of more unconverted carotene. Also, nature has not been entirely consistent in associating the orange color with provitamin A. Rutabaga, for example, is an orange-colored food, but its chief pigment is not carotene. Thus, ½ cup of cooked rutabagas yields 270 IU of vitamin-A activity, while the same amount of carrots provides 7615.

The association of vitamin-A activity with certain fats is shown in Figure 9.2 in the difference between the values for 1 cup of whole milk (350 IU) and the same amount of buttermilk made from skim milk (10 IU). In recognition of the increasing use of skim milk in the United States, it is now mandatory that not less than 2000 IU of vitamin A per quart be added to fluid skim milk and to lowfat milk. Therefore, fluid skim milk and lowfat milks sold in the United States are approximately equal to whole milk in vitamin-A value. Fortification standards for milks of different fat content are shown in Table 9.1. Fortification of dry skim milk is optional. If it is fortified, however, the product is designated as "nonfat dry milk fortified with vitamins A and D" and must contain 2000 IU of vitamin A and 400 IU of vitamin D per reconstituted quart. Federal specifications for fortified margarine require a minimum of 15,000 IU of vitamin A per pound, the approximate amount provided by butter.

More than half the foods in Figure 9.2 furnish less than 70 IU of vitamin-A activity per serving. This group includes all the muscle meats, all the fish, all the breads and unfortified cereals, the cooking fats and salad oils, sugar, and a few fruits and vegetables. These are negligible sources.

> Arrange your own list of representative foods in order of their quantitative importance as sources of vitamin-A activity by sorting your index cards or half sheets. Study the list with a view to associating kinds of foods with their vitamin-A activity.
>
> Enter vitamin-A activity values on your personal meal record. Total the vitamin-A activity for the day.
>
> Familiarize yourself with the relative vitamin-A activity within the three sources—orange-colored vegetables and orange-colored fruits, and vegetable "greens"—from Appendix K. Also note the wide difference in vitamin-A activity between green vegetables, such as green beans, and the dark green leafy vegetables, such as kale.

Stability of Vitamin A and Carotene   Vitamin A and carotene are insoluble in water and resistant to ordinary cooking temperatures. They are not lost or destroyed in boiling, for example, nor in freezing and canning processes. Vegetables, fruits, and eggs dried in air can lose much of their vitamin-A activity; those dried in a vacuum retain much of it. Fats exposed to air at warm temperatures become rancid, and rancidity destroys vitamin A and carotene.

Recommended Dietary Allowances (RDA) for Vitamin A (2)

The Food and Nutrition Board has proposed daily dietary allowances of vitamin-A activity for men and women of various ages (see the RDA table). An additional amount is recommended for pregnancy and for lactation. Progressively increased amounts of vitamin A are recommended throughout childhood. The allowances assume that the vitamin-A activity in the diet is approximately one-half the provitamin carotene and one-half preformed vitamin A.

The allowances are about double the minimal amounts required to protect against vitamin-A deficiency and are related to body weight during growth. The minimal values were doubled because of evidence that intakes above actual need are beneficial to health. Storage of vitamin A in the human liver also provides a reserve supply on which the body can draw for a considerable period of

**Table 9.2
Foods and combinations that provide
at least 4000 IU of vitamin A activity**

		Vitamin A IU
1		
liver, beef	2 oz	30,260
2		
spinach	½ cup	8,100
3		
carrots	¼ cup (½ serving)	3,808
peas, green	½ cup	480
	total	4,288
4		
apricots, stewed	½ cup	4,200
tomatoes, canned	½ cup	1,085
egg	1 medium	520
milk, whole	1 cup	350
orange	1 medium	260
lettuce, loose leaf	½ cup	525
	total	6,940

time without apparent harm, if the current diet should provide little or no vitamin A.

Meeting Vitamin-A Needs   The specimen diet in Appendix H shows how an adult can choose a diet that *appears* fairly satisfactory but that provides only about 2000 IU of vitamin-A activity. The butter or margarine and whole milk in the meals furnish about 1100 IU of the vitamin-A activity of the diet, or about half of that available from all the foods.

Examination of the items on the specimen diet shows that no rich source of vitamin-A activity was chosen from the vegetable-fruit group. The addition of a half-serving of any one of the deep yellow or deep green leafy vegetables would have more than completed the daily allowance. In terms of meal planning, this would amount to a full serving of one rich source every other day. Thus the problem of obtaining a diet with adequate vitamin-A activity lies not in scarcity of the vitamin in common foods, but in knowing and using, at suitable intervals, the excellent sources available.

The food listings in Table 9.2 show four ways in which dietary needs for vitamin A can be met. The first shows the usefulness of liver as a source of vitamin-A activity on a weekly basis; the second demonstrates how a rich vegetable source can serve on an every-other-day basis; in the third an excellent source (carrots) is supplemented with a lesser source on a daily basis; and the fourth suggests a possible combination that furnishes an ample amount of vitamin A when highly concentrated sources are omitted. The specimen diet in Appendix H illustrates the possibilities for failing to attain the allowance when no concentrated source of vitamin-A activity is included. The omission of vegetables, particularly those highest in vitamin-A activity, can be traced to the general lack of acceptance of vegetables by both adults and children, as discussed in Chapter 1.

The problem of meeting a child's needs for vitamin A is not unlike that of meeting the adult's. It is a matter of making sure that certain excellent sources are included in the diet at suitable intervals to provide for an adequate daily average intake.

What is the daily dietary allowance of vitamin-A activity for your sex-age group (see the RDA table)?

How does your intake, as shown on your personal meal record, compare with this allowance? Explain why it falls below the allowance or exceeds the allowance in terms of your selection of foods. If it falls below, how could you increase it without changing your food habits drastically?

Excesses of Vitamin A and Carotene   Despite the fact that amounts of vitamin-A activity greater than the allowances are believed to be beneficial to health, there is increasing evidence that *large* excesses are *toxic* (1, 2). Such excesses result not from eating rich food sources but from taking highly potent concentrates in liquid or capsule form (7). Children are more susceptible to toxicity than adults. Many symptoms from such excesses have been reported, including loss of appetite, irritability, bone *decalcification*, and skin lesions.

Large doses of vitamin A are frequently prescribed in the treatment of dermatological conditions. Continued intake of doses 20 to 30 times the RDA without medical supervision has led to chronic *hypervitaminosis A* in adults. There also are reports of development of vitamin A toxicity in people who have used large doses of vitamin preparations on a daily basis at the suggestion by non-professionals that large quantities of vitamins would provide health benefits (1).

Excessively large daily intakes of vegetables high in carotenoids may produce a yellow skin color, as a result of an accumulation of carotene in the blood. The conversion of carotene to vitamin A is not rapid enough to cause vitamin A toxicity, however (1). The abnormal skin coloration disappears when ingestion of carotenoids is discontinued for a time.

toxic
Harmful, poisonous

decalcification
Loss of calcium from bone

hypervitaminosis
Condition produced by an excessive intake of a vitamin

Vitamin A in the National Diet

On the basis of the vitamin-A activity available from the total United States food supply, there is potentially enough for each person to receive 8200 IU daily (6). This amount is considerably greater than the daily allowance for any age or condition except lactation. Of course, it does not represent actual intake.

A sample of household diets analyzed by the US Department of Agriculture in 1965 presents a less favorable picture. It showed that only about three-fourths of the diets met the vitamin-A activity allowance (8). A study of the diets of individuals in some of these households gave more definitive information about vitamin-A intakes by sex-age groups. The diets for several age groups of girls and women averaged 5 to 15 percent below the RDA for vitamin-A activity; the diets of elderly men and women also averaged somewhat below the RDA. For most age groups of males, the vitamin-A intakes were 10 percent or more *above* the RDA (9).

More recently, the HANES (1971-72), preliminary findings showed that mean intakes of vitamin A exceeded its standards (see Table 8.2) for all age, sex, race, and income groups except two. The mean intake of 18- to 44-year-old white females below poverty level reached 80 percent of this standard, and that of 12- to 17-year-old blacks above poverty level reached 90 percent of this standard. Without examining the data for individuals that make up these means, it might be assumed that intake of vitamin A in the United States is adequate. The mean figures include very wide ranges, however; they appear favorable partly because 20 percent of the individuals in the study had intakes more than twice as high as the standard. A large proportion of persons had intakes considerably below these standards, particularly children aged 1 to 5 years (about 40 percent below) and adults 18 to 44 and over 60 (about 60 percent below) (10).

Assessing Nutritional Status

Average intakes of vitamin A for most families and for many age groups appear reasonably reassuring. Also the national food supply is rich in the vitamin. But some individuals with low intakes of vitamin A may be deficient. Just what difference such variations make in terms of nutritional status with respect to vitamin A has been the subject of many studies of children and adults. In these studies biochemical assays of levels of vitamin A in the blood are made and individuals are examined clinically for outward signs of vitamin-A deficiencies, especially skin and eye conditions. The findings are compared with diet records of the same individuals in an attempt to discern diet-health relationships.

In general, diets routinely poor in vitamin A and carotene have been associated with low blood levels of vitamin A or carotene, or both. Such signs as roughness of the skin and inflammation of the mucous membranes of the eyes, related to vitamin-A deficiency, have been found more frequently in persons with low blood levels of vitamin-A activity than in those with satisfactory blood levels.

Among children and adults in economically deprived areas of the United States, many diets fell as much as 50 percent below the RDA for vitamin-A activity. A large percentage of individuals in these populations also showed serum vitamin A below acceptable levels (11). Age groups varied in their responses, but children of all ages showed the lowest vitamin-A serum levels. In a study confined to preschool children at all economic strata, a small percentage with least incomes showed mildly low plasma levels of vitamin A and correspondingly low intakes of the vitamin (12).

Mean serum vitamin A levels found in the HANES were higher for whites than for blacks of any age group regardless of income. In general, however, mean levels of serum vitamin A were higher in groups above the poverty level for whites and blacks alike. A particularly large proportion of black children aged 1 to 5 years had low serum vitamin-A values. The data suggested a potential problem of nutritional vitamin-A deficiency in 10 percent of these children. There was a relatively low correlation between serum vitamin A levels and dietary intake in this study. Clinical examination revealed very few eye signs characteristic of vitamin-A deficiency. Skin signs suggestive of deficiency were follicular hyperkeratosis of the arms and back, and *xerosis* of the skin (3, 10).

xerosis
Abnormal dryness of the skin of mucous membranes

VITAMIN D

Vitamin D occurs in the body and in foods in two forms: as the preformed vitamin D and as a provitamin (2, 13). The provitamin present in animals is a form of cholesterol; the one in plants is ergosterol. When exposed to the ultraviolet rays of the sun or an ultraviolet lamp *7-dehydrocholesterol* (the provitamin in animals) is changed to *cholecalciferol* (vitamin D_3), and *ergosterol* becomes *ergocalciferol* (vitamin D_2). Both forms of the vitamin seem to be equally effective in humans (2). The term "vitamin D" commonly refers to either form.

cholesterol
Fatty substance; normal constituent of blood

ergosterol
Fat-soluble substance with complex molecular structure

Functions of Vitamin D

Vitamin D is essential in human nutrition for the regulation of calcium and phosphate metabolism. It promotes the intestinal absorption of calcium and is important in the utilization of calcium and phosphorus as they function in the normal formation and maintenance of bones. This need is particularly critical in infancy, childhood, pregnancy, and lactation, but it is virtually continuous throughout life as bone is resorbed and remodeled (see Chap. 8).

metabolism
Process by which a nutrient is utilized by the body

There must be a satisfactory balance of calcium and phosphorus in the body if bones are to grow and develop properly. Vitamin D assists in maintaining the proper calcium-phosphorus level in the blood. If there is a deficiency of vitamin D, these minerals will not be deposited properly, though they are present in sufficient amounts. As a result, bones fail to calcify normally. In the young this condition is known as *rickets*. The bones bend easily and malformations, including bowed legs, are often an outcome. Faulty formation of the teeth and a delayed tooth-eruption timetable may also accompany this disorder. Premature infants and babies are more susceptible to rickets than are older children because of their rapid growth rate.

Rickets has been known as a bone disease of infants for centuries. The usefulness of cod-liver oil in controlling rickets was recognized in some countries in the 19th century, but vitamin D, the curative property in the oil, was not identified for another hundred years. After the discovery of vitamin D in 1922, its use as a dietary supplement increased rapidly. Pediatricians now prescribe a vitamin-D supplement for breastfed infants and for infants of low birth weight, and most infant formulas are fortified with vitamin D. As a result of these practices, rickets has largely disappeared in the United States. Its decline also has been attributed to the addition of vitamin D to the milk supply (2). *Osteomalacia* is the disease of the adult skeleton comparable to rickets in children. (*Osteoporosis*, another bone disease in adults, is discussed under calcium in Chapter 8.)

osteomalacia
Softening of the bone due to loss of calcium

osteoporosis
Disorder in which there is a reduced amount of bone

Vitamin D has been used in the prevention and cure of rickets and osteomalacia for many years. Only recently, however, has research provided an understanding of the manner in which this vitamin is metabolized in the body to affect bone structure and calcium utilization. Dietary vitamin D is absorbed with fat and is influenced by factors affecting fat absorption in general. The vitamin is concentrated in the liver, where it undergoes a chemical modification. It is then bound to a specific protein carrier and transported to the kidney for a final change in structure to the form that is biologically active. This is the substance that functions in the transport of calcium across the intestinal mucosa (13). It is in this form also that vitamin D, along with the parathyroid hormone, is needed for the release of calcium from the bones to maintain a normal calcium concentration in blood (see Chap. 8).

Rickets and osteomalacia are not always caused by vitamin-D deficiency. These disorders may result from metabolic abnormalities, such as inborn errors of metabolism or gastrointestinal, liver, or kidney malfunction. In such cases the disorder is not corrected by administration of vitamin D. Rickets or osteomalacia may develop even with adequate dietary intake of vitamin D, when the liver or kidney is incapable of doing its part in the conversion of the vitamin to its metabolically active form. In the United States these causes are more commonly implicated than dietary deficiency of vitamin D in cases of rickets (14).

Sources of Vitamin D

Vitamin D as such occurs naturally in few common foods, and then usually in very small amounts. Liver, butterfat, and egg yolk contain some vitamin D. Most salt-water fish are relatively good sources; the vitamin is present in body fat but is more concentrated in the liver oil. Fish-liver oils are in fact the richest natural sources of vitamin D. In strong contrast, vegetable oils are negligible sources.

Vitamin D is measured in terms of International Units (IU). Each unit is based on the activity of 0.025 microgram of pure crystalline vitamin D. Many available dietary supplements are concentrated sources of vitamin D and are standardized and labeled according to their potency. The dosage should always be prescribed by a physician. Vitamin-D fortified milk is a widely available and most practical source of vitamin D. An important asset of vitamin-D milk is the fact that it supplies the vitamin automatically in routine daily meals.

Fortification of Food Sources   When foods were found to contain little vitamin D naturally, a movement was started to fortify one staple food with this vitamin. Professional groups agreed upon milk as the most logical food for vitamin-D fortification, because of the universality of its use and its calcium and phosphorus content. Fresh, evaporated, and some dry milks are fortified with vitamin D by adding a known amount of a vitamin-D concentrate to a specified quantity of milk. The final product provides 400 IU of vitamin D per fresh or reconstituted quart. *Homogenization* distributes the vitamin evenly throughout the milk. The 400-IU yield per quart of vitamin D milk was planned to correspond with the recommended daily dietary allowances for the vitamin.

homogenization
Mechanical process of forcing milk under high pressure through very small openings to disperse fat in such fine globules that it will remain distributed throughout

Stability of Vitamin D   Vitamin D remains stable at ordinary cooking temperatures as well as in processing and storage. Heated vitamin-D milk does not lose its vitamin-D content nor does fish-liver oil lose its vitamin-D value during storage.

Recommended Dietary Allowances for Vitamin D

Allowances have been established for infants, children, adolescents, young adults, and pregnant and lactating women. There is evidence that vitamin D is needed throughout all human growth periods, but the specific quantities required at different age levels have not been determined precisely. In infants, 300 to 400 IU of vitamin D per day seem to promote optimum calcium absorption and growth (2). It has been demonstrated that the recommended level of vitamin D is sufficient for good calcium nutrition in all the age groups specified in the RDA table if calcium and phosphorus intakes are adequate.

Meeting Vitamin D Needs   The required intake of vitamin D at any age depends on the amount normally created in the body by exposure to sunlight, or more specifically, the sun's ultraviolet rays. The amount of vitamin D from this source varies widely with the potency of the ultraviolet rays that reach the skin. In the tropics, for example, where clothing is scanty, people live out of doors, and the rays of the sun are direct, rickets is little known, except where the mode of life excludes the sun. In areas where the days are shorter and the ultraviolet rays less direct, people spend much time indoors, and heavy clothing often covers the body. Here rickets has been a serious problem. The condition of the atmosphere in any climate is another important factor. A clear atmosphere free of clouds, dust, fog, and smoke permits the maximum vitamin-D activity from the sun (14).

During pregnancy and lactation, the requirements for calcium and phosphorus are greatly increased over usual adult needs to satisfy the demands of the infant's developing skeleton. Vitamin D is also required at this time to play its usual role of helping to utilize these two minerals to the fullest. Probably men and nonpregnant women need not give thought to a supplemental source of vitamin D unless they are routinely deprived of sunlight, either by occupation (such as night workers), or by clothing (such as members of some religious orders). Most adults in the United States obtain a considerable amount of vitamin D automatically from vitamin-D milk and other fortified foods. Older people, if they are closely housed, may benefit from small amounts of additional vitamin D. Attention should also be given to assuring an adequate calcium intake; increased vitamin D does not compensate for the lack of this mineral. Formula-fed infants usually obtain about 400 IU of vitamin D daily from vitamin-D milk or from commercial preparations. Because human milk is low in vitamin D, pediatricians usually prescribe a daily supplement of about 400 IU for breast-fed infants.

Storage of Vitamin D   Vitamin D is stored in the body to some extent. After it is absorbed from the intestine or formed in the body, it goes to the liver, where most of the excess is held until it is needed. Body reserves of the vitamin undoubtedly help to prevent some vitamin-D deficiencies.

Excesses of Vitamin D   Excesses of vitamin D beyond need provide no benefit in normal individuals and may be dangerously toxic (2). Because vitamin D stimulates the absorption of calcium from the intestine, a large excess stored in the body can cause blood levels of calcium to become abnormally high. In chronic *hypercalcemia*, calcium may be deposited in the soft tissues (15). Early signs of toxicity may include loss of appetite, weakness, nausea, and constipation, followed by more serious symptoms if the excess continues. Individuals vary widely in their sensitivity to an excess of vitamin D, so it is impossible to specify any amount as the minimal toxic dose. Toxic effects are seen most often in infants who have received unintentional overdoses of highly concentrated sources and in adults using excessive amounts as dietary supplements. There may be a narrow margin of safety between the requirement and a toxic dosage. Daily intakes in the range of 2000 to 3000 IU per day have been reported to cause hypercalcemia in infants and to produce evidence of toxicity in adults as well. Such findings have led the Food and Nutrition Board to recommend that vitamin-D intakes should not greatly exceed the RDA (see the RDA Table). Particularly in infancy, intakes above 1000 IU per day should be avoided (16). When large doses of vitamin D are prescribed, patients must be closely supervised by a physician (15).

hypercalcemia
Abnormally high level of calcium in the blood

VITAMIN E

Vitamin E was discovered in 1922. It is a fat-soluble vitamin named *tocopherol*. Eight naturally occurring tocopherols have been isolated but only one, *alpha tocopherol*, is considered in dietary evaluations, because of its relatively higher potency. One IU of vitamin E is equal to 1 milligram of synthetic dl-*alpha-tocopherol acetate* (2).

Vitamin E is an essential nutrient for humans and for many other *vertebrates*. It is found in many different tissues, but body stores are largely in muscle and in *adipose tissue*.

vertebrates
Animals having a backbone or spinal column

adipose tissue
Fatty tissue

Functions of Vitamin E

The precise biochemical mechanism through which vitamin E serves the body is not yet known. Vitamin E is an *antioxidant,* and its importance to the human body appears to lie largely in this property (17).

Separated food fats have long been known to require protection against oxidation in order to prevent rancidity. *Polyunsaturated lipids* that are integral parts of animal cell membranes, such as *phospholipids* and vitamin A, may also require protection from oxidative destruction (18). In the tissues vitamin E, as an antioxidant, provides this protection. It combines with oxygen, thus making the oxygen unavailable to oxidizing agents such as the peroxides from unsaturated fatty acids which cause deterioration. As the intake of dietary polyunsaturated fatty acids increases, they become more concentrated in body tissues, thus increasing the need for vitamin E. The body's requirement of dietary vitamin E is therefore closely related to the amount of polyunsaturated fatty acids consumed. Nature has provided plants containing high levels of polyunsaturated lipids with the ability to synthesize tocopherols, usually in direct proportion to the amount of lipids present that are susceptible to *oxidative deterioration* (see Chap. 5).

In one long-term study, in which adult men were maintained for 6 years on a diet low in vitamin E, there was a small decrease in the survival time of *erythrocytes.* The investigator raised the question about whether the normal lifespan of other types of cells in the body might also be shortened when the phospholipids in their cell walls are not protected by an adequate level of antioxidant (18).

A deficiency of vitamin E manifests itself in different ways in different species. All the experimentally produced effects of vitamin-E deficiency in animals are related in some way to the levels of polyunsaturated fatty acids in the diet and in the affected tissues. Pathological changes occur in the reproductive system, the muscles, the nervous system, and the vascular system.

Reproductive functions are impaired in a number of animal species when a vitamin-E deficiency occurs. There is no convincing evidence, however, that reproductive malfunctions in humans are related to increased need for vitamin E (17). Nutritional muscular dystrophy develops in certain animal species as a result of vitamin-E deficiency. The hereditary *muscular dystrophy* in humans is a distinctly different disorder unrelated to vitamin-E nutrition (17).

Children who are unable to absorb fat normally, as well as infants of low birth weight and full-size infants on low intakes of tocopherol, have lower-than-normal concentrations of vitamin E in their plasma. *Hemolytic anemia* has been reported in premature infants with low serum concentrations of vitamin E (16). Premature infants have relatively low body stores of vitamin E and diminished ability to absorb fat. For these reasons, they may require a vitamin E supplement. Patients with chronic malabsorption syndromes also need a supplement.

Many health claims have been made for vitamin E. One of these is that its antioxidant properties help slow the aging process.

antioxidant
Easily oxidized substance that protects other substances against oxidation

polyunsaturated lipid
Fatty acid containing 2 or more double bonds between carbon atoms

phospholipid
Fat molecule containing phosphate and nitrogenous groups

oxidative deterioration
Breakdown of molecule due to addition of oxygen or removal of hydrogen

erythrocytes
Red blood cells

muscular dystrophy
Disorder of skeletal muscles; progressive wasting of tissue leading to paralysis

hemolytic anemia
Decreased capacity of blood to carry oxygen due to breakdown of red blood cells with liberation of hemoglobin

The hope of finding a substance to sustain youth has been a strong one through the centuries. Aging is a very complex process, however, and it seems unlikely that any one substance will effect a change in the natural series of events that occur in people as they become older.

Results of several animal research studies suggest that vitamin E may protect against lung damage by certain oxidative components of air pollution, such as nitrogen dioxide and ozone. Experiments with rats have demonstrated that a wide range of vitamin E intake levels, along with other defense systems, appear to protect the lungs (19, 20).

Meeting Vitamin E Needs

The vitamin-E content of diets in the United States varies widely, depending primarily on the amounts and types of dietary fat consumed. The Food and Nutrition Board believes there is no evidence that vitamin E status is inadequate in normal individuals eating balanced diets. Nearly two-thirds of the vitamin E in the United States food supply comes from salad oils, shortening, and margarine; some 11 percent is supplied by fruits and vegetables; 7 percent is provided by grain products. As mentioned earlier, there is evidence (mainly from animal studies) that the requirement for vitamin E is increased with high levels of polyunsaturated fatty acids in the diet. The primary sources of these fatty acids—soybean, cottonseed, and corn oils—are also rich sources of vitamin E, so that increased polyunsaturated fatty acid intakes may automatically provide additional vitamin E (Fig. 9.3).

Ordinary cooking methods do not destroy vitamin E, but there

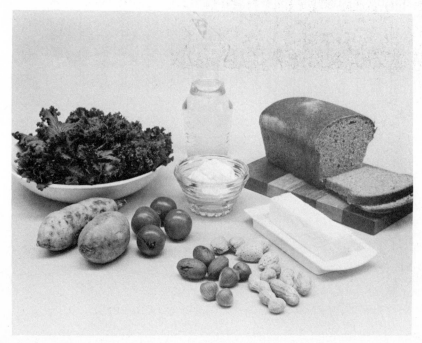

Figure 9.3
Common food sources of vitamin E. (Landon Gardiner)

are some losses in deep-fat frying, frozen storage, and in commercial processing when oxidation is involved.

The adult requirement for vitamin E when the diet contains the minimum of essential fatty acids is not known; it has been judged to be not more than 6 IU per day. (See the RDA table for the current RDA of vitamin E.) A dietary intake of vitamin E that maintains a blood concentration of total tocopherols above 0.5 milligram per 100 milliliters is believed to ensure that all tissues will contain an adequate concentration; that is, they will contain a ratio of tocopherols to polyunsaturated fatty acids that permits normal functioning of tissues and provides an allowance for possible stress situations (2).

A distinction should be made between the biological functions of vitamin E as an essential nutrient and its possible *pharmacological* action when taken in amounts many times larger than those needed to satisfy the nutritional requirement (18). Vitamin E has been taken in large doses as a supplement by many people in the United States in recent years. The vitamin has been prescribed by physicians as treatment for a wide variety of disorders and has been self-prescribed for all manner of conditions. The possible benefits resulting from clinical uses of large doses of vitamin E are now being carefully investigated.

The statement frequently has been made that vitamin E is not toxic even in large doses. Only recently, however, has a systematic evaluation of the possibility of toxicity been undertaken. A small group of adults voluntarily ingesting between 100 and 800 IU of tocopherol daily for an average of 3 years were evaluated by the performance of twenty standard clinical blood tests to assess a wide range of organ functions. It was concluded that the *megavitamin* supplements produced no apparent toxic side effects (21).

Hypervitaminosis E has recently been demonstrated in chicks fed high levels of the vitamin. Some effects were the depression of growth, of bone mineralization, and of hematocrit levels, as well as increased *prothrombin times* (22). Such evidence suggests that although adverse effects of high intakes have not been conclusively demonstrated in humans, further controlled evaluation of long-term, high-level vitamin-E intake is needed (22).

VITAMIN K

Vitamin K is essential to normal coagulation of blood, a very complex process that involves many factors. (When the clotting mechanism fails, there is danger of excessive bleeding.) Although its role in blood clotting is not fully understood, we do know that vitamin K acts in the synthesis of *prothrombin* and three other blood-clotting factors in the liver cells. These factors decrease in vitamin-K deficiency and rise to normal levels after administration of the vitamin. Defective blood coagulation is the only known sign of vitamin-K deficiency in animals (2, 23).

It appears that newborn infants normally have relatively low concentrations of prothrombin and other clotting factors. These levels decrease further during the first days of life, then rise naturally to normal concentrations. Vitamin-K deficiency, resulting in

pharmacological
Non-nutritional actions of very large doses of nutrients

megavitamin
Massive dose of a vitamin

prothrombin time
Length of time required for plasma to clot

prothrombin
Protein synthesized in liver, needed for blood to clot

hemorrhagic disease of the newborn
Vitamin K deficiency with bleeding

anticoagulant
Substance that prevents blood coagulation by interfering with the clotting mechanism

parenteral
Introduction of nutrients by vein or into subcutaneous tissues

very low plasma prothrombin levels, sometimes leads to *hemorrhagic disease of the newborn*. Vitamin-K deficiency is more common in premature infants and in infants born to mothers receiving *anticoagulants* than in normal, full-term infants (16). The Committee on Nutrition of the American Academy of Pediatrics recommends that every newborn infant receive a *parenteral* dose of 0.5 to 1.0 milligram of vitamin K as a preventive measure soon after birth (24).

In certain conditions such as coronary artery disease, the danger of *thrombus* (blood clot) formation may require anticoagulant therapy. Drugs administered as anticoagulants (Dicumarol, for example) are antagonists of vitamin K. They are believed to compete with vitamin K at the site in the liver where it functions in the synthesis of clotting factors, thus blocking normal production. This has the effect of reducing the ability of the blood to clot.

For the general population in the United States, there seems to be no reason to supplement diets with vitamin K unless there is liver injury, an abnormality in fat absorption, or some other condition for which a physician prescribes additional amounts of the vitamin.

The human requirement for vitamin K has not been determined. There are two sources of this vitamin: common foods, and the small amount synthesized by bacteria in the intestinal tract. The prevalence of vitamin K in a wide variety of green leafy vegetables, egg yolk, cow's milk, and organ meats makes a dietary deficiency rare in adults.

WATER-SOLUBLE VITAMINS

The water-soluble vitamins make up a large nutrient group, and all but one of them belong to the *B complex*. The remaining water-soluble vitamin is *ascorbic acid*, or vitamin C. For the most part, water-soluble vitamins are not stored in the body. Excesses are largely excreted, thus reducing the possibilities for toxicity that exist with overdosages of fat-soluble vitamins.

At least eleven vitamins compose the B complex. Most of them are essential in human nutrition and must be provided routinely in meals; a number of the B vitamins are included on the allowance table of the Food and Nutrition Board (see the RDA table). All the B vitamins were once thought to be a single substance, but gradually their separate identities became established. Certain overlapping characteristics and functions delayed the process of separation. For example, the fact that all B vitamins are soluble in water led to identification difficulties. All of them serve basically as *coenzymes* in converting the end products of carbohydrate, fat, and protein digestion into a form of energy the body can use.

coenzyme
Constituent of an enzyme system; usually containing a vitamin

Enzymes are proteins synthesized by living cells (see Chap. 7). They act as catalysts, for they can induce chemical changes in other substances without themselves being changed. All the B vitamins function as coenzymes; that is, each is capable of uniting with an inactive form of an enzyme to make a new compound that takes on enzyme activity. Numerous enzymes are involved in the intermediary metabolism of carbohydrate, fat, and protein in the tissues. The normal breakdown of monosaccharides, fats, and amino acids for the liberation of energy in the cells requires a series of enzyme-dependent chemical reactions. Each of the B vitamins, in its coenzyme capacity, performs in a specific way with respect to the metabolism of the nutrients. The major B vitamins are *thiamin, riboflavin, niacin, folic acid, B_{12}, B_6,* and *pantothenic acid.*

THIAMIN

Functions of Thiamin

Thiamin, in the form of *thiamin pyrophosphate*, functions in the body as a coenzyme. It is attached to a protein and is essential for the oxidation of glucose. When there is enough thiamin, the process proceeds normally, but if there is not enough, *pyruvic acid*, one of the intermediary products of carbohydrate metabolism, accumulates in the blood and tissues. This condition can lead to poor functioning of the gastrointestinal tract and to anorexia. Thus thiamin is essential to good digestion and to the maintenance of a good appetite. Growth failure in laboratory animals, traceable to a low thiamin diet, has been attributed largely to the lack of a desire to eat.

anorexia
Loss of appetite

Thiamin is also necessary for the normal functioning of the nervous system. Mild thiamin deficiency produced experimentally in human adults gradually resulted in appetite failure, nausea, and general apathy. Eventually the subjects became depressed, irritable, and moody, and their leg muscles were tender and painful. These symptoms were produced with thiamin levels that may not be far below those found in customary diets of some individuals in the United States (25).

Beriberi—Thiamin Deficiency Disease   A very low intake of thiamin leads eventually to *beriberi*, a dietary deficiency disease of the nervous system. Beriberi is characterized by degeneration of nerve tissue (especially in the arms and legs) by muscle weakness, and eventually by heart disease, edema, and paralysis. The disease has been known for centuries and plagued the Japanese Navy for many generations. Sailors on ships' rations consisting mainly of rice usually became ill, and many did not survive long sea voyages. When meats or legumes were added to the diet, beriberi was prevented or cured. For a time this favorable effect was mistakenly attributed to protein.

edema
Condition in which abnormally large amounts of water are retained in the tissues

In the late 19th century it was discovered by accident that a diet of polished white rice could produce a beriberilike disease in chickens, and that feeding the chickens polishings of the rice would cure it. A concentrate from the rice polishings brought about dramatic recovery when administered to people with beriberi. The curative property in the polishings was isolated about 40 years later and named vitamin B. In another 10 years the chemical structure of the vitamin was determined, and it was synthesized. Its official name then became thiamin (26).

Beriberi is still an important cause of disability and death in

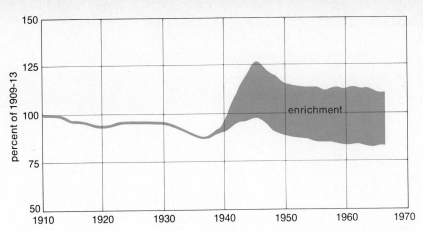

Figure 9.4
Effect of enrichment on the
thiamin content of the diet (6).

parts of the world where populations subsist on white rice that is
not enriched with thiamin. Experimental programs have shown
that mortality rates in an area can drop strikingly in a matter of
months when thiamin is added to the rice supply. Such programs
have made much headway, but beriberi is not yet conquered.

Food Sources of Thiamin

Thiamin is widely distributed in plant and animal foods, but except for a few highly concentrated sources the amounts in which it
is found are relatively small. Furthermore, whole grains, which
naturally carry significant amounts of thiamin in their outer coats
and germs, are used today in small quantities in comparison with
the more acceptable highly milled flours and breakfast foods. Recognition of these facts led nutritionists to recommend enriching
flour and bread with thiamin and certain other nutrients. (See
Chap. 8 for a brief history of enrichment and its present status in
the United States.)

The enrichment of bread and flour has been a specific factor in
raising the content of thiamin in the food supply, even in the face
of declining cereal consumption. Figure 9.4 shows graphically the
extent to which enrichment was responsible for increased thiamin
in the food supply. From 1909 to 1939 the amount of thiamin in the
United States food supply gradually decreased from about 1.7 to
1.5 milligrams per person per day. By 1945, after the enrichment
order had gone into effect, the amount of thiamin available per
person per day was more than 2 milligrams—higher than at any
time in the century. Just before enrichment (between 1935 and
1939), approximately one-fifth of the thiamin in the food supply
came from cereal grains; after enrichment, grain products furnished one-third of the supply of this vitamin (6).

The proportion of thiamin in the United States food supply that
comes from flour and other grain products remains essentially the
same today as it was in 1945—just over one-third of the total. Almost as much of the thiamin (28 percent) comes from meat, poultry, and fish; 9 percent comes from dairy products, excluding

Figure 9.5

Thiamin: Servings of representative foods in order of their thiamin content. (Each bar represents the approximate thiamin value for the foods listed below it.)

Food*	Weight or ** approximate measure	Thiamin milligrams
		▬ 0.75 mg
pork chop	1 chop	0.75
		▬ 0.25 mg
cornflakes, fortified	1 cup	0.29
peas, green	½ cup	0.22
		▬ 0.15 mg
rice, enriched, cooked	¾ cup	0.17
beans, dry, canned	¾ cup	0.15
liver, beef	2 oz	0.15
macaroni, enriched, cooked	¾ cup	0.15
sweet potato	1 medium	0.14
oatmeal	⅔ cup	0.13
orange juice	½ cup	0.12
potato, white	1 medium	0.12
		▬ 0.08 mg
bun or roll, enriched	1 bun	0.11
sausage, bologna	2 oz	0.10
bread, whole wheat	1 slice	0.09
milk, skim or buttermilk	1 cup	0.09
beef, hamburger	3 oz	0.08
bread, white, enriched	1 slice	0.07
broccoli	½ cup	0.07
frankfurter	1 medium	0.07
milk, whole	1 cup	0.07
pineapple juice	½ cup	0.07
spinach	½ cup	0.07
		▬ 0.05 mg
banana, raw	1 medium	0.06
tomato juice	½ cup	0.06
beans, green	½ cup	0.05
beef, lean chuck	3 oz	0.05
egg	1 medium	0.05
grapefruit, white	½ medium	0.05
lettuce, raw	1 cup	0.05
apple, raw	1 medium	0.04
carrots	½ cup	0.04
chicken, fried	½ breast	0.04
haddock, fried	1 fillet (4 oz)	0.04
peanut butter	2 tbsp	0.04
raisins	¼ cup	0.04
tunafish	½ cup	0.04
		▬ 0.03 mg or less
cabbage, raw, chopped	½ cup	0.03
corn, canned	½ cup	0.03
onions	½ cup	0.03
peppers, sweet, green, raw	½ medium	0.03
cheese, cottage, creamed	¼ cup	0.02
peaches, canned	½ cup	0.02
strawberries	½ cup	0.02
cheese, cheddar	1 oz	0.01
cream, half and half	1 tbsp	tr
mayonnaise	1 tbsp	tr
beverages, cola type	12 oz	(0)†
oil, salad or cooking	1 tbsp	0
sugar	1 tbsp	0
butter or margarine	1 tbsp	—

* Foods are in forms ready to eat. All meats and vegetables are cooked unless otherwise indicated.
** See Appendix K for further identification of these foods. All foods are described there more fully, and both weights and measures are indicated.
† See Appendix J.

butter; and lesser amounts are supplied by eggs and different categories of vegetables and fruits. With some reservations, the comparative thiamin yields on the representative food list (Fig. 9.5) bear out the general picture of thiamin availability. Average servings of the foods are arranged in descending order of their thiamin content.

It is apparent from Figure 9.5 that lean pork is a concentrated source of thiamin, and that several other meats, including liver, rank above enriched grain products as sources of thiamin. The point made in studying other nutrients—that regular use must be the chief consideration in making any food an important source of a nutrient—is borne out again. Breads, breakfast cereals, and other grain products are eaten at most meals and tend to overshadow the more concentrated sources of thiamin, which are eaten less often. Milk, another case in point, can contribute a significant amount of thiamin if taken daily in recommended amounts.

As with iron, we have the problem of "shopping around" for thiamin. Aside from the foods mentioned, the very small amounts of thiamin in many vegetables and fruits and the total, or almost total, lack of it in fats, oils, and sugars make it important to know where to "shop." Note that more than one serving of even the richest food sources is required to attain the adult dietary allowances (see the RDA table).

Stability of Thiamin   An additional problem in obtaining enough thiamin is that the vitamin is unstable at high temperatures (27). Some losses in cooking are therefore unavoidable. Cereals that are cooked slowly at moderate temperatures and utilize water by absorption lose little thiamin. Foods that are soaked and drained can lose large portions of the vitamin. Baked products lose roughly 20 percent, while meat losses generally vary from 10 to 50 percent or more. Some of this water-soluble vitamin remains in the meat drippings and in the liquid in which food is cooked. The utilization of cooking water and drippings therefore increases the thiamin value of the meal. The thiamin values for cooked foods given in Appendix K and elsewhere in the text take into account what appear to be normal losses from cooking processes. With careless handling foods can lose much more.

> Arrange your own list of representative foods by sorting your index cards or half sheets in order of their importance as sources of thiamin. Enter thiamin values on your meal record. Total the thiamin values for the day.
>
> What are the main sources of thiamin on the specimen diet for an adult in Appendix H? How do they differ from the sources on your own meal record?
>
> Compare the thiamin value of 1 slice of white enriched bread with the same amount of whole-wheat bread and white unenriched bread.

Recommended Dietary Allowances for Thiamin

The RDA for thiamin at all ages are related to total calorie needs, because of thiamin's function in energy metabolism (2, 26). Clinical signs of thiamin deficiency have been observed in adults when intakes are 0.12 milligram per 1000 calories or less (2). The minimum requirement for adults is considered to be approximately 0.2 milligram of thiamin for each 1000 calories. The allowance figure was set considerably higher than that amount because of large individual variations in need and the inability of the body to store quantities of thiamin. When adult energy intakes are below 2000 calories, the thiamin intake should not be less than 1.0 milligram per day. This precaution is particularly important for elderly persons who may not use thiamin efficiently. Obviously, men and older boys with higher energy allowances have higher thiamin allowances than do women and girls, except during lactation. The thiamin allowance during lactation is particularly high because the energy intake should be much higher than usual during this period (see inside cover).

> Using the values from the RDA table, prepare a graph showing the RDA for energy throughout the life cycle and another showing the RDA for thiamin throughout the life cycle. Use a solid line to represent the RDA for men and boys; a broken line for girls and women. Add separate segments for pregnancy and lactation. Compare the corresponding curves on the two charts, noting their similarity.

Meeting Thiamin Needs The specimen diet in Appendix H shows how body needs for thiamin can be met with a varied selection of foods. Cereals in all forms provide about 20 percent of the thiamin in this diet. The pork chop, a rich source of thiamin, supplies more than 50 percent of the total. If another meat—chicken for example—were substituted for the pork, the thiamin content of the day's diet would be markedly reduced to 0.74 gram rather than 1.45 grams. The small contributions made by many of the foods in the specimen diet illustrate the point made earlier—that thiamin is widely distributed in common foods but concentrated in only a few.

The food combinations in Table 9.3 show four ways in which 1.5 milligrams of thiamin or more can be obtained daily. Combinations 1 and 2 show how easily the amount can be met by eating large servings of forms of pork. Such quantities would not be appropriate, of course, for persons with relatively low energy needs. The higher the energy requirement an individual has, the larger the thiamin need. If a person has a relatively large intake of food, multiple portions of moderately rich sources of thiamin, such as enriched bread, can be assumed. Combinations 3 and 4 show the need for taking account of lesser thiamin sources when other meats are substituted for pork. In combination 3, a double serving of lamb is used; in combination 4, a single serving is used. Combinations 1, 3, and 4 also show how the use of enriched bread in quantity adds to the total thiamin intake. As with other nutrients, the fewer the

Table 9.3
Food combinations that supply 1.5 mg or more of thiamin

		Thiamin mg
1		
pork	2 chops	1.50
bread, enriched	4 slices	0.28
	total	1.78
2		
ham	6 oz	0.80
potatoes	2	0.24
milk, skim	1 pt	0.18
peas, green, frozen	¾ cup	0.33
	total	1.55
3		
lamb	6 oz	0.26
potatoes	2	0.24
peas, green	½ cup	0.22
oatmeal	⅔ cup	0.13
macaroni, enriched	¾ cup	0.15
bread, enriched	6 slices	0.42
orange	1 medium	0.13
milk, skim	1 cup	0.09
	total	1.64
4		
lamb	3 oz	0.13
potatoes	2	0.24
cornflakes	1⅓ cup	0.39
milk, skim	1 cup	0.09
beans, dry, canned	¾ cup	0.15
frankfurters	2	0.14
bread, enriched	6 slices	0.42
vegetables	4 servings	0.20
fruits	2 servings	0.10
	total	1.86

excellent sources used, the more one must depend on a larger number of less concentrated sources.

Children of different ages can obtain the thiamin they need by eating the same foods but in different quantities. This is the practical way of meeting the problem when family members eat their meals together. As children grow, their energy and thiamin needs increase simultaneously. Although milk is not a concentrated source of thiamin, it supplies a significant amount when taken in the quantities commonly consumed by children. It seems likely that in many cases milk makes the difference between adequate and inadequate thiamin intake. Serving sizes of other food sources usually are small for young children and should be increased as their needs for energy and thiamin become greater with age.

> What is the RDA for thiamin for your sex-age group? How does the allowance differ from an estimated value, based on your energy intake?
>
> How does the thiamin intake as shown on your meal record compare with the RDA for thiamin? In terms of your selection of foods, explain why your intake falls below or exceeds the allowance. If it fell below the allowance, could you adjust it easily? How?

Thiamin in the National Diet

The US Department of Agriculture reports that there would be about 1.9 milligrams of thiamin available daily for each person if the United States food supply were divided equally (6). This amount is greater than any RDA for thiamin (see the RDA table). Household diets surveyed by the US Department of Agriculture in 1965 also present a favorable picture. More than 90 percent of the diets of urban and farm families met the dietary allowances for thiamin. Farm families came nearer to meeting them than did city families in the same areas, possibly due to greater use of cereal and pork products on farms (8). Studies of individual diets in some of the same households showed that, while the diets of most age and sex groups were relatively satisfactory with respect to thiamin intake, several age groups of girls and women fell 5 to 15 percent below allowances (9).

Assessing Nutritional Status

What real evidence is there that people in the United States receive or fail to receive enough thiamin? Rarely are clinical signs of deficiency recognizable in the general population, and the dietary picture drawn above is reasonably reassuring. Remember, however, that dietary findings have more meaning when simultaneous biochemical tests support them (see Chap. 2). The Ten-State Nutrition Survey of low-income population groups reports that about 10 percent of the persons studied had lower-than-acceptable urinary excretion levels of thiamin. Diets in these same groups were also poor in thiamin (11). Low biochemical values are considered early warning signals of latent undernutrition. Thus nutritional status with respect to thiamin in some age segments of the general population, notably the elderly, may be less favorable than we have thought; poor thiamin status may also be more prevalent in low-income groups than in the general population.

Clinical moderate-risk signs of thiamin deficiency—absent knee jerks and absent ankle jerks—were reported in the HANES 1971-72 preliminary findings to be very low for persons under the age of 18. The prevalence of risk signs of thiamin deficiency was generally higher for blacks than for whites, and it increased with age. However, there were no signs suggesting that persons were at high risk of thiamin deficiency (3).

RIBOFLAVIN

Functions of Riboflavin

Riboflavin is involved in both energy and protein metabolism. It functions as a constituent of two coenzymes that are essential parts of several oxidative enzyme systems. Thus, like thiamin, riboflavin is concerned with the metabolism of energy nutrients. It contributes to the vital process of converting sources of energy into energy for body use.

When there is a mild, continuous shortage of riboflavin in humans, certain physical signs appear. Some are concentrated in the area of the mouth, lips, tongue, and nose. The mouth becomes sore and the tongue smooth and purplish in color; the lips are inflamed, with cracking at the corners of the mouth; and the skin is rough and scaly, particularly at the folds of the nose (28).

vascularization
Invasion of area with blood vessels

Other signs of riboflavin shortage pertain to the eyes. The eyelids become rough; there may be blurring of vision; and often there is sensitivity to light. *Vascularization* of the cornea has been reported to respond to riboflavin administration. Similar eye and mouth symptoms can arise for various reasons, however, including deficiencies of other vitamins. Thus a cause-and-effect relationship with riboflavin cannot always be established unless the conditions clear up as a result of restoring riboflavin to the diet.

Experiments with laboratory animals show that liberal intakes of riboflavin result in a long productive life, an extended period of adult efficiency, and vigorous health. On the other hand, animals on experimental diets low in riboflavin are retarded in growth and development; their lives are shortened; they suffer from digestive disturbances; and they display nervous symptoms and other signs, including premature aging and the eye and dermatitis symptoms.

Riboflavin Deficiency Syndrome   Clinical findings referred to as *ariboflavinosis* result from a drastic and prolonged dietary shortage of riboflavin. Some or all of the skin and eye symptoms described above may be present to an exaggerated degree. The condition usually is seen in persons who also show symptoms of other B-vitamin deficiencies, particularly of niacin. Ariboflavinosis does not have a long history like that of beriberi, with gradual identification of symptoms, eventual association with lack of a specific food as the major cause, and finally discovery of the vitamin. Actually in this case the vitamin was discovered before the deficiency disease was known. When riboflavin was finally separated from the B complex and synthesized in 1935, its functions were identified. Withholding the vitamin from the diets of laboratory animals gave the first clues of its importance, and inducing mild signs of ariboflavinosis in human subjects provided an opportunity to study uncomplicated symptoms of the disease (2, 28). Lesions of ribo-

Figure 9.6
Riboflavin: Servings of representative foods in order of their riboflavin content. (Each bar represents the approximate riboflavin value for the foods listed below it.)

Food*	Weight or ** approximate measure	Riboflavin milligrams
		2.00 mg
liver, beef	2 oz	2.37
		0.40 mg
milk, skim or buttermilk	1 cup	0.44
milk, whole	1 cup	0.41
cornflakes, fortified	1 cup	0.35
		0.15 mg
pork chop	1 chop	0.22
beef, hamburger	3 oz	0.20
beef, lean chuck	3 oz	0.19
chicken, fried	½ breast	0.17
broccoli	½ cup	0.16
spinach	½ cup	0.16
cheese, cottage, creamed	¼ cup	0.15
cheese, cheddar	1 oz	0.13
egg	1 medium	0.13
		0.08 mg
sausage, bologna	2 oz	0.12
tuna fish	½ cup	0.10
frankfurter	1 medium	0.09
sweet potato	1 medium	0.09
haddock, fried	1 fillet (4 oz)	0.08
macaroni, enriched, cooked	¾ cup	0.08
banana, raw	1 medium	0.07
bun or roll, enriched	1 bun	0.07
corn, canned	½ cup	0.07
peas, green	½ cup	0.07
beans, dry, canned	¾ cup	0.06
beans, green	½ cup	0.06
bread, white, enriched	1 slice	0.06
		0.04 mg
lettuce, raw	1 cup	0.05
potato, white	1 medium	0.05
strawberries	½ cup	0.05
carrots	½ cup	0.04
peanut butter	2 tbsp	0.04
tomato juice	½ cup	0.04
apple, raw	1 medium	0.03
bread, whole wheat	1 slice	0.03
cabbage, raw, chopped	½ cup	0.03
oatmeal, cooked	⅔ cup	0.03
onions	½ cup	0.03
peaches, canned	½ cup	0.03
peppers, sweet, green, raw	½ medium	0.03
pineapple juice	½ cup	0.03
raisins	¼ cup	0.03
		0.02 mg
cream, half and half	1 tbsp	0.02
grapefruit, white	½ medium	0.02
orange juice	½ cup	0.02
rice, enriched, cooked	¾ cup	0.02
mayonnaise	1 tbsp	0.01
beverage, cola type	12 oz	(0)†
oil, salad or cooking	1 tbsp	0
sugar	1 tbsp	0
butter or margarine	1 tbsp	—

* Foods are in forms ready to eat. All meats and vegetables are cooked unless otherwise indicated.
** See Appendix K for further identification of these foods. All foods are described there more fully, and both weights and measures are indicated.
† See Appendix J.

flavin deficiency were produced in adults on diets providing about 2000 calories per day and 0.50 milligram or less of riboflavin. Low levels of riboflavin in the urine are indicative of unsatisfactory riboflavin nutrition (2).

Food Sources of Riboflavin

Riboflavin is widely distributed in plant and animal foods, but more than 80 percent of the riboflavin in the United States food supply is concentrated in these three food groups: dairy products, excluding butter (about 45 percent); meat, poultry, and fish (25 percent); and flour and cereal products (15 percent). Riboflavin is one of the nutrients of enrichment in flour and breads (see Table 8.6). Because of the enrichment program, the proportion of riboflavin available from flour and cereal products has more than doubled from 8 to the present 17 percent. In 1941, two years before enrichment was required by War Food Order No. 1, the per capita amount of riboflavin available daily was 1.92 milligrams. In 1945, 2 years after enrichment started, the amount had risen to 2.46 milligrams. Today it is only slightly lower than this high value.

Figure 9.6 presents the riboflavin values for the foods on the representative food list. Average servings of the foods are arranged in descending order with respect to their riboflavin content. Liver is by far the most concentrated source shown. A relatively small serving of liver (2 oz) yields five times as much riboflavin as 1 cup of milk and would, at first glance, appear to challenge milk's place as the nation's primary source of riboflavin. But many people regularly consume several servings of milk foods daily, and this explains their high rank. For the same reasons, whole grain and enriched cereal products are other important sources of riboflavin.

Obtaining enough riboflavin is largely a matter of choosing a few concentrated sources, as in the cases of calcium and vitamin A. Some of the less concentrated sources of riboflavin such as leafy green vegetables can also add important amounts of the vitamin to individual diets when used regularly. Many other vegetables, most fruits, fats, and sweets are negligible sources of riboflavin (Fig. 9.6).

Stability of Riboflavin   Riboflavin is stable at ordinary cooking temperatures except in an alkaline medium. Some of the vitamin is lost in discarded cooking water and in meat drippings. Riboflavin is less readily water-soluble than thiamin, so that cooking losses are generally smaller. Nevertheless, it is important to cook vegetables quickly in a small amount of water. Soaking vegetables or simmering them can mean heavy losses of the vitamin (27). Riboflavin is unstable when exposed to direct sunlight, daylight, or artificial light. The commonly used opaque cardboard containers for milk conserve riboflavin.

> Arrange your own list of representative foods in order of their importance as sources of riboflavin by sorting your index cards or half sheets.

Enter riboflavin values on your meal record. Total the riboflavin values for the day.

Compare the riboflavin value of 1 slice of white enriched bread with that of the same amount of whole wheat bread and white unenriched bread.

Recommended Dietary Allowances for Riboflavin

Allowances for riboflavin, as for most of the vitamins, increase steadily throughout childhood and adolescence. They level off for both sexes in adult life, but at a higher point for men than for women. The allowance for pregnancy is increased to provide for the growth of the fetus and the mother's accessory tissues; during lactation, riboflavin is increased to compensate for the riboflavin secreted in the breast milk (see inside cover for RDA table).

Table 9.4
Individual foods and combinations that supply 1.7 mg or more of riboflavin

		Riboflavin mg
1		
liver, beef	2 oz	2.37
2		
milk, skim	4 cups	1.76
3		
milk, skim	2 cups	0.88
lamb	3 oz	0.23
beef, pot roast	3 oz	0.15
bread, enriched	6 slices	0.36
cereals, fortified	1 serving	0.35
broccoli	½ cup	0.16
	total	2.13
4		
cheese, cheddar	2 oz	0.26
turkey	3 oz	0.15
frankfurters	2 medium	0.18
eggs	2 medium	0.26
bread, enriched	6 slices	0.36
cereals, fortified	3 servings	0.15
potatoes	2 medium	0.10
corn	1 cup	0.14
beans, green	½ cup	0.06
orange	1 medium	0.05
apple	1 medium	0.03
	total	1.74

Meeting Riboflavin Needs The specimen diet for an adult in Appendix H provides 1.39 milligrams of riboflavin. Thus it practically meets the RDA for women 18 to 22 years of age. About 40 percent of the riboflavin is provided by the cup of milk at lunch and the ice cream at dinner; 18 percent is furnished by the breads and other baked products. The two servings from the meat group—hamburger and pork chop—contribute 30 percent of the day's riboflavin; the vegetables provide a total of about 10 percent. Another serving of milk would increase the riboflavin intake significantly. An occasional serving of liver helps to maintain a high average level of riboflavin intake, and regular use of leafy green vegetables assures maximum contribution of riboflavin from the vegetable group.

The listings in Table 9.4 show four ways of selecting sources of riboflavin, each of which would provide more than 1.7 milligrams of riboflavin. The first two examples show how this can be done by eating reasonable amounts of a single food. It is not suggested that liver be a daily item of diet, but its concentration recommends its regular inclusion in meals. Neither is it necessary for an adult to drink a quart of milk daily. As shown in combination 3, a pint of milk still makes the largest contribution among other good sources. Cheddar cheese (combination 4) and other kinds of cheese including cottage cheese can be used in place of milk to provide riboflavin, if sufficient amounts of other sources of the vitamin are added to make up the difference. When less concentrated sources of riboflavin are consumed, more servings must be eaten to attain the allowance.

> What is the RDA for riboflavin for your sex-age group (see the RDA table)? How does your riboflavin intake as shown on your meal record compare with your daily allowance for riboflavin? In terms of your food selection, explain why your intake falls below the allowance or exceeds the allowance. If it falls below, can you adjust it by making certain changes compatible with your present food habits? How?
>
> Can a strict vegetarian obtain an adequate amount of riboflavin? Plan a day's vegetarian menus (see Chap. 7). Compare the total riboflavin value of this group of foods with the RDA for your sex-age group.

For children milk alone practically meets the need for riboflavin when used daily in recommended quantities. Even a child who drinks only half the quantity of milk suggested would be unlikely to fall far short of the recommended riboflavin allowance as long as a varied assortment of other foods were included in the diet.

Riboflavin in the National Diet

The United States food supply has enough riboflavin to provide an average of 2.3 milligrams for each member of the population (6), an amount that exceeds the daily allowance for any age or condition. Considering that nutrients are not divided equally among people or according to need, actual intakes vary greatly among individuals, families, and age groups.

Household diets studied by the US Department of Agriculture in 1965 showed that about 94 percent of families, urban and rural, met the then current allowances for riboflavin (8). Diets for various sex and age groups within some of those households were adequate, for the most part, in riboflavin. However, some age groups of girls and women failed to meet the allowances (9).

Assessing Nutritional Status

The foregoing facts suggest that some people in the United States may have intakes of riboflavin below need, and certainly below amounts that foster the best riboflavin nutrition. Is there supporting evidence for these dietary data? Are there manifestations of riboflavin deficiency that correspond with these low dietary intakes? In groups studied by USDA Experiment Station investigators, physical signs were noted in relation to the dietary content of riboflavin. Comparisons of findings were made between certain states and between sections of the country. For example, among four states with the same *average* per-person intakes of riboflavin (and of vitamin A), two reported a greater incidence of skin and eye symptoms. A closer look at the dietary findings revealed that in the two states with higher incidence of physical symptoms, more than twice as many children received less than two-thirds of the recommended allowances for riboflavin and vitamin A (29).

The Ten-State Nutrition Survey, involving clinical, biochemical, and dietary assessment in low-economic areas, showed low urinary riboflavin levels in perhaps one-fifth of this population group. Analyses of the diets supported the biochemical findings, revealing low intakes of riboflavin especially among adolescents and the aged. Some eye and skin symptoms were noted (11). A nutrition survey confined to preschool children in all income groups showed no consistent dietary shortage of riboflavin. However, urinary riboflavin excretion levels were rather unsatisfactory, particularly in the lowest income groups (12).

In the HANES, 1971–72, clinical signs suggestive of high risk of riboflavin deficiency (angular lesions and scars of the lips) were seen in less than 3 percent of the individuals in any group. Moderate-risk signs (cracks at the corners of the mouth and dermatitis around the nose and lips) were seen in about 5 to 7 percent of some groups of persons aged 6 to 44 years (3).

HANES
Survey designed to measure the nutritional status of US population

There is no way of knowing from clinical symptoms how much riboflavin deficiency exists in the United States. When it does occur, it is usually complicated with multiple vitamin deficiencies. The fact that the various skin, eye, and mouth symptoms are not always specific for riboflavin deficiency makes diagnosis difficult. It is possible that some of the symptoms are attributable to long-continued low intakes of riboflavin.

NIACIN

Functions of Niacin

Niacin functions in the body as a component of two enzymes. These enzymes are concerned chiefly with *glycolysis*, with tissue respiration, and with fat synthesis. There is also a close relationship between niacin and the amino acid *tryptophan*, a precursor of niacin in the body (2, 30).

In the absence of niacin, characteristic skin lesions, inflammation of mucous membranes in certain body areas, and psychic changes develop. Routine, prolonged deficiency of niacin leads to the disease *pellagra*.

Niacin Deficiency Disease   Pellagra has been called the "disease of the three D's": dermatitis, diarrhea, and dementia. Rough and irritated skin is characterized by identical lesions appearing on opposite sides of the body—for example, on both elbows or both hands. The symptoms are aggravated when the skin is exposed to the sun. Chronic digestive disturbances, with alternating constipation and diarrhea, are common accompaniments. The mucous membranes of the gastrointestinal tract become irritated; the tongue is inflamed and swollen. If the disease continues without treatment, *dementia* ensues, and death follows.

Pellagra was known in the 18th century in southern Europe, where its cause was associated with poor diet. When pellagra was identified in the United States in the 19th century, there were various theories about its cause. The disease was seen most often in persons who lived on limited, low-protein diets including large amounts of corn meal. From this observation evolved a theory, widely accepted at the time, that it was due to an infection caused by eating spoiled corn. In 1915 this theory was disproved and the diet theory upheld. Researchers in the United States Public Health Service were able to produce pellagra in healthy male subjects (prisoner volunteers) with an experimental diet of the type commonly eaten by pellagra sufferers—corn meal, fat pork, and syrup, with no milk and only a few vegetables. Attendants who lived in the identical environment but ate an adequate diet did not develop pellagra. From then on, pellagra was acknowledged as a dietary deficiency disease, but the special factor involved still remained a mystery.

The medical and nutrition organizations of the United Nations report that pellagra occurs in many tropical areas of the world. The disease usually accompanies a gross restriction in variety of foods and a predominance of corn in the diet. Pellagra is practically unknown—even where diets are relatively poor—when an appreciable quantity of legumes or of cereals other than corn are consumed. In the early 1900s pellagra was a leading cause of death in southern areas of the United States. It is rarely seen now. Subclinical forms of the disease, which may exist particularly among low economic groups and persons allergic to certain proteins, are difficult to identify. Although niacin is the central factor in curing pellagra symptoms, treatment often calls for riboflavin to remove mouth and tongue symptoms and thiamin to clear up the neural signs completely.

Discovery of Niacin

In an effort to identify the pellagra-preventive substance, research workers learned to produce pellagra (called "black tongue") in dogs (30). Once this had been accomplished, they were in a position to test various substances for their effect on the disease in these animals. Finally, in the late 1930s, *nicotinic acid* isolated from liver proved to be the important factor. It was promptly tested on pellagra patients and effectively cleared up most of the symptoms of the disease. To avoid confusion with the nicotine of tobacco, with which nicotinic acid has no connection, the substance was called niacin, a term evolved from contractions of the original name.

As soon as the niacin values of foods became known, a puzzling question arose: Why did many people fail to develop pellagra when their diets were low in niacin? Specifically, persons whose diets were known to be low in niacin and that contained even small amounts of milk failed to develop pellagra, while those receiving more niacin but no milk developed pellagra symptoms. The answer lay in the essential amino acid tryptophan, present in milk and in other protein foods. Tryptophan was found to be a precursor of niacin in the body. In effect, foods providing tryptophan are basically sources of niacin as well.

Niacin, therefore, is available in foods and in the body in two forms: as niacin itself and as its proniacin form, tryptophan. The sum of the two is known as *niacin equivalent*. In order to arrive at niacin equivalent values, it was necessary to find out how much tryptophan it takes to provide a given amount of niacin. Experiments on human beings revealed that the human body can synthesize 1 milligram of niacin from about 60 milligrams of tryptophan. The accepted conversion factor is 60; thus tryptophan values can be converted to niacin values by simple division (mg of tryptophan ÷ 60 = mg of niacin).

Food Sources of Niacin

Nearly one-half of the niacin in the food supply of the United States is provided by meat, poultry, and fish, and about one-fourth is furnished by flour and cereal products (niacin is one of the nutrients of enrichment listed in Table 8.6). Lesser but still important sources of niacin are legumes and nuts, particularly peanuts.

Figure 9.7 gives the niacin values of foods on the representative food list. The foods are listed in order of their concentration of niacin in an average serving. Note that only eighteen of the fifty items provide 1 milligram or more of niacin per serving. No one food furnishes the RDA for an adult in a single serving (see the RDA table). Chicken, tunafish, and beef liver appear at the top of the list, each furnishing about 10 milligrams per serving. Other meats and fish, along with peanut butter, come next on the list, but on the average they furnish less than half as much niacin per serving as the first three foods. Whole grains, enriched grain prod-

Food*	Weight or ** approximate measure	Niacin milligrams	
			12 mg
chicken, fried	½ breast	11.6	
			9 mg
tunafish	½ cup	9.5	
liver, beef	2 oz	9.3	
		4 mg	
beef, hamburger	3 oz	5.1	
peanut butter	2 tbsp	4.8	
pork chop	1 chop	4.5	
beef, lean chuck	3 oz	3.8	
haddock, fried	1 fillet (4 oz)	3.5	
cornflakes, fortified	1 cup	2.9	
	1.3 mg		
potato, white	1 medium	1.6	
rice, enriched, cooked	¾ cup	1.6	
peas, green	½ cup	1.4	
sausage, bologna	2 oz	1.4	
corn, canned	½ cup	1.2	
frankfurter	1 medium	1.2	
beans, dry, canned	¾ cup	1.1	
macaroni, enriched, cooked	¾ cup	1.1	
tomato juice	½ cup	1.0	
	0.7 mg		
bun or roll, enriched	1 bun	0.9	
sweet potato	1 medium	0.9	
banana, raw	1 medium	0.8	
bread, whole wheat	1 slice	0.8	
peaches, canned	½ cup	0.8	
bread, white, enriched	1 slice	0.7	
broccoli	½ cup	0.6	
orange juice	½ cup	0.5	
strawberries	½ cup	0.5	
	0.3 mg		
carrots	½ cup	0.4	
spinach	½ cup	0.4	
beans, green	½ cup	0.3	
cabbage, raw, chopped	½ cup	0.3	
pineapple juice	½ cup	0.3	
grapefruit, white	½ medium	0.2	
lettuce, raw	1 cup	0.2	
milk, skim or buttermilk	1 cup	0.2	
milk, whole	1 cup	0.2	
onions	½ cup	0.2	
peppers, sweet, green, raw	½ medium	0.2	
raisins	¼ cup	0.2	
	0.1 mg		
apple, raw	1 medium	0.1	
cheese, cottage, creamed	¼ cup	0.1	
oatmeal, cooked	⅔ cup	0.1	
cheese, cheddar	1 oz	tr	
cream, half and half	1 tbsp	tr	
egg	1 medium	tr	
mayonnaise	1 tbsp	tr	
beverage, cola type	12 oz	(0)†	
oil, salad and cooking	1 tbsp	0	
sugar	1 tbsp	0	
butter or margarine	1 tbsp	—	

* Foods are in forms ready to eat. All meats and vegetables are cooked unless otherwise indicated.
** See Appendix K for further identification of these foods. All foods are described there more fully, and both weights and measures are indicated.
† See Appendix J.

Figure 9.7
Niacin: Servings of representative foods in order of their niacin content. (Each bar represents the approximate niacin value for the foods listed below it.)

ucts, and some of the popular fruits and vegetables can collectively provide a significant quantity of niacin when a number of servings are used each day.

Values shown in Figure 9.7 are for niacin present in food as niacin and do not take into account the amount that will be formed in the body from tryptophan. Some of the foods on the list also make important contributions of niacin in the form of tryptophan.

Sources of Tryptophan   Milk and eggs are among the better sources. Meats, legumes, and nuts represent other good sources of tryptophan, as well as of niacin. The Food and Nutrition Board estimates that most diets in the United States supply 16 to 33 milligrams of niacin equivalent per day. About half this amount is provided by niacin as such (8 to 17 milligrams); the other half, as tryptophan (500 to 1000 milligrams).

Meeting Niacin Needs   Calculating the amount of niacin actually available to the body from food is difficult, since no specific values have been established for niacin equivalents of tryptophan in foods. The specimen diet for an adult in Appendix H provides 16.2 milligrams of niacin as such. Substitution of a tunafish sandwich for the hamburger at lunch would increase the day's niacin intake to 20.6 milligrams. It may be assumed that 50 grams of good protein will yield about 10 milligrams of niacin equivalent from its tryptophan content (30). Taking this into consideration, the sample diet would probably furnish a total of about 26 milligrams of niacin equivalent. Of the 69 grams of protein in the diet, 54 are from animal sources and thus would be expected to furnish at least 10 milligrams of niacin equivalent.

If a variety of foods is selected with emphasis on niacin and tryptophan sources, there should be no danger of a dietary shortage for either adults or children. Items from which to choose include lean meats, poultry, fish, milk, eggs, legumes, and whole grain and enriched cereals.

Stability of Niacin   Niacin is relatively stable when heated, particularly in a dry medium. However, the fact that it is water-soluble makes it important to use the same care in cooking as with other water-soluble vitamins. Meat drippings and water in which vegetables are cooked should be used when feasible.

Recommended Dietary Allowances for Niacin

The Food and Nutrition Board has based the RDA for niacin on calorie intake (see the RDA table), because the human requirement for this vitamin has been shown to depend upon total energy intake. Research on both men and women established the minimal requirement of niacin needed to prevent pellagra, and this requirement served as the base line for the calculated allowances. Experimental diets that provided less than 4.4 niacin equivalents per 1000 calories led to pellagra (30). The RDA for niacin are greater during pregnancy and lactation (2).

Niacin in the National Diet

People in the United States consume relatively large amounts of animal foods—meat, poultry, fish, milk, and eggs. These foods are excellent sources of niacin, tryptophan, or both. Enriched flour and bread to which niacin has been added now make up a very large percentage of all the white bread and flour consumed in the United States.

In spite of what would seem to be an adequate amount of niacin in the United States food supply, clinical signs suggestive of persons being at risk of niacin deficiency were found in the HANES, 1971–72. The highest prevalence of symptoms considered to be suggestive of high risk (specific changes in the tongue) occurred among groups over 60 years of age. Moderate risk signs (other types of changes in the tongue) also were most prevalent among older persons and among teenage, low-income blacks (3).

FOLACIN AND VITAMIN B$_{12}$

DNA
Genetic material in the nucleus of every cell

Folacin and vitamin B$_{12}$ have interrelated functions. Coenzymes of both of these vitamins are required for synthesis of *DNA*. A deficiency of either folacin or vitamin B$_{12}$ results in the disruption of the replication process of most body cells. In bone marrow, the site of red blood cell production, an insufficiency of either vitamin causes abnormal, ineffective cells to be released into the bloodstream. The clinical result is *megaloblastic anemia* (2, 31). Certain other actions of folacin and vitamin B$_{12}$ in the body are quite different and require separate consideration.

megaloblastic anemia
Type of anemia characterized by the presence in the blood of abnormally large, immature red blood cells low in hemoglobin

Folacin

The term *folacin* designates folic acid and related compounds that exhibit the same biologic activity. *Folate* is another term referring to the group of substances that function as folacin in the body. In general use, the three terms folic acid, folacin, and folate are used interchangeably. Different foods contain different forms of the vitamin in varying amounts. The relative efficiency of absorption of the different forms of naturally occurring folates in foods is not known with certainty (2). After absorption, folacin must be converted to its coenzymatic forms to function in the cells. In addition to their action with vitamin B$_{12}$ in DNA synthesis, folacin coenzymes are involved in several amino acid conversions and other metabolic syntheses (31).

Serum levels of folate are commonly used to evaluate nutritional status with respect to this vitamin. Survey data have shown low folate values in blood serum and red blood cells among certain groups, especially premature infants, pregnant and lactating women, and alcoholics. Experimental evidence suggests that humans utilize approximately 50 micrograms of folacin each day, and that requirements for folacin are remarkably increased—perhaps doubled—during pregnancy. Lactation also increases the need for folacin, but to a lesser extent (2). On the basis of these estimates, and taking into consideration the variability of folate absorption from different foods, the Food and Nutrition Board has made its recommendations (see the RDA table).

The body's folacin requirement is directly related to its daily metabolic and cell-turnover rates; thus the need is increased whenever the metabolic rate is increased (as in infection or *hyperthyroidism*) and whenever cell turnover is increased (as in hemolytic anemia, growth of a fetus, or growth of malignant tumors). Alcohol intake increases the folacin requirement because alcohol interferes with folacin utilization (31).

Folic acid deficiency may result from insufficient dietary intake, from impaired absorption, and from abnormalities in demand for, or in the metabolism of the vitamin. *Glossitis* and diarrhea are characteristic marks of folic acid deficiency. *Anorexia,* general discomfort, and irritability may accompany or precede outright megaloblastic anemia.

hyperthyroidism
Disorder caused by excessive secretion of thyroid hormone

glossitis
Inflammation of the tongue

Food Sources of Folacin

Folacin occurs widely in nature in both plant and animal foods. Almost all foods are lower in this vitamin after cooking, but the amount of decrease varies widely. Decreases are due both to the destruction of folacin by heat and to the vitamin's leaching into the cooking water (32). Whole grains are good sources of folacin; the vitamin is concentrated in the bran and germ. Whole wheat flour contains almost twice as much folacin as white flour. Some breakfast cereals are now being fortified with folacin. Legumes are generally good sources, with roasted peanuts, cooked cowpeas, and pinto beans furnishing more than lima beans and red beans. Vegetables particularly high in folacin include spinach, beets, and broccoli. Most fruits have less folacin than vegetables have. Oranges and orange juice are among the best sources in the fruit group. Dairy products, poultry, and muscle meats of all kinds, are low in folacin. Fish are somewhat higher. Liver is an excellent source (32).

Vitamin B$_{12}$

Vitamin B$_{12}$ (*cyanocobalamin*) is a large molecule with one atom of cobalt in the center of its structure. This vitamin is necessary for the normal functioning of body cells, particularly those of the bone marrow, the nervous system, and the gastrointestinal tract.

Vitamin B$_{12}$ is absorbed from the intestinal tract by two separate mechanisms. The physiologic mechanism involves the attachment of free vitamin B$_{12}$ in the stomach to the *intrinsic factor,* normally a constituent of gastric juice. The vitamin B$_{12}$-intrinsic factor complex moves along to the *ileum* where it becomes attached to the *mucosa*. In the presence of calcium, the vitamin is released from the complex and passes through the intestinal mucosa. It enters the *portal venous blood* and is carried to the cells by a specific vitamin B$_{12}$-binding protein. An alternate pharmacologic mechanism for the absorption of vitamin B$_{12}$ is apparently by diffusion (see Chap. 5). Approximately 1 percent of any amount of the free vitamin in the small intestine is absorbed in this manner (31).

ileum
Last portion of small intestine

mucosa
Membrane lining the intestinal tract

portal venous blood
Blood flowing from the intestinal tract to the liver

Vitamin B_{12} is best known for its relationship to *pernicious anemia,* which is characterized by disturbances in the gastrointestinal, nervous, and blood-forming systems. Symptoms include megaloblastic anemia, glossitis and neurological signs such as numbness and tingling of the hands and feet, poor coordination, agitation, depression, and dim vision. The chief cause of pernicious anemia is the absence of the intrinsic factor, which has the effect of withholding vitamin B_{12} from the body (31). To correct this situation, vitamin B_{12} is usually administered by subcutaneous or intramuscular injection, thus bypassing the need for absorption—the step requiring the action of the intrinsic factor.

As described earlier, the blood picture in pernicious anemia is the same as in folic acid deficiency, and may be corrected by administration of either vitamin B_{12} or folic acid. Treatment with folic acid, however, does not alleviate the nervous system changes, which may progress to a more serious stage. As a safeguard against this masking of the symptoms of pernicious anemia by correction of the anemia with folacin, the sale of this vitamin without prescription is restricted to moderate-size doses.

Vitamin B_{12} is present only in foods of animal origin. Liver and other glandular organs are the most concentrated sources, but muscle meats, eggs, milk, and salt-water fish provide enough vitamin B_{12} to prevent deficiency under normal circumstances (2). The vitamin is relatively stable under most ordinary cooking processes.

In rare instances inadequate intake of vitamin B_{12} may be the cause of pernicious anemia, but this seldom happens in the United States because of the liberal use of foods of animal origin. Strict vegetarians who refrain from using milk and eggs as well as flesh foods may be at risk of developing vitamin-B_{12} deficiency. They are advised to include a vitamin B_{12} source in their diets (see Chap. 10).

Vitamin B_{12} is required in extremely small quantities. On the basis of research studies, it is believed that the vitamin B_{12} needs of a normal adult do not exceed 2 micrograms a day. The RDA for vitamin B_{12} provides a margin of safety above normal physiological requirements; the higher allowance during pregnancy is based on the demands of the fetus. Average amounts of vitamin B_{12} in United States diets appear to vary from approximately 5 to 15 micrograms a day (2).

VITAMIN B_6

Vitamin B_6 consists of three related chemical compounds: *pyridoxine, pyridoxal,* and *pyridoxamine.* All three compounds act in the form of phosphates, as coenzymes in the metabolism of the energy-yielding nutrients. More than sixty pyridoxal-phosphate-dependent enzymes are known. The major metabolic functions of vitamin B_6 relate to protein and amino acids—particularly tryptophan, which cannot be converted to niacin without vitamin B_6 (2, 34).

A deficiency of vitamin B_6 results in characteristic symptoms, but they are similar to those caused by a lack of other B vitamins. A vitamin-B_6 deficiency induced experimentally in adults produced

amino acids
Structural units of proteins

a dermatitis around the eyes and at the angles of the mouth, inflammation and soreness of the tongue and lips, muscular weakness, nervous disorders, depression and irritability. Some years ago, infants fed a proprietary milk formula developed nervous irritability and convulsive seizures. Vitamin B_6 in the formula had been destroyed by heat in processing. These deficiency symptoms disappeared when vitamin B_6 was added to the diet in any of its three forms (34).

Studies to determine the vitamin B_6 requirement of human adults have yielded widely varying results, depending on the amount of protein in the diet. As dietary protein increases, the requirement for vitamin B_6 appears to increase (2). An additional amount of vitamin B_6 is recommended during pregnancy to meet the fetus' need for the vitamin, and during lactation to replace the vitamin secreted in human milk (see the RDA table). The RDA for infants and children increase with age. It is believed that amounts of vitamin B_6 recommended by the Food and Nutrition Board can be supplied through basic diets. Foods rich in vitamin B_6 include liver, pork, muscle meats, vegetables and whole-grain cereals (the outer coats of the grain contain the vitamin). Few foods are poor sources. Losses of vitamin B_6 in the course of preparing foods vary with cooking times and temperatures (33).

PANTOTHENIC ACID

Pantothenic acid is essential in human nutrition, and it serves in many important ways. It functions in the body as part of coenzyme A and as such is involved in the series of chemical reactions that occur in the breakdown of carbohydrates, fats, and proteins for the production of energy (35).

Because the vitamin is so widely distributed, a deficiency has not been observed among people eating a diet of natural foods. When volunteers were fed a partially synthetic diet low in pantothenic acid and were given a substance that inhibits the action of the vitamin, the following symptoms developed: weakness, fatigue, nausea, insomnia, cramps in the legs, and some personality changes (35).

The average diet of adults in the United States probably provides between 5 and 20 milligrams of pantothenic acid per day, and a daily intake of 5 to 10 milligrams probably is sufficient for all adults (2). Many of the best food sources are those rich in the other B vitamins: liver, kidney, heart, and eggs. Lean muscle meats, legumes, and cereals are important but somewhat less concentrated sources than the glandular meats; milk and most vegetables and fruits are less concentrated sources than the muscle meats.

BIOTIN

Biotin plays a role in normal human nutrition as an essential part of several enzyme systems. It is involved in carbohydrate, fat, and protein metabolism and in the synthesis of fatty acids. There have been reports of biotin's interrelationships with folacin, with vitamin B_{12}, and with zinc. When biotin deficiency was experimentally produced in a small number of human subjects, symptoms similar to those resulting from deficiencies of other B-complex vitamins developed (36).

Biotin is widely distributed in foods and is also synthesized by intestinal bacteria. A deficiency of the vitamin due to dietary inadequacy has not been known to occur in humans, although a few cases of biotin deficiency have been reported among individuals consuming excessive quantities of raw egg white (37). *Avidin*, a protein-carbohydrate compound in raw egg white, combines with biotin and prevents its absorption and use by the body. The Food and Nutrition Board suggests that people whose diets contain 150 to 300 micrograms of biotin daily will undoubtedly obtain enough of the vitamin, and that this amount is probably provided by most diets in the United States. In addition, there is evidence that the biotin synthesized in the intestine by microorganisms is absorbed and utilized by the body (2).

ASCORBIC ACID (VITAMIN C)

Ascorbic acid is the only water-soluble vitamin not related to the vitamin-B complex. It was originally known as vitamin C. Later it was named ascorbic acid. The two names are now used interchangeably.

Ascorbic acid is a dietary essential for humans, for other *primates,* and for only a few other species of animals. Most species are endowed with enzymes to synthesize this relatively simple compound (38).

primates
Mammals of the order Primates; including monkeys, apes and man

Functions of Ascorbic Acid

Ascorbic acid is a substance of great physiological importance, and one that is apparently involved in many intracellular chemical reactions. The mechanisms by which ascorbic acid performs certain functions are well understood, while the precise role it plays in other reactions is not at all clear. The vitamin acts as a coenzyme in some situations (38).

Ascorbic acid is involved in the metabolism of several amino acids. Perhaps its most fundamental role is in the formation and maintenance of *collagen*, a protein substance that binds cells of connective tissue together. *Procollagen* molecules are synthesized by connective tissue cells, secreted into the extracellular spaces, and assembled into the larger collagen molecules. Collagen is unique in that it is the only protein containing *hydroxyproline*. Ascorbic acid is essential for the conversion of the amino acid *proline* to hydroxyproline (39).

Collagen forms the organic matrix of bone, and bone formation is known to be impaired when a lack of ascorbic acid causes a defect in collagen synthesis. Ascorbic acid has also long been regarded as a factor in hastening healing of cuts and wounds and recovery from surgery. Collagen, the cementing substance, presumably is involved in this action. Delayed wound healing has been observed in some studies in which scurvy was experimentally induced, as well as in spontaneous cases of the disease. In some other studies of scurvy, however, impaired wound healing could not be demonstrated (38). It seems clear that a deficiency of vitamin C must be quite severe before wound healing is hampered.

Ascorbic acid functions in the synthesis of *epinephrine* (adrenalin) and *hydrocortisone* by the adrenal gland. There is some evidence that it may be necessary for the utilization of vitamin B_{12} and folacin as well. Ascorbic acid may also be related in some way to cholesterol metabolism (38).

Scurvy—Ascorbic Acid Deficiency Disease (38, 39)

Scurvy has been known since the 15th century. The disease often afflicted men at sea who were deprived of fresh foods for months or even years at a time. It was not until the middle of the 18th century, however, that diet became the prime suspect as the cause. At that time a physician in the Royal British Navy attempted to discover which, if any, foods were involved. He fed several different food supplements, including vinegar, cider, sea water, oranges, and lemons, to a group of sailors suffering from scurvy. All men had the same basic diet. Two sailors receiving a daily supplement of two oranges and one lemon were the only ones who showed improvement.

As a result of this experiment, the physician in charge recommended the regular use of citrus fruits by the British navy and merchant marine. Almost 50 years later, upon the urging of another naval physician, an administrative order made it a requirement that each British seaman and marine be issued lemon or orange juice daily. Following this step, scurvy disappeared from the British Navy "as if by magic."

Through the years a number of home remedies have been used to treat scurvy. American Indians, for example, saved the lives of many early colonists by introducing them to a syrup made from pine needles that cured the disease. In conditions of war and famine, people in various parts of the world have used the syrup of rose hips (the ripened fruit of the rose bush).

The knowledge that citrus fruits, pine needles, and rose hips could prevent and cure scurvy still did not reveal the secret of their curative property. It was not until the early part of the 20th century that vitamin C was discovered. A few years later, when the vitamin was isolated from lemons and identified chemically, it was named ascorbic acid to relate it to the dietary deficiency disease, scurvy.

People with scurvy show these symptoms: general weakness; lack of appetite; brown, thickened, rough, and scaly skin; spongy, blue-red gums; and hemorrhages in body tissues. If the condition continues, death often ensues. Outright scurvy is uncommon in the United States today, although a considerable amount of subclinical ascorbic-acid deficiency may exist. Infants who are fed sterilized formulas and who do not receive a regular source of ascorbic acid sometimes develop characteristic symptoms. Soft tissues, particularly those surrounding the joints, become swollen, tender, and painful. Elderly people on limited diets deficient in vitamin C are apt to show such symptoms as swollen, spongy, and sore gums. Hemmorrhages sometimes appear as *petechiae* in areas on the body that receive even mild pressure, indicating that the walls of

petechiae
Pinpoint-sized red spots in skin caused by subcutaneous hemorrhages

Food*	Weight or ** approximate measure	Ascorbic acid milligrams

65 mg

Food	Measure	mg
broccoli	½ cup	70
orange juice	½ cup	60

45 mg

peppers, sweet, green, raw	½ medium	47
grapefruit, white	½ medium	44
strawberries	½ cup	44

22 mg

sweet potato	1 medium	26
potato, white	1 medium	22
cabbage, raw, chopped	½ cup	21
spinach	½ cup	20
tomato juice	½ cup	20

13 mg

liver, beef	2 oz	15
banana, raw	1 medium	12
pineapple juice	½ cup	12
peas, green	½ cup	11

6 mg

cornflakes	1 cup	9
beans, green	½ cup	8
onions	½ cup	8
apple, raw	1 medium	6
corn, canned	½ cup	6
carrots	½ cup	5
lettuce, raw	½ cup	5
beans, dry, canned	¾ cup	4
peaches, canned	½ cup	4

2 mg and less

haddock, fried	1 fillet (4 oz)	2
milk, skim or buttermilk	1 cup	2
milk, whole	1 cup	2
bread, white, enriched	1 slice	tr
bread, whole wheat	1 slice	tr
bun or roll, enriched	1 bun	tr
cream, half and half	1 tbsp	tr
raisins	¼ cup	tr
butter or margarine	1 tbsp	0
egg	1 medium	0
oil, salad or cooking	1 tbsp	0
peanut butter	2 tbsp	0
sugar	1 tbsp	0
beverages, cola type	12 oz	(0)
cheese, cheddar	1 oz	(0)
cheese, cottage, creamed	¼ cup	(0)
macaroni, enriched, cooked	¾ cup	(0)
oatmeal, cooked	⅔ cup	(0)
rice, enriched, cooked	¾ cup	(0)
beef, hamburger	3 oz	—
beef, lean chuck	3 oz	—
chicken, fried	½ breast	—
frankfurter	1 medium	—
mayonnaise	1 tbsp	—
pork chop	1 chop	—
sausage, bologna	2 oz	—
tunafish	½ cup	—

Figure 9.8

Ascorbic acid: Servings of representative foods in order of their ascorbic acid content. (Each bar represents the approximate ascorbic acid value of the foods listed below it.)

*   Foods are in forms ready to eat. All meats and vegetables are cooked unless otherwise indicated.
** See Appendix K for further identification of these foods. All foods are described there more fully, and both weights and measures are indicated.

the blood vessels are fragile. Moderate symptoms are difficult to diagnose because most of them can be due to other causes. The best proof of scurvy lies in the cure. If intake of pure ascorbic acid removes the symptoms, then a lack of ascorbic acid can be assumed to be the cause. The cure is usually dramatically rapid and complete.

Food Sources of Ascorbic Acid

Ascorbic acid is widely but unevenly distributed in nature. It is produced by plants in the process of growth but is not present in mature seeds. The US Department of Agriculture reports the percentage of ascorbic acid available from the food groups as follows: about 38 percent from all kinds of fruits (27 percent from citrus, 11 from all others), 54 percent from vegetables (17 percent from potatoes), and the remaining 8 percent from all other foods, chiefly milk and meat. Dry legumes, eggs, grains, sugars, and fats provide little or none (6).

Figure 9.8, which lists the representative foods, bears out the importance of fruits and vegetables as sources of ascorbic acid. The fifty foods are listed in descending order of vitamin-C concentration per serving. Note that only the first thirty-one contribute any ascorbic acid at all, and these include all the fruits and vegetables on the list. Liver is the only other kind of food that appears relatively high on the list. Among the foods that yield little or no ascorbic acid are the muscle meats, poultry, eggs, cheese, grains, fats, oils, and sugar.

It is generally well known, and is evident from Figure 9.8 and Appendix K, that citrus fruits are rich in ascorbic acid. Many of them have the added advantage of being available the year round in various forms. Half a grapefruit provides approximately three-fourths the amount of ascorbic acid as ½ cup of orange juice. Grapefruit juice furnishes about two-thirds as much ascorbic acid as orange juice; tomato juice about one-third, and pineapple juice about one-fifth. Muskmelon and strawberries are also rich in ascorbic acid. Because these fruits are seasonal in most parts of the United States, they are, on the whole, less important sources.

Apples, apricots, peaches, pears, and prunes contain small quantities of ascorbic acid per serving. These fruits are important sources only when they are eaten daily in large amounts and in forms in which the vitamin has not been lost in processing. Pineapples and bananas are slightly better sources but definitely of less value than citrus fruits, strawberries, and muskmelons.

Some tropical fruits not commonly available in the United States are very concentrated sources of ascorbic acid. The acerola cherry, which grows wild in the Caribbean area, is a good example. One or two cherries provide all the ascorbic acid required by either adult or child for a day. The camu-camu, a small fruit from Peru, may be the most concentrated natural source found. It provides up to 2000 milligrams of ascorbic acid per 100 grams of mature fruit (40). Papayas and guavas, particularly the latter, are other excellent sources (see Appendix K).

Broccoli is an outstanding source of ascorbic acid among vegetables. The leafy greens vary considerably in their concentrations of this vitamin. Collards can provide as much ascorbic acid as an equal serving of broccoli, while turnip greens have about two-thirds and spinach about one-third as much. One medium-size potato yields about the same amount of ascorbic acid as a serving of spinach. As a staple food, however, white potatoes provide almost one-fifth of the ascorbic acid in the total United States food supply. In areas of the world where potatoes are eaten at nearly every meal, an outbreak of scurvy threatens when the potato crop fails. This is another example of a food with a relatively low concentration of the nutrient being an important dietary source.

There is no way of knowing the precise ascorbic-acid value of any individual food at the time it is eaten. Its content of the vitamin is affected by many factors, which include the conditions under which it was grown, the time and temperature involved in handling it, the kind and amount of processing or cooking it has undergone, and the conditions of storage before use.

Different varieties of fruits and vegetables also vary in their ascorbic-acid concentration. Some varieties of apples, for example, have much more ascorbic acid than others, although no common varieties are particularly rich sources. It has been shown that some fruits and vegetables, such as oranges and tomatoes, develop more ascorbic acid when ripened in direct sunlight than when ripened in the shade. (Such variations have entered into the computation of average values shown in the food lists and tables in this text.)

Stability of Ascorbic Acid   Ascorbic acid is probably the least stable of all nutrients. It is particularly vulnerable to oxidation, a process hastened by enzymes present in raw fruits and vegetables, and by exposure to warm temperatures, strong light, alkalies, and copper. The latter acts as a catalyst in the destruction of ascorbic acid. Three general rules for handling vegetables, based on these facts, are:

☐ move vegetables from harvest point to the dinner table as quickly as possible;
☐ keep them cool and covered while they are moved or stored; and
☐ cook them quickly and without introducing alkali (such as baking soda in the cooking water), and in a pan free of contact with copper.

In considering the amount of ascorbic acid in the vegetables you eat, the question is not whether there has been any loss, but rather how great the loss is (41). In the interim between the harvest and the time the produce reaches your refrigerator, some loss of ascorbic acid is inevitable. If the vegetables are cooled immediately, shipped in refrigerated cars or trucks, and kept cool at the market, the loss is minimal. If, on the other hand, the produce is allowed to lie in the sun after harvesting and becomes wilted before it reaches the consumer, there is probably little ascorbic acid left. The same chances for retention or loss of the vitamin exist in the kitchen. Cool, crisp vegetables, used promptly and eaten raw, can be expected to supply the most ascorbic acid. No matter how carefully vegetables are cooked, however some loss takes place in the process. Quick cooking in a small amount of water minimizes vitamin-C loss and preserves the vegetable's original color as well (42). Because the vitamin is water-soluble, there may be a considerable amount of it dissolved in the cooking water. When vegetables are simmered for a long time in a large amount of water and the water is then discarded, the loss of ascorbic acid is great. For example, the average concentration of ascorbic acid in collards cooked in a large amount of water is only about two-thirds as much as in collards cooked in a little water. Studies have shown that for different vegetables the percentage of ascorbic acid in the water in which they were cooked or canned may vary from 5 to almost 40 percent (43).

Whole, uncut citrus fruits preserve their ascorbic acid content well when stored at room temperature. When they are cut or squeezed for juice, destruction of the vitamin is less rapid than in many other foods, because the citric acid content of the fruit affords a measure of protection. Tomatoes have a similar advantage. Nevertheless, these foods should be kept covered in glass or plastic containers for maximum ascorbic acid retention and best flavor (44).

Many fruits and vegetables are now used in frozen, canned, and dried forms. How do these rank with fresh produce as sources of ascorbic acid? A comparison of fresh and dried peas, for example, reveals that no ascorbic acid remains in the dried form. Most of the vitamin is destroyed by oxidation in the drying process. For the production of high-quality canned and frozen fruits and vegetables, it is of utmost importance that the time of processing coincide with the food's optimum stage of nutritional quality. The processes themselves, when properly carried out to protect the vitamin, do not greatly reduce the vitamin content of a food. High-temperature, short-time blanching results in the greatest retention of ascorbic acid, with steam blanching extracting only about half as much of the vitamin as water blanching (43). In modern commercial canning and freezing operations, total processing losses are seldom in excess of 25 percent (45). Some loss of ascorbic acid occurs during storage of processed foods. The higher the storage temperature and the longer the time the product is stored, the greater the loss. Considerably more ascorbic acid is retained in frozen foods at storage temperatures of 0°F and below than at temperatures closer to the freezing point (43). When frozen and canned fruits and vegetables are prepared for consumption, they are subject to essentially the same additional ascorbic acid losses as fresh forms of the same foods.

The ascorbic-acid values in Figure 9.8 and Appendix K represent the most recent and reliable data available on the ascorbic-acid content of many raw, cooked, and processed foods. It must be emphasized, however, that these values should be applied with full knowledge of the multiple opportunities for ascorbic acid destruction. It might be wise to allow for an even greater margin of loss than is assumed in the values listed. Such a precaution is particularly desirable when meals are eaten in institutions, where cooked vegetables are often held on steam tables and raw salad greens on cafeteria counters for considerable periods of time.

> Arrange your own list of representative foods in order of their quantitative importance as sources of ascorbic acid by sorting your index cards or half sheets.
>
> Enter ascorbic acid values on your meal record. Total the ascorbic acid values for the day.

Recommended Dietary Allowances for Ascorbic Acid

The daily dietary allowances for ascorbic acid are based on several factors. The starting point is the amount of the vitamin needed to prevent scurvy—10 milligrams a day. Infant requirements are based on the amount of ascorbic acid supplied daily by 850 milliliters of breast milk. As with all allowances, the Food and Nutrition Board has proposed levels for ascorbic acid to provide for considerable variation in individual need. It has also allowed for potential losses of ascorbic acid from food sources, such as those just discussed. As for most nutrients, the RDA for ascorbic acid is greater for pregnant and lactating women.

Storage of Ascorbic Acid in the Body

Adequate food sources of ascorbic acid should be included in the diet every day. Moderate excesses may be beneficial, for some ascorbic acid is retained in the body. Great excesses in intake are wasteful, however. When blood levels of the vitamin reach a certain concentration, the reabsorptive mechanism of the kidney that serves to conserve ascorbic acid "turns off," allowing it to be excreted in the urine (38). Claims that ascorbic acid supplements of 1 gram or more per day are beneficial in the prevention and treatment of the common cold and other conditions have not yet been substantiated (38, 39). Massive doses (5 to 15 g daily) may lead to gastrointestinal distress manifested as nausea and diarrhea. There have been reports that massive doses may have various other undesirable effects, including urinary stone formation, spontaneous abortion, and *conditioned deficiency*—a relative lack of responsiveness to normal doses (38).

Meeting Ascorbic Acid Needs   The specimen diet in Appendix H shows that even a diet without fruit or other highly concentrated sources of ascorbic acid can provide 40 milligrams of the vitamin. About one-third of the total is furnished by potatoes and another third by the cole slaw and green onions.

The foods and groups of foods in Table 9.5 show four ways in which 60 milligrams or more of ascorbic acid can be obtained. The first two choices, broccoli and muskmelon, illustrate that a relatively small serving of an individual food can furnish the entire daily ascorbic-acid allowance for adults. These foods are not generally recognized as dependable sources of ascorbic acid. They may be

Table 9.5
Foods and combinations that provide at least 65 mg of ascorbic acid

		Ascorbic Acid mg
1		
broccoli	½ cup	70
2		
muskmelon	½ 5″ diameter	90
3		
tomato juice	½ cup	23
strawberries	½ cup	44
	total	67
4		
pineapple juice	½ cup	12
banana	1 medium	12
apricots, stewed	½ cup	3
apple, raw	1 medium	6
potato	1 medium	22
peas, green	½ cup	11
	total	66

impractical choices under certain circumstances but can be economical if they are plentiful in the market or home-grown. Combination 3 shows that tomato juice is a good but not highly concentrated source of ascorbic acid. It can be teamed with one very good source, strawberries in this case, to provide an adequate intake for the day. Strawberries can be an economical source of ascorbic acid when they are in season, particularly if they are home-grown. Combination 4 reveals how many poor-to-good sources of ascorbic acid are needed to furnish about 65 milligrams when no excellent source is used.

Children of different ages, as well as adults, can easily meet their needs for ascorbic acid. Orange juice is an excellent, dependable source, well-liked and used daily by many.

> What is the RDA for ascorbic acid for your sex-age group (see the RDA table)?
>
> How does your ascorbic-acid intake, as shown on your meal record, compare with the daily allowance for your sex-age group? In terms of food selection, explain why it falls below or exceeds the allowance. If it falls below, how could you correct it?

Ascorbic Acid in the National Diet

Judging by the amount of ascorbic acid available per person per day from the total food supply, there is no doubt that this nutrient is plentiful in the United States. On this basis, an average of about 119 milligrams per person are available daily (6). This value is much higher than the allowance for any age or condition. But, as with all other nutrients, availability and consumption are not the same thing. It is important to know how families and individuals fare with respect to their actual consumption of ascorbic acid.

The diets of individual members of representative households in the United States in 1965 presented a favorable picture with respect to ascorbic acid intake. For most sex-age groups, average diets approached 90 to 100 percent or were above the RDA. Only one group, men 75 years of age and older, had diets that did not meet the allowance (9).

Assessing Nutritional Status

scorbutic gums
Swollen, inflamed gums due to ascorbic acid deficiency

The Ten-State Nutrition Survey in low-income areas in the United States showed that about 15 percent of the total population studied had less-than-adequate serum levels of ascorbic acid. A breakdown of data by age groups revealed values of similar magnitude from infancy to old age. In the clinical appraisals, a small percentage of the subjects were found to have *scorbutic gums*. As would be expected, their diets were low in ascorbic acid and in many cases fell far below the established dietary guidelines (11).

A nutrition survey of preschool children at all economic levels showed that approximately half of the children ingested less than two-thirds of the RDA for ascorbic acid, and 10 percent had unacceptable levels of plasma ascorbic acid. However, clinical evidence of ascorbic acid deficiency was not found (12).

In the HANES, 1971–72 mean intakes for ascorbic acid reached or exceeded the standard for all groups regardless of income level. Mean intakes were highest—almost twice the standard—for white children aged 1 to 5 and 6 to 11 above poverty level. In spite of the largely satisfactory *mean* levels of intake, a high proportion of *individual* intakes fell below the standards, especially among children aged 1 to 5, and adults between 18 and 44 or over 60, regardless of income level (10).

The clinical moderate-risk sign for vitamin-C deficiency is bleeding and swollen gums. Prevalence of this symptom was very low among children under 12 years of age. In age groups over 12 years, symptoms were generally more frequent among blacks than among whites. Blacks in the age group between 45 and 59 years had the highest prevalence for any age group regardless of income level (almost 15 percent) (3).

THE DIET AS A WHOLE IN RELATION TO BODY NEEDS

We have considered the major nutritional needs of the body one by one and have found that, for the most part, they can be met by proper selection of foods from the nutrient classes: proteins, fats, carbohydrates, mineral elements, and vitamins. You have examined your own eating habits with respect to individual nutrients and you are now ready to review your diet as a whole and to evaluate it in terms of desirable nutritional goals. A graphic summary based on your diet record makes an effective device for visualizing such information. You are in a position to make such a summary if you have kept a personal diet record. You are well aware of the inherent shortcomings in any plan that attempts to set dietary goals for an individual and to use dietary data based on estimates of food intake. But, in spite of these drawbacks, a visual record may still serve a useful purpose.

Draw a series of 12 bars all of the same size, each representing 100 percent of a desirable goal. On the first 11 bars, shade in the percentage of energy and nutrients provided by your own diet, in relation to RDA ranges shown on Table 10.2 as dietary goals (in each case, use as 100 percent the value that represents the midpoint of the range). On the 12th bar show your current body weight in relation to the desirable body weight for your height and body build.

The shaded bars will make it possible to characterize your diet as a whole. They should indicate whether your food intake is generally satisfactory or is generally poor. They should also suggest adjustments you may make to improve the nutritional quality of your meals. The final bar will tell you how well you are keeping total food intake in line with energy needs.

REFERENCES

1. O. A. Roels and N. S. T. Lui, "Vitamin A and Carotene," Chap. 5 Sect. A in R. S. Goodhart and M. E. Shils, eds., *Modern Nutrition in Health and Disease* (Philadelphia: Lea and Febiger, 1973).

2. Food and Nutrition Board, National Research Council, *Recommended Dietary Allowances,* Pub. 2216 (Washington, D.C.: National Academy of Sciences, 1974).

3. S. Abraham, F. W. Lowenstein, and D. E. O'Connell, *Preliminary Findings of the First Health and Nutrition Examination Survey, United States, 1971–72: Anthropometric and Clinical Findings,* DHEW Publication No. (HRA) 75-1229 (Washington, D.C.: US Gov. Print. Office, 1975).

4. Agency for International Development, *Vitamin A, Xerophthalmia, and Blindness,* Vol. I. W. W. Kamel, "A Global Survey of Mass Vitamin A Programs;" Vol. II. A. G. van Veen and M. S. van Veen, "Vitamin A Problems with Special Reference

to Less Developed Countries," (Washington, D.C.: Agency for International Development, US Dept. of State, July 1973).

5. J. H. Shaw and E. A. Sweeney, "Nutrition in Relation to Dental Medicine," Chap. 27 in R. S. Goodhart and M. E. Shils, eds., *Modern Nutrition in Health and Disease* (Philadelphia: Lea and Febiger, 1973).

6. S. J. Hiemstra, *Food Consumption, Prices and Expenditures,* Agric. Econ. Report No. 138 (Washington, D.C.: Economic Research Service, USDA, July 1968). (Also Supplement for 1974, published Jan. 1976).

7. K. C. Hayes and D. M. Hegsted, "Toxicity of the Vitamins," Chap. 11 in Comm. on Food Protection, Food and Nutrition Bd., Nat. Res. Council, *Toxicants Occurring Naturally in Foods* (Washington, D.C.: National Academy of Sciences, 1973).

8. *Food Consumption of Households in the United States* (Washington, D.C.: USDA, 1967, Household Food Consumption Survey, 1965–66, Report Nos. 1, 2, 3, 4).

9. *Food Intake and Nutritive Value of Diets of Men, Women and Children in the United States, Spring 1965* (Washington, D.C.: USDA, March 1969), ARS 62-18.

10. S. Abraham, F. W. Lowenstein and C. L. Johnson, *Preliminary Findings of the First Health and Nutrition Examination Survey, United States, 1971–72: Dietary Intake and Biochemical Findings,* DHEW Publication No. (HRA) 76-1219-1 (Washington, D.C.: US Gov. Print. Office, 1974).

11. A. E. Schaefer, *Statement Before Senate Select Committee on Nutrition and Related Human Needs* (Washington, D.C.: Jan. 22, 1969 and April 27, 1970).

12. G. M. Owen, K. M. Kram, P. J. Garry, J. E. Lowe and A. H. Lubin, "A Study of Nutritional Status of Preschool Children in the United States, 1968–70," *Pediatrics* 53 (April 1974), pp. 597-646.

13. J. L. Omdahl and H. F. DeLuca, "Vitamin D," Chap. 5 Sect. B in R. S. Goodhart and M. E. Shils, eds., *Modern Nutrition in Health and Disease* (Philadelphia: Lea and Febiger, 1973).

14. H. H. Sandstead, "Clinical Manifestations of Certain Vitamin Deficiencies," Chap. 20 in R. S. Goodhart and M. E. Shils, eds., *Modern Nutrition in Health and Disease* (Philadelphia: Lea and Febiger, 1973).

15. Committee on Nutritional Misinformation, "Hazards of Overuse of Vitamin D," a Statement of the Food and Nutrition

Board, National Research Council, National Academy of Sciences, November, 1974, *Am. J. Clin. Nutr.* 28 (May 1975), pp. 512-13.

16. S. J. Fomon, *Infant Nutrition* (Philadelphia: Saunders, 1974).

17. M. K. Horwitt, "Vitamin E," Chap. 5 Sect. D in R. S. Goodhart and M. E. Shils, eds., *Modern Nutrition in Health and Disease* (Philadelphia: Lea and Febiger, 1973).

18. M. K. Horwitt, "Vitamin E: A Reexamination," *Am. J. Clin. Nutr.* 29 (May 1976), pp. 569-578.

19. "Vitamin E," A Scientific Status Summary by the Institute of the Food Technologists' Expert Panel on Food Safety & Nutrition and the Committee on Public Information, *Food Technology* 31 (Jan. 1977), pp. 77-80.

20. A. L. Tappel, "Vitamin E," *Nutrition Today* 8 (July-Aug. 1973), pp. 4-12.

21. P. M. Farrell and J. G. Bieri, "Megavitamin E Supplementation in Man," *Am. J. Clin. Nutr.* 28 (Dec. 1975), pp. 1381-86.

22. B. E. March, E. Wong, L. Seier, J. Sim, and J. Biely, "Hypervitaminosis E in the Chick," *J. Nutr.* 103 (March 1973), pp. 371-77.

23. R. E. Olson, "Vitamin K," Chap. 5, Sect. C in R. S. Goodhart and M. E. Shils, eds., *Modern Nutrition in Health and Disease* (Philadelphia: Lea and Febiger, 1973).

24. Committee on Nutrition, American Academy of Pediatrics, "Vitamin K Supplementation for Infants Receiving Milk Substitute Infant Formulas and for Those with Fat Malabsorption," *Pediatrics* 48 (Sept. 1971), pp. 483-87.

25. R. R. Williams, H. L. Mason, B. F. Smith and R. M. Wilder, "Induced Thiamin Deficiency and the Thiamin Requirement of Man," *Archives of Internal Med.* 69 (May 1942), pp. 721-38.

26. R. A. Neal and H. E. Sauberlich, "Thiamin," Chap. 5, Sect. E in R. S. Goodhart and M. E. Shils, eds., *Modern Nutrition in Health and Disease* (Philadelphia: Lea and Febiger, 1973).

27. M. Bennion, *Introductory Foods* (New York: MacMillan, 1974).

28. M. K. Horwitt, "Riboflavin," Chap. 5, Sect. F in R. S. Goodhart and M. E. Shils, eds., *Modern Nutrition in Health and Disease* (Philadelphia: Lea and Febiger, 1973).

29. A. F. Morgan, *Nutritional Status, U.S.A.*, Bull. 769 (Berkeley: California Agricultural Experiment Station, University of California, Oct. 1959).

30. M. K. Horwitt, "Niacin," Chap. 5, Sect. G in R. S. Goodhart and M. E. Shils, eds., *Modern Nutrition in Health and Disease* (Philadelphia: Lea and Febiger, 1973).

31. V. Herbert, "Folic Acid and Vitamin B_{12}," Chap. 5, Sect. J in R. S. Goodhart and M. E. Shils, eds., *Modern Nutrition in Health and Disease* (Philadelphia: Lea and Febiger, 1973).

32. B. P. Perloff and R. R. Butrum, "Folacin in Selected Foods," *J. Am. Dietet. Assoc.* 70 (Feb. 1977), pp. 161-72.

33. M. L. Orr, *Pantothenic Acid, Vitamin B_6 and Vitamin B_{12} in Foods*, Home Economics Research Report No. 36 (Washington, D.C.: Consumer and Food Economics Research Division, Agricultural Research Service, USDA, August 1969).

34. H. E. Sauberlich and J. E. Canham, "Vitamin B_6," Chap. 5, Sect. I in R. S. Goodhart and M. E. Shils, eds., *Modern Nutrition in Health and Disease* (Philadelphia: Lea and Febiger, 1973).

35. H. E. Sauberlich, "Pantothenic Acid," Chap. 5, Sect. H in R. S. Goodhart and M. E. Shils, eds., *Modern Nutrition in Health and Disease* (Philadelphia: Lea and Febiger, 1973).

36. R. S. Goodhart, "Biotin," Chap. 5, Sect. L in R. S. Goodhart and M. E. Shils, eds., *Modern Nutrition in Health and Disease* (Philadelphia: Lea and Febiger, 1973).

37. R. L. Pike and M. L. Brown, *Nutrition: An Integrated Approach* (New York: John Wiley and Sons, 1975).

38. R. E. Hodges and E. M. Baker, "Ascorbic Acid," Chap. 5, Sect. K in R. S. Goodhart and M. E. Shils, eds., *Modern Nutrition in Health and Disease* (Philadelphia: Lea and Febiger, 1973).

39. R. Passmore, "How Vitamin C Deficiency Injures the Body," *Nutrition Today* 12 No. 2 (March/April, 1977), pp. 6-11, 27-31.

40. R. B. Bradfield, and A. Roca, "Camu-Camu: A Fruit High in Ascorbic Acid," *J. Am. Dietet. Assoc.* 44 (Jan. 1964), pp. 28-30.

41. "Procedures for Calculating Nutritive Values of Home-Prepared Foods," (Washington, D.C.: USDA, March 1966), ARS 62-13 (Table II: Retention of Vitamins in Cooked Foods).

42. I. Noble, "Ascorbic Acid and Color of Vegetables," *J. Am. Dietet. Assoc.* 50 (April 1967), pp. 304-7.

43. R. S. Harris and H. Von Loeseche, *Nutritional Evaluation of Food Processing* (New York: John Wiley and Sons, 1960).

44. A. Lopez, W. A. Krehl and E. Good, "Influence of Time and Temperature on Ascorbic Acid Stability," *J. Am. Dietet. Assoc.* 50 (April 1967), pp. 308-10.

45. R. E. Hein and I. J. Hutchings, "Influence of Processing on Vitamin-Mineral Content and Biological Availability in Processed Foods," in American Medical Association, *Nutrients in Processed Foods: Vitamins, Minerals* (Acton, Massachusetts: Publishing Sciences Group, 1974).

Anderson, T. A., "New Horizons for Vitamin C," *Nutrition Today* 12 (Jan./Feb. 1977), pp. 6-13.

DeLuca, H. F., "Vitamin D: New Approaches to Treatment of Metabolic Bone Disease," *Nutrition and the M.D.* 2 (Aug. 1976), pp. 1, 2.

Engler, P. P. and J. A. Bowers, "B-Vitamin Retention in Meat During Storage and Preparation," *J. Am. Dietet. Assoc.* 69 (Sept. 1976), pp. 253-57.

"Recent Developments in Vitamin D," *Dairy Council Digest* 47 (May-June 1976), pp. 13-17.

Scrimshaw, N. S. and V. R. Young, "The Requirements of Human Nutrition," *Scientific American* 235 (Sept. 1976), pp. 50-64.

Part 3
Applying the Science of Nutrition

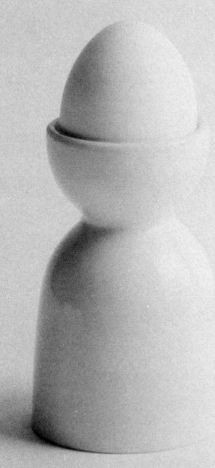

The science of nutrition is applied when it provides the foundations for intelligent food selection and sound nutritional status. Parts one and two have furnished certain scientific bases for understanding the nutrient components of an adequate diet in relation to human needs. Part three offers interpretation of this information in terms of the foods that supply the nutrients, in various concentrations, to fulfill those needs.

The emphasis now shifts from nutrients to foods and food groups, the purveyors of those nutrients. Learning to regard foods in the light of their individual and collective nutrient contributions is a first step in simplifying selection of the day's food. We will consider various nutritional guidelines for food selection—those that relate to dietary needs of young adults under usual conditions as well as those that cover the varied nutritional demands throughout the life cycle.

Nutritional Guidelines for Selecting the Day's Food

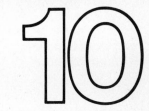

Food Selection Guides
Nutrition Labeling
Food Safety
Food Additives

It is obviously impractical to calculate the nutrient content of your food daily in order to determine whether it meets standards of nutritional adequacy. Some less complicated method must serve the purpose. In the United States and in many other countries, daily food selection guides have been devised, based on foods available in each country as well as foods to which various cultural groups may be accustomed. The scientific bases for such guides are the RDA and similar nutrition criteria discussed in Chapter 2.

A successful food selection guide is merely a ground plan or pattern for helping people to choose nutritionally adequate, varied, and satisfying meals. It is not a precise instrument. Just how well it accomplishes its objective will be explored next. Food selection guides in the United States have evolved over a period of years (1). Table 10.1 resembles the types currently in use (2). This guide takes into account the food supplies available to the United States population and is flexible enough to cover regional, seasonal, ethnic, and economic differences. It presents basic foods under four

Table 10.1
A Daily food selection guide

Foundation Foods

Milk group
2 or more servings[1] milk—adults
3 or more servings, milk—children and pregnant women
4 or more servings, milk—teenagers and lactating women
Cheeses, ice cream, ice milk and other milk-made foods can supply part of the milk (see Table 10.8 for calcium equivalents).

Meat group
2 or more servings[2]
lean meats, fish, shell fish, poultry, eggs, cheese
dry beans, dry peas, lentils, peanuts, textured vegetable proteins, nuts, nut butters

Vegetable-fruit group
4 or more servings[3]
a dark green leafy or orange-colored vegetable at least every other day
citrus fruit or other vitamin-C-rich sources daily
other fruits and vegetables, including potatoes

Grain group
4 or more servings[4]
whole-grain, enriched, fortified

Foundation foods are the nucleus of nutritionally adequate daily meals. It is often desirable to use more than the minimum choices offered within the groups.

Additional foods
Other foods may be added if individual calorie needs permit. These include: sweets, fats, dressings, sauces, unenriched grains, flavorings, condiments. They supplement but do not replace foods from the foundation groups.

Provide 400 IU of Vitamin D daily during childhood, young adulthood, pregnancy, and lactation.

[1]serving size, milk: 1 cup (½ pt) fresh fluid; reconstituted evaporated, dry milk; yogurt; buttermilk.
[2]serving sizes, meats: approximately 3 oz cooked; dry legumes: approximately ¾ cup, cooked.
[3]serving sizes: cooked vegetables, fruits: ½ cup; raw fruits: units, as one medium-size orange.
[4]serving sizes: bread, 1 slice; cooked cereal: ⅔ cup; dry cereal: 1 oz.

For more detail on serving sizes and food choices within food groups, see pp. 303–317 and Appendix K.

main groups: milk and milk products, meat and meat alternates, vegetables and fruits, and grains. A four-group plan was first suggested by nutritionists of Harvard University in 1955 as a revision of the "Basic Seven" guide then in common use (3). The seven-group plan seemed complicated, and steps were taken to provide a plan easier for people to remember and follow. In general, however, the more food groups included in a plan, the more specific and detailed the directives and the more reliable the instrument. The vegetable-fruit group is a case in point. In a seven-group guide, three groups are devoted to fruits and vegetables, and the sources of major nutrients are pinpointed specifically. In a four-group guide, these three are condensed into one group with subdivisions (see Table 10.1). Unless these subdivisions plainly indicate the choices that must be made to ensure a supply of the main nutrients provided by fruits and vegetables (notably vitamin-A activity, iron, and ascorbic acid), the four-group plan is clearly a less dependable instrument than the seven-group plan.

Food Groups—Basis of Food Selection Guides

As outlined in Part 2, certain classes of foods are similar in their nutrient content and therefore form natural groupings. The four food groups in Table 10.1 were chosen because of the significant nutrient contribution each can make to the total diet. They have thus earned the designation "foundation foods." They appear in Table 10.1 under that heading. "Additional foods" include fats, sweets, unenriched cereals, and flavorings that are commonly used in addition to the foundation foods.

Figure 10.1 shows graphically the nutrient contributions made by the four foundation food groups and by the additional foods in a general mixed diet of the type eaten by many people in the United States. (An example of such a diet is shown in Tables 10.2 and 10.3). You will notice when you examine Figure 10.1 that each

Figure 10.1
Food sources of nutrients: contributions made by food groups to mixed diet (Table 10.2)

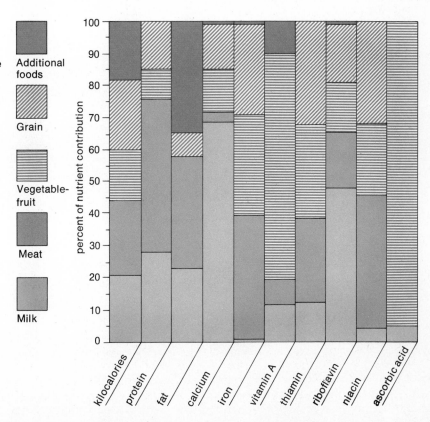

Table 10.2
Nutrients furnished by a traditional mixed diet based on the food selection guide

Foods	Measure	Kilocalories	Protein g	Fat g	Calcium mg	Iron mg	Vitamin A IU	Thiamin mg	Riboflavin mg	Niacin mg	Ascorbic Acid mg	Vitamin D IU
Foundation foods												
milk group												
milk, whole, vit. D	2 cups	318	18	18	576	0.2	700	0.14	0.82	0.4	4	200
ice cream	⅛ qt	127	3	7	96	tr	290	0.03	0.14	0.1	1	
meat group												
pot roast	3 oz	295	20	23	9	2.6	40	0.05	0.15	3.7	—*	
ham, boiled	2 oz	132	10	10	6	1.6	0	0.24	0.08	1.4	—	
egg	1 medium	72	6	5	24	1.0	520	0.05	0.13	tr	0	
vegetable-fruit group												
peas	¼ cup	28	2	tr	8	0.8	240	0.11	0.04	0.7	6	
carrots	¼ cup	12	1	tr	12	0.3	3808	0.02	0.02	0.2	3	
lettuce	2 leaves	10	1	tr	37	0.8	1050	0.03	0.04	0.2	10	
lettuce	¼ head	18	1	tr	27	0.7	450	0.08	0.08	0.4	8	
celery	1 stalk	3	tr	tr	7	0.1	47	0.01	0.01	0.1	2	
grapefruit	½ medium	46	1	tr	19	0.5	10	0.05	0.02	0.2	44	
baked apple	1 medium	120	tr	tr	8	0.4	50	0.04	0.02	0.1	3	
banana	1 medium	101	1	tr	10	0.8	230	0.06	0.07	0.8	12	
grain group												
bread, enriched	4 slices	304	8	4	96	2.8	tr	0.28	0.24	2.8	tr	
rolls, enriched	2, plain	168	4	4	40	1.0	tr	0.14	0.12	1.2	tr	
Totals, foundation foods		1754	76	71	975	13.6	7435	1.33	1.98	12.3	93	200
Nutrient goals												
RDA ranges for adults		1800–3000	44–76		800–1200	10–18	4000–6000	1.00–1.50	1.10–1.80	12.0–20.0	45–60	400
Additional foods												
butter or margarine	5 tsp	170	tr	20	5	0.0	785	—	—	—	0	
French dressing	1 tbsp	66	tr	6	2	0.1	—	—	—	—	—	
mayonnaise	1 tbsp	101	tr	11	3	0.1	40	tr	0.01	tr	—	
sugar	3 tsp	46	0	0	0	0.0	0.0	0.0	0.0	0.0	0	
Totals, additional foods		383	—	37	10	0.2	825	0.0	0.01	—	—	
Grand totals		2137	76	108	985	13.8	8260	1.33	1.99	12.3	93	200

*See Appendix J

Table 10.3
Menus based on diet in Table 10.2

Foundation foods 82% of total calories		Calories	Additional foods		Calories
Breakfast					
grapefruit	½ medium	46	+ sugar	1 tsp	15
egg, poached	1 medium	72			
toast, enriched	2 slices	152	+ butter or margarine	2 tsp	68
milk, whole	1 glass (cup)	159	coffee		
			+ sugar	1 tsp	15
Lunch					
ham sandwich					
bread, enriched	2 slices	152			
ham, boiled	2 oz	132	+ mayonnaise	1 tbsp	101
lettuce	2 leaves	10			
celery	1 stalk	3			
milk, whole	1 glass (cup)	159			
apple, baked	1 medium	120			
Dinner					
pot roast	3 oz	295			
peas, carrots	½ cup	40	+ butter or margarine	1 tsp	34
head lettuce salad	¼ head	18	+ French dressing	1 tbsp	66
rolls, enriched	2	168	+ butter or margarine	2 tsp	68
ice cream	⅛ qt	127			
			beverage		
			+ sugar	1 tsp	15
Between meals					
banana	1 medium	101			—
	total calories	1754		total calories	382
Grand total, calories for the day				2136	

foundation food group—milk, meat, vegetable fruit, grains—provides substantial amounts of certain nutrients:

Foundation foods	Nutrient contributions
milk group	protein—about one-fourth calcium—two-thirds riboflavin—nearly one-half
meat group	protein—about one-half thiamin—one-fourth iron—more than one-third niacin—more than one-third
vegetable-fruit group	ascorbic acid—practically all vitamin A activity—nearly three-fourths iron—more than one-fourth
grain group	iron thiamin } more than one-fourth each niacin

Each food group also makes important contributions of nutrients other than those they provide in abundance. Each foundation food group furnishes one-fourth or more of at least three nutrients supplied by the mixed diet. The proportion of nutrients supplied by the additional foods presents a sharp contrast to those furnished by the foundation foods (Figure 10.1). Despite the fact that the additional foods account for about one-fifth of the energy value of the diet and one-third of its fat content, the only significant nutrient contribution is one-tenth of the vitamin-A activity.

Figure 10.1 thus provides a clear indication of the relative nutritional importance of certain food *groups*. There is current interest in establishing nutritional quality ratings for *individual* foods. This calls for comparing foods singly with certain nutritional criteria to determine their nutritional status—in effect, to learn whether or not they classify as nutritious foods. Investigators have approached the process in different ways. One group has used *nutrient density* of foods—that is, nutrient content of foods within the framework of energy yield—to arrive mathematically at an *Index of Nutritional Quality* (INQ). The index rates, numerically, the relationship of nutrients present in each food to the nutritional standards for intake of those nutrients. Application of the INQ provides a precise interpretation of such adjectives as *poor, good*, and *excellent* commonly used in describing levels of nutritional quality (4). The INQ plan, with modifications, is also proposed for evaluating nutritional quality of total diets (5).

Another proposed system is called a *Nutrient Calorie Benefit Ratio* (NCBR). The ratio, like the index, is obtained by calculating the level of food nutrients present to recommended intake, taking into consideration the energy yield of the food being rated (6). The numeral derived in each case indicates the level of NCBR of a given nutrient in a specific food. In application, the nutritious quality of a food is judged by the number of nutrients of specified NCBR status in the food.

Details of these proposed systems are omitted here because some of them are still in various stages of development, and in some cases sophisticated techniques involved make application to daily meals impractical at present. Nevertheless the concept of an index or a ratio for easily identifying the nutritional quality of foods is an important one that will have increasing attention and, undoubtedly, eventual acceptance. Meanwhile, certain established guidelines continue to offer reasonable assurance of attaining dietary adequacy. These include the choice of a wide variety of foods, selected for their special assortment of nutrients, and a nutritionally sound daily eating pattern.

Assessment of the Food Selection Guide

The reliability of a daily food selection guide must be judged by its performance as a planning tool in the hands of persons with little or no knowledge of nutrition. Let us assume that a person who answers this description gives the guide a practical test. What is the outcome in terms of attaining dietary goals?

A diet plan for 1 day based on the daily food selection guide in

Table 10.1 is shown in Tables 10.2 and 10.3. The dietary goals proposed are not single values established by RDA, but rather *ranges* in nutrient values that span recommended amounts of nutrients for persons of different sex-age levels. The ranges are entered on Table 10.2 directly below the nutrient totals for foundation foods. They serve merely as general indicators in a broad frame of reference. (See also the RDA for allowances that apply to your own sex-age group.) Foods appear on Table 10.2 under the four food groups. In the milk group, for example, a serving of ice cream and 2 cups of milk are listed. In the meat group, two servings of meat and one egg make up the choices. Four vegetables and three fruits are selected for the next group, and four slices of bread and two rolls comprise the grain group. Table 10.3 shows how the day's food can be distributed into meal units and demonstrates the way the concept of foundation and additional foods can be applied to meal planning.

Totals for the individual nutrients recorded on Table 10.2 fall within the nutrient ranges set for them. The foundation foods provide about 80 percent of the food energy for the day and most of the nutrients come from the foundation foods alone. The kinds and amounts of foods chosen from within the foundation food groups can make a vast difference in dietary adequacy. As a general principle, the larger the proportion of total calories provided by foundation foods, the greater the prospects for meeting total nutrient goals. Furthermore, the lower the total energy value of the diet, the more important it is to obtain a high proportion of calories from foundation foods.

The particular foods in Table 10.2 have no special significance but merely represent one of the many ways in which the food selection guide can be interpreted. These foods are available in most communities in the United States the year round. Likewise, the meals in Table 10.3 are not meant to suggest a preferred way of distributing foods throughout the day but simply one way it can be done. The meals are shown in Figure 10.3.

Adaptability of the Food Selection Guide

A traditional diet, planned in accordance with the recommendations of the food guide, can easily meet the RDA, particularly if the guide is interpreted rather liberally, with judicious use of the "or more" provisions. There is still the question of how dependable the guide is when applied to the varied circumstances under which people eat today. In homes and restaurants more ethnic foods are served; formulated and fabricated foods have become regular meal items; people are eating food mixtures that cannot readily be identified with any of the four food groups; and many people are turning to special diets, including vegetarian diets. A strict or total vegetarian diet is one that includes grains, legumes, nuts, and fruits as well as vegetables but is free of all animal foods. It poses difficult dietary problems (7).

Can the present food-selection guide serve as a reliable pattern in choosing a nutritionally adequate total vegetarian diet? Let us examine such a diet, shown in Tables 10.4 and 10.5. It meets or

Table 10.4
Nutrient value of a total vegetarian diet †

Foods	Measure	Kilo-calories	Protein g	Fat g	Calcium mg	Iron mg	Vitamin A IU	Thiamin mg	Ribo-flavin mg	Niacin mg	Ascorbic acid mg	Vita-min B₁₂ mcg
Breakfast												
grapefruit	½	69	0.9	tr	27	0.7	147	0.07	0.04	0.4	68	—
whole wheat toast	2 slices	137	5.2	2	48	1.3	—	0.14	0.06	1.6	—	—
margarine	2 tsp	72	—	8	2	—	330	—	—	—	—	—
corn grits, cooked	¾ cup	94	2.2	tr	1	0.6	111	0.07	0.06	0.7	—	—
soy milk*	3½ oz	68	2.2	4	51	1.0	205	0.04	0.06	0.5	5	0.2
dates	¼ cup	123	1.0	tr	26	1.3	22	0.04	0.05	1.0	—	—
molasses	1 tbsp	46	—	—	57	1.2	—	0.02	0.02	0.2	—	—
cashew nuts, roasted	8 nuts	78	2.4	4	5	0.5	13	0.06	0.03	0.3	—	—
Lunch												
lentils, cooked	¾ cup	160	11.5	tr	37	3.1	30	0.10	0.09	0.9	—	—
brown rice, cooked	¾ cup	102	2.1	1	11	0.6	—	0.09	0.02	1.3	—	—
grated raw carrots	¼ cup	11	0.3	tr	10	0.2	3025	0.01	0.01	0.1	2	—
grated cooked beets	¼ cup	6	0.2	tr	3	0.1	3	0.01	0.01	0.1	1	—
grated parsnips	¼ cup	13	0.3	tr	9	0.1	5	—	0.01	0.1	3	—
vegetable oil	2 tbsp	252	—	28	—	—	—	—	—	—	—	—
lemon juice	2 tbsp	4	0.1	tr	1	—	3	0.01	—	—	7	—
whole wheat roll	1 roll	67	2.5	1	23	0.6	—	0.08	0.03	0.8	—	—
margarine	1 tsp	36	—	4	1	—	165	—	—	—	—	—
soy milk*	1 cup	163	5.5	9	123	2.4	492	0.10	0.15	1.2	12	0.5
Dinner												
spanish beans	¾ cup	177	11.7	5	57	3.6	—	0.17	0.19	1.0	—	—
whole wheat bread	2 slices	134	5.0	2	46	1.2	—	0.16	0.06	1.6	—	—
turnip greens, cooked	1 cup	29	3.2	tr	267	1.6	9140	0.22	0.35	0.9	100	—
margarine	2 tsp	72	—	8	2	—	330	—	—	—	—	—
banana	1 large	127	1.6	tr	12	1.0	270	0.08	0.09	1.0	15	—
soy milk*	1 cup	163	5.5	9	123	2.4	492	0.10	0.15	1.2	12	0.5
Totals		2203	63	85	942	23.5	14,783	1.39	1.5	15	225	1.2
Nutrient goals	RDA ranges for adults	1800–3000	44–76		800–1200	10–18	4000–6000	1.0–1.5	1.1–1.8	12–20	45–60	3

*fortified with vitamin B₁₂   †Provided by Selma Chaij Rhys, R.D. Director of Dietetic Education, Hinsdale, Illinois Sanitarium and Hospital.

Table 10.5
Menus based on total vegetarian diet

breakfast
fresh grapefruit
corn grits cooked in soy milk, served with molasses
whole wheat toast with margarine
dates and cashews

lunch
lentils on brown rice
rainbow vegetable salad with oil-lemon juice dressing
whole wheat roll with margarine
soy milk fortified with vitamin B_{12}

dinner
Spanish kidney beans
cooked turnip greens with lemon
whole wheat bread with margarine
fresh banana
soy milk fortified with vitamin B_{12}

practically meets recognized standards for an adult for 1 day (8). This diet therefore may serve as a criterion against which to judge the adaptability of the guide. A variety of plant sources are represented in the diet: whole grains, legumes, vegetables, fruits, nuts, and soy milk, along with modest amounts of vegetable oil, margarine, and molasses. There are no foods that would normally be classed in the milk group and no animal foods that belong to the meat group (Fig. 10.2).

In Table 10.6 the foods representing a traditional mixed diet and a total vegetarian diet are distributed under the four groups of the food selection guide for the sake of comparison. This distribution brings out the similarities and differences between food choices in the two types of diets. Notable characteristics of the vegetarian diet include the substitution of soy milk (fortified with vitamin B_{12}) for cow's milk; the consumption of large amounts of dry legumes for vegetable protein to supplant meat; and the use of more vegetables (especially greens) and more whole grains. The additional foods are virtually the same in the two types of diets.

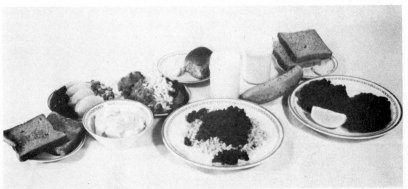

Figure 10.2
Food in a total vegetarian diet for one day (Table 10.4). (Hinsdale Sanitarium and Hospital)

Figure 10.3
Food in a traditional mixed diet
for one day (Table 10.2).
(Landon Gardiner)

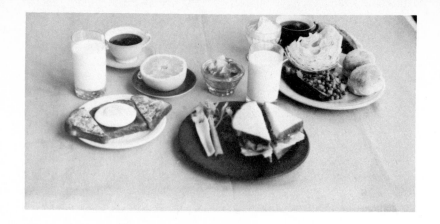

Not only must many types of vegetable foods be included regularly in the total vegetarian diet, but the ample servings indicated also must be maintained and vitamin B_{12} taken regularly, either as a separate supplement or as a fortification ingredient. Vitamin B_{12} is not present in plant foods (9). If Vitamin B_{12} is present in a fortified food, it must be clearly evident on the label. If soy milk is not included in a diet, thus eliminating it as a source of calcium, other sources of calcium must be increased. Leafy green vegetables are good sources, but to substitute for the soy milk calcium they must be eaten in very large quantities.

It is obvious that the basic four food guide requires certain adjustments to accommodate the unique demands of total vegetarian diets. These adjustments are indicated in Table 10.7 in a listing of five food categories, with the minimum daily servings of each required (Fig. 10.4) (8).

Granted that adjustments in the food guide are required to meet the severe challenge of total vegetarian diets, but are guide changes also necessary in planning *modified* vegetarian diets? The answer is *no*. These modified diets include milk, eggs, or both and are called *lacto-, ovo-,* or *lacto-ovo vegetarian diets.* The animal foods add quantity and quality of protein that permit a reduction

lacto-vegetarian diets
Diets including dairy foods as the sole source of animal protein

ovo-vegetarian diets
Diets including eggs as the sole source of animal protein

lacto-ovo-vegetarian diets
Diets that include dairy foods and eggs as sole sources of animal protein

Figure 10.4
Legumes and nuts not only
constitute one of the five
categories of a total vegetarian
diet but they are important meat
alternates on the Daily Food
Selection Guide. (Landon
Gardiner)

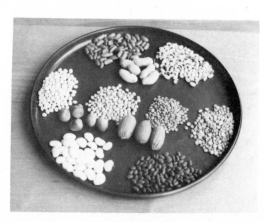

Table 10.6
Foods chosen for a traditional mixed diet and for a total vegetarian diet compared with daily food selection guide

Traditional diet Table 10.2, 2137 calories	**Food selection guide*** Table 10.1	**Total vegetarian diet** Table 10.4, 2203 calories
Foundation food groups		
	Milk group	
2 cups milk 1/8 qt ice cream	2 or more servings	no animal milk (substitute 2 1/3 cup soy milk, fortified with vitamin B_{12})
	Meat group	
3 oz beef 2 oz ham 1 egg	2 or more servings	3/4 cup lentils 3/4 cup Spanish beans 8 cashew nuts no animal protein foods
	Vegetable-fruit group	
1/2 cup carrots, peas 1/4 head lettuce, 1 stalk celery, 2 leaves lettuce 1/2 grapefruit 1 baked apple 1 banana	4 or more servings	1/4 cup raw carrots 1/4 cup beets 1/4 cup parsnips 1 cup turnip greens 1/2 grapefruit 1/4 cup dates 2 tbsp lemon juice 1 banana
	Grain group	
4 slices enriched bread 2 enriched rolls	4 or more servings	5 slices whole wheat bread 3/4 cup corn grits 3/4 cup brown rice
Additional foods		
5 tsp butter or margarine 1 tbsp French dressing 1 tbsp mayonnaise 3 tsp sugar		5 tsp margarine 2 tbsp vegetable oil 1 tbsp molasses

*cooked or processed except celery, lettuce, banana, dates, carrots, grapefruit, lemon.

in the intake of vegetable protein. Animal foods also provide vitamin B_{12}, thus eliminating the need for a supplement. Experience has shown that the regular four-group guide can be applied as successfully to modified vegetarian diets as to the general mixed diet that includes animal flesh. In general, nutritionists recommend that vegetarians include milk and/or eggs in their diets (7). Dietary allowances are easy to attain with common foods; the modified vegetarian diet itself is less spartan; and serving sizes are more in keeping with customary food habits. All these advantages augur

Table 10.7
Adjustments in the food guide for total vegetarian diets

Minimum number of daily servings*	Food group	Serving size
one serving of	nuts and seeds, including nut butters	2 tbsp
two servings of	prepared vegetable proteins fortified with vitamin B_{12}, including fortified soy milk	1 slice meat analog (meat substitute made of legumes and/or grains), or 1 cup soy milk or a vitamin-B_{12} supplement
three servings of	fruits, preferably fresh; also dried fruits and unsweetened juices	1 fresh fruit, 2 tbsp dried, or ½ cup juice
four servings of	vegetables, include one serving legumes or beans, *and* one serving green leafy vegetables	1 cup
five servings of	grains, preferably unrefined, including breads, cereals, rice, barley, corn, millet, and pasta	½ cup cooked grains or 1 slice bread

*Increase all servings by one during growth periods such as adolescence, pregnancy, and lactation, as follows: two servings of nuts and seeds, three of B_{12} fortified foods, four of fruits, five of vegetables, and six of grains.

well for a person continuing on a modified vegetarian diet. (See Chap. 7 for a more definitive consideration of quantitative and qualitative protein needs as they may apply to vegetarianism.)

Some people take exception to the food-group concept for food selection guides. They believe it is confusing to have foods assembled in groups that provide such a wide range of nutrient offerings, and that variety in food selection is sufficient guarantee of nutritional adequacy. Variety is important because no food or grouping of foods contains all the nutrients needed in sufficient amounts (10). But generalizations have their limitations. The word "variety" has different meanings to different people. Unless consumers have some knowledge of food values and nutrient needs, or certain boundaries are prescribed with respect to food choices, nutritionally important foods can be overlooked and food intake can be deficient in certain essential nutrients, even though the diet contains many different foods.

There are others who maintain that food groups do not reflect the way people really choose their food. In one study of a small number of low-income rural families, a few families obtained all their calcium from sources outside the milk group. A few families also obtained their entire supply of dietary ascorbic acid from foods outside the vegetable-fruit group (11). This is an interesting finding, but official agricultural consumption data show that people in the United States as a whole obtain about 75 percent of their calcium from milk and milk products and more than 90 percent of their ascorbic acid from vegetables and fruits. These facts substantiate the soundness of the food-group concept in food guides. The survey probably best demonstrates that there are many ways to obtain an adequate diet.

Finally, there are some people who advocate disregarding food groups entirely and going directly to nutrients. This is essentially the philosophy of nutrition labeling. We will consider labeling in light of its potential usefulness for providing guidance in meal planning through the nutrient approach.

Nutrition Labeling—An Aid to Food Selection

Certain basics of the Federal Food and Drug Administration's (FDA) nutrition labeling program were introduced in Chapter 2 in connection with the US RDA, the scientific foundation for its labeling plan. You should review these principles as a preliminary to considering the program as a food selection tool (12).

Figure 10.5 shows an actual nutrition label as it appears on a quart carton of skim milk. It illustrates the way labels provide definitive nutrient information about individual foods. It also demonstrates the way the food processor implements the requirements of the labeling program outlined in Chapter 2. First, the label identi-

Figure 10.5
Nutrition label: one quart carton skim milk

SKIM MILK
Vitamin A & D
Grade A, Pastuerized
Homogenized

Nutrition Information
per serving

Serving size	one cup
Servings per container	4
Calories	90
Protein	8 grams
Carbohydrate	11 grams
Fat	1 gram

Percentage of U.S.
Recommended Daily Allowances (U.S.RDA)

Protein	20	Vitamin D	25
Vitamin A	10	Vitamin B6	4
Vitamin C	4	Vitamin B12	15
Thiamin	6	Phosphorus	20
Riboflavin	25	Magnesium	8
Niacin	*	Zinc	4
Calcium	30	Pantothenic acid	6
Iron	*		

*Contains less than 2% of the U.S.RDA
of these nutrients
Skim milk, Vitamin A Palmitate, Vitamin D3

fies the product, skim milk, and makes the claim that vitamins A and D have been added. It then specifies that 1 cup of milk is the serving size and that there are four servings in the quart carton. The energy value of 1 cup of milk and the grams of protein, carbohydrate, and fat in that amount appear next. Eight nutrients are listed below that, with the percentages of the RDA for each supplied by 1 cup of milk. These eight—protein, vitamin A, thiamin, riboflavin, niacin, vitamin C, calcium, and iron—are the nutrients that must appear on the label if the processor engages in labeling. The remaining seven nutrients listed are among the twelve optional ones that may be added at the discretion of the processor: vitamin D, vitamin B_6, vitamin B_{12}, phosphorus, magnesium, zinc, and pantothenic acid. In this particular case, the processor has chosen not to provide optional information about cholesterol, saturated and unsaturated fatty acids, and sodium (see Chapter 2).

You can obtain a considerable amount of information about individual foods from nutrition labels. Such data are available primarily for foods sold in containers—cans, cartons, wrappers—on which information can be printed. Foods in fresh form, such as fresh vegetables, fruits, meats, poultry, and fish, do not carry nutrition labels, although efforts are being made to extend the program to foods of this type. At present, however, a large proportion of common foods are not included in the labeling program. This fact prevents consumers from depending on nutrition labels as the sole source of nutrition information about their diets. For the time being they must seek composition data for nonlabeled foods elsewhere, chiefly in government-compiled tables developed for the purpose (13).

Despite these limitations, labeling has many favorable aspects, among them the increased public awareness of the importance of foods as sources of nutrients, and consciousness among consumers of the health advantages of selecting nutritious foods. Shoppers are asking for more nutrition-labeled foods. Concern of food processors for providing nutritious products is also an outcome; more processors are entering the labeling program. Nutrition labeling thus has made a significant start. By studying labels people can see the vast difference in the nutrient contributions of foods and the need for variety in food selection if foods are to dovetail satisfactorily into nutritionally adequate diets. People are also learning to compare labels in seeking good sources of certain nutrients at reasonable prices and are noting the nutrient contributions of formulated and fabricated foods. They look for the specific nutrients their diets require, such as vitamin B_{12} in the total vegetarian diet.

Without some expertise in nutrition and great perseverance, however, one should not expect to rely on labeling information to determine the adequacy of a total diet. Nutrition labeling data are necessarily scattered and incomplete. A common problem related to the interpretation of data is the temptation to attach undue importance to the individual nutrient contributions of foods without regard for the total concept of an adequate diet. An example is the choice of a synthetic fruit-flavored drink fortified with ascorbic acid but devoid of other nutrients, in preference to a citrus fruit juice carrying ascorbic acid and several other important nutrients.

The consumer in this instance is aware of the need for ascorbic acid, but the selection of a beverage is made without regard for the nutritional completeness of the diet as a whole.

Nutrition labeling does provide an important instrument for identifying nutritive values in foods. It should become increasingly useful as more foods are labeled and people learn to adapt and interpret the specific data made available. It will become a more helpful nutritional device when consumers learn to use labeling in conjunction with a daily food selection guide that provides a reliable general pattern of eating (Table 10.1).

The guide, with its roots in the RDA, provides a general perspective on the foods that supply the day's required nutrients. Nutrition labeling, which also has its origin in the RDA, may supplement and amplify this function with nutritional data that helps to evaluate and upgrade the diet. Any single plan for dietary improvement has certain limitations. The food selection guide and nutrition labeling, when judiciously implemented, can be mutually supportive. Nutrition education of the public is important to the full success of both.

A CLOSER LOOK AT THE FOUNDATION FOOD GROUPS

In putting the food selection guide to use it is necessary to know the make-up of its food groups and the practical aspects of their use in meal planning. Let us consider each group individually.

Milk Group

The daily food guide calls for specified amounts of milk to cover nutritional needs for different ages and conditions. The amount designated may be consumed as a beverage, in combination with other foods in prepared dishes, and as an accompaniment of such foods as cereals and desserts. The amount of milk used in soups, hot chocolate, and casserole dishes, for example, may be considerable. Milk products such as ice cream and cheese can be used as alternates for milk to some extent (Table 10.8). Federal and state standards have been established for the composition of milk products, and current data provide nutritive values of dairy foods (Fig. 10.6) (14).

Milk is available in various forms: fresh fluid, evaporated, and dried. Some is whole milk, containing all of its original butterfat, while some is partially or entirely skimmed. Buttermilk, for example, may be skim or partially skim milk; dry milk may be skim or whole milk; evaporated milk is double-strength whole or skim milk. Any of these milks can be used as a sole or partial milk supply. The cartons, bottles, cans, or packages in which these milks are sold specify whether their contents are skim- or whole-milk products.

Labels also indicate what, if anything, has been added to the milk and the methods of processing involved. For example, *pasteurization,* homogenization, evaporation, and drying processes are indicated, and additions such as vitamin A and D concentrates and nonfat dry milk solids are specified with their amounts. When

pasteurization of milk
Heating of milk to 161° F and maintaining that temperature for 15 seconds (one of several equivalent time-temperature relationships)

homogenization
Mechanical process of forcing milk under high pressure through very small openings to disperse fat in such fine globules that it will remain distributed throughout

Figure 10.6
Milk group (National Dairy
Council)

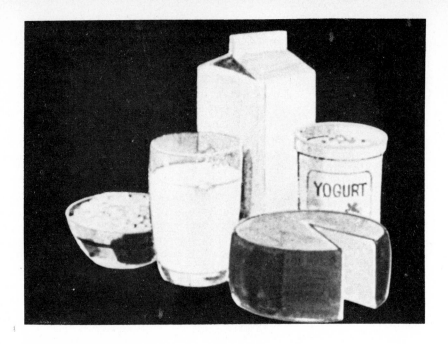

chocolate syrup is added to whole milk or low-fat milks (1 or 2 percent butterfat), the products are called chocolate milk and their
cartons are properly labeled.

   Yogurt, a widely accepted milk with the consistency of soft custard, is a fermented milk manufactured from fresh whole or low-fat
milk, often with skim milk solids added. Fermentation is accomplished by a milk culture of one or more strains of organisms. The
milk is pasteurized and homogenized, inoculated, and incubated at
a specified temperature. Research has brought forth various other
forms of milk (15). Sweet *acidophilus milk*, another fermented
milk, has been introduced in some markets. Scientists are experi-
menting with the treatment of milk with lactase from microbial
sources such as yeast to aid persons who are intolerant of lactose.

lactose intolerance
*Resulting from insufficient
lactase enzyme to digest
lactose*

   Cheeses are made from the curds of whole or skim milk; some
cheeses are hard, others are semihard or soft. When curds are
formed in making cheese, the whey is drained off and with it part
of the water-soluble vitamin content of the original milk. Thus,
while cheese is a concentrated source of many of the nutrients of
milk, its loss of whey prevents it from being a full milk equivalent.
Attempts have been made to retrieve the nutrient losses in whey
on a commercial basis. Various whey products have been developed
experimentally to enhance the nutritive value of other foods.

   Ice cream is made from cream, milk, and milk solids with stabi-
lizers, sweetening agents, flavorings, and sometimes fruits and
nuts. Under federal standards, plain ice cream contains not less
than 10 percent milk fat and 20 percent total milk solids by
weight. Obviously it contains all the nutrients of milk itself. However, the nutrients in ice cream are present in different proportions
than in milk. The addition of sweeteners reduces the proportion of

nutrients to energy value; this prevents ice cream from being fully equivalent to milk on a volume basis (Table 10.8).

Filled and imitation dairy products are on the market. A filled product is one made by combining fats or oils other than milk fat with milk solids. The resulting product resembles an existing dairy food. Canned milks that fit this description are now available. Cheese in which vegetable oils replace the milk fat have been introduced, and nondairy creamers for coffee in which similar substitutions have been made are sold in powder form. An imitation dairy product resembles an existing dairy food but contains no milk solids.

Servings   One standard cup of milk is regarded as a serving. This represents 8 ounces of fluid milk or, in liquid measure, ½ pint or ¼ quart. When the number of servings is specified in glasses, each must be large enough to contain 1 measuring cup of milk. About 1 to 1½ ounces of the hard cheeses and 2 ounces of cottage cheese (¼ c) are considered servings of these foods. For ice cream, ¼ to ⅓ pint is usually one serving.

Choosing Dairy Foods   Enjoyable, safe, economical, and nutritionally adequate meals are the ultimate objective of the daily food guide. The selection of foods within each food group should therefore be made with these points in mind. As applied to the milk group, the guidelines mean buying products of good quality as well as choosing forms of milk and dairy foods consistent with the limitations of the food budget, the food tastes of family members, and

Table 10.8
Milk equivalents

Full equivalents of 1 cup (8 oz) fluid whole milk

1 cup whole milk yogurt	
½ cup undiluted evaporated milk	+ ½ cup water
⅓ cup dry whole milk	+ ⅔ cup water
1 cup fluid skim milk	+ ¾ tbsp (1 medium pat) butter
1 cup fluid buttermilk	+ ¾ tbsp (1 medium pat) butter

Full equivalents of 1 cup (8 oz) fluid skim milk

⅓ cup dry skim milk	+ ⅔ cup water
1 cup fluid buttermilk	
1 cup skim milk yogurt	

Calcium equivalents of various dairy foods to 1 cup of whole milk

Because the milk group makes such an important contribution of calcium, the various foods in the milk group are usually equated on the basis of their calcium content:

1½ oz American or cheddar cheese	= 1 cup whole milk
2 cups creamed cottage cheese	= 1 cup whole milk
1¾ cup ice cream	= 1 cup whole milk

the nutrient values of the different products. When economy is a prime consideration, a survey of local prices of the different forms of milk will show which form, or combination of forms, constitutes the best choice.

Dairy foods purchased should be those produced, handled, packaged, and sold under the jurisdiction of officially constituted agencies. State and local governments, through their public health departments, have the legal responsibility for protection of fluid milk supplies. Sanitary standards are recommended by the Federal Public Health Service and are used in many states, counties, and municipalities as the bases for sanitary regulations. Containers and bottle caps carry a permit number issued by the local health official to each authorized dealer.

Pasteurization is recognized as the only broad-scale measure that destroys disease organisms in raw milk, if they should be present. There are small losses of water-soluble vitamins in the pasteurization of milk, but the public health advantage of pasteurization far outweighs such losses. *Ultrapasteurization* of whipping cream and half-and-half has been introduced to extend the length of time they can be stored. Sterilized half-and-half is sold mostly in individual-serving size containers.

ultrapasteurization of cream
Heating of cream to 280° F for at least 2 seconds (sterilization)

Certain manufactured dairy products are subject to grade labeling under US Dept. of Agriculture's quality-approved rating plan (16). Canned milk products are processed and handled under government supervision. The same is true of dry milks. At present, instant dry skim (nonfat dry) milk may be packed under US Department of Agriculture grade labels. The appearance of the official shield emblem on a package of such milk assures the consumer of dependable flavor, wholesomeness, and compliance with sanitary requirements.

Several firms sell cottage cheese under a US inspection emblem, and certain hard cheeses bear US grade designations (16). Grading is based on standards of flavor, body, and texture. Approved dairy plants using the grading service operate under the rules for sanitation and packing specified by the US Department of Agriculture.

Fresh fluid milk requires special care in handling after it reaches the kitchen. It should be placed in the refrigerator at once and kept there, tightly covered in its original container and isolated from foods of strong odor. Leftover milk should not be returned to the original container. These measures not only protect the milk from possible contamination but also avoid absorption of foreign flavors that lessen the enjoyment in consumption.

The food selection guide was developed with foods and eating patterns of the United States in mind. But few people today eat in strictly traditional fashion. This includes choices of dairy foods. You may therefore wish to know how some of the less familiar foods can be accommodated by the food selection guide. It is necessary to be aware of the nature of the ethnic foods involved and, if they are mixtures, to know the kinds and amounts of their major ingredients. For example, you need to know that café con leche is coffee made chiefly of milk in order to place it properly in the milk group, and that yogurt is the equivalent of other milks of similar

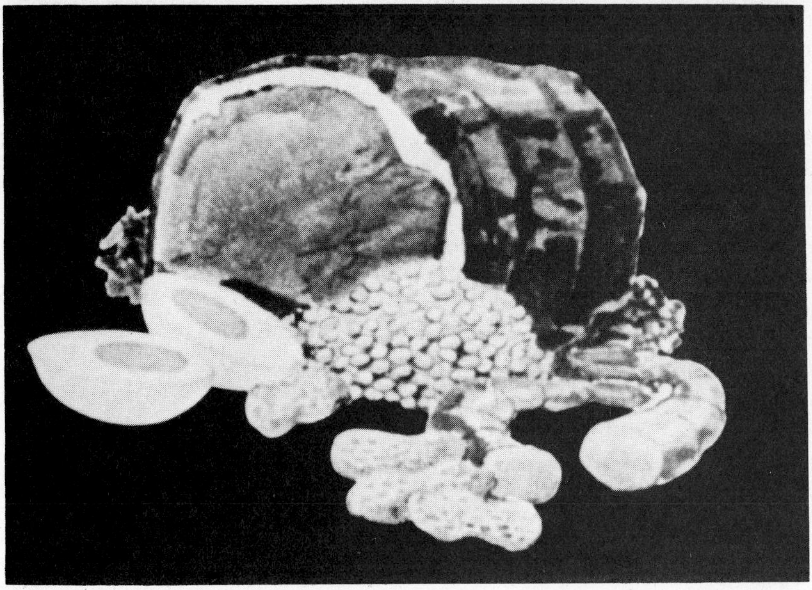

Figure 10.7
Meat group (National Dairy Council)

fat content. Another problem in dealing with the milk group is equating unfamiliar cheeses of the Near East and other areas with milk nutrients. When actual nutrient values of such cheeses are unavailable, Appendix K may be useful for estimating equivalents for products similar to those of the United States.

Meat Group

The daily food guide offers a double listing under the meat group: foods of animal origin, such as lean meats, fish, poultry, eggs, and cheese; and alternate foods of plant origin, such as dry beans, dry peas, and nuts (Fig. 10.7). These general classes offer a large number of individual foods from which to choose two or more daily servings. Lean meat, for example, can be selected from such familiar sources as beef, veal, lamb, pork (fresh or cured) and liver, as well as from the *variety meats* including heart, brains, tongue, and kidneys. Less usual are wild meat sources, such as squirrel, rabbit, bear, deer, and buffalo.

Fish choices include shellfish, fresh- and salt-water varieties of fish, and fish in fresh, dried, frozen, or canned forms. Poultry refers to any type of fowl, such as chicken, turkey, guinea hen, duck, goose, and the giblets of these birds. Game birds—pheasants, wild ducks, and grouse—are also members of this group. Less traditional forms of meat include "turkey ham," made from turkey meat but treated and smoked to look and taste like ham, and "hot dogs" made from turkey or chicken instead of the usual pork or beef.

Meats, poultry, and fish can be prepared in many different ways, thus adding to the variety in selection. They can be roasted, broiled, fried, baked, or simmered in soups and stews.

Eggs can be from any kind of fowl, but composition data used in this text are for domestic hens' eggs. Brown-shelled and white-shelled eggs are equal in nutritive value, flavor, and cooking performance. Hard cheeses and cottage cheese are considered part of the meat group because of their protein content, but cream cheese does not qualify. Eggs and cheese also can be served in a variety of ways, both alone and as ingredients of other dishes.

Plant sources in the meat group include all kinds of dry legumes, such as navy beans, lima beans, and lentils, which are usually served baked or boiled in main dishes. Cooked beans are available in frozen form in some areas but are more commonly bought in cans. Peanuts are also legumes, although they are commonly used as nuts in the United States. Also in this classification are the various kinds of split dried peas, pinto beans, black beans, black-eye peas, red kidney beans, soy beans, chick peas, and pigeon peas. Nuts, as well as nut butters, are likewise considered members of the meat group (16). Also included are the textured vegetable proteins (*TVP*)—largely soy—which may be processed to simulate in shape and flavor meat products such as sausage and bacon. These are referred to as meat *analogs*. TVP granules may be blended with fresh ground beef and thus serve as meat extenders. The federal school lunch program accepts a mixture of 30 percent TVP and 70 percent beef in the Type A lunch (see Chap. 12).

TVP
Processed vegetable proteins
analogs
Something similar to something else

The meat group thus offers almost limitless choices from among many kinds and varieties of food prepared in many different ways. As shown in Figure 10.1, this group provides significant amounts of protein, iron, and thiamin in an ordinary mixed diet. Its major contribution is protein. From our previous consideration of protein, you know that animal and vegetable sources differ in quality, and that it is desirable to consume some protein from animal sources daily unless the vegetable source is soybeans, gandules, or garbanzos, which approach lean meats in amino-acid content.

Efforts are being made to provide meats with less fat. For example, meat animals are being bred for leanness, ground beef can be purchased with different proportions of lean to fat, and meat foods such as frankfurters and luncheon meats are available with more lean and less fat than formerly. The fat content of federally inspected frankfurters and other cooked sausages is limited to 30 percent by US Department of Agriculture regulation.

Servings   About 3 ounces of cooked fish, poultry, or lean meat (without bone) are considered one serving on the daily food guide. The same meats in their raw state weigh about 4 ounces. Portions vary somewhat with the kind and cut of meat, as indicated in Appendix K.

The following quantities of other foods in the meat group are commonly considered as servings: one egg, 1 to 1½ ounces of cheese, 2 ounces of luncheon meat (such as bologna), 2 tablespoons of peanut butter, or ¾ cup canned baked beans. Remember, however, that each provides at most about half the amount of protein in a serving of lean meat, fish, or poultry. Therefore, if any one of these is to be used as a full protein equivalent, the quantity must be doubled. Serving sizes are usually controlled by the number of sources available. Fewer sources merely mean larger servings or more of them. Sizes of servings must also be adjusted for persons whose needs differ from those of the average adult. Young children need smaller servings; fast-growing, active teenagers, larger ones.

While variety is always desirable, it is possible to select adequately from the meat group even when few choices present themselves. For example, Woodlands Indians obtain sufficient protein although their sources are sometimes limited to fish or wild game (see Appendix E). Spanish-Americans find beans an adequate chief source of protein, provided the varieties chosen offer high-quality protein (see Appendixes B and C).

Ethnic Foods—Meat Group (17)   Various kinds of meats and meat alternates are staples in certain ethnic diets and must be evaluated for their eligibility to belong to the meat group. For example, salt pork and fat back, which have little or no lean portions, do not qualify as protein foods. Many of the meats classified as "soul foods" probably can not be considered as full servings of lean meats. These include pigs' feet, jowls, tails, ears, knuckles, and chitterlings. Unfortunately, there is little specific data on their nutritive yields, but protein and iron content are undoubtedly low. When such meats are prepared in combination with dry beans, however, a liberal serving of the mixed dish may well be credited as a serving from the meat group.

An acceptable selection of meat alternates may depend on the *kinds* of dry beans used. This is a problem with Spanish-American diets, some of which include more than ten times the amount of beans typically eaten in the United States. When beans of poor protein quality are used, such as red kidney or white navy beans, the addition of animal protein or beans of higher protein quality makes an important difference. When legumes such as soybeans, garbanzos, and gandules are eaten in liberal amounts, the need for animal protein is lessened. In such cases, interpretation of the food guide goes beyond the mere number of servings.

Food mixtures that include ground meat pose a problem of what qualifies as a serving. For example, Mexican tacos, a favorite food with many North Americans, consist of ground meat with shredded lettuce rolled in a tortilla. But tacos vary greatly in size. On the basis of the amount of meat in one taco, it is necessary to estimate what portion of a serving of meat it represents and how many tacos one must eat to equal about 3 ounces of lean meat. Other types of mixed dishes, such as those of South American origin, must also be evaluated. Brazil's *feijoada*—a stew of black beans and pork—fully qualifies as a member of the meat group. The same can be said of *pasta e fagiuoli*, based on pinto beans, and of *moqueca*, based on fish, which are typical Brazilian food mixtures popular in the United States.

Choosing Meats   Meats are well liked and form the basis of many meals. If economy is a consideration, it is important to know how to get the most meat for the money available. Price is not the criterion of food value, and flavor often depends more on how the meat is cooked than on its cost per pound. Choosing the right cut and cooking the meat properly ensures maximum food value and flavor in the particular dish prepared.

Considerable assistance is offered to consumers in choosing meat for its safety and quality (16). For example, federal inspection is compulsory for all meat shipped in interstate commerce. Any meat that is graded must first be inspected for wholesomeness. Meats that pass inspection carry a round purple stamp of harmless vegetable coloring bearing the legend "U.S. Inspected."

Beef, veal, calf, lamb, yearling mutton, and mutton are federally graded. These meats bear a purple stamp in the shape of a shield with the letters "USDA" and the designated grade. The federal meat grader assesses only whole carcasses or wholesale cuts. This is done in the interest of a fair and technically adequate appraisal of the entire animal. The stamp itself appears in such a way that the grade label can be seen on almost all retail cuts.

Grades have been carefully defined and are similar for most meats. Details are beyond the scope of our discussion, but the US Department of Agriculture provides such information through its consumer bulletins (16). Grades offer consumers a choice of quality and give them an opportunity to choose a less expensive cut of meat when necessary without sacrificing wholesomeness. The lower grades often have more lean and less fat (and sometimes less bone), giving more for the money than higher grades. Slight variations in beef grading guidelines are pending. These will permit buyers to select choice grade beef of lower fat content than formerly. Any good-quality beef, graded or ungraded, has a red lean portion, red bones, and flaky, light-colored fat. Poultry and eggs—and, to a more limited extent, dry beans and peas—also have their own grading systems.

The US Department of Commerce provides an official inspection service for fish. Such products can be identified by the official USDC grade or inspection shields that appear on the package. Fishery products that display these shields have been processed under continuous in-plant inspection and have met definite quality, processing, and packaging requirements.

Fresh meat, like fresh milk, needs careful handling in the kitchen if it is to stay in top condition and retain the best flavor. Meat should be covered loosely and stored in the refrigerator. Ground fresh meats and variety meats such as liver keep less well than others. These should be cooked within a day or two at most after purchase.

Vegetable-Fruit Group

Figure 10.1 shows that the vegetable-fruit group is almost the sole source of ascorbic acid in an ordinary mixed diet and provides more than two-thirds of the vitamin-A activity. However, there is great variation in the yield of these vitamins from individual kinds of fruits and vegetables. Knowing these variations makes it possible to take advantage of the higher nutrient values of certain vegetables and fruits and to avoid the limitations imposed by poor choices. The group as a whole is composed of a vast number of foods from which to select the four or more servings proposed by the daily food guide (Fig. 10.8).

Dark Green and Orange-Colored Sources of Vitamin-A Activity   The dark green (mainly leafy) vegetables eaten chiefly for their vita-

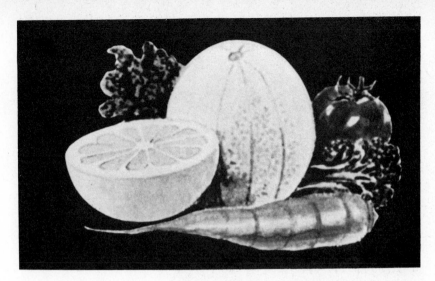

Figure 10.8
Vegetable and fruit group
(National Dairy Council)

min-A activity include beet greens, broccoli, chard, collards, cress, kale, mustard greens, spinach, turnip tops, and wild greens (dandelion and others). The orange-colored vegetables, also rich in vitamin-A activity, include carrots, pumpkin, sweet potatoes, winter squash, and yams (Fig. 9.2). A few orange-flesh fruits that represent good sources of vitamin-A activity are apricots, muskmelon, and mangoes. (For a selection of vitamin-A equivalents, see Table 10.9).

Table 10.9
Equivalents in Vitamin A activity

Each of the following common foods in the quantity designated provides approximately the same amount of Vitamin A activity as does ½ cup of carrots. This amount is more than the adult's daily dietary allowance for the vitamin. Vegetables are cooked unless otherwise specified.

| carrots | ½ cup
1 serving | Vitamin-A activity
7615 IU |
| --- | --- | --- |
| | **Approximate quantity** | **Number of servings** |
| **spinach** | ½ cup | 1 |
| **sweet potato** | ⅔ potato (orange color) | 1 (scant) |
| **muskmelon** | ½ fruit (orange flesh) | 1 |
| **collards** | ½ cup | 1 |
| **dandelion greens** | ¾ cup | 1¼ |
| **winter squash** | 1 cup | 2 |
| **mustard greens** | 1 cup | 2 |
| **apricots** | 1 cup (dried, stewed) | 2 |
| **peppers,** sweet | 2⅓ peppers (red, raw) | 4 |
| **broccoli** | 2 cups | 4 |
| **chili powder** | 6 tsp (from red peppers) | 6 |
| **tomato juice** | 4 cups | 8 |
| **peas,** green | 8 cups | 16 |
| **cabbage** | 64 cups (shredded raw) | 127 |

Table 10.10
Equivalents in ascorbic acid

Each of the following common foods in the quantity designated provides approximately the same amount of ascorbic acid as does one serving of fresh orange juice. This amount covers an adult's daily dietary allowance for this vitamin.

orange juice	½ cup (1 small glass) 1 serving	ascorbic acid 60 mg

	Approximate quantity	Number of servings
acerola cherry	½ cherry	½
guava	¼ guava	½
peppers, sweet	½ pepper (red, raw)	½
muskmelon	⅓ melon	¾
broccoli	½ cup (cooked)	1
strawberries	⅔ cup (raw)	1⅓
grapefruit	¾ fruit	1½
papaya	⅔ cup cubed fruit (raw)	1½
mangoes	1 cup cubed fruit (raw)	2
potato	2 potatoes (white, cooked)	2
cabbage	1½ cups (shredded raw)	3
tomato juice	1½ cups	3
pineapple juice	2½ cups	5
lettuce	2 heads	8
beans, green	4 cups (cooked)	8
apples	10 apples (raw)	10
apple juice	30 cups	60

Sources of Ascorbic Acid Citrus fruits widely known for their ascorbic acid content include grapefruit, oranges, lemons, and tangerines, and their juices (Fig. 9.8). Other good or excellent sources of ascorbic acid are muskmelons, strawberries, broccoli, and several tropical fruits including guavas and raw sweet green and red peppers.

Less concentrated but often significant sources of ascorbic acid include the following foods when consumed in quantity: tomatoes, tomato juice, white potatoes, dark green leafy vegetables, and other vegetables and fruits when eaten raw. (For ascorbic acid equivalents, see Table 10.10).

Other Fruits and Vegetables Other vegetables include: asparagus, lima beans, green beans, beets, cabbage, cauliflower, celery, corn, cucumbers, eggplant, kohlrabi, lettuce, okra, onions, green peas, plantain, rutabagas, sauerkraut, summer squash, and turnips.

Other fruits include: apples, avocados, bananas, berries, cherries, dates, figs, grapes, nectarines, peaches, pears, pineapple, plums, prunes, raisins, rhubarb, and watermelon; as well as the juices and nectars of many of the fruits. Vegetables and fruits are important sources of fiber. Most of those listed above furnish some vitamin A and ascorbic acid as well as minerals, and they provide a variety of color, texture, and flavor in meals and snacks.

Many fruits and vegetables are available in fresh, canned, dried, and frozen forms. In general, nutrients are retained well when foods are processed by modern methods. Therefore, fruits and vegetables with high nutrient levels at the time of processing offer the best prospects of remaining good sources of nutrients at the time of consumption.

Servings Serving sizes of vegetables and fruits vary somewhat with the kind and form of food that is served; nevertheless ½ cup is considered one serving of practically all cooked vegetables, cooked fruits, and fruit juices. In the case of most raw fruits, it is more practical to consider as one serving a single unit of the fruit, such as one banana or one potato, or some portion of a unit, such as one-half grapefruit.

The daily food selection guide specifies a dark green or orange-colored vegetable at least every other day. A person may well eat a full serving of such a vegetable every day, however. If that is not feasible, a half-serving daily or a full serving three to four times weekly can substitute. Some good sources of vitamin-A activity also provide significant amounts of ascorbic acid, as shown in Tables 10.9 and 10.10.

In choosing foods for ascorbic acid value, it is usually safer to pick one excellent source or a few very good sources daily than to depend on small amounts obtained from a number of poor sources. If less concentrated sources are chosen, it is best that they be eaten in raw form. Ascorbic acid is easily destroyed or reduced in the handling and cooking of foods. Normal losses are accounted for in Appendix K. However, there is no way of knowing the exact losses that have taken place in any given food at the time it is eaten (see Chap. 9).

Ethnic Foods—Vegetable-Fruit Group Vegetables and fruits found in ethnic diets should be evaluated to see if they qualify in ascorbic acid and vitamin-A content for the food guide. Peppers serve as a good example. Quantity is the first consideration, for you must determine whether they are served in liberal amounts, as in Mexican-American diets, or merely as seasoning or garnish, as in the traditional diet of the United States. There are many kinds of peppers with a wide range of nutritive values. In general, sweet red peppers in raw form are a good source of vitamin A and an excellent source of ascorbic acid (see Tables 10.9 and 10.10.). In canned hot chili sauce the vitamin-A content remains high, but ascorbic acid content is reduced considerably. The ascorbic acid content of chili powder made from red peppers is fairly low, but some vitamin A is retained. In general, green peppers are strikingly lower in vitamin-A content than red peppers and somewhat lower in ascorbic acid. Tropical fruits such as acerola cherries, guavas, mangoes, and papayas are excellent sources of ascorbic acid (Table 10.10).

Bamboo shoots and bean sprouts have recently become popular in the United States. Both vegetables may be counted in the vegetable-fruit group if the amounts eaten qualify as servings. Neither is a good source of vitamin A, but some types of bean sprouts in the raw state are moderately good sources of vitamin C. Some foods that grow wild, found particularly in the southwest United States are nutritionally equivalent to cultivated products. These include wild potatoes, onions, celery, spinach, cactus, berries, and yucca fruits. Prickly pear cactus can serve as a vegetable salad. Green plantain can substitute for white potato in the food selection pattern when serving sizes are comparable.

Choosing Vegetables and Fruits   The condition of fresh vegetables and fruits when they reach market makes a big difference in the food value, appearance, and flavor of these foods when served. Wilted, discolored, soft, or moldy foods probably have lost most of their ascorbic acid (see Chap. 9). In addition, there is wastage from excessive trimming. Such foods are expensive at any price.

The federal government has established grade standards for most of the fresh fruits and vegetables on the market (16). At present this has been done chiefly for the wholesaler, but consumers benefit indirectly because of the generally high quality of graded products. In addition, there are a limited number of standards developed for use at the retail level. These grades and their definitions are carefully outlined in publications of the US Dept. of Agriculture. It is important for consumers to become familiar with the characteristics that form the basis for grades. These are helpful in identifying desirable qualities of fresh fruits and vegetables that bear no grade designations. Grades have also been developed for a large number of canned, dried, and frozen fruits and vegetables.

Review the specific suggestions made in Chapter 9 for handling and cooking vegetables and fruits at home to preserve ascorbic acid. The measures taken to keep foods crisp and to preserve their attractiveness and flavor are the same measures that help to retain their nutritive values.

Estimate at local prices the costs of those foods in Table 10.9 that are equivalent in vitamin-A activity to ½ cup of cooked carrots.

Do the same for foods in Table 10.10 that are equivalent in ascorbic acid yield to ½ cup of orange juice.

Consider the feasibility of using the various foods in the amounts required as sources of these two vitamins. Make a list of fruits and vegetables that furnish significant quantities of both ascorbic acid and vitamin-A activity.

Grain Group

The grain group includes all the grains that are served in whole grain, enriched, or fortified forms: wheat, corn, oats, buckwheat, rice, and rye. It consists of several categories of foods, as follows:

☐ *breads:* yeast breads, rolls, quick breads, biscuits, buns, muffins, pancakes, waffles, crackers;
☐ *breakfast cereals:* ready-to-eat including flaked, rolled, puffed; to be cooked including whole, ground, rolled; and

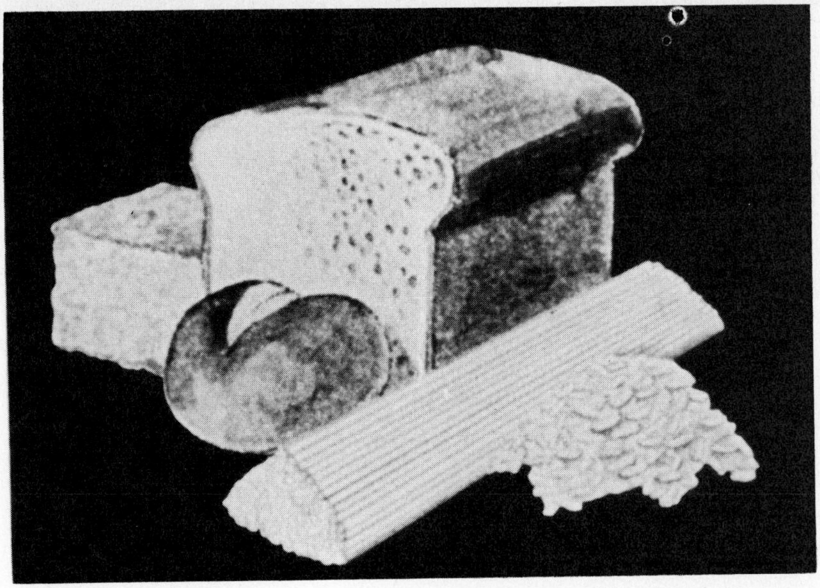

Figure 10.9
Grain group (National Dairy
Council)

□ *grain foods:* macaroni, spaghetti, noodles, flours, rice, corn-meal.

The daily food pattern calls for four or more servings of whole grain, enriched, or fortified grain products (Fig. 10.9). Whole grains are those that retain their germ and outer layers and thus the nutrients contained in those parts. Whole-grain products include whole-wheat flour and the products made from it, bulgur, dark rye flour, brown rice, and whole ground corn meal. Enriched flour and breads have been identified in Chapter 8. Essentially, enriched flour is white flour to which specified amounts of iron, thiamin, riboflavin, and niacin have been added. Fortified grain products may have enrichment nutrients and/or other nutrients added in varied amounts.

Servings   Serving sizes of grain products naturally vary with the different forms in which they are served. In breads, for example, they are designated in small convenient units, such as one slice, one bun, or one pancake. In cooked cereals, the serving is about ⅔ cup; in the lighter, ready-to-eat cereals the serving is about 1 cup. Servings of grain foods such as macaroni, spaghetti, or rice have been designated as ¾ cup when they are used as main dishes in a meal, usually combined with another food—meat, tomato, or cheese, for example. The individual variations in measures within the grain group are indicated in the separate listings in Appendix K. In general, individual servings within the group can be used interchangeably in menus as long as they adhere to the whole grain, enriched, or fortified categories and the quantities are comparable. As shown in Figure 10.1, grains eaten in amounts proposed on the food guide do not make a striking contribution of any one nutrient but supply substantial amounts of several of them.

Enrichment of flours and breads has done much to make grain products significant sources of certain nutrients in the United States food supply (see Chap. 8). These nutrients, iron and the B vitamins, are sometimes difficult to obtain in sufficient amounts. The use of recommended quantities of enriched, fortified or whole grains may in many cases be the deciding factor in achieving adequacy. Other enriched grain products are macaroni, noodles, rice, and corn meal (Table 8.6).

Grain products of all kinds, including breads, are pleasantly bland foods that people do not tire of. These foods are usually present in at least one form in almost every meal. Grain products are staple items that blend with and extend the use of many other foods, such as fruits with breakfast foods, vegetables or cheese with macaroni, and spreads on bread or crackers.

The major losses of nutrients in the commercial processing of cereals have been taken into consideration in Appendix K. Also considrered are additional losses, chiefly of thiamin, that may result when cereals are home-cooked. Small decreases of thiamin in toasted bread are taken into account as well.

Ethnic Foods—Grain Group   Grains and grain products common in ethnic diets should be examined for their eligibility for the grain group in the food guide. In order to qualify, such products must consist of whole, fortified, or enriched grains. When they qualify, foods made of corn—preferred by Latin Americans and in the southern areas of the United States—are for practical purposes interchangeable with other grains. Corn bread, corn pone, tortillas, and hominy grits—all made from corn—can substitute for yeast breads, rolls, hot breads, pancakes, and breakfast cereals made from wheat or other grains. Bulgur, a form of whole wheat, is the full equivalent of equal amounts of other whole wheat products. The starchy cassava commonly eaten in Brazil and other parts of the world is considered a substitute for common breads although it is not usually a full nutritional equivalent. Essentially the same exchanges can be made for rice, which is preferred among several ethnic groups. "Fry bread," a kind of unsweetened doughnut and a staple in the diet of many American Indians, qualifies for the grain group, as does bread of the Navajos made from their blue cornmeal (see Appendix E).

Choosing Grain Products   Consumers are assisted in shopping for grain products in two major ways: by labels on food wrappings and by federal gradings of a few products. Bread wrappers, for example, inform the purchaser of the weight of the loaf and the kind of flour or flours used, as well as the remaining ingredients listed in order of quantity. The manufacturer may also voluntarily provide certain nutrition information, including the percentage of US RDA furnished by a serving of the product. If a nutritional claim is made, or one or more nutrients added, the manufacturer is *required* to supply a nutrition label, as explained earlier. Under similar circumstances, containers for breakfast cereals must furnish the same type of information. They indicate which, if any, nutrients have been added to fortify the cereal, how much of each nutrient is present in a specified amount of the product, and what percentage they supply of the US RDA.

Federal grades have been established for both white and brown rice, and retail packages sometimes carry these grades. The grades are based on such factors as the presence or absence of defective kernels and objectionable foreign material, whether varieties have been mixed, and the general appearance and color of the rice.

Try out the food selection guide as a measuring stick with various types of diets—your own, the specimen diet (Appendix H), the Puerto Rican diet (Appendix B), and the Plains Indians diet (Appendix E). In each case distribute the day's foods among the four food groups.

Evaluate the food guide as a practical device for locating strengths and weaknesses in food selection. In your own diet, does comparison with the guide reveal essentially the same favorable and unfavorable factors as did your calculations of nutrient content?

A CLOSER LOOK AT ADDITIONAL FOODS

Additional foods are all those that do not fall within the foundation groups we have discussed. Specifically, they include sugars, honey, syrups, jams, jellies, candies, soft drinks, unenriched refined cereals such as grits, and fats. Fats are table spreads, shortenings, cooking fats, fat meats, and oils. These foods are eaten alone, in mixtures such as baked goods, casserole dishes, made desserts, and snack foods; and as additions to other foods such as butter or margarine on bread, sugar with fruits, and dressings on salads.

When additional foods are combined with foundation foods in recipes, the resulting dishes are classified in accordance with the predominate ingredients. Only if a foundation food is the chief ingredient or is supplied in sufficient quantity to provide a full serving of that food should a combined dish be classed as a foundation food. A gelatin dessert with a few slices of banana, for example, should not be considered a serving of fruit.

Additional foods are certainly a part of everyone's daily meals, even though they do not merit the emphasis given to foundation foods as sources of nutrients. Besides their contribution of energy and some nutrients, additional foods help to give meals "staying" qualities. They lend interest and variety in flavor and texture. Additional foods need not be sought, because they are already present to some extent in many foundation foods, such as fat in milk and meat and natural sugars in ripened fruits. Furthermore, calories usually are easy to obtain; every food provides some. The energy most needed are those sources providing abundant nutrients.

As shown in Figure 10.1, energy is the chief contribution of additional foods. Fat is obviously the main source of that energy. The nutrient content of additional foods is small under all practical circumstances. Rarely can real nutrient deficits be eliminated by these foods alone.

FOOD SAFETY

Food falls short of its full nutritional purpose if it is not bacteriologically safe to eat. In that context the subject of food safety is discussed briefly here (18, 19). Federal government agencies establish certain food standards that relate basically to safety (20). In addition, the FDA provides food processing plant inspection and laboratory examination services that deal directly with bacteriological safety measures. These services offer reasonable assurance that food products will be safe and wholesome because they concentrate on those production phases in which faulty processing or insanitary practices can easily result in contamination. The result is that food safety problems at the industry level have been reduced to a minimum. It is estimated however, that there are more than 20 million cases of food poisoning annually and that the majority of them are traceable to unsafe methods of handling food in post-commercial operations. Consequently special emphasis is being placed on improved procedures for handling food in homes and institutions. Recommended methods are reviewed here along with reminders of the hazards involved in consuming foods when safety measures are ignored and bacterial growth in food is uncontrolled.

Bacteria are present in all foods. Some are relatively harmless; others cause specific illnesses in human beings. The danger of the latter type lies not so much in their mere presence as in the rapidity with which they can multiply and produce toxins under certain conditions. The prevention or retardation of bacterial growth characterizes most efforts to keep foods safe to eat. The temperature at which food is held and the nature of the food itself largely determine the rate of bacterial growth. Organisms grow most rapidly in a warm atmosphere and in a *medium* that supplies suitable food for them. Under such circumstances, persons who eat the food may develop specific symptoms even though the food was safe to eat when it was brought into the kitchen or when it was first prepared. The same situation exists in institutional kitchens, where mishandling of food can affect large numbers of patrons. Food is frequently subjected to conditions favorable to bacterial growth when it is prepared in quantity and must be ready in advance of an event such as a catered meal, banquet, or picnic.

There are several types of common bacterial infections from foods (21). *Salmonellae* bacteria cause an infection called *salmonellosis*. These bacteria—actually a group of more than a thousand related types—are transmitted primarily by eating foods such as poultry, eggs, red meats, and dairy products that are contaminated with the organism. They are a widespread source of infection and difficult to control. Salmonellae live and grow in the intestinal tracts of people and animals and are passed on by infected people handling food. Foods that are neither washed nor cooked pose a particular threat. Cracked eggs are especially to be avoided. Bacterial growth in the food can be controlled by temperature. Salmonellae are destroyed by heating the food to 140°F for ten minutes or to a higher temperature, such as 155°F, for a few seconds. Refrigeration at 40°F and freezing inhibit the growth of salmonellae but do not destroy them.

medium
Substance in which a specific organism lives and thrives

Staphylococcus aureus bacteria cause a *staphylococcal* ("staph") infection, a very common type of food poisoning in the United States. The infection is transmitted by food handlers who carry the bacteria, chiefly in the nose and throat, and can also be contracted by eating foods containing a toxin produced by the bacteria. Custards, salami, cheese, and salads made of egg, chicken, or ham are most apt to be infected. The bacteria that generate the toxin are only mildly resistant to heat, but the toxin they produce is highly resistant. Again, temperatures provide the controls: keeping hot foods above 140°F and cold foods below 40°F successfully inhibits the growth of bacteria that produce the toxin. However, once the toxin is present, heating the food to a temperature of 240°F (which requires a pressure cooker) for 30 minutes or boiling it (at 212°F) for several hours is necessary to destroy it. Refrigeration and freezing temperatures inhibit the production of the toxin but do not destroy it.

Clostridium perfringens bacteria cause *perfringens* poisoning. The condition arises from eating such foods as stews, soups, gravies, or meat casseroles made from poultry or red meat heavily contaminated with the bacteria. These bacteria are spore-forming and grow in the absence of oxygen. In the spore stage, they are very heat-resistant. To prevent the growth of the bacteria in cooked foods to be eaten later, the foods should be cooked, cooled quickly, and refrigerated at 40°F or below, or maintained at a temperature above 140°F.

Clostridium botulinum organisms generate a toxin that causes botulism when it is present in foods. In an inactive state the bacteria form spores. The organisms are present everywhere—in soil, in drinking water, and in foods—but they are harmless unless subjected to conditions in which there is a lack of oxygen. This is the case in sealed canning containers. Canned low-acid foods are a major source of botulinum contamination. Without oxygen, the spores become active, grow and divide, and generate their deadly poison. Bacterial spores in foods are destroyed at very high temperatures, such as those attainable in a pressure cooker. To kill the spores at boiling temperature requires more than 6 hours. The toxin itself is destroyed by steady boiling for 10 to 20 minutes.

Bacteriologically safe food depends on scrupulously sanitary practices and personal hygiene in handling food to avoid contamination. This entails paying meticulous attention to cleanliness of dishes, utensils, and surfaces in contact with foods; serving food promptly to minimize holding time under conditions that invite bacterial growth; and maintaining suitable temperatures that inhibit bacterial development. Figure 10.10 presents a chart of temperature levels, showing how they affect bacterial growth in foods. It offers practical guidance in utilizing proper temperatures to assure a safe food supply.

High and low temperatures provide protective zones; warm zones invite danger. Continuous research in temperatures creates an ever-changing picture. Freezing once was thought to provide complete protection against bacterial growth in foods, but recent studies have indicated that salmonellae and staphylococci are only slightly reduced by freezing (22).

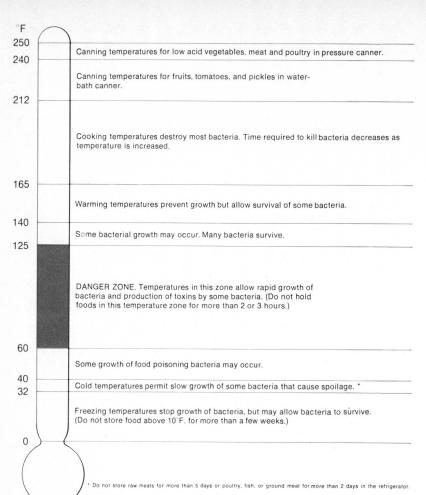

Source: US Department of Agriculture

The figure contains the following labels:

°F

250
240 — Canning temperatures for low acid vegetables, meat and poultry in pressure canner.

— Canning temperatures for fruits, tomatoes, and pickles in water-bath canner.

212

— Cooking temperatures destroy most bacteria. Time required to kill bacteria decreases as temperature is increased.

165 — Warming temperatures prevent growth but allow survival of some bacteria.

140
125 — Some bacterial growth may occur. Many bacteria survive.

— DANGER ZONE. Temperatures in this zone allow rapid growth of bacteria and production of toxins by some bacteria. (Do not hold foods in this temperature zone for more than 2 or 3 hours.)

60 — Some growth of food poisoning bacteria may occur.

40
32 — Cold temperatures permit slow growth of some bacteria that cause spoilage. *

— Freezing temperatures stop growth of bacteria, but may allow bacteria to survive. (Do not store food above 10°F. for more than a few weeks.)

0

* Do not store raw meats for more than 5 days or poultry, fish, or ground meat for more than 2 days in the refrigerator.

Figure 10.10
Temperature of food for control of bacteria

The number of persons affected by bacterial contamination of food in the United States is difficult to assess. The condition is seldom traced directly to food contamination and even when recognized is not always reported to public health authorities. Informed estimates in the mid-1970s indicated that only the common cold causes more loss of working time (23). Nausea and diarrhea are fairly common to all such infections, and often vomiting and cramps occur as well. In cases of salmonellosis, perfringens, and staphylococcal infections, symptoms frequently last only a few days unless the person is reinfected. Infants and the elderly are more susceptible and usually more severely affected than others. For botulism the situation is different. The fatality rate for botulism in the United States is about 65 percent of cases. Symptoms include respiratory paralysis, speech difficulty, and inability to swallow (21). Concern for the problem of safe food is suggested by the fact that a nationwide Food Safety Council has recently been formed by representatives of scientific groups, industry, and government. Its major objective is to develop new safety criteria for food.

FOOD ADDITIVES

Food additives are of increasing interest to persons concerned with the content of their food. General apprehensions are due primarily to a lack of understanding about what additives are and what functions they perform. Potential dangers from their use have also been widely publicized.

An additive has been described as "a minor ingredient added to a food to achieve a specific technical effect" (23). These are the so-called "intentional" additives, included in precise amounts for specific purposes. The overall intent of such additives is to extend the applicability of such basic processes as heating, drying, refrigeration, freezing, and chemical processing (used for such foods as blue cheese and sauerkraut). In other words, food additives are intended to go beyond what can be accomplished by traditional food processing steps alone. A food additive can serve many purposes, acting as a flavoring agent, a nutrient, a preservative, an emulsifier, or an antioxidant (24). The ultimate objective of additives is to ensure tasty, nutritious, safe, and attractive food that keeps well over a reasonable period of time, thus safeguarding against spoilage and waste.

The farther a consumer is removed from the source of food, the more important additives are for a varied diet. We have come to rely not only on "convenience" foods, but also on bread that does not turn moldy, cereals that resist insect infestation, salad dressings and cottage cheese that do not "separate," and ice cream that keeps its shape, color, and taste and is not icy. Such desirable attributes have been made possible by the use of food additives. There are other, more significant effects; certain antioxidant additives, for example, reduce the rate at which fats become rancid. Rancidity of fats indicates the presence of peroxides, which in turn may be carcinogenic. Suggestive evidence of a cancer link also lies in the fact that stomach cancer is apparently waning in the United States, while it is on the rise in countries where much fried food is eaten and the fat is used repeatedly, often when rancid.

Additives with preservative functions inhibit the growth of molds. Common molds grow almost everywhere: some produce carcinogenic toxins. One of these is aflatoxin produced by a mold that grows on peanuts under certain conditions. It may be significant that in parts of Africa where people eat large amounts of poor-quality, rejected peanuts untreated with mold-resistant additives, there is a high rate of liver cancer.

Table 10.11 provides a condensed directory to food additives used in the United States at the present time, grouped under several major functions (25). A few examples of commonly used additives accompany each function, as does a sampling of the foods in which they are frequently found. This table gives some understanding of the comprehensive role played by food additives in today's meals. Not included in Table 10.11 and not considered addi-

antioxidant
Easily oxidized substance that protect other substances against oxidation

carcinogenic
Cancer causing

tives in the strict sense of the definition are sugar, salt, and certain sweetening agents. These are used in far greater quantities than conventional additives.

Table 10.11
A guide to food additives

Functions in foods	Some commonly used additives	Some foods in which used
preservatives *Antioxidants* are used to prevent oxidation, resulting in rancidity of fats or browning of fruits.	Butylated hydroxyanisole (BHA), tocopherols (Vitamin E), citric acid, ascorbic acid.	Vegetable shortenings and oils, potato chips, pudding and pie filling mixes, whipped topping mix, canned and frozen fruits.
Other Preservatives are used to control the growth of mold, bacteria and yeast.	Sodium benzoate, propionic acid, calcium propionate.	Table syrup, bread, cookies, cheese, fruit juices, pie fillings.
for consistency/ texture *Emulsifiers* make it possible to uniformly disperse tiny particles or globules of one liquid in another liquid.	Mono- and di-glycerides, lecithin, polysorbate 60, propylene glycol monostearate.	Salad dressing mixes, margarine, cake mixes, whipped topping mix, pudding and pie filling mix, chocolate, bread.
Stabilizers/Thickeners aid in maintaining smooth and uniform texture and consistency; provide desired thickness or gel.	Algin derivative, carrageenan, cellulose gum, guar gum, gum arabic, pectin, gelatin.	Instant pudding mixes, ice creams, cream cheese, frozen desserts, chocolate milk, baked goods, salad dressing mixes, frozen whipped toppings, jams and jellies, candies, sauces.
acids/bases Control the acidity and alkalinity of many foods; may act as buffers or neutralizing agents.	Citric acid, adipic acid, sodium bicarbonate, lactic acid, potassium acid tartrate.	Gelatin desserts, baking powder, baked goods, process cheese, instant soft drink mixes.
nutrient supplements Mainly vitamins and minerals—are added to improve the nutritive value of foods.	Potassium iodide (iodine), Vitamin D, thiamine mononitrate, (Vitamin B₁), riboflavin (Vitamin B₂), ascorbic acid (Vitamin C), niacin (a B Vitamin), Vitamin A Palmitate, ferrous sulfate (Iron).	Iodized salt, milk, margarine, enriched or fortified breakfast cereals, enriched macaroni, enriched rice, enriched flour, instant breakfast drink.
flavors and flavoring agents Both natural and synthetic types are added to foods to give a wide variety of flavorful products without restrictions of season or geographic locale.	Natural lemon and orange flavors, dried garlic, herbs, spices, hydrolyzed vegetable protein, vanillin and other artificial flavors (mainly fruit flavors).	Pudding and pie filling and gelatin dessert mixes, cake mixes, salad dressing mixes, candies, soft drinks, ice cream, barbecue sauce.

**Table 10.11
continued**

Functions in foods	Some commonly used additives	Some foods in which used
colorings Both natural and synthetic types are used to enhance the appearance of foods. Most colors used today are approved synthetic colors since there are not enough natural colors available.	Carotene, caramel color, beet powder, artificial colors.	Margarine, cheese, soft drink mixes, candies, jams and jellies, fruit flavored gelatins, pudding and pie filling mixes.
miscellaneous additives Include anti-caking agents, anti-foaming agents, flavor enhancers, humectants, curing agents, sequestrants, and firming, bleaching and maturing agents, nonnutritive sweeteners.	Sodium silico aluminate, mono sodium glutamate (MSG), glycerine, saccharin.	Dessert mixes, soft drink mixes, seasoned coating mixes, salad dressing mixes, flaked coconut, special diet products.

Of the conventional additives, natural and synthetic flavoring agents are the most widely used. Herbs, fruit flavors, spices, and condiments are a few such additives. As we saw in Chapter 1, the flavor of foods and the taste mechanisms of individuals are important factors in the acceptance of foods. Nutrient supplements constitute the second largest group of additives. These are the substances employed in the food enrichment and fortification processes that we have discussed. Nutrients are added in specified amounts that are needed to enhance the adequacy of the United States food supply. They include iodine added to salt; iron, thiamin, riboflavin, and niacin added to grain products, including bread and flour; vitamin A added to margarine; vitamin C added to synthetic fruit drinks; and vitamin D added to milk.

A total of more than 1900 food additives are found in foods in the United States (26). The major contribution by weight (93 percent) is made by salt, sugar, and other sweeteners. Thirty additives account for 5.5 percent of the total by weight, or about 9 pounds annually per individual. These include leavening agents (such as yeast), baking soda, citric acid, vegetable colors, and the gas found in carbonated drinks. The intake of all remaining food additives (nearly 1900) amounts to only 1.5 percent of the total, by weight, estimated on the average to be about 1 pound per person per year. Considering the small total intake level of this large group of additives (which includes those currently causing much concern), individual consumption is trifling indeed—often consisting of trace amounts. However, more than the quantity of such additives is at issue. Fear persists that possible dangers to health may result from regular consumption of certain of these additives, particularly of those found to be suspect as a result of required testing procedures.

What signalizes danger in an additive? A major warning is proof that an additive causes cancer in laboratory animals when fed under carefully defined conditions prescribed by United States law. The vast majority of additives have been tested and declared safe. Those additives that fail the test, or that cause some doubt in interpretation of the results, are by due process banned or placed under restrictions. In the recent past, cyclamates and red dye No. 2 have been banned as a result of their failure to meet fully specified requirements. Nitrates and nitrites, used in curing and processing meat and some smoked fish, are under investigation. The color, flavor, and texture of ham, bacon, sausage, and "hot dogs" are attributable to nitrites. More importantly, this additive serves as a preservative to retard the growth of bacteria, particularly clostridium botulinum. The risk involved in the use of nitrites stems from the fact that they can combine with secondary amines that occur naturally in foods to produce *nitrosamines,* which have been shown to be carcinogens. While testing continues, the US Dept. of Agriculture has made a compromise ruling that nitrites be kept at a minimum level to prevent botulism, but not at a level to enhance color in meat. It is not known with certainty whether the small amount of nitrites now permitted actually combines with amines in the stomach to form nitrosamines; nor is it known to what extent nitrosamines are formed in the cured meat products and smoked fish. In the meantime, the quest for substitute additives continues.

Through its cautious procedures and increasingly refined techniques for detecting evidence of danger, the FDA continually reviews available data on additives as part of its program to protect the health of the public. Details of the meticulous process involved are beyond the scope of this text, but you may wish to pursue the topic through additional reading and inquiry (27).

REFERENCES

1. A. A. Hertzler and H. L. Anderson, "Food Guides in the United States, An Historical Review," *J. Am. Dietet. Assoc.* 64 (Jan. 1974), pp. 19-28.

2. Daily Food-Selection Guides (Posters): *A Daily Food Guide:* (Washington, D.C.: U.S. Dept. of Agriculture); *A Guide to Good Eating:* (Chicago: National Dairy Council).

3. O. Hayes, M. F. Trulson and F. J. Stare, "Suggested Revision of the Basic 7," *J. Am. Dietet. Assoc.* 31 (Nov., 1955), pp. 1103-7.

4. A. J. Wittwer, A. W. Sorenson, B. W. Wyse and R. G. Hansen, "Nutrient Density-Evaluation of Nutritional Attributes of Foods," *J. Nutrition Education* 9 (Jan.-March, 1977), pp. 26-30.

5. A. W. Sorenson, B. W. Wyse, A. J. Wittwer and R. G. Hansen, "An Index of Nutritional Quality for a Balanced Diet," *J. Am. Dietet. Assoc.* 68 (March 1976), pp. 236-42.

6. H. A. Guthrie, "Concept of a Nutritious Food," *J. Am. Dietet. Assoc.* 71 (July 1977), pp. 14-19.

7. "Vegetarian Diets," Statement of the Food and Nutrition Board, Washington, D.C.: Nat. Acad. Sciences—National Research Council, May 1974.

8. S. C. Rhys, "A Complete Diet Pattern for Total Vegetarians," *The Review* (article in press).

9. U. D. Register and L. M. Sonnenberg, "The Vegetarian Diet—Scientific and Practical Considerations," *J. Am. Dietet. Assoc.* 62 (March 1973), pp. 253-60.

10. R. M. Leverton, "Tools for Teaching Food Needs," *J. Am. Home Econ.* 65 (Jan. 1973), pp. 37-39.

11. M. Inano and D. Pringle. "Dietary Survey of Low-Income, Rural Families in Iowa and North Carolina," III, Contributions of Food Groups to Nutrients, *J. Am. Dietet. Assoc.* 66 (April 1975), pp. 366-70.

12. "Nutrition Labeling—how it can work for you," Bethesda, Maryland: National Nutrition Consortium, 1975.

13. B. Peterkin, J. Nichols and C. Cromwell, "Nutrition Labeling, Tools for Its Use," Washington, D.C.: USDA Bulletin No. 382, 1975.

14. "Composition and Nutritive Value of Dairy Foods" *Dairy Council Digest,* 47 (Sept.-Oct. 1976), pp. 25-30.

15. N. E. Roberts, "Nutrition-Related Research at USDA's Eastern Regional Research Center," *J. Am. Dietet. Assoc.* 69 (July 1976), pp. 56-60.

16. *How To Buy* Series, Individual bulletins for: dairy foods, meats, legumes, cheeses, vegetables, fruits, other. (Washington, D.C.: USDA Agricultural Marketing Service, Home and Garden Bulletins).

17. B. Montoya, "Catching the Ethnic Flavor," *Food and Nutrition* 3 (June 1973), pp. 12-15.

18. H. Bradley and C. Sundberg, *Keeping Foods Safe* (Garden City, New York: Doubleday, 1975).

19. B. C. Hobbs, "Problems and Solutions in Food Microbiology," *Food Tech* 31 (Jan. 1977), pp. 90-96.

20. Facts About Federal Food Standards, AMS—548 (Washington, D.C.: USDA, Agricultural Marketing Service, November 1976).

21. Keeping Food Safe To Eat. Home and Garden Bulletin No. 162 (Washington, D.C.: USDA, Agricultural Research Service, 1975).

22. L. D. Witter and G. G. Gengenbacher, "Freezing Does Not Kill All Bacteria in Food," *Illinois Research* (Spring 1974), pp. 6-7.

23. R. L. Hall, "Food Additives," *Nutrition Today* 7 (July/August 1973), pp. 20-28.

24. G. E. Damon, Primer on Food Additives, (FDA Consumer— May 1973) DHEW Publication No. (FDA) 74—2002, Washington D.C. US Gov. Print. Office, 1974.

25. Today's Food and Additives, General Foods Corporation (White Plains, N.Y.: 1976).

26. T. Larkin, "Exploring Food Additives," FDA Consumer, (DHEW, June 1976).

27. A. M. Schmidt, "Food and Drug Law: A 200-Year Perspective," *Nutrition Today* 10 (No. 4, 1975), pp. 29-32.

"Aflatoxins: Stopping the Trouble before It Starts" (Washington, D.C.: FDA Consumer, DHEW, Feb. 1974).

Council on Foods and Nutrition. "Improvement of the Nutritive Quality of Foods." *J.A.M.A.* 225 (Aug. 27, 1975).

J. T. Dwyer, L. D. V. H. Mayer, K. Dowd, R. F. Kandel and J. Mayer, "The New Vegetarians: The Natural High?" *J. Am. Dietet. Assoc.* 65 (November 1974), pp. 529-36.

T. H. Jukes, "Nitrates and Nitrites as Components of the Normal Environment," Parts I and II *Food and Nutrition News* 47 (May-June 1976), pp. 1, 4; 48 (Oct.-Nov. 1976), pp. 1, 4.

T. Larkin, "Natural Poisons in Food" (Washington, D.C.: FDA Consumer, DHEW, Oct. 1975).

E. M. Whelan and F. J. Stare, *Panic In The Pantry* (New York: Atheneum, 1975).

Varied Nutritional Demands in Life Cycle— Adjusting Guidelines to Nutritional Needs

11

Pregnancy
Lactation
Infancy
Childhood
Adolescence
Later Years
The Family as a Group

We know that individuals differ in dietary requirements and also that age groups, on the scale from infancy to maturity, vary in their nutritional needs. These differences, of course, are due to varied demands of the human body under changing circumstances of life. It is important to understand these demands as they relate to dietary goals. Growth, and particularly the *rate* of growth, is a basic demand in several of the periods to be considered.

PREGNANCY

The Start of the Life Cycle

Growth begins with conception; thus the newborn infant is actually 9 months old. The rate of growth of the fetus in late pregnancy exceeds that at any other period of life. During the prenatal period, the nutrients for the growing fetus must come from the food the mother eats or from her own organism (1). Her diet should be

**Table 11.1
Live births by age of mother,
United States, 1975**

Age of mother	Number of births
under 15 years	12,642
15–17 years	227,270
18–19 years	354,968
20–24 years	1,093,676
25–29 years	936,786
30–34 years	375,500
35–39 years	115,409
40–44 years	26,319
45–49 years	1,628
total	**3,144,198**

Source: Monthly Vital Statistics Report, Advance Report Final Natality Statistics, 1975.

nutritionally adequate throughout pregnancy and, ideally for the years preceding as well (2, 3). Improving the diet during pregnancy can provide many health benefits, but it cannot be expected to correct the effects of a lifetime of poor nutrition (4).

Childbearing can take place over some 30 years in a woman's life. Table 11.1 shows the distribution of ages of the mothers of live infants born in the United States in 1975. (5). Pregnancy at any age brings about changes in *hormonal secretions*, with accompanying alterations in the metabolism of the maternal organism. Changes in metabolism can, in turn, alter the nutritional status of the mother. Thus, while many factors affect the course of pregnancy, nutrition is important among them (4).

The Importance of Nutrition in Pregnancy

Pregnancy is a normal stage in the life cycle. An adequate diet during this time maintains the nutritional status of the mother at a level that conserves her own body tissues and contributes to the normal development and birth of a healthy, full-term baby (6). A backlog of research on laboratory animals and observations on human subjects of a wide age range indicates how important it is for mothers to be well nourished, both for their own well-being and for that of their infants (7, 8, 9, 10). These studies represent different approaches, and their findings are not in agreement on all points. All well-nourished mothers did not bear well-nourished infants, and all poorly nourished mothers did not bear poorly nourished infants. However, the preponderance of evidence in most of the studies showed that well-nourished mothers experienced fewer complications of pregnancy and easier deliveries. They also gave birth to stronger infants and had a lower incidence of premature births and neonatal deaths. One of the classic older studies, for example, found that most of the infants born to mothers on "good" or "excellent" diets during pregnancy were in "good" or "excellent" physical condition at birth. In contrast, many of the babies born to women

hormonal secretions
Substances synthesized by glands and transported to another part of the body to regulate specific processes

metabolism
Sum of the chemical processes taking place in the cells.

in the "very poor" diet group were in poorest physical condition (Fig. 11.1).

Size of the infant at birth is of considerable importance, for infant mortality is directly related to low birth weight. Small infants generally have a higher-than-usual risk of illness and death around the time of birth. Because of this association, a number of investigators have been attempting to identify factors contributing to low birth weight. An infant may be small for *gestational* age (having grown at a slower-than-normal rate in the uterus) or small because it is born prematurely (having had insufficient time to achieve normal size). In a study in Guatemala described in Chapter 3, when diets of moderately malnourished women were supplemented during pregnancy, the birth weights of infants increased. In this situation, the nutrition of the mother was demonstrated to be of importance in the outcome of pregnancy.

Infant mortality in the United States has declined significantly during this century. In 1915, about 100 infants of every 1000 born alive died during the first year of life. By 1940, the rate was 47 per 1000; in 1960, 26 per 1000; and by 1974, there were fewer than 17 infant deaths per 1000 live births. Reduced mortality, especially in the *neonatal* period, implies improved care of the newborn (11). Further reduction in infant death rates undoubtedly is possible in the United States, particularly since a large discrepancy exists between the infant mortality rate for white infants and that for "all other" ethnic groups; the latter is 58 percent higher (11).

Pregnancy in Adolescence

In recent years, increasing numbers of infants have been born to very young mothers in the United States. In 1966, about 8000 girls under 15 years of age gave birth; by 1975 the number had increased to more than 12,500 (5). Within certain population groups, and particularly in some urban areas, the percentage of mothers less than 18 years of age is much higher than the 1975 national average of 7.6 percent. In Chicago, for example, it was reported that 5544 babies (11.6 percent of the total births that year) were born to girls under 18; 451 of them to girls aged 14 and younger (12). In another United States city, 7.4 percent of the mothers served by

gestational age
Period of fetal development

neonatal period
First 28 days after birth

Figure 11.1
Relationship of prenatal maternal dietary ratings to the physical condition of the infant at birth (8).

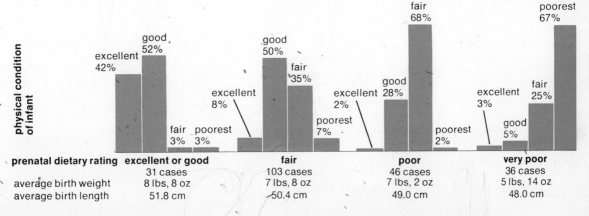

prenatal dietary rating	excellent or good	fair	poor	very poor
	31 cases	103 cases	46 cases	36 cases
average birth weight	8 lbs, 8 oz	7 lbs, 8 oz	7 lbs, 2 oz	5 lbs, 14 oz
average birth length	51.8 cm	50.4 cm	49.0 cm	48.0 cm

a maternal and infant care project were 15 years of age or younger as compared with the national average of 0.4 percent (5, 13).

Although adolescence and pregnancy are both normal life stages, each condition presents biologic and psychologic stress. The combination of the two, plus the fact that pregnancy in adolescents is often unplanned and possibly unwanted, makes for a severely stressful situation in many cases. It is not surprising that teenage pregnant girls are more at risk than are women in their twenties (4). In general, low birth weights, frequent premature deliveries, high infant mortality rates, anemia of the mother, and difficulties of labor and delivery are associated with pregnancy in the early teen years (14). Some studies have related these problems to the nutritional status of young prospective mothers (15, 16). One study that examined the dietary practices of a small group of pregnant high school girls attending maternity clinics found that most of the girls had calcium intakes—and several of them had protein and calorie intakes—less than two-thirds of the RDA. When their pregnancies were evaluated "not one of them had a completely trouble-free pregnancy" (16). In other observations on a few mothers under 14 years of age, there appeared to be a positive relationship between "probably adequate diets" of the girls during pregnancy and normal birth weights of their infants (16).

Of a group of pregnant Iowa women, nearly one-third were teenagers (17). When the *obstetrical* record of the entire group was compared with that of a similar group studied several years earlier in the same laboratory, the later group had the better record. This group proved to have diets superior to those of the first group. The obstetrical records of both groups were considered "good," but infants of the better-fed women showed improvement over the others in incidences of stillbirths, prematurity, and *congenital* defects.

Nutrition is important in pregnancy at any age, but it may be particularly so when the mother is immature. In such cases, and especially in repeated pregnancies, provision must be made for the special nutritional needs of pregnancy in addition to those of the rapidly growing girl.

Special schools and services have been provided in some areas for pregnant adolescents in an attempt to meet their particular needs, to prevent their terminating their education, and to reduce the health risks of teenage pregnancy. At one such Family Learning Center, in addition to regular school course work, girls receive instruction in health, nutrition, and child care. Prenatal care is provided at local clinics. Among 175 girls who attended this school during its first 4 years, only three had babies of low birth weight (less than 2500 grams, or 5 pounds, 8 ounces) (18).

A nutritional status study of 29 pregnant girls aged 15 to 19 attending the same Family Learning Center revealed that in general their home diets appeared to be adequate in most nutrients. However, about one-third of the girls had intakes for calcium, iron, and vitamin A below the standards adopted. Blood levels of vitamins were generally acceptable, but more than 10 percent of the girls had low blood levels of *folate* and of vitamin B_6 (18).

There were no complications at delivery for any of these 29 girls. All infants but one weighed more than 2500 grams at birth.

anemia
Deficiency in the oxygen-carrying capacity of the blood

RDA
Nutrient standards for the United States

obstetrical
Pertaining to pregnancy and labor

congenital
Existing at birth

folate
Vitamin of the B complex

The investigators interpreted the results to suggest that the age of the mother alone is not the prime determinant of the outcome of teenage pregnancy. They believed that the reasonably adequate diets maintained during pregnancy were beneficial but did not claim that the favorable outcome of pregnancy among these girls was entirely due to nutritional status. Other factors in the school situation, although they could not be measured, were believed to be contributory. Medical and social services were available to the girls as needed, as was psychiatric care. A relaxed, nonpunitive atmosphere prevailed. The girls received emotional support from the staff and from their peers. The relative freedom from psychological stress probably had a beneficial effect on nutritional status. Other studies have demonstrated that calcium and nitrogen retention were decreased in individuals under emotionally stressful circumstances. Evidence also suggests that the requirement for ascorbic acid may increase as a result of mental stress (18).

Nutrient Goals

The recommended dietary allowances for pregnancy are high (6). Energy needs are increased as a result of the mother's higher metabolic rate, which begins at about the fourth month. Basal metabolism may increase as much as 25 percent above the nonpregnant level, due to the building of uterine and mammary tissues for the mother's body, an increase in her blood volume, and the growth of the baby. The fetus increases in weight about threefold during the final trimester. Body fat stored by the mother during pregnancy provides an energy reserve needed for lactation (4). The energy cost of pregnancy has been estimated to be 80,000 calories, or an average of approximately 2000 calories per week for the 40-week gestation period. An average weight gain of 24 pounds during pregnancy is recommended for women who enter pregnancy at a normal weight for their height. Pregnant girls who have not completed their own growth are expected to gain about 24 pounds *in addition to* the increase in weight they would normally gain at that stage of maturity if they were not pregnant. Inadequate maternal weight gain is associated with low birth weight and increased risk to the newborn (4). Pregnant adolescents in a California study were found to be extremely sedentary. Their energy expenditures averaged approximately 2400 calories per day, excluding the energy required for continuance of maternal growth in the very young mothers in the group. Basal metabolic rates during pregnancy among these girls averaged 17 percent higher than *postpartum* values (19).

    The energy expenditure and energy consumption of mature pregnant women were studied by the same investigators. The mature women had somewhat higher energy needs late in pregnancy than the younger group. Basal metabolic rate increased proportionately more than body weight during pregnancy. During the latter half of gestation, average energy output was 2200 to 2300 calories per day; average daily energy intake was 1955 calories, or 28.5 calories per kilogram of body weight. Protein intake represented 17 percent of the gross energy consumed. The energy-intake level re-

trimester
Three-month period
lactation
Period of milk secretion

postpartum
After childbirth

ported by these women may not have been sufficient to maintain positive nitrogen balance (20, 21). Regardless of their energy expenditure, the energy intake of healthy women should not fall below 36 calories per kilogram of pregnant body weight—the amount of energy required for adequate protein utilization during pregnancy (6).

Increased intakes of protein, calcium, and phosphorus are recommended during pregnancy. The baby's skeleton is a major repository for these nutrients. A child's first set of teeth is well on the way by the end of the first trimester of pregnancy, and at the time of birth the crowns of all twenty of the teeth are almost entirely calcified. Additional quantities of all vitamins and minerals for which RDAs have been established are also recommended daily during pregnancy to satisfy the rapidly increasing needs of the fetus. In addition, there is an RDA for vitamin D during pregnancy (see the RDA table).

If the prepregnancy diet was adequate, the changes involved in moving to an adequate pregnancy diet can be achieved mainly by increasing intakes of basic foods. Can these increased levels of energy and nutrients be obtained in a practical way from common foods? The inclusion of more milk in the diet is suggested in Table 10.1. For example, 2 cups of milk in addition to the 2 recommended for all adults will supply not only the extra calcium and phosphorus, but also additional amounts of protein and several other nutrients that are to be increased. The milk may be in any form; the selection depends on many factors, including personal preference, cost, and caloric level.

Other foods should be chosen to supply nutrients not provided in sufficient quantities by the milk, particularly vitamins A and C and thiamin. Foods rich in iron also should be included. Iron requirements in pregnancy and good food sources of iron were noted in Chapter 8. The difficulty of obtaining adequate amounts of iron from common foods to meet the needs of pregnancy has been recognized, and supplemental iron is usually recommended. The large increase in folacin needed for pregnancy may also require a supplementary source. The physician will prescribe the supplements that are needed.

Using the day's menus given in Table 10.3 as a prepregnancy base, add enough foundation foods to build a diet adequate for pregnancy.

Turn to Table 10.2, which shows the nutrient values of the day's foods. Add the values of the extra foods you have included, and compare the new totals with the RDA for pregnancy. If necessary, make adjustments in the amounts of added foods until their nutrient values approximate the RDA for pregnancy.

Converting an *adequate* prepregnancy diet to an adequate pregnancy diet obviously presents few problems. However, women often enter pregnancy on diets of poor quality. In the Iowa study mentioned above, the teenagers and the older women had the most unsatisfactory diets (17). Calcium, iron, and vitamin A appear to be rather consistently low in the diets of young women. In a Texas study of pregnant adolescents these nutrients, especially calcium and iron, fell below RDA levels. Biochemical tests tended to support the dietary data (22). When the prepregnancy diet has been *inadequate,* converting it to a diet adequate for pregnancy is more difficult. Consideration must be given to making changes that will be acceptable to the pregnant woman. Explaining *why* changes are suggested often results in greater cooperation.

Interpreting the Food Guide in Pregnancy

Does the daily food selection guide (see Table 10.1) provide a reliable pattern for choosing a nutritionally adequate diet for pregnancy? On the basis of the above discussion, it can be assumed that if foods are eaten in the amounts specified in the guide, the RDA for pregnancy will usually be met with the possible exceptions of vitamin D, folic acid, and iron. Liberal interpretation of the "or more" clauses on the guide may be desirable in many cases. For example, more than the minimum of three glasses of milk daily is needed for adequate intake of vitamin D. The specifications about kinds of vegetables and fruits must be followed carefully for vitamin A and iron intake. To attain the iron allowance with foods alone, you will recall, excellent sources of iron must be chosen and eaten regularly in liberal amounts. These sources are dark green leafy vegetables; organ meats, such as liver; lean muscle meats; dried legumes; dried fruits; and whole grain and enriched grain products. A review of information about the incidence of iron deficiency in the United States by the Council on Foods and Nutrition of the American Medical Association indicates that iron deficiency is prevalent among infants and pregnant women (23). Because of the difficulty of obtaining enough iron from food to meet the needs during pregnancy, most obstetricians prescribe an iron supplement, and many believe it is also desirable to administer a supplement of folic acid to prevent anemia during pregnancy (4).

A simple way to meet the calcium and phosphorus requirements for pregnancy, and to add other nutrients as well is to drink three or more glasses of milk as proposed by the daily food guide. Milk is sometimes avoided because it is thought to be "fattening." If gaining excess weight is a problem, skim milk, which yields only one-half the calories of whole milk, may be substituted. It is fortified with vitamins A and D, and provides all the other nutrients that whole milk does. Occasionally, for various reasons, a calcium supplement may be used as a source of calcium. Of course it is not a substitute for milk. Calcium supplements usually are in capsule form in combination with phosphorus and vitamin D. Calcium provided as calcium gluconate or calcium lactate is efficiently absorbed and utilized.

The amount of calcium required during pregnancy has not been established, and research data are limited and variable (24). Women long accustomed to low calcium intakes seem to provide the calcium required by the fetus, as well as by the breast-fed infant, on lower levels of intake than the RDA. If vitamin D is sufficient, dietary calcium is absorbed more efficiently during pregnancy than usual.

Multiple mineral and vitamin supplements, in addition to calcium pills, are often taken during pregnancy despite the ease with which most nutrients can be obtained from a well-selected diet. Many medical authorities believe that broad-spectrum supplementation of the pregnancy diet with pills and special concentrates is ill advised. Excessive intakes above the recommended dietary allowances do not bestow protective benefits. The committee on maternal nutrition of the Food and Nutrition Board reports that there is no established evidence that diets of pregnant women require routine vitamin supplementation, particularly if the woman is eating a well-balanced diet. It is customary practice, however, to prescribe certain dietary supplements for those women whose diets are or have been substandard. The committee also points out that the cost of supplements relative to the cost of the same nutrients in foods should be taken into consideration, especially in dealing with patients of low income (4).

In general, people seem to believe they can compensate for poor food habits by taking supplements. This creates a false sense of security. Dietary supplements do not provide all essential nutrients —many can be obtained only from food. An appreciation of the interrelationships in functions among nutrients may well serve as an active deterrent to dependence on supplements. On the basis of the information presented here, any price paid for supplements is high if the mother can take and enjoy common foods. Excessive nutrients of any kind are financially extravagant, wasteful of nutrients, and, in some cases, may actually be harmful to health.

LACTATION

Adequacy of the pregnancy diet not only contributes to the mother's ability to supply nutrients to the fetus but also affects her ability to produce breast milk adequate in quantity and quality to meet the needs of the infant after birth (25). The lactation diet largely determines whether the mother can provide a continuing supply of high-quality breast milk, so important to an infant's physical development. A poor maternal diet will result in a decreased volume of breast milk. The concentration of protein, fat, and carbohydrate does not change appreciably, but the vitamin content of the milk is reduced (26, 27). Good nutrition during lactation is important also for maintaining maternal tissues and replenishing the mother's nutrient stores.

The RDAs for lactation in relation to pregnancy and prepregnancy levels can be seen on the RDA table. Additional calories proposed for lactation are in line with the quantity of milk produced; an average milk yield of 850 milliliters per day is assumed. Human milk provides about 1.2 grams of protein per 100 milliliters. This indicates the need for protein intake greater than that of the pregnancy diet. Amounts of vitamin A, calcium, and phosphorus greater than those in the pregnancy diet are also recommended to help ensure that the nursing infant obtains enough of these nutrients. Increases in RDAs for thiamin and riboflavin serve as replacements for the amounts of these vitamins secreted daily in the breast milk.

The four or more glasses of milk recommended for lactation on the daily food guide will cover the RDAs for calcium, phosphorus, and protein. This amount of milk also contributes substantial amounts of other nutrients. As in pregnancy, the food selection guide offers practical safeguards. The extra energy allowance, which permits more total food, should be used to help ensure the nutritional adequacy of the lactation diet. If the added foods are chosen chiefly from the foundation-food groups, rather than from foods providing empty calories, they will contribute a comfortable surplus of nutrients to take care of varying individual needs. Dietary supplements are to be avoided in lactation, as in pregnancy, unless a need for them has been established by a physician.

> Starting with a nutritionally *adequate* pregnancy diet, show various ways in which an adequate lactation diet can be achieved.

Preventive Program for Mothers and Young Children

Studies mentioned above and in Chapter 3 have shown a relationship between diet and the health and development of young children. Infants, young children, and pregnant women in low-income groups in the United States have been identified as being at risk of malnutrition. Their diets tend to be low in certain essential nutrients. Iron-deficiency anemia is prevalent, and infant mortality rates are higher than in the general population. For these reasons, a Special Supplemental Food Program for Women, Infants, and Children (WIC) was established (28).

Through the Food and Nutrition Service of USDA, funds are made available through the WIC program to participating State Health Departments. These funds are distributed to local public health or welfare agencies in needy areas. Local health clinics use them to carry out health and nutrition programs under which specified food supplements are provided to pregnant, nursing, and post-partum women, and to children up to their fifth birthday. The supplemental foods have been selected to provide high-quality protein, iron, calcium, vitamin A, and vitamin C—those nutrients known to be lacking in the diets of populations at nutritional risk. Specific foods include iron-fortified infant formula, fortified milk, cheeses, eggs, high-iron breakfast cereal, and high-vitamin fruits and vegetable juices. Nutrition education is a part of the food assistance program (29) (Fig. 11.2).

A medical evaluation of the WIC program has been made, and its measurable effects have been reported to include an acceleration of growth in weight and height of the infant and children participants, along with a reduction in the prevalence of anemia. Improved nutrient intakes of pregnant women participants were associated with desirable weight gains during pregnancy, a reduc-

Figure 11.2
The WIC program places an increasing emphasis on nutrition education. Women participants are taught principles of infant and child feeding and family meal planning. (WIC Program, US Department of Agriculture)

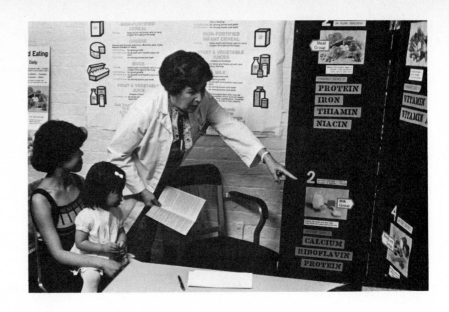

tion in the anemia rate, and an increase in the mean birth weight of babies (30).

INFANCY AND CHILDHOOD

Breast milk furnishes nutrients in amounts and forms that are well utilized by human infants. It also provides bacterial and viral antibodies that help the infant resist infections during the first few months of life. Allergic reactions to protein and to other food components are less common among breast-fed infants than among formula-fed infants. Because human milk does not provide vitamin D, iron, or fluoride in adequate amounts to meet the needs of the infant, supplements are prescribed to furnish these nutrients. Commercial formulas have been designed that contain all known nutrients in approximately the same proportions as in human milk (26).

Planning the diets of infants is the province of the physician. Whether a baby is fed from the breast or bottle, the physician will prescribe other foods to be added to the diet of milk at appropriate times. Such additions serve two purposes: they ensure the nutritional adequacy of the baby's diet, and they accustom the baby gradually to solid foods. The physician in charge indicates the foods (or supplements) to be added, when they are to be added, and the forms in which they are fed. Particular care must be taken to ensure adequate intakes of vitamin D, ascorbic acid, and iron. By the end of the first year, the baby is usually on a schedule of three to five meals daily and is eating a variety of foods covered by the food guide. By the age of 2, young children are routinely eating meals with the family, and few adjustments need be made in menus to meet their needs (31, 32).

What are the possibilities for applying the food selection guide successfully when children are old enough to eat regularly at the family table? Adapting the guide to a child's nutrient requirements through the growing years is largely a matter of adjusting a) the number of servings of milk; b) the sizes of servings of other foundation foods; and c) the quantities and kinds of additional foods needed to meet the total energy requirements. Table 11.2 gives an example of the way a family's menus can be adapted to the needs of three approximate age groups—5-, 10-, and 15-year-olds eating together and enjoying almost identical foods.

To test the adaptability of the guide to planning meals for preteens, let us use as an example the meals for 10-year-old children in Table 11.2. The foods are classified in Table 11.3 in the column on the far left into the four food groups and *additional foods*. You will see that the foods compare favorably in amount and kind with those specified on the food guide for preteens (children in this age range). These foods are combined in the accompanying menus that are shown in Table 11.4. To the right in Table 11.3 the nutrients in the foods are tabulated and the total values are compared with

Table 11.2
Sample meals* from the same menus for three ages of childhood
food selections based on the daily food guide

5 years old**	10 years old**	15 years old** (boy)
Breakfast		
orange juice: ½ cup	orange juice: ¾ cup	orange juice: 1 cup
whole-grain cereal: ½ cup	whole-grain cereal: ⅔ cup	whole-grain cereal: 1 cup
milk: ⅓ cup	milk: ½ cup	milk: ½ cup
toast: 1 slice	toast: 2 slices	toast: 3 slices
butter:† 1 tsp	butter:† 2 tsp	butter:† 3 tsp
milk: 1 glass	milk: 1 glass	jam: 2 tbsp
		ham: 1 slice
		milk: 1 glass
Lunch		
macaroni and cheese: ¼ cup	macaroni and cheese: ½ cup	macaroni and cheese: 1 cup
cole slaw: ¼ cup	cole slaw: ½ cup	cole slaw: ¾ cup
pear: ½	pear: 1	pear: 1
cookie: 1	cookies: 2	cookies: 3
milk: 1 glass	milk: 1 glass	milk: 2 glasses
Dinner		
hamburger: 1 (2 oz)	hamburger: 1 (3 oz)	hamburger: 2 (3 oz)
potato, boiled: 1 (small)	potato, boiled: 1 (medium)	potato, boiled: 1 (large)
butter:† 1 tsp	butter:† 1 tsp	butter:† 2 tsp
corn: ¼ cup	corn: ½ cup	corn: ¾ cup
butter:† 1 tsp	butter:† 1 tsp	butter:† 1 tsp
bread, whole wheat: 1 slice	bread, whole wheat: 1 slice	bread, whole wheat: 2 slices
butter:† 1 tsp	butter:† ½ tsp	butter:† ½ tsp
tomato: ½ medium	tomato: 1 medium	tomato: 1 large
baked custard: ½ cup	baked custard: ½ cup	baked custard: ½ cup
milk: 1 glass	milk: 1 glass	milk: 1 glass

*Foods for snacks may be taken from the regular meals, such as bread and butter. Fruit, or other foods may be added as proposed in Table 11.3 (apple, peanuts).
**Approximate ages.
†Or margarine.

Table 11.3
A child's diet based on the daily food selection guide—
nutrient yields compared with estimated dietary goals for preteens

Foods	Measure	Kilo-calories	Protein g	Fat g	Calcium mg	Iron mg	Vitamin A IU	Thiamin mg	Ribo-flavin mg	Niacin mg	Ascorbic Acid mg	Vita-min D IU
Foundation foods												
milk group												
milk, whole, vit. D	3½ cups	557	32	32	1008	0.4	1225	0.25	1.44	0.7	7	350
custard, baked	½ cup	153	7	7	149	0.6	465	0.06	0.25	0.2	1	—
meat group												
hamburger	3 oz	186	23	10	10	3.0	20	0.08	0.20	5.1	—	—
macaroni and cheese	½ cup	215	17	11	181	0.9	430	0.10	0.20	0.9	tr	—
peanuts, shelled	⅛ oz	187	7	18	25	0.7	—	0.11	0.04	5.3	—	—
vegetable-fruit group												
coleslaw	½ cup	60	tr	4	26	0.2	90	0.04	0.04	0.2	18	—
corn	½ cup	87	3	1	3	0.6	370	0.03	0.07	1.2	6	—
tomato, raw	1 medium	20	1	tr	12	0.5	820	0.05	0.04	0.6	21	—
potato, boiled	1 medium	122	4	tr	11	0.9	tr	0.17	0.07	2.3	30	—
apple	1 medium	80	tr	1	10	0.4	120	0.04	0.03	0.1	6	—
orange juice	¾ cup	92	2	tr	20	0.2	405	0.18	0.03	0.8	90	—
pear, fresh	1	100	1	1	13	0.5	30	0.03	0.07	0.2	7	—
grain group												
oatmeal	⅔ cup	87	3	2	15	0.9	0	0.13	0.03	0.1	0	—
bread, white, enrich.	2 slices	152	4	2	48	1.4	tr	0.14	0.12	1.4	tr	—
bread, whole-wheat	1 slice	67	3	1	24	0.8	tr	0.09	0.03	0.8	tr	—
Total foundation foods		2165	107	90	1555	12.0	3975	1.50	2.66	19.9	186	350
Nutrient goals												
Estimated ranges from RDA for ages 10–12		2400—2600	36—44		800—1200	10.0—18.0	3300—4000	1.2—1.4	1.2—1.5	16—18	40—45	400
Additional foods												
sugar	1 tsp	15	0	0	0	tr	0	0	0	0	0	—
butter or margarine	5 tsp	170	tr	19	5	0	752	0	0	0	0	—
cookies*	2	103	1	6	7	0.4	20	0.02	0.02	0.2	tr	—
Total additional foods		288	1	25	12	0.4	772	0.02	0.02	0.2	tr	—
Grand Totals		**2453**	**108**	**115**	**1567**	**12.4**	**4747**	**1.52**	**2.68**	**20.1**	**186**	**350**

*Cookies are borderline foods with respect to classification. Each food of this type should be judged on an individual basis, depending on the kind and quantity of ingredients. They are classed here as additional foods, because such foods, high in fat and sugar, usually have a nutrient dietary goals for 10- to 12-year-old boys and girls as the criteria for adequacy. The calculations for the diet in Table 11.3 show that the foundation foods alone meet or exceed the dietary goals for 10- to 12-year-old children, except for energy. The nutrient needs of growing children are proportionately higher, compared to their body size, than those of adults. However, you can see that the estimated ranges can be met with ease. Energy allowances for children give the meal planner a liberal calorie "budget" within which to operate, and the higher milk quota for children called for by the food guide makes it easy to attain the greater allowances for calcium. It is safe to assume that by adjusting quantities of foods in line with total energy needs, the nutrient allowances of 5-year-olds and 15-year-olds also would be met by the meals suggested in Table 11.2.

Table 11.4
Menus based on a preteen diet (Table 11.3)

Foundation foods		Calories	Additional foods		Calories
Breakfast					
orange juice	¾ cup	92			
oatmeal	⅔ cup	87	+ **sugar**	1 tsp	15
and **milk**	½ cup	80			
toast, enriched	2 slices	152	+ **butter**	2 tsp	68
milk, whole	1 glass (cup)	159			
Lunch					
macaroni and cheese	½ cup	215			
coleslaw	½ cup	60			
pear, fresh	1	100			
milk, whole	1 glass (cup)	159	+ **cookies** chocolate chip	2	103
Dinner					
hamburger	3 oz	186			
potato, boiled	1 medium	122	+ **butter**	1 tsp	34
corn	½ cup	87	+ **butter**	1 tsp	34
tomato, raw	1 medium	20			
bread, whole-wheat	1 slice	67	+ **butter**	1 tsp	34
milk, whole	1 glass	159			
baked custard	½ cup	153			
Between Meals					
apple	1 medium	80			
peanuts, shelled	1⅛-oz packet	187			
Total calories		2165			288
Grand total calories for the day—2,453					

Preschool (33, 34)   By the time children are 2 years old they will, ideally, have learned to know and like most of the common foods that will be available to them throughout life. They may be less interested in food than formerly, due to the somewhat slower growth rate and the many distractions at this age. A *smaller* appetite, however, should not necessarily be interpreted as a *poor* one, and a less eager eater should not be allowed to develop into a problem eater by overanxious adults.

The preschool child's meals can be chosen from the family meals if the latter are well planned. Smaller glasses of milk may be indicated in some cases, but the same meats, vegetables, fruits, and cereals eaten by other family members are usually suitable. Only the amounts and sometimes the forms of the foods need be adjusted to meet the child's needs. In Table 11.2, for example, reductions in quantities of foods are shown for the 5-year-old. Foods should be prepared simply for preschool children, for they prefer them that way, and they learn to enjoy individual foods for their own distinct flavors.

Many 2- to 5-year-old children spend regularly scheduled amounts of time in the care of someone other than a parent. Young children who attend preschools may eat their meals at home but have a snack as part of the school program. Day-care centers provide for children during variable periods of each day, often determined by the work schedules of parents. The matter of meal content and scheduling for such groups is dealt with in Chapter 12.

School Age   The meals of school-age children are merely an extension of the preschool diet (see Table 11.2). On entering school, children acquire many new interests, enjoy the regular companionship of other children, and usually take part in more outdoor activities—all of which help to create a new outlook on food. If a child eats lunch at school, this represents a new development in the day's meal schedule. Lunch should be an ample, well-balanced meal, whether the child eats it at home, carries it from home, or buys it at school. The school nutrition program, the school lunch, and/or the school breakfast may acquaint children with new foods and stimulate an interest in foods, their preparation, and their association in meals (see Chap. 12).

Good food habits at this period, however, may be difficult to maintain. A child's early and often hurried breakfast, lunch away from home, the pressure of outside activities, the diversion of television, and the consequent encroachment on sleep sometimes lead to appetite problems that may result in over- or undereating.

ADOLESCENCE

A comparison of the meals for the three age levels of childhood in Table 11.2 shows that those for 15-year-olds differ from the others chiefly in that they include more milk, larger servings of most foods (meat, vegetables, fruits, and cereals), and added foods such as a breakfast meat and jam. The additional milk is called for specifically on the daily food guide. Larger servings of all foods are required to meet the much higher energy and nutrient allowances at this period. The magnitude of these allowances can best be appreciated by comparing them with allowances for other age periods. For example, a 15-year-old-boy has a calorie allowance nearly double that of a 5-year-old child. As would be expected, the allowance for 10- to 12-year-old children falls between these. The allowances for girls present a similar picture. The need for energy varies also with body size and activity level of persons of the same age and sex. In addition, individuals vary in energy requirements for unknown or less well understood reasons than the factors mentioned above. As children grow and their energy requirements increase, foods must be carefully selected if the diet is to be of good nutritional quality. The increase in energy value of the diet should be accompanied by corresponding increases in amounts of nutrients. This means placing strong emphasis on foundation foods.

> Plan a day's menus for a teenage boy or girl of a less conventional type than shown in Table 11.2. Check the foods chosen against the daily food guide.

Surveys show that the diets of many teenagers do not meet dietary goals. In general, however, teenage boys appear to eat somewhat better than girls in the same age range. This may be due to the fact that boys usually are less concerned about gaining weight and therefore consume more food. Studies show that, for both boys and girls, high energy intakes tend to reflect satisfactory intakes of protein, minerals, and vitamins. Also, those teens who eat regular meals, usually with snacks added, are more likely to have an adequate diet than those with highly irregular meal patterns. For the most part, adolescents who eat fewer than three meals daily tend to have inadequate diets (35).

Various surveys of the foods consumed by teenagers are in general agreement about which nutrients are most often below RDA levels for this age. Calcium is one that is almost universally reported to be low in the diets of both boys and girls. In some cases, particularly in girls' diets, the intake may be 30 percent or more below RDA (36). Iron is also likely to be low, especially in the diets of girls (36, 37). Teenagers in low-income groups appear to fare even less well. For example, in the preliminary findings of one study in poverty areas, adolescents' diets were found seriously lacking in iron and vitamin A—a fact borne out by biochemical data on the subjects (38). Diets inadequate in calcium, iron, and vitamin A reflect lower-than-recommended intakes of milk, vegetables, fruits, and enriched cereals. (Chapter 12 considers meals and snacks in developing sound food habits and achieving good nutritional status.)

Adolescent boys and girls face many problems related to nutrition. First, there is great physical need for food, to provide for rapid skeletal and muscle growth. Both boys and girls are maturing and facing psychological and social pressures that affect their emotional development. It is a period of transition to adult life. These changes call for vigor, stamina, and a wholesome outlook on life, qualities that are best achieved with good nutritional health (39). As we have already seen, for girls good nutrition is also an important asset for future motherhood. The course of a girl's pregnancy, her own nutritional status, and that of her developing infant are all at stake.

Overweight and obesity, which are discussed in Chapter 13, represent another problem of adolescence. Teenage girls are often addicts of fad reducing diets. They try to live for considerable periods of time on diets drastically low in energy and nutrients. Teenagers dealing with the problem of weight control require nutrition knowledge. They may also require sensitive nutritional counseling and support during the weight-control process.

obesity
Excessive amount of body fat

Are Teenagers Well Fed? Evidence from the dietary surveys mentioned suggests that many teenagers are not well nourished. But the image of American young people is one of health and vigor, and their growth record is phenomenal (see Chap. 3). Can these two concepts be reconciled? It has been suggested that seeming deficiencies in adolescent diets may be due to excessively high allowances for certain nutrients or that the RDA are applied too rigidly. Perhaps we have been misled by the unconventional character of some teenagers' diets into thinking that they are less nutritious than they are in fact (40). Our primary concern must be for the *nutrients* provided by foods, rather than for the foods themselves. Foods and combinations that seem most unappetizing to an adult may be accepted and enjoyed by a teenager, and these same foods may be fully as nutritious as more conventional choices.

Undoubtedly, however, many teenagers are *not* well fed. Food choices may be not only unconventional but also poor from a nutritional standpoint. A succession of tidbits eaten throughout the day, added to nutritionally poor meals, is not adequate by any dietary standards. Surveys show that teenagers routinely eat more than three traditional meals a day. What can be done to reap maximum benefits from the multiple-meal practice? One obvious answer is to maintain high nutritional quality in all meal segments of the day and to regard each as a part of the day's total nutrient contribution. An important approach is through the improvement of snacks. Left to themselves, most teenagers snack on whatever is at hand. A logical step, therefore, is to stock the refrigerator with foundation foods such as fruits, raw vegetables, fruit juices, cheese, peanut butter, and milk, from which they may eat as they please, and deliberately keep to a minimum the cakes, pastries, concentrated sweets, soft drinks, and snack items high in fat and salt content (Fig. 11.3).

Teenagers need food that will satisfy their appetites and provide sufficient nutrients to support normal growth and activity. Teenagers whose meals are not satisfying are the ones most apt to eat almost constantly, and many of the popular snack foods they eat contribute little to their nutrient needs. One remedial step is to place more emphasis on well-balanced, ample meals which have "staying" qualities. When regular meals largely meet the daily nutrient needs, the adequacy of the total diet does not hinge on the

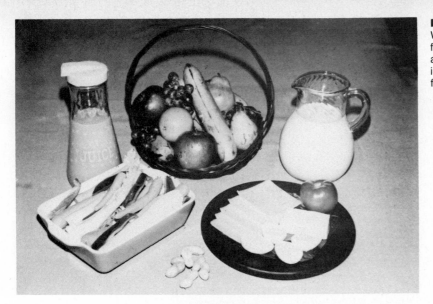

Figure 11.3
Wholesome snacks: When foundation foods are readily available, they are often eaten in the place of less nutritious foods. (Landon Gardiner)

quality of snacks; they can then assume chiefly a social, rather than a nutritional, role.

Studies show that family eating practices are among the most important influences—good and bad—on the food habits of teenagers. Family disorganization, which leaves adolescents on their own with respect to eating, fosters poor eating habits. The young people who eat most poorly are those who eat with their peers or alone; those who eat with their families usually eat better. In general, when families eat together in a relaxed atmosphere and the mealtime conversation is pleasant, they eat best (41).

Teenagers obviously need nutrition knowledge, despite their avowed lack of interest in the subject. Objective information, offered in a friendly, straightforward, nondictatorial manner that helps them understand their own nutritional problems, is the kind of guidance most acceptable to adolescents.

Diets of Teenage Athletes   For the most part, teenagers engaged in sports improve their diets under the motivation of increasing their skill in athletic performance. Many teenagers in athletic training programs are encouraged to follow a scientifically acceptable eating pattern, to eat regular meals, and to gain in weight and strength as a phase of their normal growth and development.

Unfortunately, in some cases the students' sound ideas of nutrition and good food habits become distorted when coaches advocate practices not based on scientific principles with respect to special dietary needs of athletes. Many unsound principles persist even though the theories on which they were based have been shown to be without foundation in the light of modern medical and nutrition knowledge (42). For example, feeding extremely high protein diets to athletes to replace "muscular substance" supposedly "lost" in heavy exercise is a fallacy. Needs for *energy,* not protein are increased with exercise. Young growing athletes and those just beginning training require somewhat more protein than do older athletes to provide for growth and for development of muscles. Their requirements for protein will be satisfied if the RDA for their sex-age group is met (43). Excessive dietary protein produces no known benefit, and may actually be detrimental because it causes extra work for the kidneys (43, 44, 45).

Authorities on the subject of nutrition and athletic performance generally agree that the nutritional needs of athletes, as of non-athletes, are met when they eat diets of ordinary foods based on the daily food guide. When athletes' diets are adjusted to meet their energy requirements by the addition of foods from the guide, ample amounts of all nutrients will be supplied to meet their nutrient requirements (43, 44). There are no data to support the impression that supplements of vitamins and minerals enhance athletic performance (44).

The optimal distribution of energy in the athlete's diet is the same as for the population in general: about 15 percent of total calories from protein, 35 percent from fat, and 50 percent from carbohydrate (44). This distribution should be maintained when changes are made in the energy level. Adjustment of energy intake appropriate for body size and activity is of particular importance. In most athletes in training, appetite and *satiety* automatically regulate food intake to maintain energy balance. A caloric excess will result in an increase in total body fat which decreases the quality of athletic performance and may lead to habitual overeating and obesity later in life (43).

satiety
Feeling of fullness or gratification of appetite

On the other hand, encouraging boys to adopt drastic reducing diets in order to qualify for lower-weight classifications in boxing or wrestling is a dangerous practice with negative implications for nutrition. Boys who must lose 5 to 25 pounds in a few weeks, when they normally would be gaining weight steadily, dehydrate their bodies on low fluid intake, and live on diets of 400 to 500 calories daily. Furthermore, they must maintain this reduced weight status throughout the wrestling or boxing season. Some consciously starve themselves to achieve these subnormal standards—a practice that is not only harmful to health but may even defeat their purpose by impairing athletic performance. In such a case the compelling motivation of athletics acts in reverse. Nutrition and medical authorities alike condemn this practice (46).

Some athletes believe that certain foods prepared in special ways eaten as the pregame meal give them competitve advantages. There are no data to substantiate this. The psychological effect, however, is real. General guidelines to be used in selecting a pregame meal have to do mainly with allowing for digestion and absorption of the food before the event. For short-duration events, a normal well-balanced meal should be eaten about three hours before the event; for long-duration events, three or more hours before. Fat and protein intake should be relatively low; foods that may cause flatulence should be avoided, and two or three cups of water or other beverages should be included. Athletes may need to eat or drink during long-duration events. Limited amounts of fruit juices or non-carbonated soft drinks may be given in small amounts at frequent intervals to maintain energy and prevent dehydration. Concentrated sweets should be avoided (44).

About 25 years ago, a veteran coach collaborating with scientific authorities had this to say: "In order to obtain the energy and dexterity necessary for a winning team, week after week, an adequate diet is essential not only on days of a game, but every day. Long-term conditioning is important. In brief periods of very strenuous physical exercise, muscular efficiency depends on energy reserve and training, not on composition or size of the preexercise meal . . . there are no magic foods which produce super power or agility. The same meat, milk, eggs, vegetables, fruits, enriched and whole grain breads and cereals that are fundamental to the health of every person are needed by the athlete" (47). It is interesting that almost identical statements are made by investigators today. The director of a laboratory for human performance research concluded a paper published in 1977 with these words: "Both quantity and quality of the food consumed by an athlete are important, and maintenance of a good diet should be year-round. It should be understood, however, that even a balanced diet cannot compensate for poor skill development or a poor regimen of physical conditioning." Earlier in the paper he wrote, "A balanced, ordinary diet is proper for an athlete. There are no dietary tricks that give a competitive advantage." This investigator advocated that coaches and athletes seek the counsel of a dietitian for nutritional advice (43).

Potential Drug-Related Nutritional Problems

Alcohol   Alcohol is a toxic drug. Excessive use of alcoholic beverages results in alcoholism, a problem in almost all age groups including teenagers. The subject demands consideration here because of the relationships among alcohol, food, and nutrition. It was estimated that 95 million or more people in the United States who were drinking alcoholic beverages during 1970 consumed an average of 3.9 gallons of absolute alcohol per person (48). *Cirrhosis* of the liver, strongly associated with chronic alcohol consumption, ranked seventh among the causes of death in the United States in 1974 (49).

Alcoholism can be viewed as a problem of enormous proportions that begins for many people in the teenage years, when consumption of beer often symbolizes "coming of age." The percentage of alcohol in beer is deceptively small compared to other alcoholic beverages. However, one 12-ounce container of beer contains approximately the same amount of alcohol as a 4-ounce glass of table wine or a jigger of whiskey, gin, or rum (50).

The incidence of malnutrition among alcoholics is high for several reasons. Alcohol may displace foods in the diet as well as limit funds available for purchase of food. Chronic alcohol consumption interferes with normal digestion and absorption of food by reducing the production of enzymes normally present in intestinal secretions. It also causes erosion of the gastrointestinal mucosa, thus interfering in still another manner with the absorption of nutrients. Vitamin deficiencies seen among alcoholics include folate, thiamin, riboflavin, and pyridoxine. Protein depletion may occur as the result of inadequate intake of protein foods, or of decreased protein production in the body due to liver impairment (51).

cirrhosis
Chronic disease of the liver; increased formation of connective tissue ultimately resulting in failure of liver function

enzymes
Proteins essential for stimulating reactions in the body

mucosa
Membrane lining the intestinal tract

At high intake levels, the full 7 calories per gram of alcohol are not available for body use. There is inefficient conversion of energy from the alcohol to high energy phosphate bonds—the form in which cells can utilize energy. Heat is produced without conservation of chemical energy. Fat is not oxidized normally and accumulates in the liver. The *smooth endoplasmic reticulum* adapts to the processing of excessive fat molecules and dispenses unusually large quantities of them into the blood. High blood lipid levels constitute a risk factor for coronary heart disease (49, 51).

Controlled investigations have shown that chronic consumption of alcohol leads to deposition of fat in the liver even when the diet is nutritionally adequate. Liver damage occurs at moderate levels of alcohol in the blood—below those producing the state of intoxication. Chronic use of alcohol results in progressively more severe liver damage, often leading to alcoholic *hepatitis* and cirrhosis. Treatment requires restoration of vitamin, mineral, and protein levels as well as control of alcohol intake (51, 52).

Drugs of Addiction   The misuse of drugs leading to addiction involves changes in eating habits and severely reduced nutrient intake. In one rehabilitation center for drug addicts, nutritionists became involved in evaluating the nutritional status of the clients and in providing services for them (53). Over a 2½-year period, 250 subjects were studied and treated. Most of them had been on drugs for 2 years or more when they came to the center and about three-fourths of the clients had consumed substantial quantities of hard liquor, wine, or beer daily.

Interviews with the clients revealed that, prior to their addiction, almost half of them had diets deficient in leafy vegetables, citrus fruits, and milk products. Many reported craving and consuming high-carbohydrate, low-nutrient foods such as cake, cookies, candy, sweet-flavored drinks, potato chips and pretzels. These foods are relatively inexpensive and readily available, two factors that have some bearing on their frequent consumption. Clinical and biochemical examinations showed that a few (about 5 percent) of the subjects had deficiencies of vitamin A and vitamin B_{12}. Low serum levels of vitamin C were found in 30 percent of the subjects, and more than one-fourth had seriously low folate levels; 12 percent had high serum triglyceride levels and 13 percent of the subjects had high cholesterol levels. Clinical and laboratory evidence of past or active liver disease was a common finding. A number of previously undiagnosed cases of hypertension were identified.

The investigators suggested many factors that probably contribute to the development of nutritional deficiencies in "hard" drug users. The generally disorganized life style often accompanying drug addiction is not conducive to regular meal patterns. In many cases all available funds are spent on drugs, leaving no money to buy food. There probably is a lack of interest in food during drug "highs," while the frequent occurrence of infections increases nutritional requirements.

Results of this investigation demonstrate the need for corrective nutritional programs as part of the services provided for rehabilitating drug addicts. Well balanced nutritious meals were

endoplasmic reticulum
System of channels within the cell

smooth endoplasmic reticulum
Involved with fat synthesis and transport

hepatitis
Inflammation of the liver

cholesterol and triglycerides
Fatty substances; normal constituents of blood

served at the center. The concern shown for the addict as a person by those people who provided the adequate diet was also of therapeutic value (53).

Therapeutic Drugs   Food-drug interactions are of two general types: drug-induced impairment of the absorption and/or utilization of nutrients, and alteration of the effect of a drug by specific foods or patterns of eating. Laxatives—drugs that increase gastrointestinal motility—result in nutrient losses due to the decreased time for absorption to occur. *Hypocholesteremic agents* also decrease absorption of vitamin B$_{12}$, iron and, sugar. Some drugs indirectly affect absorption of nutrients by destroying or injuring cells of the intestinal mucosa.

Drugs may alter the amount of food eaten by decreasing taste acuity; by causing nausea, vomiting, and loss of appetite due to their unpleasant taste; or by affecting the central nervous system. Tranquilizers, antidepressants, and oral contraceptives have been reported to stimulate appetite (54).

hypocholesteremic agents
Drugs used to decrease absorption of cholesterol, thus lowering serum cholesterol levels

Oral Contraceptive Agents   *Oral contraceptive agents* (synthetic sex hormones) are used by many women over extended periods of time. The possible effects of these compounds on nutritional status have been investigated. Biochemical measurements of blood and urine of women using oral contraceptives show an association of these drugs with changes in metabolic needs for several nutrients, suggesting that folic acid, and vitamins A, B$_6$, B$_{12}$ and C may be needed in larger quantities than usual. However, for the most part, clinical correlations have not substantiated needs for routine nutrient supplementation.

Increased blood levels of iron, copper, and vitamin A have been observed among women taking oral contraceptives, suggesting possible decreased needs for these nutrients. Allowances for nutrients recommended by the Food and Nutrition Board appear to provide guidelines that are adequate in most cases (see the RDA table) (55).

oral contraceptive agents
Synthetic hormones in pill form taken by mouth to prevent ovulation and conception

LATER LIFE

Aging is a biological process that extends over the entire life span. In humans aging is usually accompanied by various disease processes, so that its uncomplicated course is unknown. The term aging has been described as progressive changes in biochemical processes that alter the structure and function of tissues. Thus, the entire organism is ultimately affected (56). Most of what is known about aging was learned by studying animals and even lower forms of life. Studies at the cellular level support the conclusion that reduced efficiency of organ performance observed in older people is primarily due to cell death. Individual cells appear not to be less efficient than earlier in life, but there are fewer functioning cells in the organ (56). One result of the physiological process of aging is decreased efficiency in the absorption and utilization of nutrients in the body. Thus although the protein, mineral, and vita-

physiological
Pertaining to functions of the body

min needs of older people remain essentially the same as those of younger adults, larger dietary intakes of some nutrients may be needed to ensure that required quantities reach the cells.

Basal energy metabolism decreases slightly but steadily throughout adult life, and people tend to be less physically active with advancing years. Both of these factors contribute to lowering the body's energy requirement. Meal planning for good nutrition in older persons, therefore, is largely a matter of keeping nutrient intake high and energy intake adjusted in line with desirable body weight (57). In many instances this adjustment is not being made satisfactorily because people tend to retain food habits established earlier in life. The resulting imbalance of energy intake and output leads to overweight and obesity, which are common among middle-aged and older people, especially women, in the United States (59). Overweight is a burden to the cardiovascular system and accelerates the development of degenerative diseases (58). *Atherosclerosis*, diabetes mellitus, and hypertension, which probably have their beginnings in young adulthood, if not earlier, become manifest in later years. There is major concern about the relationship between these degenerative disease processes and nutrient intake. Many large-scale investigations have been made and others are in progress in an attempt to identify causative factors and reveal possible preventive measures.

Dietary studies conducted in the United States indicate that many older people have diets of generally poor quality with clear-cut nutrient shortages, often a result of poor food choices. Findings in a nutrition survey in low-income areas showed that among various groups of elderly people, diets were far below acceptable levels in iron, vitamin A, vitamin C, and riboflavin (38). In the first HANES, in which the population sample is representative of the entire United States, the nutrients most frequently deficient in diets of older people to age 74 were iron, vitamin A, vitamin C and calcium. Clinical signs of deficiency, however, except for those of low dietary iron, were of very low frequency (60).

In a study of elderly patients in a nursing home, dietary intakes were determined and nutritional status evaluated (61). All of the subjects, who ranged in age from 63 to 93 years, were sedentary or bedfast. Energy requirements seemed to be met by 1400 calories per day for women and 1600 for men. Nutrients provided daily by the general diet equaled or exceeded the RDAs and mean intake of nutrients approximated the RDA standards for older men and women. More individuals had low dietary intakes of calcium than of any other nutrient, although almost half of the subjects consumed more than 800 milligrams of calcium daily. About half of the subjects had intakes of less than 10 milligrams of iron per day. Hemoglobin values were classified as low or deficient in almost all of the men and in 40 percent of the women according to guidelines used in the Ten-State Nutrition Survey. Hematocrits for all men and 48 percent of the women were below acceptable values but plasma iron and *transferrin* saturation were satisfactory for almost all subjects. Plasma ascorbic acid and folic acid concentrations were normal. Bone densities were significantly lower for women than for men. Two-thirds of the women had bone densities

atherosclerosis
Thickening of linings of arteries due to deposits of fatty substances

diabetes mellitus
Disturbances of carbohydrate, fat and protein metabolism due to an inadequate supply of effective insulin

hypertension
High blood pressure

hematocrit
Percentage of red cells in the blood by volume

transferrin
Iron-binding protein in blood plasma which transports iron

osteoporosis

Disorder in which there is a reduced amount of bone

suggestive of osteoporosis. There was no correlation between the low bone densities and low intake of any particular nutrient. When the parameters of nutritional status for patients of ages 63 to 84 were compared with those for patients of 85 to 93 years, no statistically significant differences were found (61).

Interpreting the Food Guide for Older Persons

If the diet in early adult life has been nutritionally adequate, its character need not be altered sharply in later years (62). The food selection guide described in Chapter 10 may well continue to provide direction in the choice of foods. If body weight is within the desired range, the diet shown in Table 10.2 can serve as a pattern for the general content of meals. If a person is overweight and calories must be reduced, the modifications suggested in Chapter 13 offer guidelines for choosing meals high in foundation foods and low in additional foods.

Dietary studies show that older people, particularly women, often use less than recommended amounts of milk, which undoubtedly accounts for their generally low calcium intake. Inadequate intake of calcium over a prolonged period may be a factor in the occurrence of osteoporosis, which is particularly prevalent in older women (58). Some people do not use milk as a beverage. When that is the case, milk in dry or liquid form can be added to casserole dishes, soups, and desserts. Diets low in vitamin A and ascorbic acid, which are common among older people, indicate failure to use desirable amounts of vegetables and fruits. If poor condition of the teeth or ill-fitting dentures are the cause, these foods can be cooked until soft or even pureed and combined with other foods. Difficulty in chewing also may serve to curtail the use of meat. Ground or chopped meats help to circumvent this problem, and eggs, cheese, and cottage cheese provide protein alternates that are easy to eat.

Improving the nutritive quality of the diets of older people, as for people of any age, can best be achieved by increasing consumption of foundation foods. This means decreasing the intake of additional foods if calorie levels are to be maintained or lowered. Consumption of fats and high-fat mixtures can well be curtailed. As body processes slow down, the fat-digestion enzymes handle fat less well than formerly. Sweets also should be taken in small amounts, for they satisfy the appetite too easily and fail to yield the nutrients the body needs. Menus for aging individuals are planned in the same way as those for younger adults: to provide the maximum number of foundation foods compatible with attractive, edible meals.

Food versus Pills

Older people should be encouraged to enjoy ordinary foods instead of "health" foods, special dietary supplements, and nutrient concentrates in tablets and capsules. Common foods are less expensive and provide all the nutrients needed under ordinary circumstances. For some older persons with specific problems of absorption or utilization of nutrients, or problems interfering with an adequate food intake, vitamin-mineral supplements may be required. Use of supplements, however, should be based on an assessment of each individual's need. In one study, a variety of vitamin or mineral supplements was being taken by 35 percent of the aging people—usually by persons whose nutrient intakes already were adequate (63). In another situation, supplements of vitamins and minerals were prescribed by physicians; intakes of particular nutrients lacking in the diet were not necessarily supplemented (61). In general, nutrients lacking in diets can be furnished by slight adjustments in food choices.

Food Habits

An older person's state of nutrition depends on the food habits of a lifetime (57). If people have eaten poorly since childhood, the inclination to continue doing so will be strong even though there may be great need for change. Often the changes indicated are not drastic; perhaps adding milk or a regular food source of ascorbic acid to the diet is all that is needed. But good nutrition in advancing years involves more than nutrients. Decreased taste sensitivity sometimes is the problem in loss of appetite among the aged. Poor appetite can, however, be aggravated by many things: living and eating alone, which can lead to introspection and a negative outlook; the difficulty of shopping for one person and cooking in small quantities under unfavorable conditions; or managing limited funds to buy attractive foods and those requiring a minimum of preparation.

In general, the chief nutrition problem of aging persons lies not in their changing physiological needs but in their need to devise practial ways of obtaining appetizing, nutritious meals. Many older people benefit from dietetic and social consultation. In providing optimum nutrition for the elderly, diets should be planned to meet individual needs. In some cases, the diet must be modified to have therapeutic value for disease and disability states. When older persons have been oriented in health, nutrition, *gerontology* and consumer protection they are better able to cope with their financial and physiological restrictions (64). Older people require meals substantial enough to maintain their health and vigor. As far as possible these meals should be eaten in the company of others who will help them relish the food and divert their attention from real or imaginary ills. Recent arrangements in many city centers to provide well balanced, moderately priced group lunches as well as home-delivered meals (described in Chapter 12) for elderly citizens greatly enhance their enjoyment of food and improve their nutritional status (Fig. 11.4).

It must be recognized, however, that "the health and social problems of the aged can be ameliorated but cannot be abolished by good nutritional practices" (65).

Statistics show that people in the United States have a greater life expectancy now than at any time in history (see Chap. 3). This situation has resulted in a growing number of older people in the population. And, as numbers have increased, more attention has been focused on the welfare of these older men and and women.

gerontology
Study of the aging process

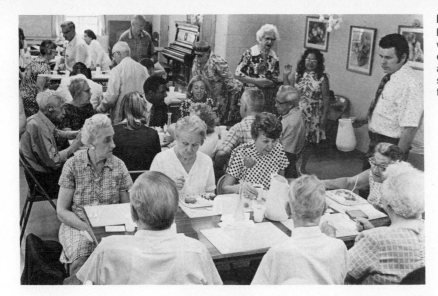

Figure 11.4
Enjoying well balanced meals with friends in a pleasant environment is an important aspect of nutrition programs for senior citizens. (Mayor's Office for Senior Citizens, Chicago)

FAMILY MEALS

Thus far we have considered nutrient needs for young adults, for aging persons, and for those who are in the growth cycles of pregnancy, lactation, and childhood. We have seen that the daily food selection guide, properly applied, results in meals that meet reasonable dietary goals in most cases. Family meals are, in effect, the summation of the meals of several individuals, all with different needs and tastes. Providing such meals successfully takes time and effort on the part of the homemaker and requires either a knowledge of nutrition or some reliable practical plan, such as the daily food guide, for use as a pattern.

Applying the Food Guide to Family Meals

The characteristics and content of a nutritionally adequate day's food supply have been explored, with particular emphasis on planning the day's menus as a unit and making foundation foods their basis. The meal planner can utilize the daily food guide in setting up skeleton menus for breakfast, lunch, dinner, and between-meal foods. Basic menu plans can be developed with the food habits of the family in mind, taking into account such individual meal needs as packed lunches and snacks. Skeleton meal plans are merely an aid in interpreting the food guide from day to day. They serve as reminders to include foods that make meals varied and nutritious, and they are flexible inasmuch as they suggest the general content of meals, not specific foods.

Table 11. 5 illustrates the adaptation of skeleton menu plans to actual menus for breakfast, lunch, dinner, and snacks. The skeleton plan is shown on the left in each double column. The menus on the right are those from Table 10.3. Such a plan is adaptable to any number of meals in the day.

The selection of foods within the framework of the daily food

Table 11.5
Skeleton menu plans applied to one day's menus from Table 10.3

Breakfast		Lunch		Dinner		Between-meal snacks	
skeleton plan	menu	skeleton plan	menu	skeleton plan	menu	skeleton plan	menu
fruit	grapefruit	main dish such as: sandwich substantial soup casserole	ham sand-wich	main dish such as: lean meat fish, fowl casserole	pot roast	fruits juices milk drinks other	banana
main dish such as: cereal egg meat	poached egg	vegetable	lettuce celery	vegetable	carrots and peas		
milk	milk, whole	milk	milk, whole	salad or relishes	lettuce salad dressing		
breadstuff (enriched)	toast	breadstuff (enriched)	bread in sandwich	breadstuff (enriched)	rolls		
beverage	coffee			beverage	coffee		
		dessert such as: fruit cookies puddings	baked apple	dessert such as: fruit cake pie frozen desserts	ice cream		

guide depends on such factors as the food preferences of the family, the ages and occupations of its members, work schedules, meal habits, and the family budget. Many households adhere more or less closely to the three-meals-a-day plan. This routine provides greater comfort and satisfaction for family members than haphazard eating. Most simple methods of food preparation preferable for children should be equally acceptable to adults. Quantities of food will, of course, be adjusted to suit individual energy and nutrient needs.

Meals planned on a daily unit basis should be projected in advance and synchronized with the shopping schedule. Preplanning for several days or a week saves time, effort, and sometimes money. It provides opportunities to anticipate which foods can be the basis for more than one meal, and still permits substituting one comparable food for another at the market to take advantage of good buys. Long-range planning presupposes a carefully developed market list, using the skeleton menu plans as a guide.

Planning to meet the recommendations of the daily food guide for each member of the family is the most challenging aspect of the job. Specifically, it involves estimating the number of servings of each food needed by each individual in the family group for a specified period and transferring the total to the market list in units to be purchased. Let us consider one simple example: if four full-size (¼ pound raw) hamburgers and two half-size (⅛ pound) hamburgers are needed for a meal, the total amount of meat to be purchased is 1¼ pounds.

Milk offers little or no problem in estimating purchases because of the specificity of the daily food pattern and the easy identifica-

Table 11.6
Low-cost food plan: amounts of food for a week[1] (67)

Family member	Milk, cheese, ice cream[2] qt	Meat, poultry, fish[3] lb	Eggs no	Dry beans and peas, nuts[4] lb	Dark-green, deep-yellow vegetables lb	Citrus fruit, tomatoes lb	Potatoes lb	Other vegetables, fruit lb	Cereal lb	Flour lb	Bread lb	Other bakery products lb	Fats, oils lb	Sugar, sweets lb	Accessories[5] lb
child:															
7 months to 1 year	5.70	0.56	2.1	0.15	0.35	0.42	0.06	3.43	0.71[6]	0.02	0.06	0.05	0.05	0.18	0.06
1–2 years	3.57	1.26	3.6	.16	.23	1.01	.60	2.88	.99[6]	.27	.76	.33	.12	.36	.68
3–5 years	3.91	1.52	2.7	.25	.25	1.20	.85	2.95	.90	.30	.91	.57	.38	.71	1.02
6–8 years	4.74	2.03	2.9	.39	.31	1.58	1.10	3.67	1.11	.45	1.27	.84	.52	.90	1.43
9–11 years	5.46	2.57	3.9	.44	.38	2.13	1.41	4.81	1.24	.62	1.65	1.20	.61	1.15	1.89
male:															
12–14 years	5.74	2.98	4.0	.56	.40	1.99	1.50	3.90	1.15	.67	1.88	1.25	.77	1.15	2.61
15–19 years	5.49	3.74	4.0	.34	.39	2.20	1.87	4.50	.90	.75	2.10	1.55	1.05	1.04	3.09
20–54 years	2.74	4.56	4.0	.33	.48	2.32	1.87	4.81	.93	.71	2.10	1.47	.91	.81	2.11
55 years and over	2.61	3.63	4.0	.21	.61	2.38	1.72	4.92	1.02	.62	1.73	1.23	.77	.90	1.16
female:															
12–19 years	5.63	2.55	4.0	.24	.46	2.17	1.17	4.57	.75	.63	1.44	1.05	.53	.88	2.44
20–54 years	3.02	3.21	4.0	.19	.55	2.34	1.40	4.17	.71	.55	1.31	.94	.59	.72	2.13
55 years and over	3.01	2.45	4.0	.15	.62	2.54	1.22	4.57	.97	.58	1.24	.86	.38	.64	1.11
pregnant	5.25	3.68	4.0	.29	.67	2.80	1.65	4.99	.95	.66	1.52	1.06	.55	.78	2.56
nursing	5.25	4.16	4.0	.26	.66	2.99	1.67	5.33	.78	.61	1.55	1.16	.76	.91	2.70

[1]Amounts are for food as purchased or brought into the kitchen from garden or farm. Amounts allow for a discard of about one-tenth of the *edible* food as plate waste. spoilage. etc. Amounts of foods are shown to two decimal places to allow for greater accuracy. especially in estimating rations for large groups of people and for long periods of time. For general use. amounts of food groups for a family may be rounded to the nearest tenth or quarter of a pound.

[2]Fluid milk and beverage made from dry or evaporated milk. Cheese and ice cream may replace some milk. Count as equivalent to a quart of fluid milk: Natural or processed Cheddar-type cheese. 6 oz.: cottage cheese. 2½ lbs.: ice cream. 1½ quarts.

[3]Bacon and salt pork should not exceed ⅓ pound for each 5 pounds of this group.

[4]Weight in terms of dry beans and peas. shelled nuts. and peanut butter. Count 1 pound of canned dry beans—pork and beans. kidney beans. etc.—as .33 pound

[5]Includes coffee. tea. cocoa. punches. ades. soft drinks. leavenings. and seasonings. The use of iodized salt is recommended.

[6]Cereal fortified with iron is recommended.

tion of serving units. Fresh vegetables probably present the greatest difficulty because of variation in the size of units (heads of broccoli, cabbage, and so on), the difference in the amount of trimming necessary before use, and the shrinkage in cooking. Facility in buying just enough, but not too much of the foods needed can best be acquired through experience. Some homemakers use a chart on which they record the number of servings that can be obtained from average market units of foods as purchased. Thus they gradually build up a body of information that serves as a convenient reference in shopping. The US Department of Agriculture publishes useful information on the amounts to buy per serving of many foods (66).

Table 11.6 was developed to ensure that enough foods from each food group are provided for every member of the family (67). This is a low-cost family food plan. Moderate-cost and liberal budget plans are also available (67), as well as a thrifty food plan (68). The plan, worked out for a 1-week period, is based on the daily food guide; properly followed, it provides the nutrients to meet the daily dietary needs of members of a family in most cases. Quantities of foods are specified for each age level, for both sexes, and for pregnancy and lactation. These amounts, expressed in market units of pounds and quarts, are essentially translations on a weekly basis of the daily servings indicated on the food guide. With this type of breakdown, a weekly shopping guide can be tailored to fit a family of any size or composition by totaling the amounts in each food group that are appropriate to the family to be served.

The amounts of foods are, of course, only approximations. Needs within age levels vary greatly. Individual variations in growth rate and activity must be allowed for in each family group. Despite slight shifting to fit specific situations, the totals in any given case will provide helpful and important guidelines for buying the raw materials for adequate family meals.

Make up a weekly shopping list for a hypothetical family of specified size and composition from Table 11.6.

Price the list on two levels: one in which the most economical kinds and forms of foods are purchased within the framework of the plan, and one in which no effort is made to economize.*

Over and above the mechanics of meal planning is the consideration of the enjoyment factor in eating. Many people suppose that nutritious foods are not enjoyable. Actually good nutrition and enjoyment of food are entirely compatible. Of course, individual preferences in foods in terms of flavor, texture, aroma, appearance, and

---

* The US Department of Agriculture issues at intervals estimates of average weekly and monthly food costs in the United States for individuals of different ages. These estimates represent current costs of providing a nutritious diet on a low, moderate, or liberal food budget. Write the Office of Information, US Department of Agriculture, Washington, DC 20250.

temperature must be taken into account. Experience soon helps in assembling meals that give pleasure and satisfaction, as well as good nutrition.

The Food Budget

Fortunately, the cost of a food does not reflect its nutritive value. Some foods are worth their cost at almost any price because of their high yield of nutrients, while others are expensive at any price because of their low nutrient yield. Such contrasts in food values have been pointed out repeatedly in the preceding pages. It is obviously never economical, nutritionally speaking, to skimp on foundation foods and overemphasize high-calorie, low-nutrient additional foods, even though the latter may cost less. Foundation foods are economical because they carry more than their share of nutrients per calorie. Some of these foods are in the higher price range. How can we reconcile these apparently contradictory facts and arrive at practical procedures for meeting dietary goals at low cost? The lower the food budget, the more important it is to plan meals carefully and shop for foods prudently. In interpreting the daily food guide, economies can be effected in several ways. A few guidelines follow:

1. Select carefully within the food groups, choosing less expensive but equally nourishing sources of food, such as economy cuts of meat, forms of milk, kinds and forms of vegetables and fruits. Take advantage of seasonal low prices. Avoid specially cooked and prepared foods; buy *foods*, not services.
2. Choose adequate amounts of foundation foods within the specifications of the daily food guide, but not to excess when money is scarce.
3. Buy breads and cereals in their most economical forms. Home-baked products and home-cooked breakfast cereals are usually the most economical.
4. Watch and compare prices; buy in quantities that permit savings on purchases but in amounts compatible with storage space and ability to use the foods while still in prime condition.
5. Take advantage of special sales on foods only if they are really bargains—that is, if the foods fit into the basic plan.
6. Control waste; prepare and store foods and leftovers carefully to make maximum use of the foods and preserve the nutrients.

The cost of food is roughly 20 percent of the total consumer income in the United States. This includes money spent for meals away from home as well as for food purchased for home meals. The percentage of indiviudal family incomes spent for food varies greatly. In general, however, it is much higher among low-income groups than among high-income groups. In other words, the poorer the family, the larger the proportion of the income that goes for food (69, 70). Despite this difference, in most cases the *actual* outlay for food is much less in low-income families. US Department of Agriculture survey results showed low-income households to have a greater return in energy and nutrients per dollar spent for food than higher income families (71). In 1975 families in the United States spent their food dollar as follows (72):

  12 cents for milk and milk products, other than butter

  37 cents for meat, poultry, fish, and eggs

  18 cents for vegetables and fruits, including juices

   7 cents for flour, cereals, and bakery products

  12 cents for fats, sweets, other foods

   6 cents for mixtures from 2 or more groups such as frozen dinners, frozen, canned and dried soups, jellies and jams

   8 cents for accessories—coffee, tea, cocoa, soft drinks, leavening agents, flavorings and condiments.
_____
100

Certain broad boundaries for food expenditures are automatically established in applying the daily food guide to family meal planning. But it is the person who plans, buys, and prepares the family's food who exercises the greatest control. There is, of course, a low-cost limit below which an adequate diet cannot be purchased, but above this limit and still well within the low-cost zone one can purchase a diet that is nutritionally adequate and as satisfying and enjoyable as one that costs far more. Knowledge and ingenuity must be applied in practicing the types of economies outlined above. Usually more physical effort is involved in food preparation; few services in the form of convenience foods can be included.

PUTTING THE GUIDE TO WORK—SAFEGUARDS IN APPLICATION: A SUMMARY

Having assessed the daily food guide under various conditions, what can we conclude about its usefulness to inexperienced meal planners? Can it be turned over to them without any specific advice or directions for its use?

It must be remembered that no food guide is infallible. Many different food combinations can result in an adequate diet; there are considerable differences in the nutrient needs of individuals and great variations in the nutrient values of foods within the food groups. The fact remains that a carefully developed food selection guide, designed with available food supplies and prevailing dietary customs in mind, is far better than hit-or-miss planning or no planning at all. Properly interpreted and applied, a food guide encourages good food habits. To derive maximum benefits from a plan, it is important to recognize its inherent weak points and take steps to strengthen them as much as possible.

In recommending the daily food guide in Table 10.1 to a person with no experience in applying such a pattern and no basis for making decisions with respect to nutritional values, the following points serve as a nucleus of suggestions:

1. *Choose more than the minimum number of servings of foundation foods.* The "or more" phrase on the guide indicates that

more than the minimum number of servings is nutritionally desirable. The larger the proportion of energy supplied from foundation foods, the greater the prospects for obtaining an adequate diet.

2. *Select foundation foods carefully.* Some nutrients are more difficult to obtain than others, chiefly because they occur in small amounts in most foods or they are easily destroyed. Here are a few good rules to observe in obtaining them: Use organ meats frequently, perhaps once a week; make lean pork a weekly or semiweekly item; include dark green leafy vegetables for vitamin-A activity and iron.

3. *Allow for cultural preferences in foods.* The guide is flexible regarding foods that qualify within the groups (see Chap. 10).

4. *Adapt food choices to the food budget.* There is wide variation in costs of foods within the four food groups.

5. *Count only full servings.* Estimate the number of servings correctly. Do not count as servings trivial amounts such as a leaf of lettuce, a radish, or a slice of apple. Note serving sizes indicated on the food guide in Chapter 10 and in Appendix K. Large servings may count as two servings if the amount warrants it.

6. *Use foundation foods as a framework for daily meals.* Think of the day as a unit in planning meals. Build meals around the foundation foods; enter these foods first in developing menus. Complete the menus for each day with additional foods within the limits of the energy allowance.

7. *Use additional foods judiciously.* Include additional foods to round out meals, to lend variety in flavor and interest. Additional foods are insignificant sources of nutrients in relation to their high yield of calories and should therefore not be allowed to dominate the diet. Rather, they must be kept in line with the body's energy needs for activity and growth.

8. *Plan on variety in meals for food value and enjoyment.* Avoid monotony in food choices. Variety in itself does not assure nutritional adequacy, but the likelihood of including some of the hard-to-get nutrients is greater when the choice is not confined to a random few foods. Variety in foods and food combinations adds interest and pleasure to meals.

Analyze the eight summary statements above. Criticize the suggestions. What would you delete? How would you alter them?

What suggestions would you add to assure that the user of the daily food guide obtains adequate amounts of nutrients?

REFERENCES

1. E. M. Widdowson, "Nutrition of the Foetus and the Newly Born," *Proc. Nutr. Soc.* 28 (1969), pp. 17-24.

2. E. M. Gold, "Interconceptional Nutrition," *J. Am. Dietet. Assoc.* 55 (July 1969), pp. 27-30.

3. H. N. Jacobson, "Diet in Pregnancy," *N. Engl. J. Med.* 297 (Nov. 10, 1977), pp. 1051-53.

4. Committee on Maternal Nutrition, *Maternal Nutrition and the Course of Pregnancy* (Washington, D.C.: National Academy of Sciences-National Research Council, 1970).

5. Advance Report Final Natality Statistics, 1975. Monthly Vital Statistics Report. (HRA) 77-1120, Vol. 25, No. 10 Suppl. Dec. 30, 1976. DHEW, Public Health Service.

6. Food and Nutrition Board, National Research Council, *Recommended Dietary Allowances* 8th revision (Washington, DC: National Academy of Sciences, 1974).

7. J. H. Ebbs, F. F. Tisdall and W. A. Scott, "The Influence of Prenatal Diet on the Mother and Child," *J. Nutr.* 22 (Nov. 1941), pp. 515-20.

8. B. S. Burke, S. S. Stevenson, J. Worcester and H. C. Stuart, "Nutrition Studies During Pregnancy," *J. Nutr.* 38 (Aug. 1949), pp. 453-67.

9. P. C. Jeans, M. B. Smith and G. Stearns, "Dietary Habits of Pregnant Women of Low Income in a Rural State," *J. Am. Dietet. Assoc.* 28 (Jan. 1952), pp. 27-34.

10. W. J. McGanity, et al, "The Vanderbilt Cooperative Study of Maternal and Infant Nutrition," *Am. J. Obstet. and Gynec.* 67 (March 1954), pp. 491-500.

11. M. E. Wegman, "Annual Summary of Vital Statistics: 1975," *Pediatrics* 58 (Dec. 1976), pp. 793-99.

12. "Health Board Data Cited: 11% of '75 Births to Girls Under Age 18," *Chicago Tribune* (April 29, 1977).

13. N. I. Huyck, "Nutrition Services for Teen-Agers," *J. Am. Dietet. Assoc.* 69 (July 1976), pp. 60-62.

14. *11 Million Teenagers—What Can Be Done About the Epidemic of Adolescent Pregnancies in the United States?* (New York: Planned Parenthood Federation of America, 1976).

15. M. G. Phillips, *Food for the Teenager during Pregnancy,* DHEW Publication No. (HSA) 76-5611 (Washington, D.C.: US Gov. Print. Office, 1976).

16. H. N. Jacobson, "Pregnancy in School Age Girls," *Food and Nutrition News,* Part 1, 41 (May 1970), pp. 1, 4; Part 2, 41 (June 1970), pp. 1, 4.

17. H. A. Stevens and M. A. Ohlson, "Nutritive Value of the Diets of Medically Indigent Pregnant Women," *J. Am. Dietet. Assoc.* 50 (April 1967), pp. 290-96.

18. C. M. Hansen, M. L. Brown and M. Trontell, "Effects on Pregnant Adolescents of Attending a Special School," *J. Am. Dietet. Assoc.* 68 (June 1976), pp. 538-41.

19. M. L. Blackburn and D. H. Calloway, "Energy Expenditure of Pregnant Adolescents," *J. Am. Dietet. Assoc.* 65 (July 1974), pp. 24-30.

20. M. W. Blackburn and D. L. Calloway, "Basal Metabolic Rate and Work Energy Expenditure of Mature, Pregnant Women," *J. Am. Dietet. Assoc.* 69 (July 1976), pp. 24-28.

21. M. W. Blackburn and D. H. Calloway, "Energy Expenditure and Consumption of Mature, Pregnant and Lactating Women," *J. Am. Dietet. Assoc.* 69 (July 1976), pp. 29-37.

22. W. J. McGanity, et al, "Pregnancy in the Adolescent," *Am. J. Obstet. and Gynec.* 103 (March 15, 1969), pp. 773-88.

23. Council on Foods and Nutrition, "Iron Deficiency in the United States," *J. Am. Med. Assoc.* 203 (Feb. 5, 1968), pp. 407-12.

24. R. W. Hillman and R. S. Goodhart, "Nutrition in Pregnancy," Chap. 23 in R. S. Goodhart and M. E. Shils, eds., *Modern Nutrition in Health and Disease* (Philadelphia: Lea and Febiger 1973).

25. I. G. Macy and H. J. Kelly, "Food for Expectant and Nursing Mothers," *Food—The Yearbook of Agriculture* (Washington, D.C.: USDA, 1959), p. 273.

26. S. J. Fomon, *Infant Nutrition* (Philadelphia: Saunders, 1974).

27. L. J. Filer, Jr., "Maternal Nutrition in Lactation," *Clinics in Perinatology* 2 (Sept. 1975), pp. 353-60.

28. "National School Lunch and Child Nutrition Act Amendments of 1973," Public Law 93-150, 93rd Congress, H.R. 9639, *Fed. Reg.* (Nov. 7, 1973).

29. M. Bendick, Jr., T. H. Campbell, D. L. Bawden and M. Jones, *Efficiency and Effectiveness in the W.I.C. Program Delivery System*, Misc. Pub. No. 1338 (Washington, D.C.: USDA, Sept. 1976).

30. Select Committee on Nutrition and Human Needs, United States Senate, *Medical Evaluation of the Special Supplemental Food Program for Women, Infants and Children*, (Washington, D.C.: US Gov. Print. Office, 1976).

31. V. A. Beal, "Dietary Intake of Individuals Followed Through Infancy and Childhood," *Am. J. Pub. Health* 51 (Aug. 1961), pp. 1107-17.

32. M. E. Lowenberg, "Philosophy of Nutrition and Application in Maternal Health Services," *Am. J. Clin. Nutr.* 16 (April 1965), pp. 370-73.

33. E. Kerrey, S. Crispin, H. M. Fox and C. Kies, "Nutritional Status of Preschool Children," *Am. J. Clin. Nutr.* 21 (Nov. 1968), pp. 1274-84.

34. M. McWilliams, *Nutrition for the Growing Years* (New York: John Wiley and Sons, 1975).

35. R. L. Huenemann, L. R. Shapiro, M. C. Hampton and D. W. Mitchell, "Food and Eating Practices of Teen-agers," *J. Am. Dietet. Assoc.* 53 (July 1968), pp. 17-24.

36. *Food Intake and Nutritive Value of Diets of Men, Women and Children in the United States, Spring, 1965* (Washington, D.C.: USDA, Agric. Res. Service 62-18, March 1969).

37. M. C. Hampton, R. L. Huenemann, L. R. Shapiro and B. W. Mitchell, "Caloric and Nutrient Intakes of Teen-agers," *J. Am. Dietet. Assoc.* 50 (May 1967), pp. 385-96.

38. A. E. Schaefer and O. C. Johnson, "Are We Well Fed? The Search for the Answer," *Nutrition Today* 4 (Spring 1969), pp. 2-11.

39. M. Balsley, M. F. Brink and E. W. Speckmann, "Nutritional Component in Some Problems of Adolescence," *J. Home Econ.* 60 (Oct. 1968), pp. 648-52.

40. R. M. Leverton, "The Paradox of Teen-age Nutrition," *J. Am. Dietet. Assoc.* 53 (July 1968), pp. 13-16.

41. M. C. Harrington, "Give Them the Knowledge They Need," *J. Am. Dietet. Assoc.* 52 (April 1968), p. 307.

42. American Alliance for Health, Physical Education and Recreation, *Nutrition for Athletes: A Handbook for Coaches* (Wash-

ington, D.C.: Am. Assoc. for Health, Phys. Educ. and Recreation, 1971).

43. E. R. Buskirk, "Diet and Athletic Performance," *Postgrad. Med.* 61 (Jan. 1977), pp. 229-36.

44. D. M. Huse and R. A. Nelson, "Basic, Balanced Diet Meets Requirements of Athletes," *The Physician and Sportsmed.* 5 (Jan. 1977), pp. 52-56.

45. "Are We Eating Too Much Protein?" *Med. World News* 15 (Nov. 8, 1974), p. 106.

46. American College of Sports Medicine Position Stand on "Weight Loss in Wrestlers," *Sports Med. Bull.* 11, No. 3 (July, 1976), pp. 1-2.

47. B. S. Upjohn, J. Shea, F. J. Stare and L. Little, "Nutrition of Athletes," *J. Am. Med. Assoc.* 151 (March 7, 1953), pp. 818-19.

48. A. Fisher, "How Much Drinking is Dangerous?" *New York Times Magazine* (May 28, 1975).

49. C. S. Lieber, "The Metabolism of Alcohol," *Scient. American* 234 (March, 1976), pp. 25-33.

50. L. E. Lamb, *Metabolics: Putting Your Food Energy to Work* (New York: Harper and Row, 1974).

51. C. S. Lieber, "Alcohol and Nutrition," *Nutrition News* 39, No. 3 (Oct. 1976), pp. 9, 12.

52. F. L. Iber, "In Alcoholism, the Liver Sets the Pace," *Nutrition Today* 6, No. 1 (Jan.-Feb. 1971), pp. 2-9.

53. R. T. Frankle and G. Christakis, "Some Nutritional Aspects of 'Hard' Drug Addiction," *Dietetic Currents* 2 (July-Aug. 1975), pp. 1-4.

54. E. A. Hartshorn, "Food and Drug Interactions," *J. Am. Dietet. Assoc.* 70 (Jan. 1977), pp. 15-19.

55. "Oral Contraceptives and Nutrition," Statement, Committee On Nutrition of the Mother and Preschool Child, Food and Nutrition Board, National Academy of Sciences, *J. Am. Dietet. Assoc.* 68 (May 1976), pp. 419-20.

56. D. M. Watkin, "Nutrition for the Aging and the Aged," Chap. 25 in R. S. Goodhart and M. E. Shils, eds., *Modern Nutrition in Health and Disease* (Philadelphia: Lea and Febiger, 1973).

57. P. Swanson, "Nutrition for the Later Years," *Food and Nutrition News* 35 (April 1964), pp. 1-4.

58. A. A. Albanese, "Nutrition and Health of the Elderly," *Nutrition News* 39 (April 1976), pp. 5, 8.

59. S. Abraham, F. W. Lowenstein and D. E. O'Connell, *Preliminary Findings of the First Health and Nutrition Examination Survey, United States, 1971-1972: Anthropometric and Clinical Findings,* DHEW Publication No. (HRA) 75-1229 (Washington, D.C.: US Gov. Print. Office, 1975).

60. S. Abraham, F. W. Lowenstein and C. L. Johnson, *Preliminary Findings of the First Health and Nutrition Examination Survey, United States, 1971-1972: Dietary Intake and Biochemical Findings,* DHEW Publication No. (HRA) 76-1219-1 (Washington, D.C.: US Gov. Print. Office, 1974).

61. C. L. Justice, J. M. Howe and H. E. Clark, "Dietary Intakes and Nutritional Status of Elderly Patients," *J. Am. Dietet. Assoc.* 65 (Dec. 1974), pp. 639-45.

62. *Food Guide For Older Folks,* Home and Garden Bull. No. 17 (Washington, D.C.: USDA, 1974).

63. R. C. Steinkamp, N. L. Cohen and H. E. Walsh, "Resurvey of an Aging Population—Fourteen Year Follow-up," *J. Am. Dietet. Assoc.* 46 (Feb. 1965), pp. 103-10.

64. D. M. Watkin, "Nutrition for the Elderly of Today and Tomorrow," *Nutrition News* 38, No. 5 (April 1975), pp. 5, 8.

65. D. M. Watkin and G. V. Mann, "Nutrition for the Aged: A Summation," *Am. J. Clin. Nutr.* 26 (Oct. 1973), pp. 1159-62.

66. B. Peterkin, *Your Money's Worth in Foods,* Home and Garden Bull. No. 183 (Washington, D.C.: USDA, Sept. 1976).

67. B. Peterkin, "Food Plans and Family Budgeting," *Family Economics Review* (Washington, D.C.: USDA, ARS-NE-36, Spring 1975), pp. 3-10.

68. B. Peterkin, "Dietary Guidance for Food Stamp Families," *Family Economics Review* (USDA: ARS-NE-36) Winter 1976, pp. 18-25.

69. N. S. Barrett and A. Driscoll, "The Impact of Inflation on Families," *Family Economics Review* (Washington, D.C.: USDA, ARS-NE-36, Spring 1976), pp. 20-24.

70. D. A. Jolly, "Food Cost, Farm Policy and Nutrition," *J. Nutr. Educ.* 8 (April-June 1976), pp. 56-58.

71. *Household Food Consumption Survey, 1965-66,* (Washington, D.C.: USDA, ARS 62-18, July 1969).

72. C. Cromwell and R. Kerr, "How Food Dollars were Divided, 1965 and 1975," *Family Economics Review* (Washington, D.C.: USDA, ARS-NE-36, Summer 1977), pp. 12-16.

Meals— and Between

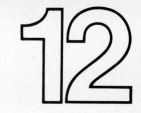

Meal Frequency
Breakfast
Lunch
Home-Delivered Meals
Fast-Food Meals
Snacks

The preceding chapters have placed major emphasis on the day's total nutritive needs. The recommended dietary allowances (RDA) and the US RDA are based on the day as a unit, and the food selection guide recommends foods to be included in the day as a whole. Nutrition standards for the content of individual meals are largely lacking. However, the increase in government nutrition programs that emphasize individual meals and changing customs with respect to the content and spacing of meals make it desirable to give more attention to meals as units. This chapter focuses attention on meal structuring and meal frequency as they influence eating patterns and affect dietary goals.

MEAL FREQUENCY

In the United States, the three-meals-a-day pattern is traditional. During the Colonial period and the early days of the Republic, all three meals were substantial in terms of the amounts and kinds of foods eaten. More recently, the eating pattern has come to consist of two light meals, breakfast and lunch (or supper), and one heavy meal, dinner. For many people this practice in turn has gradually given way to a pattern of multiple small meals throughout the day. Experiments with humans and laboratory animals have given some favorable support to the theory that eating more frequently, but consuming the same total amount of food, may result in better utilization of nutrients and a lessening of the tendency to store fat (1).

With or without scientific backing, the public has moved toward a multiple meal regime. Adults at work have regular food "breaks" and snacks are provided for children in official child nutrition programs. In practical application, multiple-meal regimes require careful planning. Nutrients should be distributed as equally as possible throughout the day's feedings, and calories should be rigidly controlled to prevent undue weight gain.

Structured meals have an important place in the day's total intake of food; they can be the pivotal points around which smaller meal segments are planned. It should be remembered that conventional meals do not function for physical satisfaction alone; the social aspects of eating have great importance.

More and Different Foods   Not only are people eating on a different time schedule, but they are also eating different foods (or foods in different forms) and are consuming them in different settings. The US Department of Agriculture reported in 1976 that about 60,000 different food items are available to consumers. In one recent year, food companies introduced 7200 new food products. Many of the new foods are mixtures (formulated foods), and a growing number are classified as convenience foods, which, according to USDA, are foods "in which significant amounts of preparation time, culinary skills, and energy inputs have been transferred from the kitchen of the food service outlet to the food processor and distributor" (2). Convenience foods, also widely used in homes, usually are more expensive than their home-prepared counterparts, but this is not consistently true (3).

About 60 percent of convenience food items are frozen. These items are used in homes, hospitals, restaurants, and schools. In institutions, they simplify operations and reduce personnel. Some of the significant developments that make foods convenient take place in the area of packaging, such as foil cans, pop-tops, portion control trays, and individual serving packs. Convenience foods are not necessarily the best solution from the standpoint of good nutrition or of food acceptance on the part of patrons, however.

Convenience foods have permeated the total pattern of eating in the United States. They are eaten as meals and snacks, included as ingredients in preparing other foods, and served along with traditional food items in meals eaten at home or elsewhere. Our focus here, therefore, is not primarily on convenience foods as such, but on the structure and content of meals, "mini-meals," and snacks as they relate to good nutrition for people of all ages. Breakfast is a logical place to start.

Breakfast

The Need   The nutritional importance of breakfast is generally recognized, but it is a meal often poorly selected, containing inadequate amounts of food, or skipped entirely. Studies show that children who miss breakfast lessen the chance that they will have an adequate diet that day (4). It is difficult to compensate in other meals for the nutrients not obtained in breakfast. Early studies showed that, as the quality of children's breakfasts declined from excellent to poor, the quality of the total day's diet declined in direct proportion (5).

Unfortunately, published evidence of the advantages of a good breakfast in terms of productivity is scarce. One well-known study, conducted at the University of Iowa over a period of 10 years, surveyed subjects of different ages (6). The work performance of the subjects—male and female office workers—was measured on a bicycle ergometer (Fig. 3.12). All subjects did significantly more work in the late morning hours when they had started the day with a good breakfast than when breakfast was omitted.

Another segment of the Iowa study was devoted to schoolboys 12 to 14 years of age. Maximum work rate and maximum work output in the late morning hours were definitely better when the boys had eaten a basic breakfast than when they had eaten none. Also, according to teachers' records, most of the boys showed better attitudes and better scholastic achievement during the period when they ate breakfast, than when it was omitted. On the other hand, reactions to certain tests proved negative. For example, omitting breakfast produced no effect on maximum grip strength, and grip-strength endurance (6).

Improved behavior and better scholastic performance have usually followed the implementation of school breakfast and lunch programs, according to subjective reports. Many such reports come from anecdotal records of teachers and comments by parents. The findings suggest that a good breakfast decreases the apathy of children, which in turn leads to improved attitudes and awareness and greater school accomplishments. Apparently, the hungry child is frustrated when confronted with difficult tasks. One nutritionist points out that "hunger may influence learning and behavior primarily in terms of ability to concentrate, rather than of structural change in the brain and central nervous system" (7).

Breakfast Habits   Breakfast has changed in recent years (8). It has become more of an individualized meal than formerly, with family members often preparing their own food and eating alone at their own convenience. The meal also tends to be a smaller one, with fewer but different items: consumption of eggs and breakfast meats has declined; that of ready-to-eat cereals and toaster products has increased (9). In one study, the eleven most popular options available to Americans at breakfast time were considered; coffee alone was chosen by 5 percent and no breakfast at all by 13 percent (10).

Ready-to-eat cereals with milk are reported to be the most frequent at-home breakfast choice. This combination is included in about 25 percent of all breakfasts (8). Children particularly are heavy consumers of breakfast cereals. The sugar content of presweetened ready-to-eat cereals is a matter of concern, however, for these make up about one-third of the volume of all ready-to-eat varieties. An analysis of the sucrose and glucose content of 78 ready-to-eat cereals was made in 1974 (11). Only eight had less than 5 percent sugar. At the other extreme 24 of the 78 cereals contained 25 to 50 percent sugar and 11 had more than 50 percent, with one as high as 68 percent sugar and 2.8 percent glucose. Even the "natural" cereals (commercial granolas) were found to contain 10 to 25 percent sugar (11).

Many surveys have been made in an effort to assess the breakfast habits of people of various ages. In a study of preteen boys and girls in a poverty area, 27 percent of the breakfast score ratings were unsatisfactory and 28 percent were only relatively satisfactory. The number of unsatisfactory breakfasts increased almost directly with age—among the girls more markedly than among the boys. At 9 years of age 60 percent of the girls had satisfactory breakfast, in contrast to only 29 percent at 13 years of age (4).

A 24-hour dietary recall on a sample of 80,000 school children in Massachusetts revealed that only 5 percent of them ate a good morning meal on that day; 13 percent ate *no* breakfast, and 24 percent came to school with an inadequate breakfast (18).

In a study of teenagers, both girls and boys in the lowest economic group ate fewer breakfasts than those in higher economic groups (12). Those who skip breakfast give many reasons for the practice: they are not hungry in the morning; there is no time to eat; they do not like the food for breakfast; or, in the absence of other family members, they do not like to prepare their own meals and eat alone.

Another reason people often give for skipping meals is that they want to cut down on calories and thus control body weight. The likelihood of accomplishing just the opposite has been documented. A midmorning snack may more than compensate for the "saved" calories. A well-balanced breakfast that supplies about one-fourth of the daily calorie allowance will usually discourage morning snacking.

National School Breakfast Program   The original purpose of the School Breakfast Program (SBP) was to provide breakfast at school for children from needy homes and/or children traveling long distances to school. The program originated in 1966 with the passage of the Child Nutrition Act, which provided for a 2-year pilot program. The SBP has been continued from time to time by a series of legislative extensions. Public Law 94-105 1975 reaffirmed Congressional support of SBP (13). Since 1973, the funding ceiling has been removed and the opportunity to apply for the program has been granted to all public and nonprofit private schools of high school grade and under where needed to provide adequate nutrition. The growth of the program has been phenomenal. Perhaps the most important long-range benefit is the formation, in childhood, of the habit of eating a nutritious breakfast regularly. The program is administered by the Food and Nutrition Service of the US Department of Agriculture.

School breakfasts must meet nutritional guidelines set by the USDA. With certain stated exceptions, each meal must include at least a specified amount of milk, fruit or full-strength fruit juice or vegetable juice, and enriched bread or cereal. Table 12.1 shows the USDA breakfast pattern (14). If breakfast is served in their schools, students from needy families are eligible for a free or reduced-price meal. Other pupils can buy the breakfast at a reasonable price. Some USDA-donated commodities are provided to the participating schools. (Fig. 12.1).

Exceptions to the regular school breakfast pattern relate to the formulated grain-fruit products that have had the approval of the USDA when a school has limited or no kitchen facilities. These formulated "cakes" are of several types, all highly fortified to supply 25 percent of the RDA for specified nutrients when served with ½ pint of milk. These formulated products are questioned on nutritional grounds. In 1977, the USDA proposed that the breakfast cakes be withdrawn. Major concerns focus on the possibility that certain as-yet-unidentified *micronutrients* may be lacking, or that the nutrients present may be in imbalance. A further criticism relates to the high sugar content of some of these formulated products. In addition, nutrition educators point out that children who have been accustomed to eating a fortified sweet cake at the school breakfast may be confused and come to regard all cakes as equally nutritious, thus defeating the educational aspect of the school breakfast.

micronutrients
Nutrients present in minute amounts

Lunch

The Need   Lunch, like breakfast, is needed to provide its share of the day's nutrients. When lunch is skipped or slighted, there is little likelihood that other meals of the day will supply the day's total requirements. The afternoon may well be a period of poor performance in the absence of an adequate meal at noon.

Table 12.1
The breakfast pattern (14)

> **fluid milk:** ½ pt (fortified with vitamins A and D) as a beverage or on cereal.
>
> **fruit or vegetable or fruit or vegetable juice:** ½ cup of fruit or vegetable; or ½ cup full-strength fruit or vegetable juice.
>
> **bread or cereal:** one serving of bread or ¾ cup (1 oz) of cereal, or an equivalent combination.
>
> **meat or meat alternate:** to help meet children's nutrition needs, breakfast should contain as often as possible a 1-ounce serving (edible portion) of meat, poultry, or fish; or 1 oz of cheese; or one egg; or 2 tbsp of peanut butter; or an equivalent amount of any combination of these foods.
>
> In addition, supplements, such as honey, fortified margarine, butter and jam, add nutrients, satisfy appetites and appeal, and should be served frequently.
>
> Also plan to include vitamin C foods frequently and foods for iron each day.

Figure 12.1
School breakfasts meet nutritional guidelines. When a school serves breakfast, the meal is available free or at a reduced price for students unable to pay the full amount. (US Department of Agriculture)

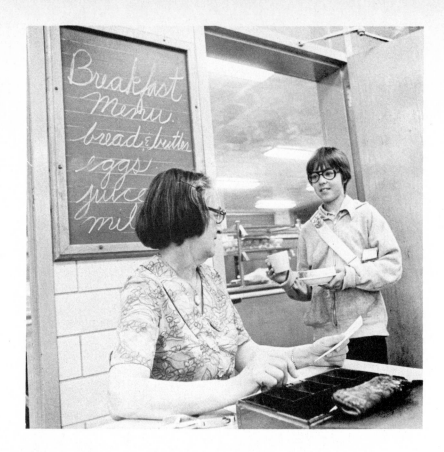

Sources of Lunch   Lunch is the meal most often eaten away from home, which creates the difficulty of controlling its content. Lunch differs from other meals in the variety of settings and circumstances under which it is eaten. These include restaurants, school and industrial cafeterias, lunch counters, fast-food operations, and on-the-job locations, to mention only a few. Lunches are often eaten in groups—business conferences, committee meetings, and social gatherings, for example—with one lunch menu planned for all. Facilities for lunch offer an equally wide range, from a full-scale lunchroom serving a complete hot meal to a vending machine bay where only snacks are available. Many people prefer to bring their lunch from home to school or work (Fig. 12.2).

Lunch Habits   With so much variation in the facilities for obtaining lunch, it is difficult to characterize lunch habits. In general, lunch is a light meal in the United States. In cases where a plate lunch is available for a package price, the meal is probably adequate in energy, if not always satisfactory in nutrient content. Surveys of lunches have been made chiefly among young people. In a study of preteens in a poverty neighborhood (4), the overall lunch-eating patterns were poorer than the breakfast patterns. There was no school lunch program. Among the children, 33 percent had two or more unsatisfactory lunches in 4 days of record-keeping, and lunch scores were poor at every age from 9 to 13 years. There were more satisfactory lunches among whites than among blacks. In the survey of teenage diets, lunch proved to be the meal most often skipped (12).

There is evidence that a nourishing diet is related to work capacity, efficiency, and morale (see Chap. 3). Hot noon meals were introduced into industrial plants to protect the health of employees and to maintain work schedules. Some evidence was produced, particularly in wartime operations, to indicate that production records were improved when hearty meals were served on the premises. Many plant-operated lunchrooms are now being supplanted by caterer-operated services and vending machines, with the latter playing an increasing role.

School Lunches as a Nutrition Measure   The school lunch was originated for the sole purpose of improving child nutrition. It had its beginnings in Germany, France, and England. In the United States, the school lunch began in the early part of the 20th century with the supplementary feeding of hungry children in poor sections of some cities. Its scope was gradually broadened, and it was soon introduced as a hot meal in urban high schools and in rural consolidated schools where children lived too far away to go home at noon. At first the lunch was strictly a feeding operation; until 1925 little or no thought was given to making it an educational experience.

Gradually lunchroom managers with home economics and dietetic training were employed to plan and supervise the preparation of the lunches. Eventually efforts were made, here and there, to

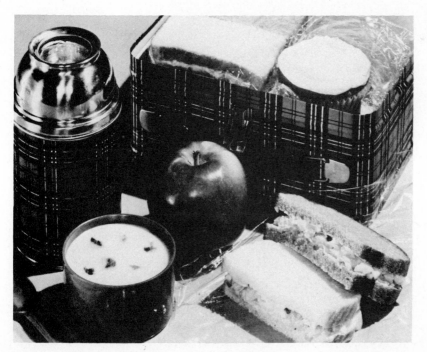

Figure 12.2
Lunch carried from home is the choice of people of all ages who prefer their favorite foods, eaten in a restful atmosphere and at a substantial saving in cost. (United Dairy Industry Association)

use the lunch as a means of teaching good eating practices. Federal assistance to school lunch operations began in 1933 with provision for labor costs and trained management personnel. By 1935, with the enactment of Public Law 320, additional assistance was made possible in the form of donated commodities. Step by step the school lunch moved toward the huge operation it is today.

National School Lunch Program

Legislation   The present National School Lunch Program (NSLP) operates under a series of Acts of Congress beginning in 1946. Permanent authorization was provided by the National School Lunch Act and the Child Nutrition Act of 1966. Amendments were enacted in October 1975 under Public Law 94-105 (13). School lunch legislation provides for a grant-in-aid program under the direction of the Secretary of Agriculture and authorizes annual ap-

Table 12.2
The Type A lunch pattern (15)

As specified in the National School Lunch Regulations, a Type A lunch shall contain as a minimum each of the following food components in the amounts indicated:

fluid milk: ½ pt of fluid milk (fortified with vitamins A and D) as a beverage.

vegetables and fruits: ¾ cup serving consisting of two or more vegetables or fruits or both. A serving (¼ cup or more) of full-strength vegetable or fruit juice may be counted to meet not more than ¼ cup of this requirement.

meat and meat alternate: 2 oz (edible portion as served) of lean meat, poultry, or fish; or 2 oz of cheese; or one egg; or ½ cup of cooked dry beans or dry peas; or 4 tablespoons of peanut butter; or an equivalent of any combination of the above-listed foods.

To be counted in meeting this requirement, these foods must be served in a main dish or in a main dish and one other item.

bread: 1 slice of whole-grain or enriched bread; or a serving of other bread such as cornbread, biscuits, rolls, or muffins, made of whole-grain or enriched meal or flour.

Add other foods not part of the lunch requirement as needed to complete lunches, to help improve acceptability and to provide additional food energy and other nutrients.

To help ensure that all Type A lunches meet the nutritional goal, it is recommended that lunches include: a vitamin-A vegetable or fruit at least twice a week, a vitamin-C vegetable or fruit several times a week, and several foods for iron each day.

It is also recommended that fat in the Type A lunch be kept at a moderate level and that iodized salt be used in preparing lunches.

The nutritional goal for school lunches is to furnish at least one-third of the RDA for children of various age groups, with the meals to consist of a suitable assortment of common foods in designated quantities. The Type A lunch requirements provide the framework for nutritionally adequate school lunches. The kinds and amounts of foods listed in the Type A pattern are based on the 1968 RDA for 10- to 12-year old boys and girls (15).

propriations in amounts to carry out the purposes and objectives of the Act.

Legislation specifies that "school lunches shall consist of a combination of foods and shall meet minimum nutritional requirements prescribed by the Secretary of Agriculture on the basis of tested nutrition research." With this mandate, the Type A lunch pattern was developed to serve as a framework for planning and choosing school lunches (Table 12.2). The pattern was designed to yield a suitable proportion of the Recommended Dietary Allowances (RDA) for the day's nutrients.

Administration   The National School Lunch Program is a joint responsibility of the federal government, state governments, and local communities and their schools. The program is administered by the Food and Nutrition Service (FNS) of the US Dept. of Agriculture. All public and nonprofit private schools of high school grade and under—as well as public and licensed nonprofit private residential child-care institutions—may participate in the program. Schools that agree to participate must conduct the food program on a nonprofit basis for all children regardless of race, color, or national origin; furnish free or reduced-price meals to children unable to pay full price without discrimination against or identification of these children; and provide lunches that meet established nutritional criteria (16).

Implementation   Efforts to improve the quality and acceptance of school lunches continue. The law has authorized a National Advisory Council on Child Nutrition, which addresses itself to many basic school lunch problems. At regular intervals the Council oversees the testing by chemical analysis of the nutritional content of school lunches and recommends any adjustments to be made in the Type A pattern, based on the findings. The Type A pattern increasingly takes account of the needs of children of different age levels, in terms of the quantities of foods specified. In the recent past there has been an effort to displace the Type A food pattern with nutrient standards. However, independent studies sponsored by USDA report that no significant nutritional differences have been found between meals planned with the Type A pattern as a guide and those planned directly by nutrient standards (17).

Studies also are conducted to find effective feeding systems for schools without physical facilities. In some cases, catered meals are the solution, or lunches prepared in central kitchens, packed in insulated cases, and transported by truck to *satellite schools* that lack kitchens. In other cases individual lunches may be delivered to children in *cup-cans*, which combine the components of a Type A lunch in a stew or other mixture; canned or frozen convenience foods also may be used when the situation dictates. When meals are transported, held, and reheated, however, there must be concern not only for the bacteriological safety of the foods, but also for the retention of nutrients and the attractiveness and flavor of the foods.

There have been certain departures in the school lunch pattern itself. For example, up to 30 percent of textured vegetable protein

satellite schools
Those subordinate or dependent

Figure 12.3
School lunches meet nutritional guidelines. Maximum benefits are achieved when the day's schedule permits students to enjoy a leisurely lunch with friends. (US Department of Agriculture)

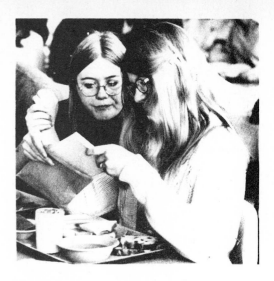

products may now be combined with meat and other animal foods in meeting the minimum requirement of 2 ounces of cooked meat specified for the Type A school lunch. The substitution has been questioned on the nutritional grounds that the replacement may not constitute full substitution. There is also an increase in the variety of milks allowable in the lunch choices. Instead of whole milk only, school lunchrooms may now offer plain skim milk, low-fat milk, cultured buttermilk, as well as flavored milks (Fig. 12.3).

Outcomes   It is impossible to measure the full nutritional impact of the school lunch on the children of the United States, although there are many indications of its benefits. In most cases, especially among needy children, it may be supposed that a school lunch consistently provides a more nearly adequate meal than does lunch from other sources. This was borne out in a survey of 54,000 children in grades 4 through 12 in Massachusetts schools: 72 percent of the children who ate the Type A lunch at school consumed a meal rated adequate in contrast to 42 percent of those who brought their lunches from home, 28 percent who went home for lunch, 23 percent who bought *à la carte* lunches in school, and 21 percent who ate in the neighborhood store (18).

a la carte lunches
Lunches purchased as separate foods, rather than as "package" lunches

It also has been demonstrated that the Type A lunch contributes to good nutrition in terms of the proportion of daily nutrients provided. In the Ten-State Survey the lunch was found to supply 30 to 50 percent of daily nutrients in low-income-ratio states and 20 to 40 percent in high-income-ratio states. Black children, presumably in greater need, received proportionally higher nutrient contributions from the school lunch than did white children (19).

Certainly the increasing numbers of schools, lunch programs, and participating children alone offer practical measures of progress. In 1944, it was estimated that approximately one million Type A lunches were served daily. In 1976, more than 26 million children participated in the National School Lunch Program—an impressive record of growth. These figures are more significant in light of the fact that the proportion of free and reduced-price lunches advanced steadily throughout the period.

Despite evidence of progress, the school lunch program faces serious problems in terms of realizing fully its purpose of contributing to the nutritional welfare of children. A major concern is for excessive plate waste at all grade levels. So deep is the government's concern for the control of food waste that Public Law 94-105, 1975 authorized a broad-scale inquiry into the reasons why children reject the food (13). Many reasons have been proposed, and it seems likely that multiple—and perhaps related—factors are involved, including absence of an effective program of nutrition education, unacceptable menus, poorly prepared and unattractive food, careless and impersonal service, unsuitable size of food portions, and an atmosphere of haste and pressure in the lunchrooms.

One official attempt to reduce plate waste allows high school students to narrow their selection to any three of the five items in the Type A lunch pattern. This plan, which eliminates two components of the pattern and thus their accompanying nutrients, will undoubtedly result in more clean plates. However, it evades, rather than meets, a fundamental challenge of the school lunch—to improve food practices. Rejection of foods in the Type A pattern emphasizes the need for greater efforts to provide well-planned meals that children will enjoy: well-cooked, tasty, and freshly prepared food, attractively served in friendly surroundings and a relaxed atmosphere. Active student participation in all phases of the lunch program and the combined efforts of interested, involved teachers, food service personnel, and parents are features of programs in which plate waste is kept to a minimum. Vigorous, practical nutrition education at all grade levels, and related to the lunch program is essential in such a plan.

The enthusiasm with which young people enjoy fast-food meals, to be discussed presently, has prompted food service managements in some secondary schools and colleges to introduce similar foods and meal combinations. Reports have stressed the wholehearted acceptance of the foods and the disappearance of the plate waste problem. In some situations the fast-food type combinations have been modified to meet the nutrient requirements of The Type A lunch formula without lessening the popularity of the meals. Such experiences would seem to offer fresh incentives for providing acceptable foods that at the same time carry their fair share of nutrients needed for the day.

"Junk" foods sold in the school are considered by many to be a major competitor of the Type A school lunch. The responsibility for regulating the sale of such foods in the school has been transferred from US Dept. of Agriculture to state and local school officials. Competitive foods often are available to children at the same hours and in essentially the same setting as the school meals. Nutritionists have urged that all foods served in the school be under the supervision of persons knowledgeable in the field of child nutrition. Arrangements should be made to prevent children from spending lunch money for miscellaneous snacks, which makes it impossible to buy the full, planned lunch. If competitive foods are to be al-

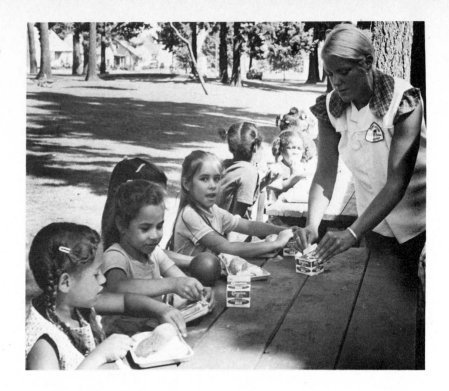

Figure 12.4
Summer meals and snacks meet nutritional guidelines. The food is available to school-age children from May to September in a planned vacation program. (US Department of Agriculture)

lowed in the school, the choice of items and the conditions under which they are sold should be rigidly controlled in the interest of conforming to the basic nutritional purpose of the school lunch program.

Food Programs for Children

Summer Food Service Programs   Summer food service programs, conducted for school-age children in districts in economic need are strengthened by Public Law 94-105, 1975. Federal assistance consists of cash reimbursements and commodity food deliveries to public and nonprofit private institutions serving school-age children. These include settlement houses, recreation centers, residential camps, summer day camps, orphanages, and homes for the mentally retarded. A notable addition to the law is the new interpretation of the word "school" as "any public or licensed nonprofit private child care institution" (13). This represents a considerable extension of the benefits of the school lunch program. To participate, institutions are no longer required to conduct educational programs. Individual children may receive breakfast, and/or lunch, and/or dinner, and/or between-meal snacks, depending on how long they spend at the site. Meals are served without charge to the children (Fig. 12.4).

The objective of the program is to raise the nutrient intake levels of children in nonschool, largely nonresidential situations, particularly of children from low-income areas where many mothers work outside their homes. To support this objective, the US Dept. of Agriculture has established certain minimum guidelines for the meals and snacks. This program has the potential of providing children with 100 percent of their daily dietary allowances if they consume all or nearly all of the food offered to them. The aim of the summer food program is to continue the benefits of school feeding in a structured vacation schedule of recreation, crafts, and study.

Child Care Food Program The concept of this year-round program, largely for preschool children, is to meet the health, nutrition, and social needs of young children in group care. Provisions of Public Law 94-105, 1975 broadened the services so that the program no longer is confined to very needy children. All public and private day-care facilities can join if they are nonprofit and are licensed to operate by a designated state agency. Staff members must meet state requirements for training and experience for working with preschool-age children. Nutrition counseling is often provided by outside agencies. Institutions approved for participation, including family day-care homes, Head Start Centers, Settlement Houses, recreation centers, and institutions providing day care for handicapped children, are expected to implement essentially the same guidelines as those for the school lunch and breakfast programs. Money and food are provided for breakfasts, lunches, suppers, and snacks. The meals, served free to needy children, include specific types of foods in at least minimum amounts in accordance with the ages of the children (13).

Tasty, attractive, nutritionally adequate meals, served in a relaxed environment, with the children seated comfortably, adds to the enjoyment of the meals and to their educational potential. Participation by children in preparing or serving the meal and some opportunity to make choices of their lunch often help to create interest in food and eating. Many day-care facilities provide for parental participation in the program as a means of relating the children's activities to life in their own homes. Thus, group care at its best does far more than provide physical care for children (20) (Fig. 12.5).

Special Milk Program   The special milk program makes it possible for all children attending a school or institution to purchase milk at a reduced price, or if they are needy, to receive it free. Institutions and schools that participate in other federal-state child nutrition programs may also participate in the Special Milk Program. The milk program, however, is particularly helpful in those schools that have no other food service.

HOME-DELIVERED MEALS

A totally different concept of providing meals to a segment of the public is that of home-delivered meals. Sometimes referred to as "meals on wheels," this service is designed particularly to aid ill and elderly persons who are unable to prepare their own food. The meals are delivered to the homes of the recipients who, in many cases, have been recently discharged from hospitals. Individual

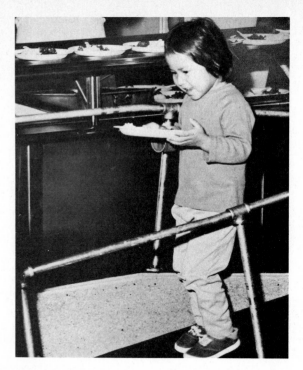

Figure 12.5
A Navajo Indian girl enjoys two meals and a snack daily at a day care center in Shiprock, N. Mex., while her mother works. (US Department of Agriculture)

programs establish guidelines for selecting clients (21, 22).

The meals are delivered 5 or 6 days a week at the noon hour. Each delivery usually consists of a hot meal to be eaten immediately and a cold meal to be eaten later as supper. Most of the meals are simple combinations of well-accepted foods. Meal planning and preparation is often under the direction of dietitians, and in some cases therapeutic diets are provided on the prescription of a physician. Volunteers usually deliver the meals and visit with or assist the patients briefly (Fig. 12.6).

Home-delivered meals are handled in different ways in different localities. Frequently, the operation is coordinated and the food prepared in a local hospital, although many other facilities are used. The volunteers are often from community and church groups composed of both men and women. Costs of the meals generally are based on the recipient's ability to pay. Despite the great need for such a service, it has been discontinued in some localities because of the expense. Those who are most in need often have insufficient income to pay for the service, or, if they are on public assistance, their meal allowance is inadequate to cover the cost of the home-delivered meals. Despite these handicaps, the movement appears to be growing. Federal, state, and local assistance with food and/or operating costs makes it possible in many cases to provide meals to needy persons at little or no cost to them.

FAST FOOD MEALS

Changes in life styles and new food marketing patterns have created new service outlets for meals. In the mid 1970s, people of

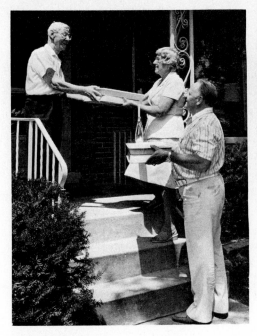

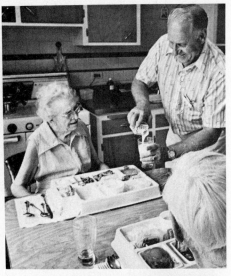

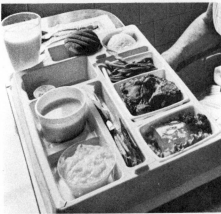

Figure 12.6

(Above) Husband and wife volunteer team deliver specially packed hot food to the home of an elderly couple.

(Above right) Volunteer puts the final touches on the attractive and ample meal.

(Right) Close up of meal. (Courtesy Lutheran General Hospital, Park Ridge, Ill.) (Ernest Tisil)

the United States used one-third of all the money they spent for food on restaurant meals. A growing number of restaurants—perhaps a third—are fast-food outlets that serve a limited number of prepared food items separately and in meal combinations. It is predicted that the number of fast-food restaurants will nearly double in the United States before 1980 (23). The success of the fast-food business is attributed largely to its swift and convenient service of foods the public likes and to such technological developments as disposable packaging, new package coatings, and the concept of portion control.

With increased patronage of fast-food places, concern has developed for the nutritional values of the foods and meals sold. Are the individual foods nutritious, and do they and the "mini-meals" contribute substantially to daily nutrient needs? The McDonald Corporation undertook to shed some light on these questions by arranging for a reputable scientific research organization to make a nutrient analysis of their major food items and meals. Later, working with the corporation, USDA compared the findings with the

Figure 12.7
Hamburger, french fries and chocolate shake. This is one of the fast food meal combinations, the nutritive yields of which are shown on Table 12.3. (McDonald's Corporation)

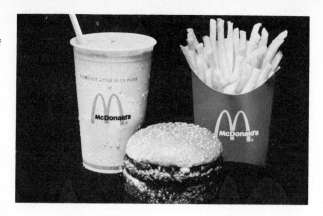

US Recommended Daily Allowances (US RDA) and considered the costs of fast-food meals. The results, confined to nutritive values, are shown in Tables 12.3 and 12.4 (24) (Fig 12.7).

Table 12.3 presents seven commonly offered meal combinations, with their nutritive values stated as percentages of daily standards for energy and certain nutrients. USDA points out that of the seven fast-food meals, five furnish 20 percent or more of the US

Table 12.3
Nutritive values of meal combinations from fast food restaurant

Food	% of food energy*	\multicolumn{8}{c}{% of US Recommended Daily Allowance}	% of food energy from fat
		Protein	Vitamin A	Thiamin	Ribo-flavin	Calcium	Iron	Ascorbic acid	
hamburger, french fries, soft drink	22	24	3	19	24	6	16	21	32
hamburger, french fries, chocolate shake	30	42	3	25	57	47	21	21	31
hamburger, french fries, soft drink, apple pie	32	28	3	20	26	8	19	24	38
cheeseburger, french fries, soft drink	24	29	6	21	32	15	15	21	35
"Big Mac," french fries, soft drink	33	45	4	25	40	17	23	23	44
¼-lb hamburger, french fries, soft drink	28	45	5	23	39	8	24	20	36
fillet of fish, french fries, soft drink	28	28	2	23	23	10	11	17	40

Source: Nutritive values from "Nutritional Analysis of Food Served at McDonald's Restaurants" based on a study by the WARF Institute, Madison, Wis., January 1973, for McDonald's Corporation. (Adapted from Table 1, ref. 24.)

*An allowance arbitrarily set at 2600 kcal. Recommended Dietary Allowance (1974) set by the National Academy of Science-National Research Council is 2100 kcal for a teenage girl and 3000 kcal for a teenage boy.

Table 12.4
Nutritive values of individual menu items in fast food meals

Food	% of food energy*	% of US Recommended Daily Allowance							% of food energy from fat
		Protein	Vitamin A	Thiamin	Ribo-flavin	Calcium	Iron	Ascorbic acid	
hamburger	10	20	3	12	21	5	14	6	36
cheeseburger	12	25	6	13	30	14	13	6	41
"Big Mac"	21	40	4	18	38	16	21	8	52
¼-lb hamburger	16	41	5	15	37	7	21	5	41
fillet of fish	16	24	2	15	21	9	9	2	49
french fries	8	4	**	7	2	1	2	15	42
apple pie	10	3	**	**	2	2	3	3	51
chocolate shake	12	17	**	5	33	41	5	**	20
soft drink†	4	**	0	0	0	0	0	0	0

Source: Nutritive values from "Nutritional Analysis of Food Served at McDonald's Restaurants" based on a study by the WARF Institute, Madison, Wis., January 1973, for McDonald's Corporation. (Adapted from Table 2, ref. 24.)
*An allowance arbitrarily set at 2600 kcal. Recommended Dietary Allowance (1974) set by the National Academy of Science-National Research Council is 2100 kcal for a teenage girl and 3000 kcal for a teenage boy.
**Insignificant amount of nutrient present.
†No nutritive value for soft drink available from McDonald's. Values used were from "Nutritive Value of Foods," HG-72.

RDA for protein, thiamin, riboflavin, and ascorbic acid. On the other hand, the meals are notably low in vitamin A, and the only meal containing a milk shake exceeds 20 percent of US RDA for calcium. The fat content of the meals is relatively high but not excessive: the percentage of food energy from fat ranges from 31 percent to 44 percent. Nutritionists recommend that fats provide about 35 percent of total calories, but fat in the American diet yields about 42 percent. The meals in Table 12.3 provide a larger share of the US RDA for food energy than for some of the nutrients when 2600 calories is used as a daily energy standard.

Table 12.4 presents nine individual menu items that, in various combinations, constitute fast-food meals and snacks of the type shown in Table 12.3 (Fig. 12.8). Their nutritive values are expressed as percentages of daily standards for energy and for certain specified nutrients. It is apparent from Table 12.4 where the nutritive strengths and weaknesses lie in the individual foods and how, with proper selection, certain of them can supplement each other

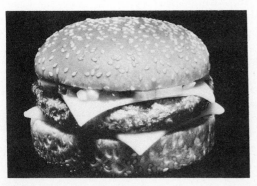

Figure 12.8
A cheeseburger is one of the several popular individual fast food items listed with their nutritive values in Table 12.4. (McDonald's Corporation)

in improving the nutritive values of meals. This system is not useful in the case of vitamin A because there are no good sources of this vitamin among the foods listed, and it has less application in the case of calcium because only one food on the list (chocolate milk shake) makes a significant contribution of calcium. Ascorbic acid is low in all individual menu items except french fries, and the potatoes are responsible for raising ascorbic acid values in all the meal combinations (Table 12.3). Thus, under the food choices available here, all food combinations would be low in vitamin A and only meals with milk as a beverage would be apt to provide considerable amounts of calcium. If such fast-food meals were to be eaten regularly, special attention should be given to obtaining vitamin A and calcium at other meals of the day. McDonald's makes its milk shakes with a nonfat dry milk base, which furnishes more calcium and less milk fat (less vitamin A) than would a shake made of whole milk and ice cream.

Of what practical significance are these calculated data for people who patronize fast-food restaurants? Two hundred eighty customers in two different outlets of one fast-food chain introduced reality when they responded to a verbal questionnaire regarding their experiences in eating fast foods. Both men and women in a wide age range were queried as they left the premises after eating at one or the other of the two restaurants. Their food choices were evaluated for energy content and for seven nutrients on the basis of published analyses of the food (25). Results showed that vitamin A and calcium were the nutrients least often consumed in amounts equal to one-third of the RDA—in the case of vitamin A, because no good sources of the vitamin were available on the menu, and in the case of calcium, because of failure on the part of patrons to choose a good calcium source.

In this actual situation, two important considerations were explored: whether the customers regarded their food choices as meals or merely as snacks, and how frequently they patronized the restaurants. If food choices represent meals, obviously their nutritive content takes on more importance. Likewise, if patronage is regular and frequent, the concern for nutritional adequacy increases. Slightly more than one-half of the customers in the two groups questioned considered the food combinations they had purchased to be meals; the remainder called their choices snacks. On the matter of frequency of patronage, the majority of customers questioned ate at the fast-food restaurants no more than one to three times a week, and of this group 61 percent categorized the foods they bought as snacks. This would suggest that these foods were eaten in addition to regular meals.

The investigators in the study suggest that improvement of fast-food meals and snacks might well proceed along two lines: encouraging fast-food businesses to provide rich sources of all nutrients among their menu items, and educating their customers to make wise food choices. Need for nutrition education was exhibited on the day of the survey by the fact that milk and milk shakes were on the menus at both restaurants and either item, if added to a meal combination, could have provided one-third of the RDA for

Table 12.5
Nutritive value of individual breakfast items from a fast food restaurant

Food	% of food energy*	% of US Recommended Daily Allowance							% of food energy from fat
		Protein	Vitamin A	Thiamin	Ribo-flavin	Calcium	Iron	Ascorbic acid	
"Egg McMuffin"	14	30	6	25	35	20	20	2	50
hot cakes, butter, syrup	18	10	4	20	25	15	10	**	17
scrambled eggs	6	25	10	4	35	4	10	**	67
pork sausage	7	20	**	15	6	**	4	**	85
english muffin, buttered	7	10	2	15	8	10	8	**	28
whole milk, 8 oz	6	15	6	4	25	30	**	4	45
orange juice, 6 oz	3	**	6	10	**	**	**	140	0

Source: Nutritive values from "Nutritional Analysis of Food Served at McDonald's Restaurants" based on study by WARF Institute, Madison, Wis., 1977 for McDonald's Corporation. (Adapted from Tables III and V, ref. 26)
*An allowance arbitrarily set at 2,600 kcal. Recommended Dietary Allowance (1974) set by the National Academy of Science-National Research Council is 2,100 kcal for a teenage girl and 3,000 for a teenage boy.
**Insignificant amount of nutrient present.

calcium in most cases. However, among the 280 meals and snack purchases, only 19 milk shakes and 13 orders of milk were reported, in contrast to 115 orders of soft drinks and 80 cups of coffee (25).

On the matter of providing rich sources of all nutrients, many fast-food restaurants have already taken steps in the direction of increasing the number of foods offered on their menus. One rather general development is the provision of foods suitable for breakfast combinations. In addition, some of the restaurants have included more flavors of certain items such as milk shakes, and whole milk, ice cream, and orange juice are usually available. Such foods lend variety and food value to many different meal and snack combinations. Table 12.5 lists several of the breakfast items added most recently by one of the fast-food chains (26) (Fig. 12.9). Thus the offerings are broadened, giving the customer more choices from which to formulate meal combinations. More choices add to the customer's opportunity to select nutritionally adequate meals.

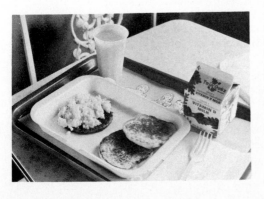

Figure 12.9
Orange juice, scrambled eggs, english muffin and milk is one of the breakfast combinations that can be chosen from the individual breakfast items shown with their nutritive values on Table 12.5. (McDonald's Corporation)

Assemble meals and snacks from the individual food items on Tables 12.4 and 12.5 by choosing combinations that achieve the maximum in total nutritive values and those that achieve the least. (Proceed by adding the percentages of US RDA for each nutrient supplied by the individual foods in the combinations you have chosen.) Your totals, in relation to 100%, will indicate the success you have achieved and which single foods have contributed most or least to total nutritive values.

How often do you eat meals at fast-food restaurants? snacks? Have fast foods affected your habits of eating? How? Does your appetite for fast foods tend to wane as you eat them more frequently?

Price the menu items on Table 12.4 and 12.5 (purchased or homemade). Which is the most expensive item in terms of nutritive yield? The most economical?

Develop a meal formula (similar to the Type A Lunch pattern) based on fast-food items, which would ensure about one-third of the US RDA for the nutrients shown on Table 12.3. What foods would you include in your formula to ensure adequate amounts of vitamin A? of calcium?

FOODS FROM VENDING MACHINES

The variety of foods available from vending machines has grown from chiefly snack items to include many substantial components of meals. Vending machines are of increasing importance in providing lunch for workers in office buildings and factories, largely as a result of the installation of microwave ovens for use in conjunction with vending machine products. Vending and food service contracting companies furnish the ovens. Customers can purchase a refrigerated sandwich or entree from the vending machine and heat it in the microwave oven to provide a hot meal or snack. The combination of refrigerated and heating equipment has been responsible for increased sales of vended foods which are best when eaten hot. This service also has been conducive to the sale of cold foods that accompany hot meals, such as salads and desserts.

Products suitable for the dispensing machines are constantly being developed. The newer machines accommodate a variety of packages, and a wide range of foods.

SNACKS

Snacks are difficult to define, as we have seen in previous discussions in this chapter. Nevertheless, snacks cannot be ignored as suppliers of energy and nutrients. The quantities of snacks that people consume vary greatly, but many consume large amounts. The Ten-State Survey, for example, reports that teenagers obtain nearly one-fourth of their total calories from snacks. Table 12.4 shows the

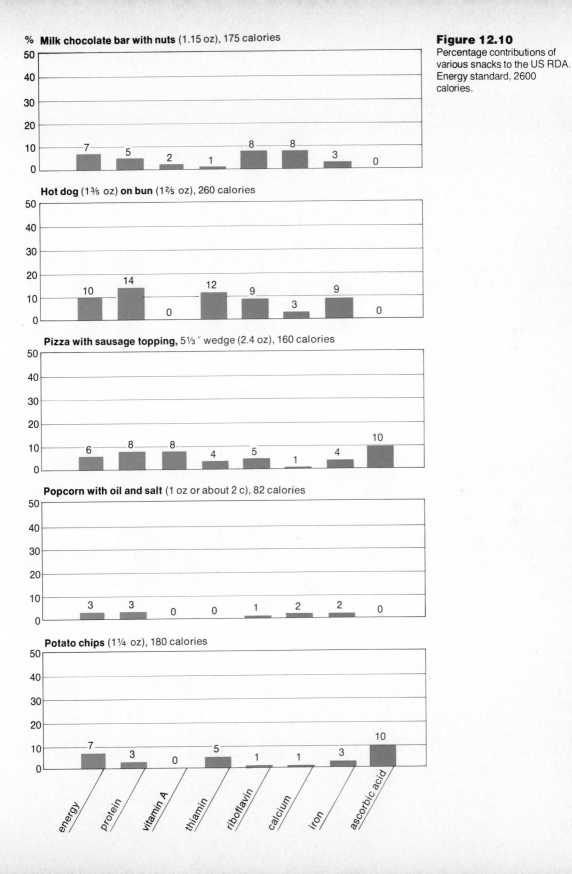

% Milk chocolate bar with nuts (1.15 oz), 175 calories

7, 5, 2, 1, 8, 8, 3, 0

Hot dog (1⅗ oz) **on bun** (1⅖ oz), 260 calories

10, 14, 0, 12, 9, 3, 9, 0

Pizza with sausage topping, 5⅓″ wedge (2.4 oz), 160 calories

6, 8, 8, 4, 5, 1, 4, 10

Popcorn with oil and salt (1 oz or about 2 c), 82 calories

3, 3, 0, 0, 1, 2, 2, 0

Potato chips (1¼ oz), 180 calories

7, 3, 0, 5, 1, 1, 3, 10

energy, protein, vitamin A, thiamin, riboflavin, calcium, iron, ascorbic acid

Figure 12.10
Percentage contributions of various snacks to the US RDA. Energy standard, 2600 calories.

Figure 12.11
Percentage contributions of various beverages to the US RDA. Energy standard, 2600 calories.

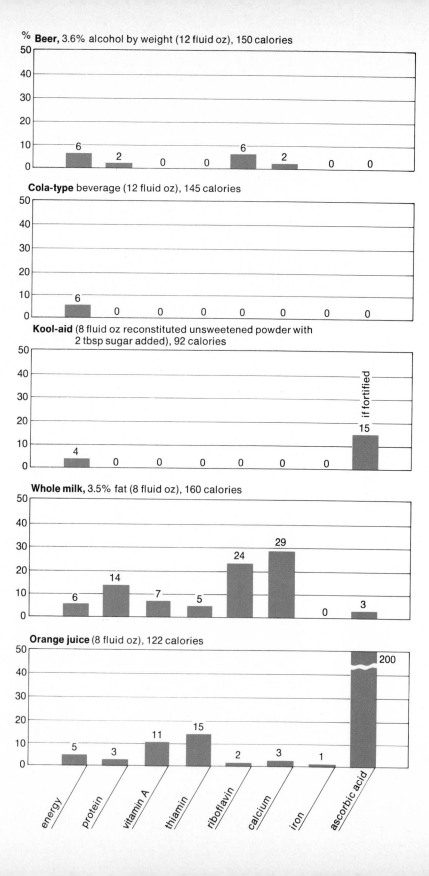

nutritive contributions of nine foods commonly eaten as snacks. Figure 12.10 shows graphically the nutritive contributions of an additional five snacks. All are obtainable from vending machines (27) or are sold at snack bars and other eating places. The information on Table 12.4 and Figure 12.10 is comparable. All data are expressed as percentages of the US RDA and of 2600 calories as the chosen energy standard. The percentages of energy supplied by the foods in Table 12.4 tend to run higher than for the foods in Figure 12.10. Serving sizes and the proportions of fat in the foods on the two lists are largely responsible for these differences. In choosing snacks for nutritive value, it would be well to study the nutrient contributions of the individual foods analyzed in Table 12.4 and Figure 12.10. If cost must be considered, the various snacks should be priced and compared in light of the the nutrients available for the money.

BEVERAGES

Beverages of all kinds are a part of meals and snacks. Figure 12.11 shows the nutritive contributions of five popular beverages. The beverages can be compared with each other for nutrient yields. Two of the beverages make distinctive contributions—milk provides calcium and orange juice ascorbic acid. Some beverages (again milk and orange juice) make multiple contributions, while others (such as colas and Kool-Aid) are essentially devoid of nutrients. Twelve ounces of beer provide 2 percent of the protein and calcium standards and 6 percent of the riboflavin standard, inconsequential amounts in light of total nutrient need. All of the beverages provide 4 to 6 percent of the energy standard. Again, a comparison of nutrient yields in relation to cost provides a satisfactory basis for judging values.

Beverage Consumption Patterns   Beverage consumption patterns in the United States are varied. People drink many different beverages and in different amounts. For most beverages per capita consumption is on the increase. This fact is demonstrated in Table 12.6, which compares per capita consumption of major beverages in 1965 and 1975, using as the index 1955=100. In the 10-year period between these dates, only fluid milk and coffee consumption declined, while tea and cocoa consumption increased 14 percent, beer 33 percent, soft drinks 44 percent, certain hard liquors 44 percent, and fruit and vegetable juices and drinks 62 percent. Analysts of the data commented that some of the consumption trends shown have been of even longer standing. For example, in the past 20 years, tea and cocoa combined rose 35 percent, fruit and vegetable juices and drinks went up nearly 80 percent, and soft drinks, beginning in the early 1960s more than doubled. Also, in the 20-year interval, alcoholic beverages rose more than nonalcoholic beverages. Beer increased nearly 40 percent, while wine, whiskey, gin, and rum rose about 90 percent. The increase for beer and wine has been chiefly in the last 10 years, but hard liquor has been rising for 20 years.

Table 12.6
Comparison per capita beverage consumption in the United States 1965 and 1975

Product	Per capita consumption*		Percentage difference
	1965	1975	1965/1975
milk	95	88	− 7
soft drinks	164	236	+44
coffee	100	85	−15
tea and cocoa	117	135	+14
fruit and vegetable juices and drinks	110	178	+62
beer	103	137	+33
wine	111	192	+73
whiskey, gin, rum	130	187	+44

*Index: 1955=100
Source: *National Food Situation*. NFS-160, June 1977. Economic Research Service, US Dept. of Agriculture. Adapted from "What Americans Drink", pp. 28-29.

Narrowing the comparisons to four beverages consumed commonly by many people in the United States, Figure 12.12 shows graphically trends in their per capita consumption since 1960. The pronounced upward spurt of soft drinks is demonstrated, as well as the tendency of tea to rise and coffee to fall, while fluid milk shows a slight decline in per capita consumption.

Beverage consumption patterns vary among sections of the country and even within states. This latter fact was borne out by an interview study conducted in New York State, using a 24-hour recall procedure to learn beverage habits of individuals between the ages of 12 and 65 years (28). For all adults, coffee and tea were the beverages most drunk. For all age groups, milk was consumed more heavily upstate, while soft drinks and fruit juices were more

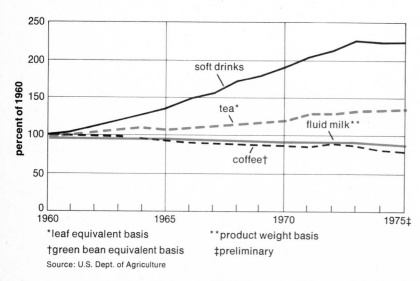

*leaf equivalent basis   **product weight basis
†green bean equivalent basis   ‡preliminary
Source: U.S. Dept. of Agriculture

Figure 12.12
Trends in beverage use in the United States: consumption of selected beverages per capita.

popular in the city. Among upstate teenagers, milk was the major beverage, while the comparable age group in New York City drank more soft drinks. With respect to beverage choices at meals, the majority of upstate teenagers preferred milk at all meals; in New York City soft drinks were the major beverage for teenagers at lunch and dinner; young adults preferred soft drinks with their evening meal.

The phenomenal increase in consumption of soft drinks has raised several questions. One concerns the tendency for such drinks to supplant milk and fruit juices. Another is the hazard of excess sugar consumed in the soft drinks. Beverages now comprise the largest single industry use of refined sugar in this country (29). As the per capita consumption of soft drinks doubled between 1960 and 1975 (from 109 to 221 16 oz-containers), the per capita consumption of refined sugar from that source has also doubled from 11.3 pounds to 21.5 pounds. This represents about one-fifth the average annual per capita consumption of white sugar in the United States. The large amount of phosphorus in soft drinks also has been questioned by nutritionists. The concern is that high phosphate content of the diet may decrease the absorption of calcium by the formation of an insoluble calcium complex.

More recently the caffeine content of cola beverages, which account for more than two-thirds of the soft drink consumption, has had increasing attention on the basis of possible health risk. Concern is expressed primarily for children whose major source of caffeine is probably cola drinks, but for adults who may be consuming large additional amounts of caffeine in tea and coffee, there also may be a health hazard. *Caffeine* has been used for generations in medicine, but knowledge of its exact actions in the body remains incomplete. Connections between caffeine and ulcers, bladder cancer, and heart disease have been reported but with insufficient evidence to classify caffeine as a risk factor in these diseases (29). Meanwhile research of a fundamental nature is underway. Progress reports indicate that caffeine may interfere with certain basic body functions at the cellular level and that it is of critical importance that such investigations continue until these important relationships are better understood and their signficance clarified (30, 31).

caffeine
Found especially in coffee, tea and kola nuts and used medicinally as a stimulant and diuretic

REFERENCES

1. "Influence of Different Feeding Frequencies on Nutrition," *Dairy Council Digest* 38 (July-Aug., 1967), pp. 19-22.

2. *Food and Home Notes* (Washington, D.C.: USDA, Sept. 20, 1976).

3. C. Cromwell and D. Odland, "Cost of Consumer-Packaged Convenience Entrees," *Family Economics Review* (Summer 1974).

4. Myer, M. L., S. C. O'Brien, J. A. Mabel and F. J. Stare, "A Nutrition Study of School Children in a Depressed Urban District," *J. Am. Dietet. Assoc.* 53 (Sept. 1968), pp. 226-33.

5. V. Sidwell and E. Eppright, "Food Habits of Iowa Children: Breakfast," *J. Home Econ.* 45 (June 1953), pp. 401-05.

6. W. W. Tuttle, "Work Capacity With No Breakfast and a Mid-Morning Break," *J. Am. Dietet. Assoc.* 37 (Aug. 1960), pp. 137-40.

7. M. S. Read, "Malnutrition, Hunger and Behavior, II. Hunger: School Feeding Programs and Behavior," *J. Am. Dietet. Assoc.* 63 (Oct. 1973) pp. 386-91.

8. E. B. Hayden, "Breakfast and Today's Life Styles," *J. School Health* 45 (Feb. 1975), pp. 83-87.

9. "Consumption of Eggs, Pork and Beef" (USDA, Economic Research Service, *National Food Situation,* May 1974).

10. *Market Research Corporation of America. 1974,* "Fourth National Household Menu Census," (Chicago, Ill.: July 1972-June 1973).

11. I. L. Shannon, "Sucrose and Glucose in Dry Breakfast Cereals," *ASCD J. of Dentistry for Children* (Sept.-Oct. 1974), p.18.

12. R. L. Huenemann, L. R. Shapiro, M. C. Hampton and B. W. Mitchell, "Food and Eating Practices of Teen-Agers," *J. Am. Dietet. Assoc.* 53 (July 1968), pp. 17-24.

13. Public Law 94-105, National School Lunch Act and Child Nutrition Act of 1966, Amendments of 1975, 94th Congress, H. R. 4222, (Oct. 7, 1975).

14. *School Breakfast Menu Planning Guide* (Washington, D.C.: USDA, NS 7, May 1976).

15. *A Menu Planning Guide for Type A School Lunches,* (Washington, D.C.: USDA, Program Aid No. 719, May 1974).

16. J. Pearson, "Child Nutrition Programs of The Food and Nutrition Service, US Dept. of Agriculture," *Nutrition Program News* (Washington D.C.: May–June, 1973).

17. R. J. Jansen, J. M. Harper, A. L. Frey, R. L. Crews, C. T. Shigetomi and J. B. Lough, "Comparison of Type A and Nutrient Standard Menus for School Lunch III: Nutritive Content of Menus and Acceptability," *J. Am. Dietet. Assoc.* 66 (March 1975), pp. 254-61.

18. *Focus on Nutrition: You Cannot Teach a Hungry Child,* Bureau of Nutrition Education and School Food Service, Mass. Department of Education, 1970.

19. US Dept. of Health, Education and Welfare: Ten-State Nutrition Survey 1968-70. V. Dietary. DHEW Publ. No. (HSM) 72-8133 (Washington D.C.: Supt. Doc., Gov. Print. Office, 1972).

20. R. A. Cook, S. B. Davis, R. A. Hulburt, F. H. Radke and M. E. Thornbury, "Nutritional Status of Head Start and Nursery School Children," Parts I and II. *J. Am. Dietet. Assoc.* 68 (Feb. 1976), pp. 120-32.

21. W. McAllister, "Implementing a Portable Meals Program," *J. Am. Dietet. Assoc.* 66 (April 1975), pp. 375-77.

22. S. T. Greenblatt, "Home Delivered Meals—Serving People in Health Care Settings: Special Situations". *J. Am. Dietet. Assoc.* 69 (July 1976), p. 78.

23. *Food and Home Notes* (Washington, D.C.: USDA, Jan. 17, 1977).

24. P. Isom, "Nutritive Value and Cost of 'Fast Food' Meals," *Family Economics Review* (Fall 1976).

25. C. P. Greecher and B. Shannon, "Impact of Fast Food Meals on Nutrient Intake of Two Groups," *J. Am. Dietet. Assoc.* 70 (April 1977), pp. 368-72.

26. Wisconsin Alumni Research Foundation, *Nutritional Analysis of Food Served at McDonald's Restaurants* (Oakbrook, Ill.: McDonald's Plaza, 1977).

27. J. A. Hruban, "Selection of Snack Foods from Vending Machines by High School Students," *J. School Health* 47 (Jan. 1977), pp. 33-37.

28. C. B. Cook, D. A. Eiler and O. D. Forker, "Beverage Consumption Patterns in New York State," *J. Am. Dietet. Assoc.* 67 (Sept. 1975), pp. 222-27.

29. *Dietary Goals for the United States,* US Senate, Select Committee on Nutrition and Human Needs (Washington, D.C.: US Gov. Print. Office Feb. 1977).

30. "Caffeine: Commentary—a Series of Reviews of recent research on effects of consumption of caffeine," *J. Home Econ.* 69 (March 1977), pp. 2-6.

31. P. E. Stephenson, "Physiologic and Psychotropic Effects of Caffeine on Man," *J. Am. Dietet. Assoc.* 71 (Sept. 1977), pp. 240-47.

Control
of Body Weight

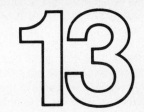

Prevention of Overweight
Behavioral Approach
   to Weight Control
Characteristics of Sound
   Weight-Control Diets
Obesity

Excess body weight is a serious nutrition problem in the United States. There are two major, related reasons for the overweight condition: too much intake from a "rich" and plentiful food supply, and too little energy expenditure in the form of physical work or exercise. The pattern of overeating often starts in childhood and continues throughout life. We live in an age of ample meals, of snacks, coffee breaks, and cocktail hours. Energy intake and output are not balanced. There is little need for physical effort at any period of life in the United States and other highly mechanized nations; 20th-century people live in an energy-sparing society. Overweight creeps up as energy needs are lessened with age due to the gradual decline in basal metabolism and decrease in physical activities. A practical problem for many individuals is that of consciously balancing energy intake and expenditure by engaging in a reasonable program of activity and diet that prevents the accumulation of excess body fat.

Although potential dangers of overweight have been well publicized, this information has not served to reverse significantly the upward trend of the problem. Some life insurance companies regard overweight persons as greater risks than persons of desirable weight and charge them higher rates accordingly. Evidence indicates that extreme overweight is associated with the onset or aggravation of certain major disease conditions, which will be discussed later in this chapter. Maintaining desirable weight results in a trim, maneuverable body that stands the best chance of functioning in maximum health and efficiency.

In considering normal energy needs and expenditures in Chapter 6, you became acquainted with desirable weight ranges for men and women of different body builds and developed your own weight chart (see Appendix I). In view of the unfavorable health picture presented for the overweight person, it is advantageous to stay within the weight range or zone indicated for one's height and body build. In terms of longevity, moderate underweight is not a health handicap but may even be desirable. For adults, patterning food habits and physical activities to maintain body weight within the desired weight zone is the preferred type of weight control.

Prevention of Overweight

It is easier to *keep* extra pounds off than to *take* them off. If your weight is within the range desirable for you but you are gaining steadily, you should look for the reasons for the increase in weight.

Recheck your calorie intake for a representative day or two. Have you inadvertently added extra foods that may be causing weight gain?

Recheck your activity schedule for a representative day (see Chap. 6) Have you dropped an activity that has lessened your energy needs?

Are you skipping meals to cut down on total calories? Studies show that this plan often works in reverse.

Have you been indulging in favorite, high-calorie foods to offset anxieties?

Do you come from a family that tends to overeat? Are your parents overweight?

Are you continuing to keep a weight chart? This provides the best proof of the effectiveness of preventive measures.

Prevention of weight gain is a realistic goal if you raise and answer questions such as these and then do something about what you learn from them. This may mean cutting out a bedtime snack, omitting dessert at lunch or dinner, or walking up a few flights of stairs daily instead of taking the elevator. Any or all of these measures are easier than trying to lose excess fat once it has accumulated.

Weight Control

Unfortunately, many people can add a few extra pounds before they realize it. Our purpose here is to consider simple modifications of a normal diet that will help a person return to the desirable weight range if this happens. It is assumed that the need for reducing calories is due merely to a mild maladjustment between intake of energy-yielding foods and energy expenditure by the body. If a real overweight problem exists, a physician should decide if weight reduction should be attempted, how much weight should be shed, and how rapidly it should be lost.

Controlling a tendency to gain weight requires dedication. One must be seriously motivated to make the initial effort—and to continue with it consistently until results are achieved. Motivations may be of many types, but all must stem from a strong conviction that desirable weight is essential to one's well-being. A compelling motive, particularly for women, is personal appearance—the unsightliness of accumulated fat. Underlying concerns may have to do with the fit of clothes, social acceptance, and qualifications for jobs. Health reasons—"doctor's orders"—serve as another effective motive. But whatever the motive, it must be sufficiently strong to carry a person through a period of adjustment to an energy level that will ensure desired weight. A weight-loss program is more apt to be successful if the person quietly determines to lose weight and goes about it without fanfare. Success in weight reduction is itself a powerful motivator. The reward of conscientious dieting is tangible evidence of weight decline, and one way to sustain interest in hewing to the diet line is by weighing yourself regularly and keeping a weight chart.

Behavioral Approach to Weight Control

Some individuals seem better able to control their weight when aided by the professional counseling of a nutritionist. Others are more successful in a structured group setting, in which a nutritionist or dietitian is the leader. The latter plan has the added advantage of serving more people in a given time. Most group plans involve behavior modifications of eating patterns, exercise and activity programs, and nutrition education (1). Some phases of the group approach have been adapted to the special needs of overweight university students. Recently, some graduate students in nutrition have been involved in conducting such programs (2, 3).

The behavioral aspects of weight control programs involve a specific regimen consisting of the following activities: recording in a weight-food diary one's daily weights, the type and amount of food eaten, the time and place of its consumption, and any stimuli preceding its ingestion; eating all food from a unique place setting in a designated area; making eating a single activity; and rewarding small units of weight loss (4). (The same procedures are adaptable to an individual self-controlled program.) Nutritionists in a group-leadership role should be trained in behavior-modification techniques, and subjects who are to practice these techniques in a weight-control program should in turn be briefed on the essential procedures. One study compared the results achieved when behavioral techniques were applied by nutritionists lacking such special training, with results observed when nutritionists as therapists were trained by, and in continual consultation with, a behavioral clinical psychologist (5). Differences in terms of weight control were not clear-cut. The first group showed small weight losses, not well-sustained. Those in the second, the behavioral stimulus control group, achieved weight losses equal to those of the first group and maintained their losses somewhat better. The investigators believe that specific behavioral guidelines are advantageous in dealing with weight loss, but that weight-reduction programs should be lengthened beyond 2 to 4 months to enable subjects to remain under treatment until their weight goals are attained (5).

Implementing a Moderate Weight-Control Diet

Table 13.1 presents a moderately low-energy diet (about 1200 calories), with suggested menus for 1 day as in Table 13.2. Nutrient goals are RDA ranges for adults. Only the calories have been reduced. The diet is based on the food guide (see Chap. 10) and for the most part meets desirable daily dietary goals for adults, with the exception of calories. The menu for this diet is almost identical to Tables 10.3 and 13.2. The meat, eggs, and vegetables are essentially the same in kind and amount, with differences chiefly in form and quantity of other foods. It should be emphasized that Table 13.2 is not a prescribed diet, but is merely one example of the many ways the daily food guide can be interpreted in meeting acceptable nutrient standards.

All sound low-calorie diet plans designed to bring about safe weight reduction have certain characteristics in common. Table 13.1, is examined below in light of these generally accepted qualifications.

Characteristics of Sound Weight-Control Diets

1. *Calorie yield must be low enough to cause weight loss.* When foods supply less energy than the body needs, the body uses its own stored fats as fuel. This is the principle upon which reducing diets are based. It is only by holding to a diet with a moderate calorie deficit until excess body fat is used up that a weight-control regime can be successful. Of all the characteristics of a weight-control diet to be discussed here, the low-calorie feature is the most exacting.

The amount of weight to be lost depends on how much one varies from desirable weight. Let us assume that, originally, your weight was within normal range for your height and body build (see Table 2.1) on a little over 2100 calories a day (Table 10.2). Later you began to gain weight, and now you are several pounds above the upper limit of your desirable range. This may not represent a serious excess at present, but if the upward trend continues,

Table 13.1
A low calorie diet developed from Table 10.2

About 1000 calories are cut from the diet in Table 10.2 to achieve a moderate daily weight reduction diet of about 1200 calories.

Foods	Measure	Kilo-calories	Protein g	Fat g	Calcium mg	Iron mg	Vita-min A IU	Thiamin mg	Ribo-flavin mg	Niacin mg	Ascorbic acid mg
Foundation foods											
milk group											
milk, skim	2 cups	176	18	tr	592	0.2	20*	0.18	0.88	0.4	4
meat group											
pot roast	2½ oz	246	17	19	8	2.2	33	0.04	0.13	3.1	—
ham, boiled	2 oz	132	10	10	6	1.6	0	0.24	0.08	1.4	—
egg	1 medium	72	6	5	24	1.0	520	0.05	0.13	tr	0
vegetable-fruit group											
peas	¼ cup	28	2	tr	8	0.8	240	0.11	0.04	0.7	6
carrots	¼ cup	12	1	tr	12	0.3	3808	0.02	0.02	0.2	3
lettuce	2 leaves	10	1	tr	37	0.8	1050	0.03	0.04	0.2	10
lettuce	¼ head	18	1	tr	27	0.7	450	0.08	0.08	0.4	8
celery	1 stalk	3	tr	tr	7	0.1	47	0.01	0.01	0.1	2
grapefruit	½ medium	46	1	tr	19	0.5	10	0.05	0.02	0.2	44
apple, raw	1 medium	80	tr	1	10	0.4	120	0.04	0.03	0.1	6
grain group											
bread, enriched	2 slices	152	4	2	48	1.4	tr	0.14	0.12	1.4	tr
roll, enriched	1 plain	84	2	2	20	0.5	tr	0.07	0.06	0.6	tr
Totals, foundation foods		1059	63	39	818	10.5	6298	1.06	1.64	8.8	83
Nutrient goals											
RDA ranges for adults		(1200)	44–56		800–1200	10–18	4000–5000	1.00–1.50	1.10–1.80	12–20	45–60
Additional Foods											
butter or margarine	2 tsp	68	tr	8	2	0	313	—	—	—	0
mayonnaise, low cal.	1 tsp	8	tr	1	1	tr	13	tr	tr	tr	—
french dressing, low calorie	1 tbsp	15	tr	1	2	0.1	—	—	—	—	—
Totals, additional foods		91		10	5	0.1	326				
Grand Totals		1150	63	49	823	10.6	6624	1.06	1.64	8.8	83

*It is mandatory in the United States that fluid skim milk be fortified with not less than 2000 IU of vitamin A per quart.

Table 13.2
Menus based on diet in Table 13.1

Foundation foods 92 percent of total calories		Calories	Additional foods		Calories
Breakfast					
grapefruit	½ medium	46			
egg, poached*	1 medium	72			
toast, enriched	1 slice	76	+ **butter or margarine**	½ tsp	17
milk, skim	1 cup	88	**coffee or tea,** if desired		
Lunch					
ham sandwich (open face)					
bread, enriched	1 slice	76			
ham, boiled	2 oz	132	+ **mayonnaise**	1 tsp	8
lettuce	2 leaves	10	(low-calorie)		
celery **	1 stalk	3			
apple, raw**	1 medium	80	**coffee or tea,** if desired		
Dinner					
pot roast	2½ oz	246			
peas and carrots	½ cup	40	+ **butter or margarine**	1 tsp	34
head lettuce salad	¼ head	18	+ **french dressing** low cal.	1 tbsp	15
roll	1 roll	84	+ **butter or margarine**	½ tsp	17
			coffee or tea, if desired		
Between meals					
milk, skim	1 cup	88			
	total	1059†		total	91†
Grand Total, calories for the day—**1150**					

*Equivalent calories in lean meat, cheese or vegetable protein sources may be alternated.

**Some or all of these foods may be taken between meals if the person dieting is better satisfied when he eats more often.

†It should be understood that such specificity in recording energy values is not practical in the application of diets, either as pertains to dietary standards or to the energy yield of foods. Exact numbers are used here and elsewhere in the text merely to be able to maintain checkable data.

it can lead to an amount that will be increasingly difficult to lose.

A modest goal for weight reduction is advised, and a reasonable objective is 1½ to 2 pounds a week. One pound of body fat has the value of approximately 3500 calories. However weight loss is not attributable to fat loss alone. Variable amounts of protein and water are lost as well as the fat. It is because the precise composition of tissue losses is unknown that calculations here are confined to fat losses. A daily deficit of 500 calories would theoretically result in a 3500-calorie deficit in one week (500 calories × 7 days). If a 2-pound weekly loss is the goal, the daily diet should be curtailed

Table 13.3
Changes made in a regular diet (Table 10.2) **to reduce energy value to about 1200 calories** (Table 13.1), using essentially the same foods and without sacrificing nutrient content unduly

Changes made	Calories "saved"
skim milk substituted for whole milk, 2 cups	142
pot roast reduced in amount from 3 oz to 2½ oz	49
raw apple substituted for sweetened baked apple	40
banana omitted as a snack	101
bread cut from 4 to 2 slices	152
rolls cut from 2 to 1 roll	84
dinner dessert omitted	127
butter or margarine cut from 5 to 2 tsp	102
French dressing, changed from regular to low-calorie, 1 tbsp	51
mayonnaise cut from 1 tbsp to 1 tsp; low-calorie substituted for regular	93
sugar omitted from beverages and fruit, 3 tsp	46
Total calories "saved"	**987**

Figure 13.1
How calories were reduced
(see Table 13.3)

By omitting foods (tray on left):
  banana
  dinner dessert
  sugar from dessert and fruit

By reducing quantity of foods
(center tray):
  pot roast   ½ oz.
  bread   2 slices
  rolls   1 roll
  margarine   3 tsp.

By modifying content of foods
(tray on right):
  whole to skim milk
  baked to raw apple
  french dressing to low calorie
  mayonnaise to low calorie and
      amount reduced
(Landon Gardiner)

by about 1000 calories for a weekly deficit of approximately 7000 calories. That would mean cutting the 2100 calorie diet to about 1200 calories daily. Such a diet is one on which a person can live comfortably, and it can assure nutritional adequacy. How one can make a reduction of that magnitude in the day's food intake, and yet continue to eat from the same menu, is shown in Table 13.3. This table lists the changes made in Table 10.2 to modify its calorie yield to that of Table 13.1—a difference of 987 calories daily (Fig. 13.1).

If it is adhered to faithfully, the diet in Table 13.1 should result in a loss of approximately 1½ to 2 pounds in body weight per week. The amount will vary from week to week and may tend to lessen as the desired weight level is approached. Variation in water retention is often a factor in irregular weekly weight loss, particularly at first—even on a consistently low-energy intake. The calorie-deficit plan can be applied to the regular diet at any energy level. However, this should be done judiciously, for there is a calorie limit below which it is impossible to maintain dietary adequacy. Only with nutritional knowledge, skillfully applied, can an adult meet nutrient needs on a diet of less than 1000 calories daily.

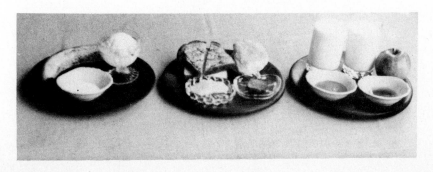

Crash reducing diets, which promise dramatic weight losses, are to be avoided. Fasting regimes have no place in moderate weight-reduction plans. If it is done at all, fasting should be closely supervised by a physician who is directing the reduction program. On a total fast, the body loses not only fat, but also some of its lean muscle tissue.

Note that noncaloric sweeteners are not listed on Table 13.3 as a means of "saving" calories. They were omitted partly because of the uncertainty of the fate of saccharin, but also to demonstrate that they are not necessary components of diets designed for weight loss. Noncaloric sweeteners have been used in increasing quantities in the United States in recent years, with the annual average per capita consumption in 1975 equivalent in sweetness to 7 pounds of sugar (6). The search continues for noncaloric sweeteners safe for use in the quantities consumed in food items such as soft drinks. The United States Department of Agriculture has developed and tested a product derived from grapefruit peels which is several hundred times sweeter than table sugar. Its sweetness is pleasant and long-lasting. Other sweeteners with negligible calorie yield are also being tested for safety, stability, and acceptability.

Make a list of foods from Appendix K that would qualify as low-calorie desserts. Group them by approximate calorie values to suggest the types most suitable for weight-control diets.

Select the apple desserts from Appendix K. Arrange them in order of their calorie value per serving, from fresh raw apple to apple pie. Indicate how the calorie value of each has been increased above that of the fresh apple. How could the calorie value of each be increased still more? Consider the relative usefulness of these apple dishes in weight-control diets.

---

2. *The diet should be built around familiar and appetizing foods.* The more nearly meals resemble those a person is accustomed to and likes, the longer he or she will be willing to continue a weight-control diet. Unless the dieter is willing to continue, the effort may not last long enough to measure its success in terms of weight loss. Keeping the new diet similar to the old one does not mean that no changes need be made. The degree of change that will be necessary depends on the quality of the food habits prior to the weight-control regime.

Table 13.1 has been developed from Table 10.2 to show how a person already eating a good diet can reduce calorie intake and yet continue to eat customary foods at home or in a restaurant. Actually, the changes are almost imperceptible to the casual observer.

For the person with poor food habits who wants to start a weight-control diet, there may be many changes. If, for example, a person is accustomed to consuming sweetened beverages and high-calorie desserts, in meals low in foundation foods, the appetite must be retrained. It has long been thought that overweight individuals prefer these types of foods. The theory was tested in a study to determine whether obese persons have the same eating patterns as people of normal weight. In a cafeteria situation, food choices were monitored unknown to the patrons. The patrons were categorized by visual appraisal according to sex, body build, height, and age. Servings of food were estimated visually and classified either as protective, with good contributions of nutrients in proportion to calories, or as high-calorie, low-nutrient choices. There was a definite tendency for the obese persons to choose more foods and more servings of food from the high-calorie, low-nutrient group (7). Even recognizing this tendency, effort should be made to retain the best features of the original diet and to preserve a nucleus of favorite dishes. Food is comforting; familiar foods are like old friends. As far as possible, eating a reducing diet should be a pleasure, not a chore. More than usual care should be taken to make the food attractive and tasty.

The practice of retaining familiar foods in weight-control diets has general application, but for ethnic groups with strong emotional ties to homeland foods, the need is heightened. There are some important implications for weight-control programs with such groups in a study of adult city residents. The findings indicate not only that the condition of overweight existed in ethnic groups, but that it was six times more common among women of low socioeconomic status; and the shorter the time a woman's family had been in the United States, the more likely she was to have an overweight problem (8).

The countless fad reducing diets that consist of two or three foods are not recommended. Limited combinations, such as tangerines and clams or lamb chops and grapefruit, soon pall. Diets restricting food intake to just one kind of food in a day, changing to another the following day, are also unsatisfactory. The considerable quantity of each food that must be eaten daily makes these diets unpalatable, and the reducing regime usually ends soon. The individual foods in such restricted diets may be appetizing in themselves and contribute their nutrient share to a varied diet, but, whether used alone or with one or two other foods, they are not nutritionally adequate or satisfying. Variety, rather than sameness, is just as desirable in low-calorie diets as in regular diets. The very monotony of extreme, unnatural diets is responsible in part for their short duration. When they are abandoned, the inclination is to return to the same food patterns followed earlier on which weight gains were made.

The diet plan with the greatest potential for ultimate success is the one based on well-accepted foods on which the dieter can live contentedly and efficiently until the desired weight loss has been realized. This type of plan may well form a new pattern of eating to be followed throughout life.

Moderately curtailed but nutritionally adequate meals, eaten day after day at the family table or elsewhere in a pleasant atmosphere, probably constitute the most effective approach to permanent weight loss.

> Calculate one of the fad reducing diets composed of two or three foods. If possible, display several such diets, using actual foods or food models.
>
> Evaluate the diets presented on such bases as nutritional adequacy, palatability, and probable length of time an individual could remain on the diet happily.

3. *Meals should be satisfying.* Successful reducing diets must be satisfying: they must allay hunger. If they do not, the dieter is constantly unhappy and periodically "breaks over." Diet breaks may be so costly in terms of added calories that the effects of the diet itself are nullified.

Testing reducing diets on adult subjects has revealed some ways of making low-calorie diets satisfying. One is to divide the food fairly evenly among the three or more meals of the day. This means a substantial breakfast, which is something chronic dieters seldom enjoy. Many omit breakfast routinely. Protein foods at breakfast help to sustain satisfactory levels of blood sugar following the morning meal. In children, post-breakfast blood glucose levels proved to be higher after a protein-rich meal than after a carbohydrate-rich meal (9).

Proteins, with their relatively slow rates of digestion, absorption, and metabolism, apparently contribute to a steadier supply of glucose to the blood than do carbohydrates. Low blood sugar is associated with hunger, fatigue, weakness, and inability to concentrate. A good breakfast is important irrespective of the total calorie level of meals for the day, but it has special significance in sustaining vigor and efficiency during a reducing regime when total daily calorie intake is below energy expenditure. A comparison of the breakfasts in Table 10.3 and Table 13.2 show that they follow the same menu pattern. Each provides a liberal amount of animal protein in the form of milk and eggs, and each would be considered a substantial meal.

Diets moderately liberal in fat and protein have also been found to be more satisfying to reducers than ones low in these two nutrients. However, there is no evidence that a diet that varies greatly from the normal, well-balanced diet in proportions of calories supplied by protein, fat, and carbohydrate offers any advantage in achieving weight loss.

There are many ways to ensure dieters of maximum satisfaction from their meals and at the same time to avoid overconsumption. These include prolonging the meal period, always eating meals at the table, confining the meal period to eating (not watching TV or reading, which divert attention from food), eating small portions, eating slowly, and enjoying each morsel. It has been assumed that obese people eat rapidly, swallow their food without savoring it, and as a result tend to eat more than those of normal weight. A comparative study has explored these possibilities. A dietitian observed 14 obese and 16 nonobese subjects eat four meals on consecutive days. The obese persons spent significantly less time eating their meals and chewing each mouthful of food than did the nonobese subjects. There was no significant difference between the two groups in the number of mouthfuls per meal (10).

Some dieters are better satisfied with their reducing regime if a portion of their food is reserved for between meals or at bedtime when they crave something to eat. This arrangement has been suggested in Table 13.2. Snacks may be substantial foods, such as a portion of the day's milk or fruit, or they may be foods (such as celery) that furnish almost no calories but provide satisfaction in chewing and swallowing, plus a temporary relief from hunger. At all times the wisdom of moderate servings should be remembered. Regardless of how few calories a serving of any food may yield, a smaller serving of that same food will always yield less (11).

The current trend for restaurants to offer smaller than usual portions, at somewhat reduced prices, should serve not only as a means of cutting energy intakes for the obese, but also as a preventive measure for those avoiding weight gains.

Suggest ways of increasing the fat level on Table 13.1 moderately without altering total calories or lessening other nutrient values significantly. Repeat for protein level.

---

4. *The diet should be nutritionally adequate*. A nutritionally adequate diet with lowered calorie yield can mean improved health and a greater sense of well-being for the overweight person. On the other hand, weight-control diets that are too low in calories and inadequate in nutrient content are a hazard to health. Individuals who remain on them for prolonged periods of time lose strength and vitality, and some become ill. The diet in Table 13.1 falls within the RDA ranges for adults, except for a planned calorie deficit and for niacin. While niacin intake itself fails to meet the dietary goal, additional niacin from the conversion of tryptophan assures an adequate intake (see Chap. 9).

About 90 percent of the calories in Table 13.1 are provided by foundation foods. In Table 10.2, which yields about 1000 more total calories, 80 percent of the calories come from foundation foods. This difference demonstrates the point made in Chapter 10: the lower the total calorie level of the diet, the larger the proportion of calories that must be provided by foundation foods if the diet is to be nutritionally adequate.

This fact and many others related to weight control were brought to light by a longitudinal study of food intake and weight of women over a 37-year period, starting in their college days. In 1973, the investigators had consecutive records at four intervals on 87 of the women. On admission to college, 77 of the number were within normal limits of desirable weight, 6 were questionably obese, and 4 were moderately obese. By 1973, 23 of the 87 were obese by any standard, and another 23 were in the upper range of normal. Except for iron and magnesium, mean intakes of nutrients equaled or exceeded the RDA. In general, the diets followed the basic four pattern for *kinds* of food. Thus the meal patterns reflected the qualitative aspects of nutrition basics, but the quantitative aspects were followed less carefully. The women whose weights remained within normal limits and those who had lost weight had made simple adjustments in their customary food intake when necessary to avoid weight gains. In general they used less fat and sugar; they ate a half-slice less bread than did the obese women and used about 50 percent more whole-grain products. Their meals were regular and structured. About an ounce less meat was used per day, but more milk and cheese were included to bring the total intake of milk solids to the equivalent of a daily pint of milk. This change in menu pattern, and the addition of orange and green vegetables, resulted in a well-balanced nutrient mixture for the successful dieters (12).

Empty calories must be kept to a minimum in a satisfactory reducing diet. The nutrient differences in food combinations and in individual foods and beverages, as indicated in tables and figures in Chapter 12, demonstrate how similar amounts of foods—often with essentially the same energy yield—can vary greatly in nutrient content. Servings of a cola beverage and of orange juice offer a good example (see Fig. 12.11). The cola provides 145 calories in 12 ounces—all energy derived from added sweeteners—and no other nutrients. The orange juice, on the other hand, furnishes 122 calories in 8 ounces with the energy derived from protein as well as the carbohydrate of the orange. In addition, orange juice supplies significant amounts of several vitamins and twice as much ascorbic acid as called for by the US RDA. It is apparent that in choosing foods for a weight-control diet one must know not only their calorie values but also their nutrient values. In a study of a group of women trying to lose weight, the successful ones not only managed to keep their calories low but maintained high nutrient quality in their diets as well (13).

The additional foods in Table 13.1 are confined to those that enhance the palatability of the foundation foods, largely fats. Concentrated sweets, such as jellies, jams, candies, rich desserts, and sweet sauces, are omitted. When the desired weight loss has been accomplished, such items can be added cautiously in small amounts to determine what quantities, if any, can be added without gain in weight.

Protein, useful in the ways already mentioned, is also needed to prevent losses of nitrogen from the body. When total energy intake is low and proteins must be used for energy, nitrogen is sacrificed in the process, and the frequent result is a negative nitrogen balance. Amounts of protein sufficient in a normal diet should therefore not be lowered when total calories are reduced, if nitrogen requirements are to be met.

How would you change the diet in Table 13.1 to meet your own food preferences more nearly without lessening its nutritive value or changing radically the proportion of calories provided by foundation foods?

Develop a series of suggestions for reducing weight for the person who eats away from home: a) in a dormitory or other

> institution where there are planned meals; b) when there is free choice of foods, as in a restaurant; c) in the case of a recent migrant from Puerto Rico or Mexico (see Chap. 1 and Appendixes B and C).

Exercise

Modern scientific weight-control programs are based on a judicious balance of proper diet and exercise—*subtracting* food energy and *adding* exercise. The more energy expended in physical activity the less the energy intake need be restricted. Both procedures contribute to weight loss. One study has sought to identify and measure the specific benefits derived from each (14). Three groups of obese college women volunteered to try, for an experimental period of 6 weeks, to reduce their weight by three different prescribed methods: one group with a 1200-calorie diet plus a planned exercise program; a second group with the diet alone; a third with the exercise alone. A fourth group served as the control. As would be expected, the first group—diet plus exercise—achieved the largest average weight loss; the diet-only group had a slightly smaller weight loss; and the exercise-only group had a much smaller weight loss. On tests of serum cholesterol levels, the diet-exercise group showed the greatest average reduction, the diet-only group showed the next greatest reduction, and the exercise-only group showed no clear-cut change. Reduction in serum triglyceride followed a similar pattern. The investigators concluded that "a combination of regular dynamic exercise and caloric restriction work together for greater weight loss, a greater feeling of physical well-being, better control of water retention, a more positive mental attitude, and a more pronounced reduction of serum triglyceride and cholesterol levels" (14).

Other studies have reported that exercise may increase basal metabolic rate and is instrumental in lowering blood pressure. An investigation of the effect of physical activity on weight reduction in obese middle-aged women has demonstrated that several benefits may result (15). A number of measurements were made on the previously sedentary subjects, aged 30 to 52, at the initiation and at the end of the exercise program. A standard electrocardiogram test revealed no abnormalities that would be considered a contraindication either to exercise testing or to participation in a regular program of physical activity. Twice a week for 17 weeks the women participated in a flexibility training session, followed by 19 minutes of intermittent jogging and brisk walking. On 2 other days of the same weeks the subjects had 1-hour body mechanics classes, during which they engaged in calisthenics, stretching, and joint flexibility exercises. Many subjects reported that they walked, swam, played tennis and bicycled in addition to the regimes associated with the program. These additional activities, of course, increased their energy expenditure. No specific dietary procedure was prescribed. Once a week the group had a 1-hour session with a college counselor for the purpose of increasing awareness of possible causes of overeating and to promote self-initiated change. In general, changes in diet were moderate.

Body composition showed significant change over the test period. There were highly significant reductions in mean total body weight, fat body weight, and percentage fat. There were no significant differences in mean values of serum cholesterol nor other serum lipid fractions.

Results from this study, as well as from others, suggest that there is a greater proportion of fat lost for a given total body-weight loss when the energy deficit is achieved by increased exercise, in addition to dietary energy restriction, than by dietary restriction alone. The program described above also provided the women with increased self-confidence, a sense of accomplishment, and—with their increased physical work capacity—the ability to participate in and enjoy various forms of regular physical activity they had previously avoided. Many of the women seemed to have modified their behavior as a result of this program. The energetic and enthusiastic group leader was credited with bringing about much of the success by motivating the participants and encouraging them (15).

To treat physical activity as an important factor in preventing or dealing with obesity requires some knowledge of the relative energy costs of common activities. Such information has been assembled, accompanied by the energy equivalents of food calories expressed in minutes of time spent in walking, bicycle riding, swimming, running, and reclining (16) (Fig. 13.2). The energy costs of the various activities used in developing the physical-energy equivalents of food energy were based on the data in Table 13.4.

Figure 13.2
Maintaining desirable body weight is one of the benefits of regular exercise.

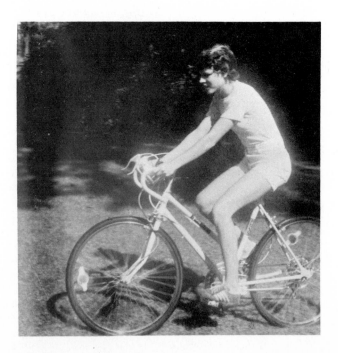

Table 13.4
Energy costs of some activities (16)

Activity	Energy cost calories per minute
walking	5.2
bicycle riding	8.2
swimming	11.2
running	19.4
reclining	1.3

> Using the energy costs of the various activities in Table 13.4 and calorie values of foods in Appendix K, calculate the energy equivalents in food calories of several common foods, expressed in minutes of activity.
>
> How much longer does it take to "walk off" a piece of apple pie than it does a fresh apple? What advantage is there in running over walking?
>
> Draw up several practical suggestions for balancing energy intake and expenditure that you think would work for you in controlling body weight.

Maintenance Diets

Loss of excess body weight is just one aspect of weight control. *Maintenance* of desirable weight, once achieved, also requires diligent attention. Adherence to diet and exercise patterns that resulted in the weight loss will serve to prevent regaining the unwanted weight. Usually the supply of calories can be somewhat more liberal than the weight-control diet afforded, but still it must be less than was supplied by the diet that permitted the weight gain. Added foods should still be in the moderate calorie range, if appetite training is to result in food habits that assure continued desirable weight.

This is the time to remember that weight gains result not only from eating large quantities of extra food. Lost pounds can also return with the steady, day-to-day consumption of very small amounts of food above one's energy need. This fact has been dramatized by a compilation of weight-gain equivalents, giving the time required to gain a specified amount of weight with a given amount of food (17). To discourage overeating, the report presents data on weight-gain equivalents of selected foods. A table illustrates the body weight gains to expect when eating a single portion of a food above daily maintenance requirements for varying periods of time. For example, eating one brownie daily—if in excess of energy need—could result in a body weight gain of 1 pound in 20 days. A toasted cheese sandwich, eaten under the same conditions, could achieve the same gain in half the time; a medium orange would take twice as long. The authors of the study emphasize that the weight-gain equivalent values are average, predicted figures and are not intended as precise values. However, the information does illustrate how weight can be gained or regained—almost imperceptibly—with very minor additions of single foods.

Building-Up Regimes

The preceding discussion of weight control has been devoted largely to the problem of unwanted weight gains, because overweight—not underweight—is a health problem in the United States. Yet there are many underweight people, and they need to know how to plan a diet in which energy intake *exceeds* energy expenditure. Only by living on such a diet, at least temporarily, can an underweight person store enough body fat to arrive at the desirable weight range. Obviously, nutrient intakes should remain high enough to meet or approach recommended levels. Energy intake must be increased. A person who wishes to gain about 2 pounds a week should add approximately 1000 calories daily until the weight goal is achieved. Thus we have the reverse of the reducing diet.

Modifying a 2000-calorie diet *upward* instead of *downward* means adding, rather than subtracting, sources of food energy. How can this be done without throwing the diet out of balance? Eating larger servings of foundation foods and more spreads, sauces, and dressings; using whole milk instead of skim milk; adding simple desserts—these are good ways to start. A person who has difficulty gaining weight often has appetite and capacity problems as well. In that case, small and frequent meals may help to accomplish the purpose of the build-up diet. An adequate diet and good food habits are still the long-term objectives.

> How would you add 1000 calories to Table 10.2 to achieve a total of 3000 calories? Re-plan the day's meals and snacks in Table 10.3 to make a practical plan for gaining weight.
>
> What proportion of the calories in your build-up diet is provided by foundation foods?

OBESITY

Up to this point in the chapter, the subject of body weight has been considered chiefly as a mild tendency to overweight, and simple measures to deal with it have been suggested. Obesity, as explained in Chapter 2, is a complex problem of body fat, often called the most prevalent form of malnutrition in the United States.

The very definition of obesity presents numerous difficulties, including selection of techniques and instruments, as well as criteria for the evaluation of the condition. There are as yet no universally accepted standards for obesity. Attempts to estimate prevalence of obesity in any society are also fraught with problems relating to the selection of people to be examined, and whether they are representative of larger populations. Thus, widely varying figures are seen, based on body weight, estimated degrees of fatness, and mathematical expressions derived from body measurements (18).

A person is generally considered to be obese who weighs more than 20 percent above the desirable weight for his or her height and age. It has been estimated that one-fifth of all people over 30 years of age in the United States are seriously overweight, but body weight alone is not the criterion of obesity. The existence of obesity is established by actual measurement of the amount of body fat. A person may be overweight without being obese. In other words, excess weight may be due to large bone size or unusual muscle development, rather than to excess fat. Methods of determining the amount of body fat have been considered in Chapter 2.

Causes of Obesity

Basically, obesity occurs as a result of imbalance in energy supply and expenditure, but this is an overly simplified statement of the case. The condition has many facets and many underlying origins, some of them only indirectly related to diet. Contributing factors to obesity include heredity, inactivity, environment, and metabolic and psychological problems.

Hereditary Influences.   Obesity in parents may suggest a genetic basis for stocky body build in sons and daughters. It has been projected that obesity is probably genetically transmitted. Studies using laboratory animals have demonstrated that the obese trait is transmitted in a systematic, genetic way. In humans, however, the identification of such a pattern is enormously difficult and thus far has not been clearly evident. In exploring the nature/nurture question, identical twins—ordinarily found to have very similar body weights—have been studied. Identical twins reared apart showed somewhat larger weight variations than those reared together, but still were more similar in weight than fraternal twins or siblings. Thus, correlation of parent-child weights is believed to be due partially to genetic factors, but it seems to be dominated by environmental influences such as family eating patterns (19).

Physical Inactivity   Inactivity, due to a sedentary mode of life and lack of regular, vigorous exercise, results in an energy imbalance when energy expenditure is less than energy intake from food. Increase in physical activity can act to reverse the process. Exercise, by increasing the basal energy rate, can raise energy expenditure even beyond that required for the specific activity undertaken (20).

It seems likely that obese individuals might have a disinclination to engage in physical activity because of the effort involved in moving their larger bodies. The more sedentary they become as a result of obesity, the more weight they are likely to gain—a vicious circle.

Environmental Factors   Social factors are major determinants of obesity in modern urban society. This conclusion has been reached through research on the influence of environment on the control of eating (21). A marked inverse relationship between the prevalence of obesity and socioeconomic status was found in a study of adult subjects in New York City. Obesity was present in 2 percent of the highest economic class studied and in 37 percent of the lowest economic class. Ethnic background was another social variable with striking influence upon the prevalence of obesity. There were considerable differences among nine ethnic groups, but in all groups the largest proportion of obese people was in the lowest economic group. All social variables tested were related to the prevalence of obesity. These included social mobility, number of generations in the United States, and religious affiliation (21).

Metabolic Abnormalities   In cases of metabolic obesity, there are abnormalities in the metabolism of fats and carbohydrates (22). Clinicians have recently uncovered several different metabolic defects in obese persons. A major fault lies in the metabolism of fat. Persons who do not break down fatty acids as well as others are more likely to become obese, for they produce triglycerides more rapidly than they can use them up. Experimental animals with metabolic obesity produce more fat than normal animals do even though they may not overeat, or indeed even when they are fasting.

Psychological Problems   Psychological disturbances undoubtedly contribute to the overeating that causes some people to become obese. There is ample evidence, however, that psychological factors are not involved in the etiology of all cases of obesity, also that being obese may itself lead to psychological problems. Disturbances may arise from frustrating efforts at weight reduction. Social pressures on obese persons, notably adolescent girls, may increase such psychological symptoms as undue obsession with their physical image. Obesity is an aesthetic problem—and thus can be a psychological one—for those who live in a society that disapproves of fatness in people (22).

In some cases of obesity, contributing factors appear to act separately; in other cases two or more factors interact. Sometimes they serve as causes of obesity, but at other times they may be the effects of obesity and tend to perpetuate the condition as well.

One can be obese at any stage in the life cycle, from infancy to old age. Childhood and adolescent obesity generally continues into adulthood, although it is the nature of the problem, rather than the length of time it has existed, that determines its persistence. Adults who have been obese from childhood appear to have more difficulty losing fat, and maintaining fat losses, than do those who become obese as adults.

Obesity in Early Childhood

Increasing attention is being directed to obesity in infancy and early childhood for two reasons: the observed tendency for childhood obesity to continue into later life, and the concern that childhood obesity may increase the likelihood of chronic disease development later in life. A study has shown that the mean time for an entire group of normal infants to double their birth weight was 119 days, or 3.8 months, rather than the generally accepted 5- to 6-month period. The mean time for bottle-fed babies to double their weight was 113 days, as opposed to 124 days for breast-fed infants in the study group. The authors of the study suggested that closer supervision of infant feeding practices was indicated, in the interest of preventing obesity in early life (23).

A clear understanding among parents of normal growth patterns in childhood, and of children's decreased needs for energy beginning in the second year of life, might also help to reduce the prevalence of childhood obesity. Identification of obesity-prone children is a primary step (24). Such children are sought in families with histories of obesity, among children of stocky build and those who shun physical activity and association with others, and among children with medical problems that may be aggravated by obesity. Tendencies to obesity can be detected by noting unusual weight gains, measuring excess body fat, and observing habits of overeating. In dealing with an obesity-prone child, a careful balance between the energy value of the diet and the child's physical activity should be maintained. Nutritional needs for growth must be fully met.

Obesity in Preadolescence and Adolescence

Medical examinations required by schools often help to identify obesity, or incipient obesity in students. Schools can also assist in dealing with these conditions through such avenues as consultation services, weight-control clinics, provision of nutritious low-calorie lunches, and classes for grooming, which often involve exercise programs. Improved appearance is frequently a compelling motive in eliminating tendencies to obesity.

Personal responsibility is an important element in the adolescent's move to prevent or treat obesity. The adolescent who has a good relationship with a physician may learn to see the problem of overweight in perspective, even if weight losses are not spectacular. Or, if a counselor has helped an adolescent to move toward his or her emotional, physical, and social goals, the boy or girl has laid the groundwork for success in dealing with such problems as weight control. The student must learn what nutrition means personally in terms of better living—not just as a way of losing weight —and must see the wisdom of cultivating interests that divert one's thoughts from food and eating. Motivated students will consciously acquire the habit of regular physical activity (25).

Adolescents can learn to live within the framework of a diet that provides the needed nutrients for growth but does not permit them to become or to remain obese. In general, the principles outlined earlier in the chapter for dietary control of weight apply here. At all times weight-loss goals should be moderate, and health and strength should be maintained. Present habits of living must be recognized and taken into account (26). In persistent cases of obesity, the adolescent should have the interest, sympathetic under-standing, and support of parents and professional counselors. Keep in mind that obesity is a complex medical and social problem that requires knowledge, skill, and perseverence in its solution. Re-member also that changing the food habits of another person under any conditions is something to be approached with caution. If emo-tional problems are a factor in obesity, they should be considered before dietary adjustments are attempted.

Obesity in Adult Life

The adult population of the United States is preoccupied with body weight, particularly with *over*weight. This is not surprising in a society where leanness is considered the ultimate in physical at-tainment. Justification for this preoccupation lies in the fact that "... statistical data available indicate a substantial prevalence of obesity at every age in both sexes, no matter how obesity might be defined" (22).

Obese adults should be considered in two groups: those who be-come obese in adult life, and those who have been obese since childhood. The first situation is simpler to deal with. Weight gains in adult life usually begin when the normal physical activity of youth subsides, while appetite and food-consumption patterns con-tinue. Weight spurts are also associated with specific situations such as pregnancy or breaking the habit of smoking. Whatever the cause, recognition of the tendency to gain weight, in its incipient stage, offers the best prospect for dealing with it successfully. Cor-rective measures largely consist of suitable exercise and a mildly restrictive diet, a combination that should gradually bring energy input and outgo into balance.

For adults who have been obese for many years, professional guidance is usually indicated. The predisposing factors to estab-lished obesity have already been discussed. Exercise of the type and degree recommended by the consultant and suitable dietary limitations are still basic tools with which to deal with obesity, even of the long-standing type (20). Gradual weight reduction is the preferred procedure.

Obesity-Health Relationships

There seems little doubt of an association between obesity and cer-tain disease conditions. Obesity appears to create an extra hazard for people who are otherwise healthy. For example, there seems to be a greater risk of hypertension and coronary heart disease for those who are obese. Established diseases, such as diabetes, re-spond favorably to weight reduction. While a causal relationship has not been established in such cases, there is an association that suggests the wisdom of controlling body weight. Other health-obe-sity relationships are generally accepted. For example, obesity is regarded as a hazard in pregnancy and as a risk in surgical cases. Gross overweight is believed to place a burden on the circulatory system, and it imposes painful pressures on arthritic joints (22).

Important elements in the program of prevention or treatment of obesity include the following:

an attractive, nutritious, moderately low-calorie diet, designed to establish good food habits;

a program of activity, suitable in kind and amount, that helps to balance energy intake and give muscle tone and a sense of physical fitness;

development of hobbies or other pursuits that will generate absorbing interests;

realistic, attainable goals for weight loss without imposing hardship; and

understanding guidance of medical and other personnel, which provides professional service and psychological support.

REFERENCES

1. A. Blake, "Group Approach to Weight Control: Behavior Modification, Nutrition, Health Education," *J. Am. Dietet. Assoc.* 69 (Dec. 1976), pp. 645-49.

2. K. O. Musgrave and M. E. Thornbury, "Weight Control Program for University Students Conducted by Nutrition Seniors," *J. Am. Dietet. Assoc.* 68 (May 1976), pp. 462-66.

3. C. L. Sloan, D. L. Tobias, C. A. Stapell, M. T. Ho and W. S. Beagle, "A Weight Control Program for Students Using Diet and Behavior Therapy," *J. Am. Dietet. Assoc.* 68 (May 1976), pp. 466-68.

4. D. R. Brightwell and C. L. Sloan, "Graduate Students and Faculty Learn Behavior Therapy of Obesity," *J. Nutrition Education* 8 (Apr.-June 1976), pp. 71-72.

5. B. K. Paulsen, R. N. Lutz, W. T. McReynolds and M. B. Kohrs, "Behavior Therapy for Weight Control: Long-Term Results of Two Programs with Nutritionists as Therapists," *Am. J. Clin. Nutr.* 29 (Aug. 1976), pp. 880-88.

6. *Sugar and Sweetener Situation,* Economic Research Service, SSS-2 (Washington D.C.: USDA, Nov. 1975).

7. J. C. Gates, R. L. Huenemann and R. J. Brand, "Food Choices of Obese and Non-Obese Persons," *J. Am. Dietet. Assoc.* 67 (Oct. 1975), pp. 339-343.

8. P. B. Goldblatt, M. E. Moore and A. J. Stunkard, "Social Factors in Obesity," *J. Am. Med. Assoc.* 192 (June 21, 1965), pp. 1039-44.

9. I. Arvedson, G. Sterky and K. Tjernström, "Breakfast Habits of Swedish School Children," *J. Am. Dietet. Assoc.* 55 (Sept. 1969), pp. 257-61.

10. M. Wagner and M. I. Hewitt, "Oral Satiety in the Obese and Nonobese," *J. Am. Dietet. Assoc.* 67 (Oct. 1975), pp. 344-46.

11. R. M. Leverton, "Food Needs and Energy Use in Weight Reduction," *J. Am. Dietet. Assoc.* 49 (July 1966), pp. 23-25.

12. M. A. Ohlson and L. J. Harper, "Longitudinal Studies of Food Intake and Weight of Women from Ages 18 to 56 Years," *J. Am. Dietet. Assoc.* 69 (Dec. 1976), pp. 626-31.

13. K. J. Lewis and M. D. Doyle, "Nutrient Intake and Weight Response of Women on Weight Control Diets," *J. Am. Dietet. Assoc.* 56 (Feb. 1970), pp. 119-25.

14. A. K. Dudleston and M. Bennion, "Effect of Diet and/or Exercise on Obese College Women," *J. Am. Dietet. Assoc.* 56 (Feb. 1970), pp. 126-29.

15. S. Lewis, W. L. Haskell, P. D. Wood, N. Manoogian, J. E. Bailey and M. B. Pereira, "Effects of Physical Activity on Weight Reduction in Obese Middle-aged Women," *Am. J. Clin. Nutr.* 29 (Feb. 1976), pp. 151-56.

16. F. Konishi, "Food Energy Equivalents of Various Activities," *J. Am. Dietet. Assoc.* 46 (March 1965), pp. 186-88.

17. F. Konishi and S. L. Harrison, "Body Weight-Gain Equivalents of Selected Foods," *J. Am. Dietet. Assoc.* 70 (April 1977), pp. 365-68.

18. G. Christakis, "The Prevalence of Adult Obesity," in G. A. Bray, ed., *Obesity in Perspective* (Washington, D.C.: DHEW Pub. No. (NIH) 75-708, 1975).

19. G. V. Mann, "The Influence of Obesity on Health," (Part One of Two), *New Engl. J. Med.* 291 (July 25, 1974), pp. 178-85.

20. R. B. Bradfield, "The Relative Importance of Physical Activity for the Overweight," *Nutrition News* 31 (Dec. 1968), pp. 13-14.

21. A. J. Stunkard, "Environment and Obesity: Recent advances in our Understanding of Food Intake in Man," *Federation Proceedings* 27 (Nov.-Dec. 1968), pp. 1367-73.

22. *Obesity and Health,* US Public Health Service, Pub. No. 1485 (Washington, D.C.: DHEW, 1966).

23. C. G. Neumann and M. Alpaugh, "Birthweight Doubling Time: A Fresh Look," *Pediatrics* 57 (April 1976), pp. 469-73.

24. Committee on Nutrition, "Obesity in Childhood," *Pediatrics* 40 (Sept. 1967), pp. 455-64.

25. M. S. Read and F. P. Heald, "Symposium on Adolescent Obesity," *J. Am. Dietet. Assoc.* 47 (Nov. 1965), pp. 411-13.

26. R. L. Huenemann, "Consideration of Adolescent Obesity as a Public Health Problem," *Public Health Reports* 83 (June 1968), pp. 491-95.

Part 4
Nutrition in Action
Around the World

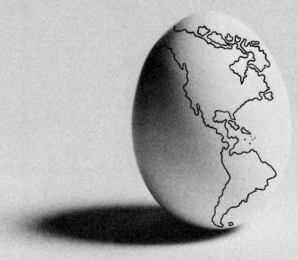

This final part of the text considers world nutrition problems and ways of dealing with them. Just as individuals are sensitive to conditions of good and poor nutrition, so also do people of the world's nations respond in terms of body size, body structure, body performance, and length of life. Awareness of this fact has grown with advances in knowledge of all the health sciences. Communities, states, nations, research groups, and international bodies are all increasingly concerned today with identifying major nutrition problems as a basis for educational and action programs to improve the quality of human life.

Nutrition problems vary in different parts of the world. Some nations are underfed; others are overfed. Each country needs to examine its own strengths and weaknesses in relation to accepted nutritional standards and to face its own shortcomings. Local, national, and international groups—private and public—must also join in concerted efforts to eliminate nutritional faults. Activities, plans, and programs toward that end are considered in the chapters that follow.

Chapter 14 summarizes major nutrition problems of the present as they exist in the world, and those that loom in the future. These are considered primarily in relation to abundance and scarcity of food supplies and to the overriding problem of population growth.

Chapter 15 outlines the myriad plans, programs, and movements designed to improve the nutritional health of all peoples. It shows how tremendous resources of knowledge, technology, and programming are being marshaled in applying the science of nutrition in behalf of human health around the world.

World Nutrition Problems

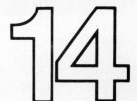

In Areas of Scarcity
In Areas of Plenty
Nutrition-Related Health Problems
 in the United States
Proposed National Dietary Goals
 for the United States

NUTRITION PROBLEMS—WHERE FOOD SUPPLIES ARE SCARCE (1)

A major nutrition problem of two-thirds of the inhabitants of the world is that of obtaining enough food for normal health and activity. These people live in the developing or less-developed nations that lie mainly in southeast Asia and in large portions of Latin America and Africa. Some constantly fend off actual starvation, while others suffer from less acute, chronic undernutrition. The problem is most critical in areas where climate, soil, and water supplies are unfavorable to farming; where entrenched beliefs and eating customs are often contrary to the principles of good nutrition; and where frequent natural disasters precipitate famines. Regardless of the circumstances, undernutrition is traceable to various types of nutritional inadequacies that involve both amounts and kinds of foods.

Nutritional Inadequacies

Protein-Calorie Malnutrition   The most widespread nutritional disease among children in developing countries is protein-calorie malnutrition (2). It is not only a leading cause of death, but it may also inflict permanent impairment of physical and mental growth on those who survive. An analysis of more than 100 community surveys in 59 developing countries in the decade preceding 1971 indicated that not less than 100 million children under 5 years of age were affected by moderate to severe protein-calorie malnutrition. Disabilities ranged from mild impairment of growth to kwashiorkor or marasmus (see Chap. 3). The necessity of protein for good nutrition is known, and educational programs for developing countries have urged special measures to assure adequate protein intakes, especially in childhood. Recently, however, it has been noted that low protein intakes are commonly associated with low-calorie diets, and that increasing levels of total food to meet energy needs usually results automatically in meeting protein requirements as well (see Chap. 7). This is the case when cereals and legumes are staples in a country's food supply, and it applies to adults and older children. It does not hold true for infants and preschool children because of their limited food capacity; foods of higher protein concentration are needed at those periods (2).

kwashiorkor
Severe protein deficiency disease

marasmus
Emaciation due to lack of food

Other Nutritional Deficiency Conditions   As we saw in the mineral and vitamin chapters (Chaps. 8 and 9), various conditions are recognized as nutrition problems in developing countries. *Xerophthalmia* is a major cause of blindness in many of them. In the Far East alone, it is estimated that more than 100,000 children go blind each year due to a deficiency of vitamin A in their diets. *Iron- and folate-deficiency anemias* in developing (and developed) countries cause ill health and result in a decreased ability to lead an active life. *Endemic goiter,* often accompanied by *endemic cretinism,* is still found in substantial numbers in some countries. In certain geographical areas, especially North Africa, *rickets* is still a serious nutritional problem, as are *pellagra* and *zinc deficiency* (2).

xerophthalmia
Dry lusterless condition of the eye

endemic
Prevalent in a particular locality

goiter
Enlargement of thyroid gland

cretinism
Arrested physical and mental development due to severe deficiency of thyroid hormone

pellagra
Niacin-deficiency disease

rickets
Vitamin-D deficiency disease

Mild Chronic Poor Health   Also related to the nutritional nature of the customary diet is mild, chronic poor health. The food supply may be low in one or more nutrients, depending upon the region, and energy yields may be inadequate. The energy value of diets in regions affected is about two-thirds that of diets in the developed regions (about 2200 and 3100 calories, respectively), and nutrients are present in widely varying amounts in relation to need. People living on such diets usually do not develop outright deficiency diseases, but they may be undersize, underweight, and beset with lack of vigor, inefficiency, short life spans, and high death rates. Poverty is the underlying cause of mass malnutrition. Expanded food production is essential, but there is also need for more equitable distribution of the food already available (3).

Decline of Breast Feeding   The decline in breastfeeding of infants in developing nations is seen as a nutritional hazard. Early weaning, under the conditions that prevail in those areas, is regarded by nutritionists as a main cause of infant malnutrition. It deprives infants of a safe, dependable food supply in their critical early months. Furthermore, home preparation of the proprietary formulas usually substituted for breast milk introduces added dangers. In the judgment of medical authorities, "for the impoverished masses who live in an environment that presents constant infectious hazards (flies, garbage, excreta, animals, dirty hands, crowded living, lack of clean water, absence of immunization and medical services), breast feeding can mean the difference between life and death for the child" (1).

Local Food Production Problems

Lack of Enough Locally Grown Food   Inadequate food production is a major nutrition problem in developing countries. Increased production of basic crops and better facilities for effectively distributing and using food supplies are thus primary means of combating malnutrition. A fundamental step is the application of agricultural procedures that have been proved sound and practical. In general, such basic measures include achieving higher crop yields per acre through use of fertilizers and irrigation; introducing fast-growing, disease-resistant crop varieties; introducing specially developed grains of relatively high protein content as a way of improving diet quality; and controlling pests and diseases of plants and animals that curtail production. These are principles upon which successful agricultural programs are based in *any* country. The precise ways in which they are applied vary from country to country, depending on local conditions.

Developing countries have low crop yields. These countries are being aided to increase local food production through national and international education programs that stress modern agricultural technologies (see Chap. 15). Agencies conducting such programs are increasingly aware that results are more promising when scientific methods are judiciously adapted to, rather than superimposed on, traditional farming procedures in those countries. Blending the new with the old, when suitable, invites the cooperation of the farmers and encourages personal involvement and the acceptance of new methods (4). In some areas this approach has led to the establishment of "village technology" units (Fig. 14.1). They call for individual and community participation in the development of ingenious, inexpensive devices to implement some of the new agricultural procedures (5). Such efforts contribute to the increase in yields of crops and give momentum to the overall objective of raising food production in developing countries. "If the people of the poor countries are to be fed, the food will have to come from their soil, their resources and their farm economies. . . . [M]ost of the developing countries are better endowed for agricultural progress than for any other kind of economic advance. . . . [F]ood indepen-

Figure 14.1
In Kenya, a village technology unit has developed a two-man bicycle-driven irrigation pump. (UNICEF/Thorning)

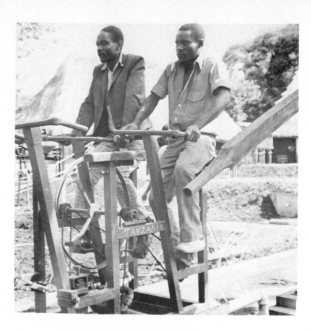

dence is an internal affair (of developing nations) and if agricultural development is given priority, it can lay the foundation for modernizing an entire economy. . . . [I]t calls for massive transfer of technology . . . from rich to poor countries" (6).

Conservation of Supplies   The conservation of food supplies on hand is one important way to make more local food available. When the quantity of food is already limited, post-harvest losses through spoilage, waste, pests, and poor storage methods are particularly pertinent to the nutritional well-being of populations. Unfortunately, losses through such avenues are large. International

Figure 14.2
(Left) Inadequate storage: traditional granary in Kenya unprotected against rodents and dampness is the cause of heavy post-harvest crop losses.

(Right) Adequate storage: A granary with the straw basket plastered with mud and an insect free spout is a food conservation measure. (UNICEF/Thorning)

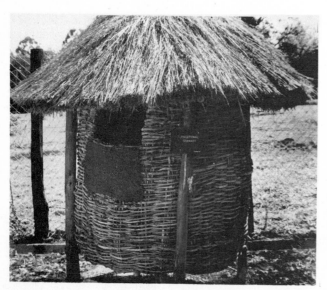

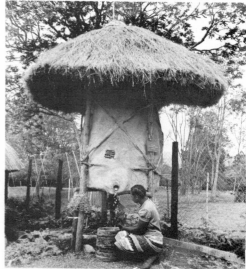

health agencies estimate a 40-percent loss of crops in Latin America from weeds, pests, and plant diseases, a 50-percent loss of sorghum in certain areas of Africa from pests eating away the crop, large losses in the Pacific and elsewhere due to consumption of foods by rats, and reduction in crop production in many areas of the world due partly to soil erosion (Fig. 14.2). Protection against such food losses thus becomes an essential aspect of the effort to provide maximum amounts of food (1, 7, 8). Conservation programs to offset food losses are underway on a worldwide basis.

New Sources of Nutrients   The search for ways to expand economical food sources of nutrients is exemplified by efforts to increase supplies of fish. The annual potential yield of conventional marine species of fish, crustaceans, and mollusks has been estimated at well over 100 million tons. The world catch in 1972 was about 50 percent of the potential. Problems include excessive "takes" of familiar fish, difficulties in marketing less familiar types, and the need to introduce modern fishing techniques, as well as marketing and distribution procedures. Supplies could be increased also by reducing waste, estimated at several million tons annually. Some fish now discarded could be marketed, and improvements could be made in handling, preserving, and storing fish. International agreements that could lead to rational management are essential, especially since most conventional types of fish will be exploited to the limit by 1985 (1). Increasingly, attention is being directed to the *cultivation* of fish. Present production from *aquaculture* of fish, crustaceans, and mollusks amounts to roughly 10 percent of world fish production. In the immediate future, the best prospects for increased output lie in tropical areas of Africa and Asia, particularly the latter, where aquacultural practice is well established and the species cultivated consumed by low-income groups (1).

aquaculture
Cultivation of certain species of seafood to provide a continuing source

Population Growth   The most serious complicating factor in the nutritional outlook for underfed countries has been their large and growing populations, brought about primarily by the control of human disease and resultant declining death rates. It is ironic that, as the population of a country mounts and its total needs increase, land that was used for growing food must be taken out of production to provide additional living space. Steps are being taken to curb population growth, particularly in developing countries. Results thus far give reason for optimism, but the problem is yet to be solved. Figure 14.3 shows the trends in population growth between 1955 and 1975 in developed countries (mostly those in the western world) and in developing countries, largely those in Southeast Asia, parts of Africa, and segments of South America. The data in this figure have special significance in any consideration of the nutritional status of peoples in the countries involved.

Population and Food Production—A Nutritional Challenge

Population Control   The most serious challenge to adequate nutrition in the world is increasing food production sufficiently to keep

Figure 14.3
Population has grown at a
much faster rate in developing
countries than in developed
countries (12). (USDA)

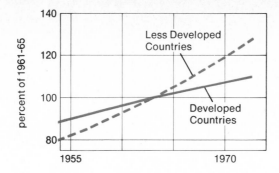

pace with population growth. Populations have grown from the beginning of time, but the recent alarming *rates* of growth are a com-
paratively new phenomenon (9). For example, it required one half
million years to reach the world's 1977 population level of slightly
more than four billion people. At recent rates of increase, that
number could easily be doubled in the next 25 years. Fortunately,
active programs for population control conducted throughout the
world in the past 10 years give promise of reducing rates of population growth significantly, particularly in developing countries (10).

In 1965, the United States began providing assistance to developing countries with programs relating to population growth.
These programs operate through several international agencies, as
well as on a bilateral basis. In the interim, most nations have removed restrictions on the provision of family planning information
and contraceptive devices. A number of nations have set up their
own programs, and some have largely accomplished their objectives (Fig. 14.4). An encouraging aspect is the relatively short time
within which progress can be seen in the areas where there are
successful programs. The compilation in Table 14.1 reflects the
demographic situation in 1965 and 1974 on a world basis, which
includes nations active and inactive in fertility control (10). The
1974 data contain some approximations, but they indicate a small,
definite decline in world birth rate of 5.8 points and in death rate

Figure 14.4
A basic problem in developing
countries is how to control
population growth. In many
countries, effective family
planning programs are
underway. (Agency for
International Development)

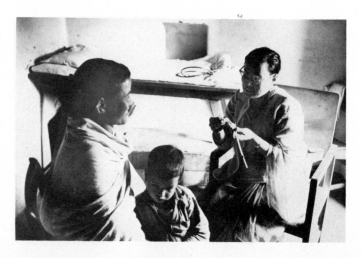

Table 14.1
Population: comparison of 1965 and 1974 demographic statistics (10)

	1965	1974
world population total	3.2 billion	3.88 billion
average world birth rate	34 per 1000	28.2 per 1000
average world death rate	14 per 1000	11.8 per 1000
annual population growth rate	2%	1.63%
annual increment in people	66 million	63 million

of 2.2 points, attained in about one decade. The resultant annual decline in world population growth rate from 2 percent to 1.63 percent reverses the historical upward trend, and—if it continues and accelerates—it forecasts decreases in population that eventually will have practical significance in terms of more nearly adequate amounts of food available per capita. Experience suggests that, even in populous developing countries, it should be feasible to reduce the birth rate to 20 per 1000 or less in an additional 10 years, and to bring the world annual population growth rate to below 1 percent. If this is accomplished, by the year 2000 the world population should be less than 5.5 billion (10).

Food Production Records (11, 12) As has been suggested, food production and population growth are inseparably linked with nutrition. Figure 14.5 shows graphically that developed countries in 1954 and 1973 produced more food, of greater monetary value, for a smaller population than did the less-developed countries. Developed countries in 1973 accounted for about one-third of the world's population and produced upwards of three-fourths of the world's food, whereas the less-developed countries, with about two-thirds of the world's population, produced about one-fourth of the world's food. On an annual basis from 1955 to 1970 in the developed countries, food production increased 1.5 percent per year; while in developing countries it increased only 0.4 percent.

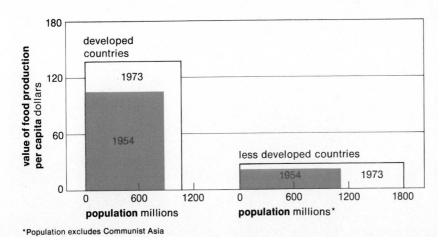

*Population excludes Communist Asia

Figure 14.5
Population and food production: in this chart the *area* of each rectangle, determined as the product of population (measured on the horizontal axis) times value of food production per capita (in dollars on the vertical axis), *represents* the total *value* of food production in million dollars for an indicated group of countries at a specified time. All four rectangles may be compared in height, in width, and in area. (Values computed at 1961-1965 average prices.) (11).

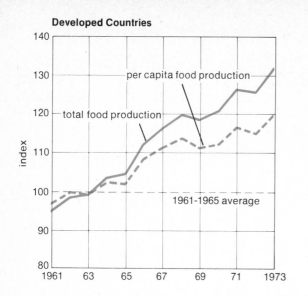

Developed Countries

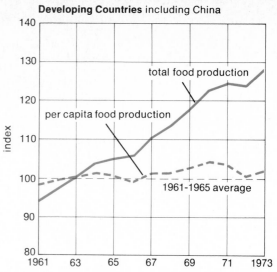

Developing Countries including China

Figure 14.6 shows the trends in total and per-capita food production in developed and developing countries between 1961 and 1973. On both the left and the right side of the figure the upper curves represent total food production; the lower curves represent per-capita food production. The per-capita production lines, in each case, provide the significant information in terms of the ability of nations to feed their peoples. The flattened lower curve on the right indicates that food production has not kept pace with need in developing countries, due to the large and growing number of persons to be fed.

Trends in per-capita food production in specified regions of the developed and less-developed countries from 1955 to 1975 are shown in Figure 14.7. The curving lines on individual segments of the chart contrast the food production situation per capita between developed and less developed areas and among the regions within the two areas. Obviously, as a consequence of differential rates of population growth, the peoples do not fare equally well. The extent to which the curves remain relatively level suggests the degree to which food supplies in developing countries are failing to meet average individual needs. The curves representing the situation in developed countries, on the left, are generally upward, which reflects a more favorable situation. In each of the developed regions, the index of food production per capita reached or exceeded 110 at least three times in the 20 years covered by the figure, whereas in none of the regions among the developing countries did the index reach 110, and Africa has actually shown a downward trend since 1961 (11, 12).

Figure 14.6
Total and per-capita food production in developed and developing countries, 1961-73 (12).

NUTRITION PROBLEMS—WHERE FOOD SUPPLIES ARE PLENTIFUL

People who live in parts of the world where the food situation is relatively favorable have diets that in the main, are varied in character and yield the needed energy. This includes North America, Western and Eastern Europe, Australia, and sections of other continents where gross forms of dietary deficiency diseases are largely nonexistent. The people in most of these areas have increased in body size from generation to generation, and their life spans have been lengthened. The abundance and quality of food supplies have undoubtedly been major factors in such changes. But, despite the encouraging outlook, nutrition problems do exist in these privileged areas. There is considerable malnutrition in certain segments of their populations. Nutritional problems in the United States have been pointed out in earlier chapters. They include suboptimal growth in poverty areas; widespread dental decay; the anemias, especially prevalent among infants, young children, and

Figure 14.7
Food production per capita in developed and in less developed countries (11).

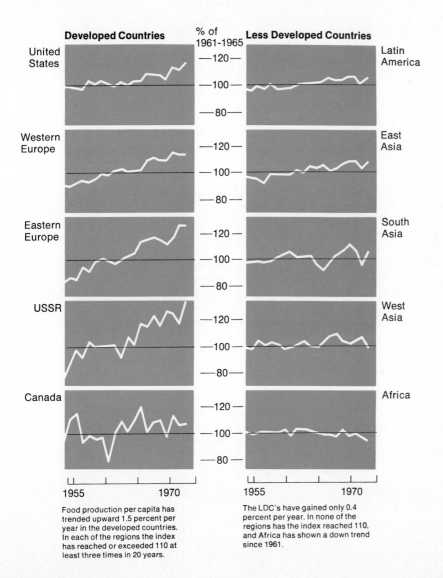

Food production per capita has trended upward 1.5 percent per year in the developed countries. In each of the regions the index has reached or exceeded 110 at least three times in 20 years.

The LDC's have gained only 0.4 percent per year. In none of the regions has the index reached 110, and Africa has shown a down trend since 1961.

pregnant women; obesity in all sex-age groups; and the degenerative diseases that are linked to nutrition.

Production and Plenty

The ample food supply of the United States is due largely to the efficiency of its agricultural operations (13) and to its moderate population increases. Greater production of food through the years is the result of improved yields rather than the use of more land. In the last four decades, farm production has increased phenomenally, using fewer acres, fewer farm workers, more mechanical power, more fertilizer, and greatly improved knowledge. In 1776 a farmer produced enough food for three people. In 1977, the amount of food produced by one farmer fed 57 people. By the year 2000, each farmer should grow food for 78 people, on about one-fifth less land than was farmed in 1977 (14). Since 1950, the amount of work per person per hour in agriculture has increased at a rate of nearly 6 percent a year.

The bases for continued increases in production lie primarily in three areas: in research that gives rise to new technologies; in conservation practices that preserve national resources such as soils and water; and in the application of research findings to the practical operations of growing, handling, and marketing foods.

Figure 14.8 shows the trends in food consumption and population growth in the United States from 1967 to 1976. Table 14.2 provides supporting data by years over the same period of time (15). It is apparent that total food consumption (food available) ran sufficiently above population growth to denote a sufficiency of food. The lowest curve on Figure 14.8 wavered generally downward from the population curve from about 1970 to 1975, when it began moving upward. The downward trend indicated a slight decline in average amount of food consumed per capita in the United States at that period. In affluent nations, where many people are already eating well above their energy needs, a mild lowering of the per

Figure 14.8
Trends in total food consumption, population growth and per capita food consumption in the United States, 1967-1976 (15).

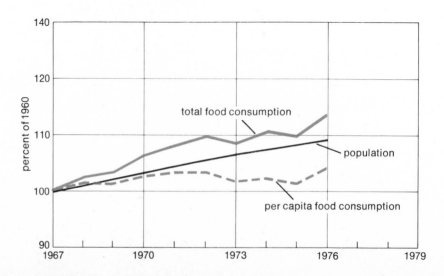

Table 14.2
Trends in civilian population growth, total food consumption and per capita food consumption in the United States, 1967–1976 (15)

Year	Population* number million	Population* index 1967 = 100	Food consumption index** total 1967 = 100	Food consumption index** per capita 1967 = 100
1967	195.3	100.0	100.0	100.0
1968	197.1	100.9	102.1	101.2
1969	199.1	102.0	103.4	101.5
1970	201.7	103.3	106.2	102.8
1971	204.2	104.6	108.0	103.3
1972	206.5	105.7	109.6	103.7
1973	208.1	106.6	108.5	101.9
1974	209.7	107.4	110.2	102.6
1975	211.4	108.2	109.9	101.6
1976†	213.0	109.1	113.8	104.3

*Population as of July 1; includes Alaska and Hawaii.
**Individual food items are combined in terms of 1957–59 retail prices.
†Preliminary.

capita curve may usually be regarded as a desirable trend. This is particularly true in the United States, where the diet is composed of a mixture rich in fats, sugars, and refined foods of high density, which is concentrated in energy value and carries more of some nutrients, such as fat, than needed.

Nutrition-Related Health Problems in the United States

Over- and Undernutrition Despite a generally varied and abundant food supply in the United States, there is evidence that many people are not well fed. Availability of food has not proved to be a guarantee of dietary adequacy. As we have seen in previous chapters, there are disadvantaged sex, age, racial, and economic segments that do not get enough and/or the right kinds of food to enjoy good nutrition. These people are underpar, grow inadequately, and suffer nutrition-related ill health. At the other extreme there are those who habitually overeat. Over consumption, coupled with reduced energy expenditure, creates an energy imbalance that results in excess body fat in a considerable segment of the population of the United States (see Chap. 13). The dangers of obesity lie mainly in its relationships with nutrition-connected degenerative diseases. Thus, nutrition problems of a serious nature can arise in the midst of abundance, from *under-* or *over*nutrition.

Diet-Health Relationships There has been increasing concern among nutritionists in the United States that its abundant food supply and the eating patterns of the population may be related to some of its most serious health problems. Research is under way to determine to what extent this may be a cause-and-effect relationship. Production-consumption trends have changed radically in character during the past half-century (see Chap. 4). There have been increases over the years in the use of fats (16), sugar, salt, and alcohol, and a decline in consumption of fruits, vegetables, and whole-grain cereals. The diet is increasingly concentrated in factors that have come to be associated with some major causes of death in this country: heart disease, cancer, *cerebro-vascular* disease, *arteriosclerosis*, diabetes, and cirrhosis of the liver.

Nutrition as a Preventive Measure   The United States has looked to medical science alone to deal with these nutrient-related diseases. However, with the realization of the limitations of cures and a new recognition of the essential relationship of nutrition to these diseases, prevention assumes greater importance. In 1971, USDA authorized a special staff committee to assess the benefits of applying the findings of human nutrition research to dietary practices (17). Among the benefits the committee listed as attainable by improved diets were: better health; a longer, active life span; and greater satisfaction from work, family, and leisure time. The report pointed out that advances in nutrition knowledge and its application have already played a major role in reducing infant and maternal deaths and deaths from infectious diseases, (particularly among children) and extending the life span and life expectancy (see Chap. 3). For the future, "a vast reservoir of health and economic benefit can be made available by research yet to be done" on human nutrition, and a more complete application of existing knowledge would result in substantial gains in dealing with the major diet-related diseases (17). The report postulated that most of the health problems underlying leading causes of death in the United States can be modified by improvements in diet, and estimated the nature and magnitude of the benefits to be expected in a number of the diseases. Preventive nutrition holds the potential of deferring, or modifying, the development of a disease so that a clinical condition would not develop, according to the report. Also, a basic change of diet would be shared by each age, sex, ethnic, and geographic segment; people at lower economic levels and nonwhites would have the greatest advantage from effective application of current nutrition knowledge.

Changing Eating Habits   The application of nutrition research, as proposed by the USDA committee, calls for major dietary changes in the eating habits of the public. This would not be easily accomplished. The problem of changing food practices has long concerned nutrition educators. (Elements of the process of habit change are considered in Chapter 1.) Strong motivation to change is a basic requirement. If there is a compelling incentive to accomplish a specific health objective, and if the necessary dietary changes are accepted as logical steps toward that accomplishment, the prospects of effecting dietary change are promising. These qualifications for success are implicit in the *Dietary Goals for the United States,* issued by the Select Committee on Nutrition and Human Needs of the United States Senate (18). Warnings by the Committee of the risk factors in the present United States diet should provide strong

cerebro-vascular
Pertaining to blood vessels of the brain

arteriosclerosis
Thickening and hardening of artery walls with loss of elasticity interfering with blood circulation

cirrhosis
Chronic disease of the liver; increased formation of connective tissue ultimately resulting in failure of liver function

motivation for change. The precise dietary goals proposed, backed by a rationale that supports the diet-health relationship, should encourage implementation.

The Select Committee has based its proposals on: 1. the July 1976 hearings of the Committee on the relationship of diet to disease and its 1974 National Nutrition Policy hearings, 2. guidelines established by government and professional bodies in the United States and other nations, and 3. a variety of expert opinion. With respect to the application of the dietary recommendations, the Committee believes that, "Although genetic and other individual differences mean that these guidelines may not be applicable to all, there is substantial evidence indicating that they will be generally beneficial" (18). The proposals are stated here as dietary goals.

Proposed Dietary Goals for the United States

The Select Committee on Nutrition and Human Needs of the United States Senate has condensed to several brief directives the dietary goals it advises (18):

Increase carbohydrate consumption to account for 55 to 60 percent of the energy (calorie) intake.

Reduce overall fat consumption from approximately 40 percent to 30 percent of energy intake.

Reduce saturated fat consumption to account for about 10 percent of total energy intake and balance with *polyunsaturated* and monounsaturated fats, which should account for about 10 percent of energy intake each.

Reduce cholesterol consumption to about 300 milligrams a day.

Reduce sugar consumption by almost 40 percent to account for about 15 percent of total energy intake.

Reduce salt consumption by about 50 to 85 percent to approximately 3 grams a day. See Figure 14.9 for a graphic representation of the dietary goals proposed above.

To achieve these dietary goals, the Select Committee recommends the following changes in eating patterns:

Increase consumption of fruits, vegetables, and whole grains.

Decrease consumption of meat and *increase* consumption of poultry and fish.

Decrease consumption of foods high in fat and *partially substitute* polyunsaturated fat for saturated fat.

Substitute nonfat milk for whole milk.

Decrease consumption of butterfat, eggs, and other high cholesterol sources.

Decrease consumption of sugar and foods high in sugar content.

Decrease consumption of salt and foods high in salt content.

Plan for Implementing Proposed Dietary Goals

To encourage the achievement of these dietary goals, the Select Committee recommends that Congress provide money for a public education program in nutrition based on the foregoing or similar

saturated
Holding as many hydrogen atoms as possible; no double bonds in fatty acid carbon chain

polyunsaturated
Containing 2 or more double bonds between carbon atoms in fatty acid chain

cholesterol
Fatty substance; present in animal tissue

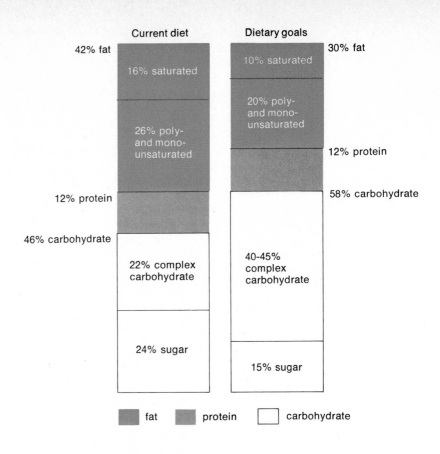

Figure 14.9
US Dietary Goals expressed graphically (18). Sources for current diet (19). (Proportions of saturated versus unsaturated fats based on unpublished Agricultural Research Service data.)

Current diet

42% fat

16% saturated

26% poly- and mono-unsaturated

12% protein

46% carbohydrate

22% complex carbohydrate

24% sugar

Dietary goals

30% fat

10% saturated

20% poly- and mono-unsaturated

12% protein

58% carbohydrate

40-45% complex carbohydrate

15% sugar

☐ fat   ☐ protein   ☐ carbohydrate

goals. The initial minimum period for the promotion of these dietary goals should be 5 years. Five functional areas are emphasized: health and nutrition education in the classrooms and cafeterias of schools, nutrition and health education for school food service workers, nutrition education in federally funded food assistance programs, nutrition education conducted by the Extension Service of the US Department of Agriculture, and extensive use of television to educate the public in the potential benefits of following certain dietary goals.

The Committee also suggests that Congress require food labeling for all foods to enable the consumer to make informed comparisons between foods. The following information should be included: percent and types of fats, percent of sugar, milligrams of cholesterol, milligrams of salt, caloric content, a complete listing of food additives.

Congress is requested to provide money to the Departments of Agriculture and Health, Education, and Welfare to conduct joint studies and pilot projects that would develop new techniques in food processing and institutional and home meal preparation aimed at reducing risk factors in the diet. Increased funding is also suggested for human nutrition research in the Department of Agriculture, in accordance with the plan of the Agricultural Research Service, and Congress is asked to establish a committee for the coordination of human nutrition research undertaken by the Departments of Agriculture and Health, Education, and Welfare.

Acceptance and Implementation of the Dietary Goals

Understandably there is not complete agreement in the scientific community with respect to the content of the proposed dietary goals. All agree that the public needs dietary guidance. Some approve of the present recommendations; others reject them in whole or in part. All urge that decisions be based on scientifically sound criteria and that they be made by qualified scientists. There are honest differences of opinion among nutrition scientists about the interpretation of the research on which the goals were established. There are also differences in judgment as to the suitability of urging the general public to adopt goals that seem to some, unnecessary or unwise and that perhaps promise too much in terms of improved nutrition-related health conditions.

Meanwhile the statements of goals and accompanying recommendations are reaching the public. How will it accept the goals? Will it be guided by them? Will significant changes in eating patterns be effected? Some of the goals may be modified eventually, others may be added or dropped. Advancement toward these goals is, and should be a continuing effort. The goals represent a major step toward the achievement of a National Nutrition Policy. Such a policy is now in the making; it will be considered next in Chapter 15 as the framework for a comprehensive nutrition education program in the United States.

REFERENCES

1. *The State of Food and Agriculture, 1974* (Rome: Food and Agriculture Organization, 1975).

2. *Food and Nutrition Strategies in National Development*, Ninth Report of the FAO/WHO Expert Committee on Nutrition, Dec. 1974 (Rome: Food and Agriculture Organization, 1976).

3. J. Mayer, "The Dimensions of Human Hunger," *Scientific American* 235 (Sept. 1976), pp. 40-49.

4. H. P. Burn, "A Truly African Green Revolution: Blending Old Traditions with New Technology," *UNICEF News* 90/1976/4, pp. 16-19.

5. The Village Technology Unit, *UNICEF News,* 90/1976/4, pp. 24-26.

6. W. D. Hopper, "The Development of Agriculture in Developing Countries," *Scientific American* 235 (Sept. 1976), pp. 197-205.

7. *Food Losses, The Tragedy . . . and Some Solutions* (Rome: Food and Agriculture Organization, 1969).

8. E. M. Martin, *Nutrition Problems of the World,* in report, Johns Hopkins University Centennial Symposium on Nutrition and Public Health (Baltimore: Nov. 11, 1975).

9. J. D. Coffey, "World Food Supply and Population Explosion," *J. Am. Dietet. Assoc.* 52 (Jan. 1968), pp. 43-48.

10. R. T. Ravenholt, "Gaining Ground on the Population Front," *War on Hunger* X (Feb. 1976), pp. 1-3, 13.

11. *The World Food Situation and Prospects to 1985* (Washington, D.C.: USDA, Foreign Agricultural Economic Report #98, 1974).

12. *World Agricultural Situation* (Washington, D.C.: USDA, Economic Research Service, Dec. 1973).

13. E. O. Heady, "The Agriculture of the US," *Scientific American* 235 (Sept. 1976), pp. 107-27.

14. *Food and Home Notes* (Washington, D.C.: USDA, Jan. 10, 1977).

15. *Food and Home Notes* (Washington, D.C.: USDA, Feb. 28, 1977).

16. C. A. Chandler and R. M. Marston, "Fat in the US Diet," *Nutrition Program News* (May-August, 1976).

17. C. E. Weir, *Benefits from Human Nutrition Research* (Washington, D.C.: USDA, Science and Education Staff, Aug. 1971).

18. US Senate, Select Committee on Nutrition and Human Needs, *Dietary Goals for the United States,* (Washington, D.C.: US Gov. Print. Office, 1977).

19. B. Friend, Changes in Nutrient in US Diet Caused by Alterations in Food Intake Pattern (Washington, D.C.: USDA, 1974).

READINGS

H. R. Cottam, "The World Food Conference," *J. Am. Dietet. Assoc.* 66 (April 1975), pp. 333-37.

B. Friend, *Changes in Nutrients in the U.S. Diet Caused by Alterations in Food Intake Patterns* (Washington, D.C.: USDA, 1974).

E. George, "Africa's Population Problem," *War On Hunger* XI (March, 1977,) pp. 13-14.

R. S. Harris and E. Karmas, eds., "Nutritional Evaluation of Food Processing," (Westport, Conn: AVI Publishing 1975).

J. McDowell, "Sunshine or Darkness (Blindness from Vitamin A Deficiency)," *UNICEF News* 90/1976/4, pp. 11-13.

US Senate, Select Committee on Nutrition and Human Needs, National Nutrition Policy: *Food Security and Availability,* (Washington, D.C.: US Gov. Print. Office, 1974).

H. L. Sipple and K. W. McNutt, eds. *Sugars In Nutrition* (New York: Academic Press, 1974).

That We May Eat, The Year Book of Agriculture, 1975 (Washington, D.C.: US Gov. Print. Office, 1975).

P. L. White and N. Selvey, eds. *Nutritional Qualities of Fresh Fruits and Vegetables* (Mt. Kisco, N.Y.: Futura Publishing Co., 1974).

Programs to Deal with World Nutrition Problems 15

A National Nutrition Policy
A National Nutrition Program
International Nutrition Programs
Common Goals for Better Nutrition

As major nutrition problems are identified throughout the world efforts are being made to deal with them. Some problems are being approached on an international scale; others at regional, national, and local levels. Agencies and organizations serving under many different auspices undertake these tasks. Their purposes and scopes differ widely, but all are concerned in some measure with the betterment of human nutrition.

It is important for citizens to know of such movements and their objectives. An informed public, convinced of the importance of improved nutrition to human welfare, is one very important factor in approaching the solution to nutrition problems. This chapter covers nutrition programs throughout the world, beginning with the United States.

A NATIONAL NUTRITION POLICY FOR THE UNITED STATES

The need for a national nutrition policy in the United States is increasingly evident. Such a policy should ensure concerted, purposeful effort in nutrition planning and programs, both at home and in international commitments (1,2). The growing number of separate agencies and organizations dealing with nutrition problems has accentuated the need for a unifying policy, as has our increased recognition of the significant role that other scientific fields play in nutrition programs and services. Individuals and groups in the field of nutrition are concerned not only with the status of national health, but also with guiding agricultural, economic, social, and educational policies, since these are inseparably associated with production, distribution, and use of food (3,4). Together they represent broad, significant dimensions of nutrition today. There is at present no overall federal policy in the United States designed to coordinate these forces toward achieving optimum nutritional health for the population, but a start has been made.

National Nutrition Consortium

Gradually a framework for a national nutrition policy for the United States is emerging (1). Guidelines and goals have been developed and are being expanded, and programs are being proposed by the National Nutrition *Consortium*, representing major scientific, nutrition-oriented societies in this country. The concept of the Consortium is to provide "a common voice and coordinated action to help guide the application of food and nutrition knowledge to the common good."

consortium
Association of agencies with a common purpose

A statement of the need for a national nutrition policy has been developed by the Consortium, listing nutritional goals and the programs needed to achieve those goals. The need and goals are outlined here in condensed form (1).

Need for a Stated Nutrition Policy   A stated nutrition policy is necessary to ensure that food will be available to provide an adequate diet at a reasonable cost to every person in the United States. Food to provide good nutrition is a fundamental need of every member of society. Individuals also must have some basic understanding of food and nutrition in relation to requirements for health.

The nutrient requirements of the population should be translated into terms of food in developing plans for food production at the agricultural and manufacturing level. Nutrient contributions of foods, as well as their economic importance, must receive consideration; agricultural and nutrition policies should be coordinated; production of sufficient food must be accompanied by adequate distribution systems; and the quality and safety of the food supply must be assured.

A national nutrition policy is needed to fulfill the United States' commitments—in cooperation with other nations and international organizations—in planning adequate food for the expanding world population. This policy should allow for maintenance of adequate world reserves of food, technical assistance, participation in world trade, and provision of foods in emergency situations.

Goals of a National Nutrition Policy (1)   The national nutrition policy, as outlined by the Consortium, should meet the following goals:

to assure an adequate, wholesome food supply to meet the needs of all the segments of the population and to be available at a level consistent with people's means;

to maintain food resources sufficient to meet emergency needs and to fulfill a responsible role as a nation in meeting world food needs;

to develop a level of sound public knowledge and responsible understanding of nutrition and foods that will promote maximal nutritional health;

to maintain a system of quality and safety control that justifies public confidence in its food supply; and

to support research and education in foods and nutrition with adequate resources and logical priorities to solve important current problems and permit exploratory basic research.

The measures and programs needed to achieve these goals were conceived and presented in the form of recommendations for action in December 1969. The Consortium has endorsed and expanded these recommendations. In effect, they represent preliminary steps toward a national nutrition program for the United States.

A NATIONAL NUTRITION PROGRAM FOR THE UNITED STATES

Many of the elements of a national nutrition program have been in operation in the United States for a number of years. However, it was not until December 1969 that a concerted effort was made to coordinate the many forces concerned with such a project. The occasion was the White House Conference on Food, Nutrition and Health called by the President of the United States to convene in Washington, D.C. (5).

The purpose of the conference was to lay the foundation for a national nutrition policy and to advise the President on the best methods of eliminating malnutrition in this country. Goals had to be defined, existing programs coordinated, unnecessary duplication avoided, and an effective national nutrition education program created. It was thought that people in the United States were not well enough informed on nutrition, and that perhaps as much as 10 percent of the population was economically unable to buy an adequate diet.

A considerable body of information about diets and habits of food selection reinforced that belief. It showed that some essential nutrients were low in many diets; that other nutrients were low in the diets of certain sex-age categories; and that deficiencies were most likely to occur among low economic groups. These findings regarding dietary intakes have been documented in preceding chapters. However, less was known of the nutritional status of the people. Many studies on various segments of the population had indicated relationships between diet and nutritional status, and a National Nutrition Survey provided clinical and biochemical evidence that some malnutrition existed in measurable degree in areas where diets were poor and most of the people were economically deprived. With such background data on which to base nutrition policy, members of the White House Conference, working in panels supported by task forces, developed recommendations for policy and action in many important areas. The members of the panels represented a cross-section of people involved in nutrition, from the research scientist to the producer and consumer of foods. From their recommendations emerged broad outlines for the development of nutrition programs. While many of the programs await initiation, others chiefly require extension of present efforts and their coordination into an effective whole with a united approach (5).

Now, almost a decade later, it should be interesting to look back and to evaluate progress made over that period. In the interim, scientific organizations, the educational community, and government resources have been directed toward implementing the recommendations (6). While considerable headway has been made in some areas, other fields are virtually untouched. Much remains to be done.

A few basic recommendations made by the White House Conference are reviewed here with brief reminders of subsequent events (many of them described in previous chapters) that appear to have been motivated by these recommendations.

1. A Comprehensive Nutrition Education Program. The recommendation for a comprehensive nutrition education program envisioned formal nutrition teaching in schools, from early years through advanced academic instruction in universities. A curriculum developed at the grass-roots level would ensure a unified, sequential nutrition education program in elementary and high schools. State departments of education would be urged to require a nutrition course in the training of elementary classroom teachers and of secondary teachers whose subject matter specialties—such as biology, health, chemistry, and physical education—lend themselves to the inclusion of nutrition instruction. Similar training in the principles of nutrition would be required of teachers in service. The services of a professional person responsible for coordinating nutrition education and nutrition services would be available to every school or school district.

In the interval since the White House Conference on Food, Nutrition and Health, there are indications of progress in attaining the objectives outlined in the foregoing paragraph (7). Steps have been taken, for example, to examine and evaluate present school curriculum guides in nutrition and to establish sounder approaches that recognize modern educational concepts and apply the laws of learning. Efforts have also been made to upgrade standards of education and experience for persons aspiring to supervisory positions in nutrition education at state and local levels. There is evidence of a new awareness that elementary teachers in service should have some training in foods and nutrition. At least one government grant program provides workshop training and experience with an experimental approach to the challenge of inservice teacher education in nutrition. Likewise, at least one innovative preservice education program in nutrition has been inaugurated experimentally. These are merely indications that could forecast future developments; they reflect a certain momentum and direction that has not been observed previously. This does not mean that a more vigorous and effective type of nutrition education is already implemented in the schools. Rather, it suggests that some sound foundations are being laid for the future.

The White House Conference recommended that less formal methods of nutrition education be carried on in communities to create public concern for the nation's nutrition problems, to foster understanding of nutrition, to disseminate information regarding food programs, and to promote better food habits. These programs would be conducted by local agencies concerned with food, nutrition, health, and welfare, and they would be directed primarily to families with limited incomes (5).

There are a number of such programs in operation. One example is the Expanded Food and Nutrition Education Program (EFNEP) of the United States Department of Agriculture Extension Service. This project was designed to teach low-income homemakers how to feed their families more nutritious meals. The instruction is conducted by paid aides, trained for the task but not professionally educated in nutrition. The program has grown dramatically since 1970.

The White House Conference further recommended that health departments, school systems, departments of public welfare, and voluntary agencies be adequately staffed with nutrition consultants. Efforts would also be made to reach disadvantaged groups through mass media techniques. Study of radio and television viewing habits of these groups, and of methods of motivating their interest in nutrition, would precede such programs. Popular nutrition education would also relate to misinformation and would help to protect the public from food fallacies and deception in nutritional claims.

Progress in implementing such recommendations is difficult to document. For example, the number of nutrition consultants has probably increased, although exact numbers are not known. Efforts are being made to upgrade the training of such consultants in nutrition subject matter and in educational techniques. Reaching disadvantaged groups with nutrition education through mass media in radio and television has not generally been marked with success and, unfortunately, misinformation about nutrition appears to be increasing despite some organized programs to counteract it.

2. Continuous Surveillance of Nutritional Status. In order to be constantly aware of nutrition problems in the United States, it was recommended that nutritional status studies be conducted on a continuing basis, especially for target groups in low-income areas. Methods of identifying malnutrition would be reviewed regularly. Procedures for biochemical, clinical, and anthropometric appraisals —and the standards applied in their use—would be evaluated con-

tinuously. Nutritional status assessment data would be used to identify specific nutritional problems and to indicate need for remedial programs. In all evaluation procedures priority would be given to vulnerable groups.

Such surveillance is now underway. The National Center for Health Statistics (NCHS) is the designated agency. The Health and Nutrition Examination Survey (HANES) collects the data. Included is clinical, biochemical, and dietary information based on a probability sample of the United States population, 6 to 74 years of age, of varied incomes. The data are collected in time cycles to provide a national surveillance system for measuring nutritional status and monitoring changes over a period of time. Preliminary findings have been published and are referred to throughout this text. The second cycle, HANES 2, has begun.

The White House Conference recommended that household and individual diet surveys, made under government auspices at intervals, be continued, broadened, and coordinated with nutritional status surveys. A 5-year sequence was recommended.

This goal is becoming a reality. USDA has announced its sixth nationwide food consumption survey, launched in April 1977. This survey will require 1 year for collection of information and an additional 2 years for analysis of the data. In addition to checking food consumption by households and by individuals in different sex-age categories, it will include two supplemental collections. In one, consumption data will be gathered in Alaska, Hawaii, and Puerto Rico; in the other, a survey will be made in 5000 households that include elderly members.

3. Special Consideration Recommended for Vulnerable Groups. All current data point to the fact that certain segments of the population are more vulnerable to nutritional deprivation than others. In general, the vulnerable groups are those with high nutritional needs. Included are those in the growth cycle—pregnant and nursing women, infants, children of all ages, and adolescents—as well as the aged and the ill.

The WIC program (Women, Infants, Children) described in Chapter 11 is a notable example of specific services to vulnerable groups, in this case pregnant and nursing women, and infants and children until their fifth birthday. Other examples are the extension of the school breakfast program, the growth of the school lunch program, the broader interpretation of eligibility of sponsors for summer feeding of school-age children, and of year-round child care programs for preschool children. These have all contributed to meeting the needs of these vulnerable groups (Ch. 12).

Aging members of the population would be aided with foods, with help in meal planning, and with service of group meals. The ill would have assistance with therapeutic diets and with programs for rehabilitation.

Considerable progress has been made in meeting these goals, especially with respect to group meals for senior citizens (see Chap. 11). In some localities the food needs of elderly incapacitated persons, especially those living alone, are met with a home-delivered Meals on Wheels program (see Chap. 12).

4. Improving Nutritive Values of Foods was Recommended.

Supportive of education and service programs would be concerted ef-forts to provide foods of maximum nutritional value. A basic step is the assessment of nutrient content of traditional foods on a contin-uing basis in relation to nutritional needs of the population. The White House Conference recommended that the need for increased enrichment and fortification of certain foods in specific nutrients be considered. It also recommended that special efforts be made to pro-vide vulnerable groups with nourishing foods, giving due attention to nutrient-fortified items.

In the years since the White House Conference, enrichment standards for bread have been raised, and standards for macaroni and noodle products have been added (see Chap. 8). The additon of specified levels of vitamin A to fluid low-fat milk, fluid skim milk, and low-fat dry milk identified as "fortified," have been made man-datory; the same is true for vitamin D in evaporated milk and for-tified nonfat dry milk. In general there has been an upsurge in for-tification of many foods, particularly dry breakfast cereals. Foods for special feeding programs such as WIC are enriched and fortified whenever there is a choice.

The White House Conference urged that efforts be enhanced to improve the protein content of cereal grains through genetic manip-ulation and to produce meat with more lean and less fat by breeding meat-producing animals for that characteristic. Nutritional guide-lines should be offered to the consumer for such characteristics as the amount of fat provided by individual products. Maximum fat levels would be established for high-fat foods. Grading standards in foods would reflect nutritive value, thus allowing leaner cuts of meat, for example, to qualify for higher grades.

There is considerable popular support for recommendations of this type, and there has been some progress in all areas mentioned. The protein content of grains has been improved through hybridi-zation (especially important in foreign nutrition programs); some steps have been taken to lower the fat content of ground meats, notably the limitation of fat in hot dogs to 30 percent and the offer-ing of low-fat ground beef; and there is some tendency to breed for leanness in food animals and to lower the grading priority previ-ously given to meats highly marbled with fat. In general the nutri-ent content of foods has been highlighted by providing consumers with more information, not only on fat content but on several other nutrients in many packaged and canned goods as well through FDA's nutrition labeling program (see Chap. 10).

5. *Implementing a National Nutrition Program.* The foregoing recommendations, though only a small part of the total program, suggest their comprehensive nature. They offer a challenge and goals toward which to aim. Significant progress has been made in some areas; in others, only token advancement is visible; and in many respects no developments can be reported.

A nutrition program of the magnitude proposed by the White House Conference on Food, Nutrition and Health would require centralized direction of nutrition policy. It would call for coordi-nated effort of federal, state, and local nutrition agencies—public and private. In view of this fact, *panels of the conference were unanimous in urging that the present widely diffused nutrition pro-*

grams be brought together under the competent guidance of an able administrator.

Despite the fact that this point of view has been endorsed by nutrition leaders throughout the country, so far no action has been taken to consummate such a plan. Meanwhile, existing nutrition programs and services of official and nonofficial agencies and groups form the foundation for much of the current nutrition activity in the United States.

What evidence is there in your locality of nutrition programs and activities of the types recommended by the White House Conference on Food, Nutrition and Health?

Which programs, in your opinion, have made the greatest progress: the school nutrition program, the School Breakfast Program, the WIC program, or some other program?

Do you have a home-delivered meals program in your area? How is it organized and financed? What part do volunteers play in it?

GOVERNMENT PROGRAMS

Among the agencies in the United States concerned with nutrition are certain departments of the federal government. These include the US Department of Health, Education and Welfare (DHEW), with its Public Health Service, Maternal and Child Health Service, Food and Drug Administration, National Institutes of Health, National Center for Health Statistics, and Office of Education; and the US Department of Agriculture (USDA) with its Food and Nutrition Service, Agricultural Research Service, Economic Research Service, and Extension Service. The research, publications, and program services of these departments, as they relate to nutrition, have been cited repeatedly in preceding chapters. USDA, for example, has provided several of the tools used throughout the text, such as data on the nutritive values of common foods (see Appendix K) and information on the eating patterns of households and individuals in different regions. DHEW, through FDA, has introduced nutrition labeling. These and other such aids are essential instruments in developing action programs for improved nutrition.

The Food and Nutrition Board of the National Academy of Sciences-National Research Council is a quasi-governmental group composed of leaders in nutrition from various scientific fields. It is largely concerned with nutrition policy and the development of specialized materials for professional use. The board also serves in an advisory capacity in the field of human nutrition to national and international groups. One of the early tasks undertaken by the board, which continues today, is the development of the Recommended Dietary Allowances (RDA) that have been referred to throughout the text.

There are also many state, county and local organizations and agencies, within the governmental framework, that are occupied in some degree with nutrition education. These include health and education departments, schools at all levels, and official welfare services. Semiofficial groups are the nutrition committees and councils in many states and major cities, which conduct varied programs of nutrition education in their areas.

NONGOVERNMENTAL PROGRAMS

Professional societies of nutritionists strengthen national and international programs through their official support and participation. The American Institute of Nutrition and the American Society for Clinical Nutrition are such organizations. Universities and colleges prepare nutritionists for teaching and other fields and carry on nutrition research through their departments of nutrition, biochemistry, medicine, and home economics. Private foundations for research and education, food industry associations and individual food companies sponsor nutrition research, and make their findings available to scientists, to action groups and to the public.

Many nongovernmental organizations, professional or educational in character, give a measure of attention to nutrition. They are national in scope, but most of them have active local affiliates. Such organizations include: the American Public Health Association, the American Dietetic Association, the Society for Nutrition Education, the Institute of Food Technologists, the American Home Economics Association, the American School Foodservice Association, and the American Nurses Association.

UNITED STATES NUTRITION PROGRAMS GEARED TO PROBLEMS ABROAD

The United States has cooperated with other nations in helping to raise the level of nutrition and health throughout the world. Three departments of the federal government are the chief contributors to nutritional phases of international programs: the Departments of State; of Health, Education and Welfare; and of Agriculture.

Department of State—Agency for International Development (AID) The Agency for International Development took the name of the Act that created it and eventually became known as AID. The basic Act, with amendments, was continued in the Mutual Security Act of October 10, 1951. These acts declared that it was the policy of the United States to aid the people of underprivileged areas in improving their economies by the exchange of technical knowledge and skills, as a means of raising the standards of productivity and living. The Foreign Assistance Act of 1961 laid the groundwork for establishing AID as an agency in the Department of State. Much of AID's work has been in agriculture. The overall objective has been to achieve a better-nourished people and thus to build stamina and health toward stronger nations. It has made skills-training available, but the transfer, adaptation, and practical application of those skills has rested largely with the people aided. Training has been provided in two ways: as "on-the-job" training, whereby trainees are hired in their own countries and assigned to work with technicians sent there from the United States; and as advanced training, given to technicians who could benefit by studying in the United States.

Nutrition education activities go hand-in-hand with the agricultural programs. AID develops patterns of procedure for planning nutrition education programs where needed; conducts investigations, conferences, workshops, and tests; and assembles data to determine directions for progress in such areas as breast feeding, nutrient fortification of staple cereals, and vitamin-A deficiency problems. Results of the AID programs are enhanced by effective cooperation with agencies in the United States government (USDA, DHEW), with UN specialized agencies, and with a host of agricultural and other agencies of international origin or of individual developing nations.

Department of Health, Education and Welfare (DHEW)   The Department of Health, Education and Welfare participates in international nutrition programs largely through its Institutes of Health (NIH) and its Maternal and Child Health Services (MCHS). The Activities of NIH are chiefly of a research nature. This agency has sponsored, for example, a major long-term research study in Guatemala to clarify relationships between malnutrition and intellectual development in children (see Chap. 3). MCHS activities are consultative and advisory in character. MCHS cooperates with AID to sponsor program planning conferences, to implement nutrition activities, and to publish nutrition education materials.

Figure 15.1
On the left, an improved variety of wheat grown in Pakistan, developed from high-yielding seed from Mexico, produces triple the crop of the traditional variety on the right. (Agency for International Development)

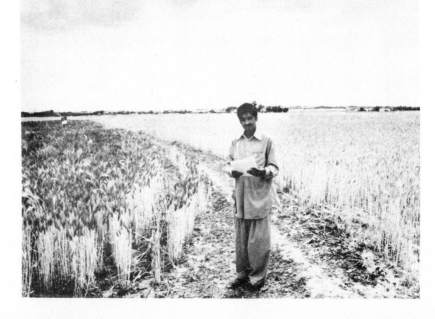

Department of Agriculture (USDA) The Department of Agriculture functions in international nutrition programs through many avenues, chiefly under two main divisions: Agricultural Research Service (ARS) and Economic Research Service (ERS). ARS develops basic information in its regional research laboratories and state experiment stations. It provides data and practical procedures for increasing crop yields and cross breeds certain cereal grains for higher protein content. Research with hybrid varieties of corn is mentioned in Chapter 7; work with other grains is discussed later in this chapter. ERS focuses on worldwide food supply-and-demand conditions; provides direct assistance and coordinates USDA's overall program to aid agricultural development in low-income countries; furnishes AID with such technical services as evaluation of its nutrition programs; and directs field tests for acceptance of newly developed foods.

Private foundations in the United States are also making significant research contributions to the betterment of world nutrition (8). These include the Ford Foundation, the Rockefeller Foundation, and the International Rice Research Institute, supported by the Ford and Rockefeller Foundations. Working in the Philippines, the Institute has developed strains of rice that have more than doubled yields per acre in Asia and increased protein content substantially (6). Similarly, the Rockefeller Foundation has developed disease-resistant, fast growing strains of wheat and corn in Mexico. These can add considerably to the food supply in underdeveloped areas, and similar programs are being carried out with other cereal grains (Fig. 15.1). This development became known as the "green revolution" (9) and, while it suffered many setbacks, in actual practice it has demonstrated the potential for providing greater quantities of food in needy nations. Foundations and AID have helped to broaden the outlook for long-term, continuing nutritional improvement by joining a worldwide movement to revolutionize agriculture in terms of basic knowledge and its application to specific situations and areas. Eight international centers are now functioning in South America, the Philippines, Mexico, India, and Africa (10) (Fig. 15.2).

Characteristic of this world-wide movement is its cooperative nature, its concept of continuity in education and service, and its recognition of and application to current nutritional and agricultural problems. One such center—in Nigeria—serves as an example. Its support is provided by AID along with the Ford and Rockefeller Foundations, the Canadian International Development Agency, the Overseas Development Ministry of the United Kingdom, the International Bank for Reconstruction and Development, the UN Environment Program and the governments of Nigeria, West Germany, Belgium, the Netherlands, and Iran (11).

Voluntary Service Organizations (12)

Privately supported organizations, which render nutrition services in developing countries, are chiefly of two types: denominational church organizations, such as Catholic Charities, American

Figure 15.2
In Nigeria, portable displays
explain the potential of
improved seeds to farmer
groups. Selected farmers are
provided with kits of improved
seeds and fertilizer to
demonstrate to their neighbors
the greater yields that can
result. (Agency for
International Development)

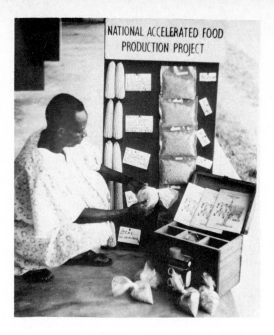

Friends Service Committee, and Lutheran World Relief, which
have foreign service commitments; and community-supported
groups, such as CARE, World Education, Save the Children Foundation, International Red Cross, and Salvation Army.

United States voluntary organizations in foreign service have
traditionally participated in nutrition programs mainly by helping
distribute government-donated foods, aiding refugees, and dispensing disaster relief. Such cooperation continues as needed, but gradually voluntary agencies have enlarged their scope. United States
legislative action has extended the ways in which food relief may
be utilized and has made it possible to expand voluntary nutrition
services into various community activities.

INTERNATIONAL AGENCIES AND PROGRAMS

The vast problems of malnutrition in the world cannot be met by
any one country, or even by a small group of countries. The task
requires combined efforts. Joint concern for the nutritional welfare
of the peoples of the world stems from World War I, when the
League of Nations was formed and a nutrition division was added
to its small health section. The League sought to find in nutrition
the solution to a situation that created food surpluses in one part
of the world and hunger in others. World War II halted this effort.

With the onset of World War II came a new perspective on nutrition. There was an awareness of the prevalence of inadequate diets in the world and of the consequences that follow. The war gave
researchers the opportunity to study the nutritional status of
adults and children under stress conditions and to observe the outcomes. The findings brought renewed realization of the need for

Table 15.1
Agencies of the United Nations—international programs involving nutrition*

UN Agencies	Origin and development	Nutritional objectives	Nature of nutrition programs
FAO **United Nations Food and Agriculture Organization**	1945, first session convened in Quebec Secretariat includes five technical divisions: agriculture, economics, fisheries, forestry, and nutrition. Three organizations that are outgrowths of FAO: 1963—Freedom From Hunger Campaign (FFHC) 1964—Young World Appeal (YWA) 1968—Young World Development (YWD)	Overall: to raise the nutritional level of the people in developing countries; infants, children, adolescents, expectant and nursing mothers to receive special consideration. To deal with nutrition in relation to production, distribution and consumption of food. To work with health, nutrition, agricultural specialists in the countries being served, to bring to each country specific needed help To strive for increased food production; better management; improved training of leaders.	Nutrition programs with local governments: Technical assistance to establish projects: materials, supplies, equipment, experts to aid. Research to develop and exploit high-nutrient, high-yield grains. Educational activities to improve nutrient intakes: supplementary feeding programs for mothers and young children; school feeding; home food management. Training and educational programs for local personnel: on-the-job training, travel-study grants, regional institutes.
WHO **World Health Organization**	1948, WHO launched at International Health Conference in New York. WHO recognizes nutrition as an essential element in concept of health; a nutrition section was established early. 1949, a Joint Committee on Nutrition with FAO was organized. Pan American Health Organization (PAHO) is the regional office of WHO for governments of the Western Hemisphere.	Overall: to achieve positive health, not merely combat disease. To assist member nations to assess their own health and nutrition needs; to plan nutrition services; to implement programs to meet needs. To direct programs toward improved general health and the prevention and elimination of dietary deficiency diseases.	Conduct surveys in member countries to determine levels of health, extent of nutritional deficiencies. Provide educational training in nutrition for medical, public health and para-professional personnel serving mothers and children. Sponsor and conduct research to assess the nature of nutritional deficiencies. Center program efforts on: nutritional anemias, endemic goiter, protein-calorie malnutrition, xerophthalmia.
UNICEF **United Nations International Children's Fund**	1946, UNICEF was created by the General Assembly of the UN, to meet emergency health needs of children. 1953, it was accorded permanent status as a UN agency. It is the only agency concerned solely with the welfare of mothers and children. UNICEF is supported by voluntary contributions of governments, groups and individuals. Local governments served provide matching funds.	To improve the quality of life for needy mothers and children throughout the world. (80% of the budget now assigned to permanent programs) To provide food as well as nutritional services when disaster strikes. To pursue objectives of the country assisted, not of UNICEF. Local governments must request aid, and for projects *they* think are important. To prepare governments to take over and continue programs when UNICEF withdraws.	Works with other agencies and with local governments to monitor the nutriture of populations, especially the children. Aids local nutrition programs with UNICEF personnel, administrative direction and with equipment and supplies needed for child care centers and health clinics. Trains local personnel to work with mothers, children and families; fosters community gardens and school feeding programs.

Table 15.1
continued

UN Agencies	Origin and development	Nutritional objectives	Nature of nutrition programs
UNESCO **United Nations Educational Scientific and Cultural Organization**	1946, UNESCO was launched when 20 countries had signed its constitution. It is an independent body with its own membership and budget; it receives from the UN appropriations for technical assistance activities.	Overall: to wipe out illiteracy as a first step in raising the standard of living throughout the world. To help people everywhere acquire an understanding about the world's food and ways they can help make it available to all.	Establishes educational centers: Trainees at centers are school teachers from countries served by UNESCO; Teachers are taught how to apply methods in their own countries. Teaches reading: Reading is taught in connection with food, homemaking and agriculture to provide knowledge for improved community life. UNESCO programs are conducted in cooperation with other UN agencies and with various organizations. There is an international exchange of personnel.

* Publications from agencies described in Table 15.1 are available as follows: UNICEF: 331 East 38th St. New York, N.Y. 10016; UNESCO and FAO: UNIPUB Inc. Box 443 New York, N.Y. 10016; WHO, Geneva, Switzerland.

nations to work together. The obvious solution was the establishment of international organizations that could deal competently with the food situation on a worldwide basis. This was accomplished by setting up agencies for that purpose within the United Nations, which was then being organized. Table 15.1 lists these major international agencies and describes their origin and development, their nutritional objectives, and the nature of their nutrition programs. The United States has played an active role in these agencies from their beginnings.

Agencies of the United Nations

The Food and Agriculture Organization (FAO) was the first of the UN subgroups to come into existence (1945). One of its five technical divisions is devoted exclusively to nutrition. In general, FAO programs deal with nutrition in relation to production, distribution, and consumption of food. On this broad base FAO works with the health, nutrition, and agricultural authorities in the countries being served, to bring to each the specific help it needs to achieve higher nutritional status for its people (Table 15.1). Its outgrowth organizations have practical, and sometimes local, implications. For example, the purpose of the Freedom From Hunger Campaign (FFHC) epitomizes the working philosophy of FAO, by helping disadvantaged and malnourished peoples help themselves. Major efforts are directed toward teaching farmers and homemakers the skills that are basic to increased production and better use of food. Training programs for teachers and for community workers are an essential aspect of this plan. Young World Appeal (YWA) involves young people in improving world conditions, including the alleviation of hunger. Youth and student groups and religious organizations vigorously support projects in other lands as well as in their own. They provide aid in such forms as educational materials, money for teachers' salaries, training institutes, and vocational demonstration projects.

The World Health Organization (WHO) came into existence in 1948 and at its inception established a section on nutrition. The agency recognizes nutrition as an essential element in the total concept of health. Its overall objectives are outlined in Table 15.1. Since the beginning, WHO has maintained, jointly with FAO, a Committee on Nutrition to deal with problems of mutual concern. The program of WHO is involved with broad aspects of human health related to nutrition, including the extent of malnutrition in populations, the development of programs for prevention of malnutrition, the training of health personnel, and research in causes and treatment of nutritional disorders.

The Pan American Health Organization (PAHO) is the regional office of WHO for governments of the Western Hemisphere, particularly those of Latin America.

Institute of Nutrition for Central America and Panama (INCAP) is an organization for nutrition research and service for the six countries of Central America.

The United Nations International Children's Fund (UNICEF) was created in 1946. UNICEF has the distinction of being the only UN agency concerned solely with the welfare of children and mothers. This group's chief purpose is to stimulate permanent programs regarded as important by local governments (Table 15.1). One phase of its activity is devoted to nutrition in a broad program of health and social welfare. In almost all major activities UNICEF cooperates, not only with local governments, but also with other UN agencies, particularly FAO and WHO.

The United Nations Educational, Scientific and Cultural Organization (UNESCO) also originated in 1946. UNESCO is the United Nations agency primarily concerned with education. The stated purpose of this group is to contribute to peace and security by promoting collaboration among the nations of the world through education, science, and culture. Its more specific relationships to food and nutrition are stated in Table 15.1.

Cooperative Activities of International Agencies   Each of the agencies of the United Nations has its specific program area, but cooperation strengthens the overall effort. A major activity of the joint nutrition committee of FAO and WHO has been the establishment of daily dietary standards for energy and for several nutrients (Table 2.2). It also sponsors research on critical nutrition problems of developing nations. Another joint activity is the conducting of seminars, workshops, and institutes with regional nutrition organizations in different sections of the world. Such seminars may consider a wide variety of nutritional problems common in the area, or they may concentrate on one topic, such as school feeding. Representatives from countries in the host region present data on local conditions. Ideas are exchanged; desirable procedures are considered; and plans are developed. These sessions inform and give direction to prospective programs. National trade policies, as they relate to food supplies and the nutritional status of populations in the countries represented, are sometimes influenced by recommendations formulated at such seminars.

INTERNATIONAL PROFESSIONAL INTERCHANGE

An increasing number of nutritionists and persons in related professional fields are establishing scientist-to-scientist contacts through international organizations. The International Dietetic Association and the International Home Economics Association are two such organizations that hold joint meetings periodically and carry on cooperative programs designed to raise the levels of their professions in member countries. The International Union of Nutritional Sciences, one of sixteen unions comprising the International Council of Scientific Unions, is a sponsor of international congresses of nutrition, held every 3 years. The movement is composed of hundreds of nutritionists representing nearly every country. Exchange fellowships and the regular scientific meetings of members have proved to be powerful devices for the interchange of knowledge and for promoting understanding of worldwide nutrition problems.

A unique professional relationship has also been established between universities in the United States and those in developing countries. Under this plan, a United States university selects a counterpart institution with which to engage in cooperative teaching, writing, and research subjects. Nutritionists have a significant role in this undertaking. Activities vary greatly in different locations, but a more intimate grasp of nutrition problems in the world is an important result.

Thus we have a worldwide network of agencies, organizations, programs, and activities, all of which seek to deal with phases of nutrition and nutrition education. Each program has its own objectives and its own procedures for working toward them. Success in approaching the total goal of better nutrition for the world's peoples depends on how well these procedures can be channeled along parallel lines. Knowing about and working on nutrition problems other than one's own is an important step in appreciating and achieving the overall objective.

IMPROVED FOOD HABITS—AN INTERNATIONAL GOAL

A basic objective in international health programs is improved food habits. A unifying factor in achieving this goal is the establishment of nutritional standards (allowances) that serve as guidelines in food selection. These standards, expressed in terms of nutrients, are customarily translated into patterns of eating in terms of foods available and eaten regularly by the various populations served. Such eating patterns are known around the world as food selection guides. (see Chapter 10, for United States guide)

Origin of Food Selection Guides in the World

Table 2.2 presents a compilation of dietary standards adopted by a number of countries. Nations that do not develop their own standards often use those of FAO and WHO, shown at the top of the Table. Here the dietary standards are confined to those for men and women, but standards for other age groups are available from the original source given at the close of the table. Once scientists in a country have adopted appropriate dietary standards for their people, they proceed to develop a corresponding food selection guide that takes into consideration food supplies and the preferences and meal habits of the people. Similarities in guides used throughout the world lie in the broad groups of foods known to be important for nourishing the body in specific ways. The chief differences lie in the number of divisions in the guides and the kinds of foods within the divisions. Certain food groups are common to most of the guides, notably meat, milk, vegetables, fruits and cereals. But foods within these groups vary not only in kind, but also in the emphasis given them by the different countries. They demonstrate the fact that there are many ways to obtain an adequate diet and that there is no one right way.

Food Selection Guides of Different Nations

The differences in food selection guides is best demonstrated by examining carefully two guides from different parts of the world where food supplies and eating habits vary greatly. This is done here by comparing the food selection guide of São Paula State, Brazil with that of the United States. The former was developed in 1974 by representatives of organizations working in nutrition education.* The movement was sponsored by the Section of Nutrition, Health Institute, Coordination of Specialized Technical Services, São Paulo State Department of Health. The similarities and differences in the two guides can be seen by comparing them in Table 15.2.

Table 15.2 is organized under the four food groups suggested in the United States food guide presented in the first column on the left. In the second column are examples of common foods of the United States that are considered representative for regular use. The third and fourth columns list the corresponding groups from the São Paulo State food guide. Similarities and differences in the lists for the two areas are evident immediately. Each of the corresponding groups contains many of the same or similar foods. The lists are different, however, in two important respects: the São Paulo State food groups include several foods that do not appear on

---

* Aspects of Brazil's food habits as discussed in this section were provided by Maria Helena Villar, Professor of Nutrition Education, Chief of the Subdivision of Studies and Health Education, DMS, SESI, São Paulo State, and Rosa Nilda Mazzilli, Nutritionist, Assistant Professor, Nutrition Department, Public Health School, University of São Paulo. They had the assistance of nutrition and health authorities in universities and other educational institutions throughout Brazil.

Table 15.2
A closer look at daily food guides of the United States and São Paulo State, Brazil

Four food groups US food guide	United States Recommended foods	São Paulo State Recommended foods	Food groups São Paulo State food guide*
milk group	milk and cheeses	milk and milk products except butter	Milk and milk products group
meat group	lean meats— beef, pork, lamb, veal poultry fish eggs legumes (dry), nuts	beef fish poultry pork eggs legumes (dry)	meats, eggs, legumes group
vegetable-fruit group	green and orange (vitamin A)—"greens," carrots, apricots	"greens"—lettuce, kale, spinach green beans, peppers, tomatoes, pumpkin, carrots and so on	vegetables group
	citrus and others (ascorbic acid)— oranges, grapefruit, tomatoes, strawberries	oranges, bananas, papaya, pineapple, guava, avocado, grapes	fruits group
	others—potatoes, beets, peas, apples, bananas		
bread-cereal group	breads breakfast foods cereal foods	breads corn flour noodles potato, sweet potato, cassava, yam	cereals and starchy roots group

*The São Paulo State Food Guide contains an additional group, for fats and oils, also sugar and sugar dishes as marmalades and sugar confections.

the United States list, and there is a different emphasis in the use of some of the foods common to both countries. The Brazilian foods that are eaten less commonly in the United States are easily identified: cassava, guava, papaya, corn flour, and pumpkin. In Brazil, cassava is a basic carbohydrate food. In some regions, beans, rice, and cassava flour are mixed until a paste is formed, the foods being combined on the plate during the meal. Cassava ranks second in Brazil's food production, with sugarcane ranking first. By contrast, cassava (as tapioca) plays a minor role in the United States, chiefly as a thickening agent for puddings and fruit pies. Pumpkin is used mainly for pie fillings in the United States. As a basic vegetable in Brazil, it is cooked with salt, oil, garlic, and onion. Guava is a familiar fruit commonly eaten in Brazil, while in the United States it is a specialty item more apt to be served as a treat. Avocado is used mainly for dessert in Brazil, in salad in the United States.

Milk is not a regular item in Brazilian meals, as suggested by the examples shown in Table 15.3. Average daily consumption of milk is about 200 grams (4/5 cup), mainly used by children. The low consumption of milk in Brazil is due in part to the fact that milk is traditionally considered a child's food. Adults rarely use it in their meals. People in some rural areas who produce milk sell their entire supply, reserving none for family use. The price of milk is not prohibitive. In Brazil, as in most parts of the world, it costs less than an equal amount of soft drink. Strong black coffee is a favorite beverage for meals and for after lunch and dinner. It is the custom to offer visitors a demitasse in homes and offices.

Table 15.3
Sample meals that might be selected from the food patterns of the United States and Brazil*

United States	Brazil
Breakfast Coffee, tea or milk, plus Toast, rolls or doughnut or Breakfast cereal, fruit juice or Bacon, egg, toast, jelly, fruit	Coffee or coffee with milk, plus: White bread or corn bread with butter or margarine and sometimes a cheese or meat sandwich or Puba, tapioca, cuscuz or beiju** or Sweet potatoes, cassava or yam

Lunch
 	
Hamburger on bun, relishes, fresh fruit, milk
or
Soup or chowder, crackers, pie, coffee or tea
or
Tuna salad sandwich, cole slaw, soft drink, cookies
	Beans and boiled rice, plus cassava flour or not,
	   depending on origin of the individual, plus
	A choice of beef, fish, pork, poultry: braised, fried or
	   roasted
	One or two choices of vegetables as lettuce, potato,
	   kale, green beans, peppers, tomato served as
	   salad or braised
	A choice of fruits, mainly bananas, oranges, papaya,
	   pineapple, or sometimes marmalade with cheese
	Fruit juice or soft drink, sometimes
	Coffee

Dinner
 	
Pot roast, potato, cooked onions, celery, gelatin dessert
or
Chicken, rice, corn, lettuce salad, ice cream
or
Macaroni and cheese, peas, sliced tomatoes, cake
(With each dinner: a beverage—milk, coffee, tea or soft
drink; a bread stuff—rolls, bread, muffins, biscuits, with
butter or margarine)
	A meal similar to lunch or:
	Soup of meat or poultry with vegetables, noodles or
	   legumes
	or
	Coffee or coffee with milk, fruit juices, soft drink plus
	   sandwiches or sweet potatoes, cassava or yam
	or
	Lunch leftovers

Snacks
 	
Choices from: Milk, milkshake, yoghurt, coffee, tea, fruit
juices, soft drinks, beer; Apples, bananas, raisins, nuts,
carrot sticks; Ice cream bars or cones, cheese wedges;
Sandwiches, tacos, pizza, french fries, potato chips,
pretzels, cookies, candy bars.
	Coffee, milk, or coffee with milk, plus breads with
	   butter, margarine or marmalade or plus sandwiches
	   or plus sweet potatoes, cassava or yam. Fruit juices
	   or soft drink, sometimes.

*These data were collected through a questionnaire answered by nutrition experts of the States of Pará, Pernambuco, Bahia, Rio de Janeiro, Brasilia D.F., São Paulo, and Rio Grande do Sul.
**Puba, tapioca, cuscuz, and beiju are typical food dishes derived from cassava, usual in the north, northeast, and middle west regions of Brazil.

Men prefer black coffee, but coffee and milk are often mixed in proportions to suit individual tastes. The mixture is sometimes served for breakfast or for snacks, particularly for children.

Breast feeding is on the decline. When infants are breast-fed, it is for a short period, usually 3 months or less if at all. Highly publicized commercial infant formulas are taking the place of breast feeding. Strong claims are made for the formulas' superior nutritional quality and the need to replace the milk of poorly-nourished mothers. The convenience and dependability of the product for mothers employed outside their homes are also stressed. Brazil hopes to reverse this trend with its active campaign to restore the practice of breast feeding.

Family Meal Patterns—The United States and Brazil

Table 15.3 shows sample meals that might be selected from food patterns of the United States (on the left) and Brazil (on the right). The foods in each meal represent combinations of flavors and textures that are pleasing to the peoples in their respective countries. The Brazilian meals would look quite different from corresponding meals in the United States, but if the nutrient values were compared they would be surprisingly similar. The way foods are prepared, their grouping in meals, and even the manner in which they are eaten epitomize the eating customs that are unique to a country. These characteristics, taken together, make the native food habits of one country distinctive from those of another. Foods are never "typical" in any country for all seasons and for all situations. Table 15.2 takes into account foods that are produced and available in different parts of Brazil at different times of the year and that form the basis for the traditional Brazilian diet. As in other countries, Brazilian homes today are influenced by international contacts that have their effect on eating practices as well as other living habits.

Brazil is a vast country of more than 8 million square kilometers, with more than 100 million inhabitants. It is only slightly smaller than the entire United States. It is not surprising, therefore, that foods differ and eating patterns vary in different sections of Brazil. Soil, ecological, ethnic, and climatic differences are responsible for the great variety in crops. Colonization and cultural adaptation have also played an important part. Brazilian foods and cookery today originated in food habits of the Portuguese colonizer, the black slave, and the native Indian. Brazil is the only country in Latin America where the official language is Portuguese. *Feijoada* and *moqueca,* two traditional Brazilian dishes, date back to Brazil's colonization. *Feijoada,* inherited from the slave, is a mixture of beans now cooked with cured and smoked meats, pork tails, pork ears, and sausages (Fig. 15.3). *Moqueca,* based on fish, was inherited from the Indians of the Amazon region. The consumption of cassava is common for the entire country. Cassava flour and cassava root are boiled, fried, toasted, or roasted and can appear in any Brazilian meal. Brazil has the greatest cassava production in the world—33 million tons in 1974. It is also the largest

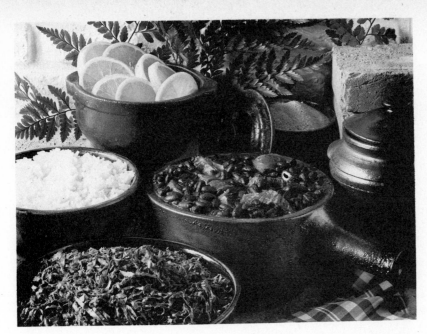

Figure 15.3

A Brazilian meal. Feijoada (center) is a traditional lunch dish in Brazil. Black beans, cured meats—pork and beef, smoked sausages, smoked pork tenderloin, bacon, cured pork tongue, foot, ears and tails—are cooked until tender and seasoned with garlic and onion fried in lard. The dish is served with boiled rice (left), cassava flour (right rear), kale (foreground)—sliced and cooked, seasoned with garlic and onion fried in lard or oil, and a special sauce made with the liquid of the feijoada, hot pepper, minced parsley and sliced onion. To complete the meal, serve with peeled, sliced oranges. (Nestlé Home Economics Center, São Paulo, Brazil)

producer of beans, as well as the largest consumer of its home product.

Later in the history of Brazil, migratory streams of Europeans —mainly Germans and Italians—brought new dishes to southern Brazil, giving this region food characteristics that differ from those of other regions. Germans introduced potatoes, sauerkraut, and frankfurters; the Italians brought spaghetti, macaroni, noodles, pizza, and polenta. Breakfast in the south region is richer than in the north. Sausages of different varieties, ham, and jelly are added and bread has replaced cassava products.

Studies of Eating Habits and Health in Brazil

Research on nutritional status, food habits, and food consumption of rural and urban population groups in Brazil show deficiencies in calorie and protein intake and deficits in vitamins (mainly vitamin A, riboflavin, and ascorbic acid) and calcium. There is insufficient consumption of energy-yielding foods. Obesity is not a public health problem in Brazil. Consumption of beef, fish, poultry, eggs, and milk is low, and intake of vegetables and fruits inadequate.

Research with school children throughout the country showed that beans, rice, bread, and coffee are the foods with highest consumption. Surveys on the same groups of school children showed, however, that the children preferred milk, cheese, beef, eggs, fish, and oranges. These foods—as well as fruits and vegetables—are generally not eaten by the poor classes in Brazil. Children have first priority on milk. Vegetables and fruits are not popular with children or adults, and consumption is low. Nutrition education efforts in Brazil are mainly directed toward increasing intakes of milk, vegetables, and fruits.

Nutrition Education Program in Brazil

Brazil is establishing a National Program on Food and Nutrition called *Pronan* (13), for the purpose of solving the serious nutritional problems of the country in an appropriate and realistic manner. The nation is attempting simultaneously to stimulate the system of food production and distribution through the use of incentives and actions to rationalize its performance. The program is based on the evidence that nutritional deficiencies stem from an extensive group of variables within which Pronan will act, emphasizing the factors that are most critical and most directly correlated with its area of competence.

Pronan concentrates on three broad streams of action:

food supplementation to pregnant women, nursing mothers, children under 7 years old, school children from 7 to 14, and workers;

rationalization of the System of Food Production with emphasis on the stimulation of the small producer; and

complementary support activities, designed basically to combat specific nutritional deficiencies through fortification of currently consumed foods, the support of studies and research in the area of food and nutrition, the qualification and improvement of human resources, and the development of an adequate infrastructure for the distribution of foods.

This overall focus stems from the principle that the improvement of the nutritional conditions of the population depends on the reduction of cost of production and trade of basic foods, as well as on a better distribution of income.

FOOD—A COMMON DENOMINATOR AMONG PEOPLES

Many factors affect people's eating habits. They tend to prefer the foods they have known and liked since childhood and they are not easily diverted from them. Familiar foods have deep significance for entire populations as well as for individuals. Adhering to long-established eating customs tends to create a feeling of permanence and solidarity among the people of a country. It often symbolizes security in the face of other basic changes, and the very importance that individual countries attach to their own native foods and eating customs enhances a common worldwide interest and concern for food.

As rapid transportation and communication have made neighbors of all peoples, the average citizen better understands the way families in remote places eat and live. Many persons are making these discoveries for themselves as a result of world travel or service overseas in various capacities, and through the myriad cultural-exchange programs under which people live, study, and work in countries other than their own. Such firsthand experiences have helped to demonstrate that basic nutrition needs are similar everywhere and that essentially the same kinds of foods nourish all peoples, even though the foods themselves may look and taste unlike those eaten at home.

Eating together is a symbol of goodwill in every culture. This simple rite tends to remove barriers to friendship that are often resistant to more ambitious efforts. Appreciation of the foods of other cultures should be encouraged, but this is not to suggest that national food customs should be abandoned and that eventually all people should learn to like and eat the same foods—quite the contrary! It does suggest the importance of increased acceptance and respect for the distinctive features of the diets of nations other than one's own. Such understanding is an essential element in recognizing world nutrition problems and a long step toward solving them.

LOOKING AHEAD

What is being accomplished by the many national and international efforts in behalf of better nutrition around the world? What, if any, are the signs of improvement?

Many reasons for encouragement have been cited in the preceding pages, and world leaders in nutrition have indicated some cause for optimism. One has pointed out, as a major advance, the mere recognition of the nature and distribution of main nutritional disorders in the world and organized efforts to do something about them. Another has declared that we are the first generation that has dared to think in terms not only of enough food but food of adequate nutritional quality for the world's people.

Research in all fields touching world feeding problems has increased enormously, and programs to interpret and disseminate the findings have made great progress. But the efforts and actions of many concerned people working together have perhaps provided the ingredient most needed for looking ahead confidently.

REFERENCES

1. US Senate Select Committee on Nutrition and Human Needs National Nutrition Consortium, *Guidelines for a National Nutrition Policy* (Washington, D.C.: US Gov. Print. Office, 1974).

2. US Senate Select Committee on Nutrition and Human Needs, *National Nutrition Policy, Nutrition and the Consumer—II* (Washington, D.C.: US Gov. Print. Office, 1974).

3. J. Mayer, ed., *U.S. Nutrition Policies in the Seventies* (San Francisco: W. H. Freeman Company, 1973).

4. J. Mayer, "Toward a National Nutrition Policy," *Science* 176 (April 1972), pp. 237-41.

5. White House Conference on Food, Nutrition and Health, 1970. *Final Report* (Washington, D.C.: US Gov. Print. Office).

6. US Senate Select Committee on Nutrition and Human Needs, *Dietary Goals for the United States* (Washington, D.C.: US Gov. Print. Office, Feb. 1977).

7. E. A. Martin and V. A. Beal, Chapters 9, 10 in *Roberts' Nutrition Work with Children* (Chicago: U. Chicago Press, 1978).

8. See Annual and Special Reports for the Ford and Rockefeller Foundations.

9. D. L. Rhoad, "Of Seed and Man—Sparking the Revolution," *War on Hunger* 10 (March 1976), pp. 1-14.

10. D. L. Rhoad, "Of Seed and Man I," *War on Hunger* 10 (March 1976), pp. 1-5.

11. A. Schuler, "Of Seed and Man II," *War on Hunger* 10 (June 1976), pp. 1-4, 11-13.

12. B. Snead, "The Voluntary Role of Foreign Aid," *War on Hunger* 10 (July 1976), pp. 5-9.

13. Pronan: Food and Nutrition National Program—Brazil, S.A., 1976–1979. Documento Técnico, Inan–6/76.

READINGS

The AID Nutrition Program Strategy (Washington, D.C.: Dept. of State, US Agency for International Development, 1973).

Board of Science and Technology for International Development, Commission on International Relations, *Food Science in Developing Countries: A Schedule of Unsolved Problems* (Washington, D.C.: National Academy of Sciences-National Research Council, 1974).

EFNEP . . . Accomplishments and Future Needs, USDA [Washington, D.C.: The Economic Research Service, HE-89 (7/75)].

Ganzin, M., "Food for All," *Food and Nutrition* (FAO), No. 3, 1975, pp. 2-7.

Jelliffe, D. B., "Thought for Food—The Social and Cultural Aspects of Malnutrition," *UNICEF News* 71 (March 1972).

Jelliffe, D. B. and Jelliffe, E. F., eds., *Nutrition Programmes for Preschool Children* (Zagreb, Jugoslavia: Institute of Public Health, 1973).

McNaughton, J., "Applied Nutrition Programmes," *Food and Nutrition* (FAO) Vol. 1, No. 3, 1975, pp. 17-23.

Nutrition Education in Child Feeding Programs in Developing Countries [Washington, D.C.: Dept. of State, US Agency for International Development (AID), 1974].

Obert, J., *Community Nutrition* [New York: John Wiley and Sons, (In Press)].

Appendixes

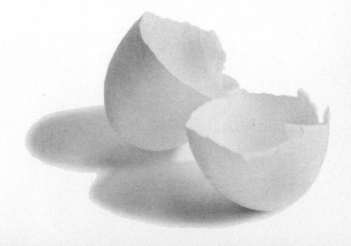

Appendix A
Sample Form for Three-day Meal Record

Instructions

First day — sample day's meals, Chap. 4			Second day			Third day	
Meals	Amount of food	Additional information	**Meals**	Amount of food	Additional information	**Meals**	Amount of food
Breakfast			**Breakfast**			**Breakfast**	
doughnut	1 plain	enriched flour	prunes				
coffee			egg				
sugar	2 tsp		toast				
			butter				
			cocoa				
Morning snack			**Morning snack**				
none			apple				
Lunch			**Lunch**				
hamburger	1 3-inch	broiled	hotdog				
bun	1	enriched	bun				
pickle	1 tbsp	relish	mustard				
catsup	1 tbsp	tomato	green-				
mustard	1 tsp	prepared	pepper				
onion	2 green	raw	onion				
milk	1 cup	whole	milkshake				
Afternoon snack			**Afternoon snack**				
soft drink	12 oz.	cola-type	cookies				
Dinner			**Dinner**				
pork chop	1 loin	broiled	chicken				
potato	½ cup	mashed	potato				
			butter*				
corn	½ cup	canned	carrots				
			butter*				
coleslaw	¼ cup		tossed salad				
rolls	2	enriched	bread				
butter*			butter*				
ice cream	1 slice	plain	rice pud-				
cookies	2	chocolate chip	ding				
Evening snack			**Evening snack**				
potato	10	medium	pizza				
chips							

* or margarine

Suggestions for recording meals

Draw up three blank forms like the sample. Adapt meal order to your own habits.

1. List all the foods you eat for a period of three days.

   Record everything you put into your mouth and swallow.

   List foods as soon after eating as possible, preferably at the table. Do not trust your memory.

   Provide additional information for each food (see form). This is needed to identify foods properly for calculation.

   Include all extras: snacks, butter for bread, butter or sauce for vegetables, dressings for salads, jelly, jam, nuts, etc. Include vitamin pills or other concentrates.

   List separately the different foods that compose one diet item, such as the makings of a hamburger (see sample first day), or cereal with milk and sugar. Indent accompanying foods for ease in interpreting the menu.

2. Measure or estimate quantities of foods.

   Measure foods in standard measuring cups or spoons. Learn to visualize quantities.

   Examine measures of foods in Appendix K to assist you in recognizing denominations of foods to be used in calculating their nutritive content. For equivalents in weights and measures and for abbreviations, see Appendix F.

3. Select one day's meals from the three recorded to be used as a basis for calculating calorie and nutrient values.

   Choose the day most representative of your regular eating habits. Weekend meals are often atypical.

   Avoid, as far as feasible, a day with several complicated food mixtures. They introduce errors because of the difficulty in estimating quantities of ingredients.

   Set up your chosen day's meals on the form used for the specimen diet in Appendix H.

Appendix B Puerto Rican Diets

I CHARACTERISTICS OF NATIVE PUERTO RICAN DIETS *

Diet core—staple items eaten daily by almost everyone in Puerto Rico

rice
beans (habichuelas)
viandas (starchy vegetables and unripe starchy fruits)
lard, used traditionally for cooking; vegetable fats and oils on increase

Regular accompaniment: Café con leche (coffee with milk)

Daily Meals in Puerto Rico

Rural family, low income	Urban family, middle income	Comment
Breakfast		
café con leche	café con leche	Prosperous families
cocoa for children	cocoa for children	especially those who
bread or soda crackers	bread, margarine	know nutritive values,
	egg, or cereal with	often add fruit juice
	milk	or nectar to breakfast;
		they may also use small-
		er amounts of rice and
		viandas and more meat
		at the other two meals
		than do middle-income
		urban families.
Lunch		
viandas (plateful)	rice and beans	In industrial and busi-
sometimes with dry	meat, small amount	ness areas, a lunch
salt codfish (bacalao)		away from home might
or sausage		be a hamburger or hot-
(rice and beans sub-		dog with soft drink
stituted when		or milkshake.
viandas are scarce)		
Dinner		
rice and beans	rice and beans	
viandas	viandas (such as fried	
no dessert	plantain in small	
	amounts)	
	ground meat, small	
	amount	
	bread, butter	
	dessert (may be stewed	
	fruit or guava paste)	

---

* Rosa Marina Torres, "Dietary Patterns of the Puerto Rican People," *Am. J. Clin. Nutr.* 7 (May-June 1959), pp. 349–55. Current facts on Puerto Rican diets were provided by Professor Lillian Reguero of the University of Puerto Rico. Professor Sylvia Santiago, a colleague on the University's nutrition staff, read the Reguero information and made valuable additions.

The native dishes, preferred foods, cooking methods and customary meal practices of people in Puerto Rico are outlined first as background for understanding food problems of migrants when they arrive in cities on the mainland. This information is intended primarily for persons helping migrant families interpret their food needs in light of their traditional diet. Major food problems encountered by the migrants and ways to approach their solution are also considered briefly.

Between-meal Snacks

native fruits	potato chips	Snacks in second
fruit drinks	pastelillos (fried turn-	column eaten especially
soft drinks	overs)	in business and
black coffee	other fried starchy	industrial areas
	foods	
	candy, pop	
	hot dogs and ham-	
	burgers	
	ham and cheese sand-	
	wiches	
	ready-to-eat cereals	
	pizza	

Rice and Beans

Rice and beans are always served together in a meal but they can be cooked separately or together; they are eaten once or twice daily by most Puerto Ricans.

Average daily per capita consumption of rice is about 4 ounces, of beans 1.3 ounces. These amounts represent decreases in recent years.

Rice is cooked in boiling salted water, with lard, vegetable fat or oil added for seasoning.

Beans are boiled until tender or bought boiled or canned and then cooked with sofrito (see seasonings) and a small portion of calabaza or potato.

Viandas

There are fifteen or more kinds of viandas:

white sweet potato (batata blanca)	potato (papa)
yellow sweet potato (batata amarilla)	ripe plantain (plátano maduro)
deep yellow sweet potato (batata	unripe plantain (plátano verde)
mameya)	white tanier (yautía blanca)
dasheen (malanga)	yellow tanier (yautía amarilla)
unripe banana (guineo verde)	cassava (yuca)
white yam (ñame blanco)	arracacha (apio)
breadfruit (panapén)	
yam (ñame)	

Viandas are usually eaten twice daily, although consumption has decreased because of price. They are boiled whole or in large pieces and served with oil and vinegar; they are often served with salt codfish or meat, boiled, as a one-dish meal. Frying viandas in thin slices for serving with meat is a popular cooking method in middle income and prosperous homes. Tostones are slices of plantain, fried, flattened and refried.

Methods of Cooking

Puerto Rican foods are largely cooked on top of the stove: boiling, simmering, stewing or frying. In very low income families, in rural areas only, cooking is sometimes done over an open fire.

Preferences within Food Groups

Meat, fish, poultry, eggs

chicken: the meat most frequently used in low income homes but it is favored by all income groups and the intake is increasing.

Meat: liked very much especially pork but all meat is used sparingly in low-income rural homes due to cost. Consumption of meat has increased significantly especially since the start of the government food stamp program.

Eggs: well-liked, sometimes home produced. They are used frequently by all income groups, the amount varying with the economic status of the family.

Fish: dry salted codfish is popular but consumption is curtailed by price; fresh fish and shell fish consumption is on the increase.

Legumes (granos): red kidney beans are preferred. Chick peas (garbanzos), navy beans, pigeon peas (gandules), and dried peas are used but less frequently.

Milk   Milk is well liked. Two to three cups are reported as daily intake, the quantity varying with the family income. Per capita consumption is increasing. Cheese and fresh, evaporated and powdered milk forms are used. Much of the milk is used in coffee and in cocoa and chocolate drinks. The coffee is made by adding a small amount of strong coffee brew or concentrate (tinta) to a cup of hot milk. Traditionally children were given café con leche (a few drops of tinta), and from it obtained most of their milk. In recent years there has been a shift from coffee to cocoa and chocolate drinks for children. Children drink plain milk or cocoa with milk with their school lunch.

Vegetables

Tomato: most commonly used vegetable in Puerto Rico, eaten largely as tomato sauce.

Viandas: used as starchy vegetables before they ripen. Unripe bananas and plantain are preferred varieties. Other kinds used frequently include sweet potatoes, ripe plantain, white yam, breadfruit and white tanier. White potato consumption is on the increase. White sweet potatoes are preferred to yellow because they do not disintegrate in boiling. Typical additions made to viandas are: codfish, meat, avocado, hard boiled eggs, and onions.

Calabaza: a yellow vegetable—a type of squash—is used extensively but in small amounts, as in preparation of soups and stews.

Other vegetables: green beans, lettuce, cabbage, green peas, whole kernel corn, carrots, okra and beets are eaten commonly but "greens" are used very little. Locally produced and imported canned and frozen vegetables are used increasingly.

Fruits   Home-grown tropical fruits are often available for the picking or at small cost; all are important sources of vitamin C.

The acerola (a West Indian cherry): very concentrated source of vitamin C.

Citrus fruits: oranges, grapefruit, and tangerines are grown in Puerto Rico and large amounts are also imported.

Other fruits: bananas, papaya, mangoes, guava, and pineapples all are grown on the island. Imported canned and frozen fruits and juices are highly esteemed in Puerto Rico. Amounts consumed are on the rise.

Cereals

White rice (arroz blanco): preferred to other rice. It must be enriched with thiamin, niacin and iron according to Puerto Rican law. In preparing rice dishes, other foods sometimes added are: legumes, sausage, chicken and codfish. Several gourmet dishes in Puerto Rico are made with rice and chicken, such as asopao.

Wheat flour: used largely in the form of bread, crackers, spaghetti and macaroni. Consumption of wheat products is on the rise as vianda consumption declines.

Cornmeal: cooked into a mush with milk; sometimes served as a substitute for rice.

Oatmeal: well-liked, served as a breakfast food, always cooked with milk.

Fats Oil is used in serving viandas and in salad dressings. Solid fats and oils are used liberally in cooking rice and for frying many foods.

Sweets Desserts are not necessarily a part of regular meals in Puerto Rico. Typical desserts for festive occasions may be made with fruits cooked in syrup or rice cooked with or without coconut milk, and with sugar and spices. Coconut milk is an ingredient of certain favorite desserts, such as bien mesabe. Sugar is used liberally in coffee, chocolate, cocoa, fruit drinks, and synthetic beverages.

Beverages Consumption of soft drinks, colas, refrescos de frutas, beer and other alcoholic beverages has increased greatly in recent years. Malt beer is a favorite drink for women and children. It is often given to lactating women in the erroneous belief that it induces milk production; it is sometimes given to children to increase weight. The basic brew used in café con leche is made from a mocha variety of coffee. It is a dark roast and finely ground so that the infusion made is very concentrated. It has a distinctive flavor unlike that of the coffee blends on the mainland.

Seasonings Garlic, onion and vinegar are preferred. Sofrito—a sauce made by sauteing chopped tomato, onion, garlic, coriander, bits of smoked ham and salt pork and green pepper, in fat—is used as the basis of flavor in much Puerto Rican cooking. It is usually colored with annato seed (achiote) or tomato sauce. Commercial versions of sofrito are being used in urban areas.

II FOOD PROBLEMS OF PUERTO RICAN-AMERICANS IN MAINLAND CITIES OF THE UNITED STATES

In Buying

in allocating food money when all food must be purchased and when the amount of money is limited.

in making the food money cover a satisfactory diet when traditional foods (such as preferred kinds of viandas and beans) are disproportionately high in price.

in learning to buy foods in season. Puerto Ricans on the island are accustomed to fresh, homegrown oranges much of the year. Frozen juices are very popular. Canned orange juice is not a favorite but other canned juices are well liked. The latter should be enriched to ensure vitamin C content.

In Making Substitutions

Puerto Ricans have a strong preference for their traditional foods and do not accept substitutes easily. For example, many reject pumpkin or yellow winter squash as a substitute for calabaza. Canned tomatoes are reluctantly used in place of fresh ones, even when the latter are out of season. Mainland coffee is not wholly accepted even when their preferred brand is costly.

In Meal Planning

The time schedule for meals may be disrupted in the city if the home-maker works outside her home. The character of meals may change to a heavier meal in the evening when the husband has noon lunch at work. These changes tend to bring about alterations in the number of home meals and in the choice of foods and may result in no planned meal at noon. It is possibly significant that Puerto Rican-American teenagers, with working mothers, ingested less vitamin C and iron and ate fewer times per day than those whose mothers did not work outside.*

In Food Preparation

Many traditional Puerto Rican dishes require long preparation and cooking. This presents a problem for homemakers on the mainland who take jobs outside their homes. Puerto Ricans in small towns on the island are accustomed to coming home for hot meals, and any curtailment of this practice is often a hardship.

Retail meats are cut differently on the mainland than in Puerto Rico. Homemakers have difficulty in identifying cuts that they can use in their preferred dishes.

Variations in recipes for preparing native dishes, such as beans, are not usually acceptable to Puerto Ricans. They do not care for bean dishes without sofrito. Rice must be prepared so that it is not "mushy"; rice prepared with milk is considered to be for sick people.

III SUGGESTIONS FOR ADAPTING TRADITIONAL PUERTO RICAN FOOD PATTERNS TO CITY ENVIRONMENTS ON THE MAINLAND

General Recommendations

Puerto Rican food customs should be respected. The basic diet is not adequate, but it needs relatively few additions to make it so.

Encourage Families

to retain their basic food pattern—beans, rice and viandas, but substitute white potatoes for viandas when latter are expensive.

to continue café con leche and other home-made milk drinks as a means of increasing milk intake.

to continue the custom of cooking cereals in milk.

---

* See reference, Chapter 1. (Duyff et al, J. Nutr. Ed. 1975) to use government food stamps to diversify meals and improve nutritional adequacy.

Suggested Additions

More deep yellow and deep green vegetables for iron and vitamin A. (Carrots and sweet potatoes may be used in part for the yellow viandas to which Puerto Ricans are accustomed.)

More citrus fruits and juices in inexpensive form for vitamin C, as well as nectars and juices of other fruits, enriched with vitamin C.

More milk for all and especially for children, to provide calcium and high quality protein. Dry skim milk can be used to reduce cost. Food demonstrations for reconstituting dry milk and for incorporating it dry into recipes are recommended.

Cereals that are enriched, especially rice and breakfast foods, for B vitamins and iron.

More white potatoes in place of pastas to provide vitamin C.

In general a more varied diet. Intake studies indicate that diversified diets supply nutrients often low in the restricted Puerto Rican diet.

Suggested Substitutions

Frequent use of raw vegetables, such as cabbage, in place of cooked forms.

Canned tomatoes for fresh tomatoes when the latter are out of season.

Low cost fish and economy cuts of meats for costlier ones. Food demonstrations to show representative fish and less expensive cuts of lean meats and methods of preparing them are recommended.

Discourage

Soft drinks, especially served to children at meal times as substitutes for milk.

High calorie–low nutrient snack foods, particularly starchy foods fried in fat.

Appendix C Mexican Diets

I CHARACTERISTICS OF NATIVE MEXICAN DIETS[1]

Staple Items of Diet in Home Land

Dry Beans	Basic source of protein Often eaten more than once daily Beans often combined with other foods and highly seasoned
Chili Peppers	Many kinds from mild to very hot Eaten as vegetable and as seasoning Used in main dish combinations and in sauces
Corn	Tortillas—thin, flat, unleavened bread, cooked on hot griddle Used as bread and as bread base for Mexican main dishes

Methods of Cooking

Most foods are stewed or fried in mixtures with other foods.

Preferences within Food Groups

Meat, Fish, Poultry, Eggs   Foods in this group are eaten sparingly except when income permits or foods are home-produced. They are rarely eaten as separate foods in meals. Small amounts of meat and chicken are combined with peppers and other foods in main dishes. Lack of adequate refrigeration has dictated a limited use of perishable foods.

Meat: beef is usually included in mixtures with chili peppers, seasoned with garlic. Various organ meats are used often. Pork is well liked and is sometimes substituted for beef. Rabbits are often grown for food.

Fish: eaten chiefly as part of religious ritual; sea foods are eaten near the coast.

Poultry: chickens are often grown for market and for home use.

Eggs: limited number eaten. Their flavor is extended by combining them with other foods such as in huevos con migas (small pieces of corn tortillas scrambled with egg).

Dry Legumes   Many kinds of dry beans (frijoles) are used. Pinto beans (red), calico beans, and garbanzos (chick peas) are favorites. Beans are boiled with seasonings and served as such; or, more often, cooked to the soft stage, mashed with hot fat, and simmered to medium thickness (fried beans). "Refried beans" are cooked by adding fried beans to hot fat in a pan and frying them until the fat is completely absorbed.

---

[1] The traditional dishes, food preferences, customary methods of cooking, and meal habits of Mexicans in their native land are described here first as background for understanding food problems of migrants when they arrive in cities of the United States. The information is intended chiefly as a baseline for those persons helping Mexican-Americans to achieve a satisfactory diet built around the best of their native food practices. Some of the food problems encountered by the migrants are indicated, and possible ways to approach their solution are considered briefly.

474

Milk Fresh milk is not a common beverage in Mexico. It is scarce in some areas, and refrigeration is often inadequate to care for it. Evaporated milk is used, particularly for infants. Recipes call for little milk in cooking. Cheese is well liked and is used more often than milk. Native cheese is a low-fat, fine-curd variety resembling cottage cheese. A hot, sweet, chocolate drink made with milk is flavored with cinnamon, coffee, vanilla and nutmeg.

Vegetables

Chili peppers: as a group, the most widely used vegetable in the Mexican diet. There are many kinds of peppers; they range from the large varieties mild in flavor, to the small, hot varieties. Peppers are used whole, chopped, mashed, or dried and ground as chili powder.

Tomatoes: mostly added to prepared foods; stewed tomatoes and tomato puree are used frequently, especially in meat and chili combinations and in basic chili sauces. Fresh tomatoes are sometimes served in salads with lettuce.

Lettuce: used shredded in small amounts in such dishes as tacos.

Wild greens: eaten in rural areas of Mexico.

Fruits Commonly Available Bananas, papayas, chayotes (cactus-like fruit), mangos, oranges, tangerines, and grapes are available in Mexico, eaten between meals usually.

Cereals

Corn: traditionally has been the basic cereal. Corn is used to prepare masa—a mixture of dried corn that has been soaked in lime water, then washed and worked into a stiff dough. Masa is the dough from which tortillas are made.

Tortillas are thin, flat, unleavened bread made of corn (corn tortillas) or wheat (flour tortillas). Wheat is replacing lime-treated corn in making tortillas, thus reducing somewhat the calcium content of diets.

Tacos consist of corn tortillas folded in half with a filling of seasoned ground beef, then fried on both sides. They may be seasoned with onion, garlic, oregano, chili sauce. Grated white cheese and shredded lettuce may be sprinkled over the filling (called a cold sandwich).

Enchiladas are rolled tortillas with a filling of grated cheese and chopped onion, served with sauce made from chili and topped with grated cheese (called a hot sandwich).

Tamales are corn dough (masa) spread on corn husks. Spicey ground meat, or other filling, is placed in the center, the husks are rolled and tied, then they are steamed until the filling is thoroughly cooked.

Tamale sauce is made with red chilis and spices.

Posole is hominy stew, made by simmering corn, pork, red beans and red chilis.

Fats Most Mexican foods are fried. Many food mixtures such as fried and re-fried beans have large amounts of fat added to the recipe. Lard is a popular fat.

Sweets   Desserts traditionally are not a major item in the Mexican diet. Sweetened soft drinks have made inroads however. "Pan dulce" is a crisp sweet roll popular in middle and upper-income families.

Seasonings   Much Mexican food is highly seasoned. Spices often overshadow the food flavor. Hot chili peppers of many kinds are used to season specific foods, and onion, garlic, oregano, and salt are used routinely.

Beverages   Black coffee, heavily sweetened, is used by families, often including the children. Pulque, the fermented juice of the maguey (a cactus plant) with a low alcoholic content, is used in some areas. Bottled soft drinks and sweetened powders for making home made drinks, along with many other snack foods, have affected traditional eating patterns.

Transition to US Scene

Food practices of Mexican-Americans vary greatly depending on:

How long they have lived north of the border and how far they live from the border (accessibility of native foods). How interested they are in maintaining their identity with Mexico and their traditional food habits often varies with the ages of the migrants.

In many cases migrants make few changes in the family diet. Staple foods of Mexican-Americans of low or marginal income continue to be beans and tortillas. As they can afford more, they add meat, eggs, fruits and vegetables. Even migrants of two or three generations retain some of the traditional dishes along with the new, thus achieving a mixture. As an example, with respect to bread, a family might have toast for breakfast, bread sandwiches for lunch and tortillas for the evening meal. Gradually migrants tend to assume food practices of the area where they live.

Circumstances dictate change. Modern competitive foods—processed and carry-out items—are available and eaten regularly despite their high prices. Such traditional dishes as corn tortillas, tamales and enchiladas are made less frequently in homes and now are largely enjoyed on special occasions. The daily use of soft drinks and fried snack foods further distorts the dietary pattern and takes the money needed for meat, milk, vegetables and fruit required to make the diet adequate.

II FOOD PROBLEMS OF MEXICAN-AMERICANS IN CITIES OF THE UNITED STATES

Limited Income, Higher Prices

The high cost of foods tends to limit the amounts and kinds that can be bought, and the cost of fuel prevents long cooking of some native foods, such as beans. Accustomed foods are often unavailable (particularly certain kinds of peppers), except in neighborhood grocery stores where prices may be prohibitive.

Working Mothers

Children may be left to shift for themselves for meals. Working mothers have insufficient time to prepare traditional foods.

Changes in Character of Diet in the New Location

Often there are more sweets. Candy, sweet beverages and sweet rolls replace more nutritious foods. French fries and other deep-fat fried foods add to fat content of diet. If families shift from lime-treated corn tortillas to wheat flour tortillas, the calcium content of the diet is reduced.

Nutritional Bases for Making Better Food Choices

Milk vs soft drinks as sources of calcium and other nutrients

Citrus fruit vs other fruits as source of vitamin C

Chili peppers—fresh and canned vs dried, powdered chili as sources of vitamin C

White potatoes vs pastas as source of vitamin C and other nutrients

Whole grain and enriched cereals vs milled, unenriched cereals for B vitamins and iron

Leafy green and deep yellow vegetables vs others, for vitamin A.

III SUGGESTIONS FOR ADAPTING TRADITIONAL MEXICAN FOOD PATTERNS TO CITY ENVIRONMENT IN THE UNITED STATES

Retain Basic Food Pattern

Beans, chili peppers, and dishes made of corn can serve as the nucleus of a varied diet.

Encourage moderate increases in amounts of economical cuts of lean meats in fillings for tacos.

Endorse continued use of beans as economical alternate sources of protein.

Retain tortillas as a basic bread source; discourage regular use of sweet rolls.

Encourage continued use of organ meats.

Retain habit of limiting desserts.

Desirable substitutions

Fresh and canned chili peppers for dried and powdered forms, for vitamin C.

Bell peppers for chili peppers when latter not available or too expensive.

Milk for soft drinks, especially for children.

Broiled and baked foods for fried foods.

Fruit for concentrated sweets.

Low-fat milk for whole milk, if weight control is a problem.

Dry skim milk for fresh milk if price is an item.

Recommendations for Strengthening the Diet

Add dark green and deep yellow vegetables and red chilis to the diet to increase vitamin A content.

Include more wholegrain and enriched flour and cereals to increase iron and B vitamins.

Use more milk and cheese especially for calcium, riboflavin, high quality protein.

Add inexpensive sources of vitamin C, such as canned and frozen forms of citrus fruits and juices, canned tomatoes and raw vegetables, to supplement the contribution of chili peppers.

Use fewer fried foods, soft drinks and sweets.

Appendix D   Diets of Blacks

I CHARACTERISTICS OF DIETS OF BLACKS IN THE RURAL SOUTH*

Staple items of diet

> pork, fish, chicken
> sweet and white potatoes
> vegetable "greens"
> hot breads
> corn breads
> hominy grits

Methods of cooking

Frying is the preferred method for cooking meat, fish poultry, eggs and some breads and vegetables. White potatoes, sweet potatoes and whole corn are the vegetables usually fried. Stewing is used for some meat-vegetable combinations. Vegetables such as greens, cabbage, dried beans, green beans and blackeye peas are usually boiled for a long time with fat meat. The pot liquor (the liquid in which the greens are cooked) is often drunk or used in soups.

Preferences within Food Groups

Meat, fish, poultry, eggs   Foods in the meat group are popular. Preferred meats are those high in fat.

> Meat: pork: chops, roasts, spareribs, sausage, ham, bacon, fat back, "streak of lean," salt pork, hog jowls, pigs ears, tails, feet, maws, neck bones, ham hocks, chitterlings; beef: pot roast, hamburger, oxtails, organ meats; rabbit, squirrel, racoon, opossum, quail and other wild meat.

> Fish: catfish, buffalo, perch and other local fresh fish are popular. Canned fish including mackerel and sardines are used. Crabs, clams and crayfish are sometimes available. (Fresh fish is usually coated with cornmeal and fried).

> Poultry: chicken, turkey, goose, duck. Chicken, where plentiful, often serves as a budget dish. Regional preferences for methods of preparation: fried, stewed, smothered. Giblets and bony parts are used.

> Eggs: eaten frequently with sausage, bacon or other meat at breakfast.

Dry Legumes   Dry beans—navy, pinto and red kidney—are used. Boiling with fat meat is the preferred method of preparation. Peanuts are commonly eaten when grown locally. Canned legumes of various kinds are used.

Milk   Sweet milk and buttermilk are used sparingly. Evaporated milk is used especially in cities. Cheeses, including cottage cheese are used little. Ice cream is popular as a dessert and for snacks. (Soft drinks used by adults with meals and as snacks often contribute to low milk consumption.)

---

* Southern dishes and eating habits are described first in some detail as a basis for considering ways to help blacks who migrate from the rural South to industrial cities to adjust to new living conditions and yet retain many of their accustomed foods. Some of the food problems encountered by the migrants and possible ways to meet them are discussed briefly.

Vegetables Fresh vegetables, especially greens, are eaten in large quantity, particularly if homegrown, but home gardening is on the decline.

Greens: collards, mustard greens, turnip tops, kale, dandelion greens, spinach. They vary in popularity by region.

Starchy vegetables: sweet potatoes, yams, and white potatoes. Sweet potato, the most commonly used deep yellow vegetable, is baked, pan fried in lard or baked in sweet potato pie. White potatoes are fried or eaten in potato salad. Macaroni sometimes serves as a potato substitute.

Other vegetables: corn, blackeye peas (cow peas) in fresh form, green peas, lima beans, snap beans, okra, rutabagas, cabbage, turnips, tomatoes, cucumbers, radishes are eaten routinely; carrots and winter squash used little.

Raw vegetables and salads: not popular.

Fruits Homegrown and wild fruits are popular. Raw fruit is eaten chiefly as snacks and total fruit consumption is generally low. Citrus fruit is eaten where the fruit is locally grown. Bananas, watermelon and other melons, figs and peaches are especially liked.

Cereals

Wheat flour (white) is used to make biscuits. They are baked or fried, and often eaten for breakfast. White loaf bread (yeast) is used more in cities than elsewhere.

Cornmeal is used for making cornbreads. Variations are many: corn-pone, hoe cake and hush puppies. Cornbreads are baked or fried. White cornmeal is preferred to yellow cornmeal in many areas. Hominy grits, made from corn and seasoned with butter or other fat, are served at breakfast along with egg, bacon or sausage.

Rice is served as a vegetable in place of white potatoes in some areas where it is grown commercially.

Other cereals include oatmeal and wheat products, dry or cooked, and often eaten with milk and sugar. Pancakes with syrup are eaten for breakfast.

Fats Salt pork and other fat meats are sometimes fried and eaten as a main dish. They are also boiled with vegetables. Drippings from frying fat meats, ham, or bacon, are served on vegetables. Lard and drippings are used for preparing breads and for cooking vegetables.

Sweets Molasses, sorghum and sugar cane are used as well as syrups, sugars, jellies, pies, cakes and other sweet desserts. Candy and soft drinks are often bought even on very low budgets. Fried pies are common in some areas.

Beverages Bottled soft drinks of all kinds are consumed liberally throughout the south. Lemonade, sweetened ice tea, and drinks made from sweetened powders are popular. Fruit juices are consumed in quantity in some areas.

Seasonings Fat pork cuts cooked with vegetables serve as seasoning; catsup, gravies, and meat drippings are used regularly.

Soul Foods Certain foods traditionally enjoyed by southern blacks and "southern" foods prepared in special ways are known as "soul foods." Such foods are associated with enjoyment of home and family, with comfort and emotional satisfaction. As blacks migrate to cities, soul foods are important in creating a familiar atmosphere in the new environment. The use of soul foods is thus to be encouraged, for they are chiefly nutritious foods that have long been the mainstay of the southern diet of blacks. There is some disagreement as to just which foods classify as "soul," but some are unquestioned. These include: chitterlings (chitlins), pigs feet, knuckles, tails and ears; black-eye peas; "greens" of many types; cornbread and homemade biscuits; and squirrel. Chicken is soul food if it is highly seasoned and fried in bacon fat. Pork chops are soul food when coated with seasoned flour and fried in a liberal amount of shortening.

Meal Patterns

Families are accustomed to two meals a day, with a snack in between or in place of supper if dinner is eaten at noon. Soft drinks are usually included in the meals of adults. Breakfast is commonly a substantial meal with eggs, bacon or sausage and toast. In general, meals are limited in the number of items served and the variety—usually one or two foods with bread. Cornbread and greens is a favorite combination but one that calls for the addition of a protein food. Snacks consist of the various types of beverages described above as well as the wide range of "junk" foods available.

Buying Patterns

Food is purchased in neighborhood stores and in supermarkets, the latter mainly in industrial areas.

II FOOD PROBLEMS OF BLACKS FROM THE RURAL SOUTH WHO MOVE TO INDUSTRIAL CITIES

Change in Pattern of Living

Move from house to apartment; no place for a garden.

Apartment far from employment; transportation problems; meal patterns disrupted.

Inadequate storage space for foods which could well be bought in quantity.

No facilities for processing fresh foods for later use.

Often shift from role of producer-consumer to consumer only: involves frequent shopping; managing cash expenditure; dealing with inaccessibility of stores.

Difficulty of Maintaining Traditional Food Practices for Health, for Satisfaction, and for Sense of Security

Cost of all foods often higher.

Favorite foods, particularly fresh greens, are expensive, unavailable, or inferior in quality to their homegrown product.

Difficult to maintain family meal schedules; members separated by distance, working hours.

Meal disruption results in problem of serving foods and combinations which have special meaning for family members.

Competition with multiple sources of ready-prepared foods at pick-up stations, with their added cost; fried foods, sandwiches, hamburgers and hot dogs.

Ready availability of sweetened beverages of all types and the general acceptance of their universal use.

Constant attraction to the endless number of crisp fried foods and concentrated sweets which compete for the migrant's food dollar.

The combination of interfering forces provide serious problems in maintaining adequate diets.

III SUGGESTIONS FOR ADAPTING TRADITIONAL SOUTHERN FOOD PATTERN TO CITY ENVIRONMENT

Retain Basic Food Pattern

Urge the continued use of greens, corn and meat with modifications, especially toward leanness in meats. (greens are a rich source of vitamin A and iron)

Advise the use of frozen greens when the fresh form is of poor quality and expensive; have a kitchen garden when possible; continue to use pot liquor for drinking and for cooking.

Encourage economy cuts of lean meats; advise fish and poultry as alternates for fat meats; use less fat meats for seasoning.

Use whole-grain and enriched forms of cornmeal and other cereals, for iron, B vitamins.

Retain traditional southern dishes and menu patterns, including a substantial breakfast.

Desirable Substitutions

Raw vegetables for some of the cooked vegetables, to increase vitamin C.

Potatoes for pastas, to increase vitamin C.

Vegetables cooked a short time, instead of those cooked long with fat meat.

Lean meats and poultry for some of the fat meats.

Baked and broiled foods for some of the fried foods.

Fruit juices for soft drinks and kool-ades.

General Upgrading of Diet

More milk for the family, especially for mothers and children. (displace soft drinks at meal time). Vitamin D milk is important; inexpensive forms of milk should be encouraged. Low-fat milk especially desirable for weight control.

Fruits and fruit juices (especially citrus in economical forms) as sources of vitamin C.

Legumes, peanut butter and organ meats as good sources of protein.

Calorie limitation with fewer fried foods and less fat in cooking.

Appendix E
American Indian Diets*

I EATING PATTERNS OF AMERICAN INDIANS ON RESERVATIONS[1]

SOUTHWEST INDIANS**
Basic Diet

Dry pinto beans, chili peppers, stews.

Cereals, both cooked and dry, oven bread, "fry" bread and tortillas, made from white enriched flour.

Meat eaten regularly, in varying amounts depending on whether they have flocks and the economic situation.

In general, with improved transportation and availability of food from various sources in the region, Indian diets are becoming similar to those of the general population at the same economic level. Likewise, certain foods and dishes of the Indians are being adopted by the general population.

Variations in Eating Patterns

While many of the same basic foods are commonly used by Indians throughout the Southwest, quantities differ and food practices vary from region to region, from tribe to tribe and from family to family. Conditions cited above have tended to narrow such differences and in the main, similarities have become greater. It seems permissable therefore to offer certain conservative generalizations of food habit patterns, with exceptions noted when distinctive differences exist between tribes.

Customary Uses within Food Groups

Animal Sources

Beef, pork, mutton, lamb, chicken, lunch meat, canned meat, bacon, canned tuna and sardines are foods in the meat category commonly eaten; Navajos are partial to mutton. Stew meat and ground meat are bought frequently. Meat, for economy reasons, is often combined in

---

* Dorothy M. Porter, Assistant Nutrition and Dietetics Consultant, Billings Area Office, Indian Health Service, rendered invaluable service in collecting the information on Indian food habits. She served as liaison to the authors in assembling from her colleagues, who are also working directly with Indians in different areas of the United States, reports which served as the basis for Appendix E.

[1] Customary foods, food preferences, methods of cooking, and meal patterns are presented for Indian tribes on reservations in three geographic areas. This information is intended as background for persons seeking to help migrant Indians, from different areas, retain the best of their traditional food customs while adapting to new situations in cities. Some of the food problems that confront the migrants and ways they may be approached are considered briefly.

** The following specialists reported on the food patterns of Indians on reservations in the *Southwest*: Patricia F. Roseleigh, Chief Nutrition and Dietetics Branch, Navajo Area Indian Health Service, Window Rock, Arizona; Hazelle N. Walker, Chief Nutrition and Dietetics Branch, Phoenix Area Indian Health Service; and Margaret Ann McCarthy, Chief Nutrition and Dietetics Branch, Albuquerque Area Indian Health Service (Pueblos). Miss McCarthy compiled contributions from: Viola Fisher, Public Health Nutritionist, Santa Fe; Sarah Lujan, Nutrition Technician, Santa Fe Service Unit; Margaret Blackman, Director of Dietetics, and Pat Mead, Clinic Dietitian, Albuquerque Public Health Service Hospital.

small amounts with other foods. Organ meats are liked and eaten when available. Horse meat is seldom used; canned meat has largely replaced it. Chicken and eggs are favorites, eaten frequently. Venison, rabbit and other game and fowl may be included when available. Venison is often dried in strips as jerky.

Milk. When milk is used as a beverage, fresh milk is the choice. Canned milk occasionally is added to coffee, and nonfat dry milk is sometimes an ingredient in making oven bread and tortillas. Yellow cheese is used in cooking and for sandwiches.

Bread and Cereals

Blue or white cornmeal is cooked in water and served as gruel or mush, or is fried. The Hopi grow white, yellow, blue and red corn.

White flour tortillas, home baked oven bread, bakery bread, corn bread and fry bread are regular diet items. The Apaches use no oven bread. The Hopi use Piki bread, usually made from blue cornmeal. It is baked in large tissue-thin sheets and rolled up like a newspaper.

Rice, macaroni and spaghetti are combined with other foods in preparing main dishes. Rice is sometimes used in desserts.

Vegetables

Dry pinto beans are used liberally in family meals but less consistently than previously. This change is particularly true of the Pueblos. Navajos eat less of the beans in summer because of the long cooking time required by their high elevation.

White potatoes are a staple of the diet. They are fried, boiled or used in potato salad.

Red and green chili peppers are eaten in large amounts by many Southwest Indians. Green peppers are not used in quantity by the Navajos. Apaches make limited use of chilies.

Onions, hominy, corn, squash, pumpkin, tomatoes, celery, green beans, green peas, carrots, spinach and cabbage, are used commonly. They are usually fresh or canned, some raw. The Navajos prefer cabbage cooked.

When available, wild vegetables are gathered for food: celery, spinach, asparagus and onions.

Fruits

Melons are enjoyed in abundance in season.

Also in season, apples, oranges and bananas are used.

Eaten too are dried fruits and canned fruits, particularly peaches and fruit cocktail.

Nuts

Piñon nuts, and roasted sunflower and pumpkin seeds are eaten.

Fats   Lard and vegetable shortening serve in frying foods and in making breads and tortillas. Margarine, butter and peanut butter are used as spreads.

Sweets   Consumption of cakes, cookies, candies, jams, jellies, syrups, sweet rolls, doughnuts and ice cream is increasing; jello and sweetened canned fruits are sometimes served as dessert.

Beverages Coffee, tea, soft drinks, artificially flavored sweet drinks and fruit drinks are used frequently. Non-dairy creamers are often added to coffee. Powdered orange drink is served by some families.

Seasonings Indian salt (a coarse salt obtained from a local lake) is collected and used.

Snacks Snacks are popular. They include most of the foods listed above under sweets and beverages with the addition of pop corn, beer, potato chips, corn chips and wine.

Additional Sources of Food Families may have small gardens, particularly if, as in the case of the Pueblos, they can irrigate. Produce grown consists mainly of beans, melons, corn, squash, potatoes and pumpkins. Some have fruit trees that contribute to the food supply. The Federal Food Stamp Program is available and benefits many families.

Tribal Celebrations

On the day a deer is killed, the Pueblos cook the entire head and serve it as a stew with beans, corn, piñon nuts, pumpkin seeds, watermelon seeds; red or green chili can be added.

Some of the other foods traditionally served by Pueblos on special occasions are: Indian pie (flat fruit pie), tamales (corn meal and meat stuffed in corn husk), chili balls (ground meat and chili), dortas (beaten egg whites and yolks mixed with flour, fried and cooked in chili sauce).

Methods of Cooking

Food is boiled, stewed or fried on top of stove. Frying is the most common form of cooking among many Indians. Oven bread is baked in an outdoor beehive oven. Meat and potatoes are frequently fried together.

(Refrigeration and freezing facilities vary greatly but both are on the increase.)

Nutritive Values

The calorie value of Indian diets is probably adequate in most cases. Protein intake may be low when income is limited and lean meat, pinto beans and other protein sources are available in inadequate amounts.

Iron intake would probably be low in cases of protein shortage unless green leafy vegetables, and whole grain and enriched cereals were used liberally.

Calcium intake is undoubtedly low due to limited milk consumption, particularly among adults. Moderate use of cheese increases the calcium intake somewhat.

The levels of vitamins A and C may vary from season to season depending on the selection of fruits and vegetables. Vitamin A intake may be low when red pepper consumption is low. This situation calls for larger amounts of green leafy and deep yellow vegetables.

Vitamin C is probably adequate during seasons when green peppers, citrus fruits and certain melons are available. Large quantities of white potatoes furnish a moderate year-round source of vitamin C.

Basic Diet

Traditional foods of Plains Indians were: meat—buffalo, elk, antelope, and many smaller game, which were eaten in large quantities; a wide range of wild greens, roots and seeds; and wild fruits, berries and rose hips. With the disappearance of the buffalo, the establishment of and confinement of people to Indian reservations, and the extensive loss of river bottom land in connection with water control programs, sources of wild foods became limited.

At present, Plains Indians depend largely on foods purchased at grocery stores. Government commodities are being rapidly replaced by the Federal Food Stamp Program.

Staple purchases include: meat, potatoes, onions, macaroni, rice, flour, bread, breakfast foods, coffee, bakingpowder, salt, lard, bacon, fat back and sugar. Increasing amounts of fresh meats are available, and fresh fruits and vegetables are obtainable, particularly in season.

A Day's Meals Might Include:

Breakfast
Cereal, hot or cold (younger generation)
Fried meat, potatoes (older generation)
Coffee (canned milk sometimes is added)
Sugar
(Weekend breakfast may provide hot cakes, eggs.)

Lunch
Meat: hamburger, hot dogs
Potatoes, fried
Vegetables—canned corn is popular
Bread with margarine or butter
Beverage: coffee or tea
(in summer—ice tea, kool ade)

Quick Lunch
Canned soup with
Crackers or bread
or
Soup and sandwich

Evening meal
Meat: roast, stew, steak or pork chops
Potatoes, boiled
Vegetables (infrequently served)
Bread
Beverage: coffee or tea

School Lunch

A nutritious lunch is provided children at school but if they do not like the menu they often purchase hamburgers, french-fries and soft drinks, from local quick-service restaurants.

Between Meals

Children frequently purchase snacks, which include candy, pop and chips.

Tribal Celebrations

On important occasions, various foods and combinations are customarily served. They might include, for example:

⋆ The following specialists contributed information on the diets of Indians in Plains areas: Dorothy M. Porter, Assistant Nutrition and Dietetics Consultant, Billings Area Office, Indian Health Service; and Minna Gutsch, Chief, Nutrition and Dietetics Branch, Aberdeen Area Office, Indian Health Service.

Cheyenne Celebration: boiled meat, potato salad, fry bread, crackers, apples, oranges; *Fort Peck* Reservation Celebration (Assiniboine and Sioux tribes): beef steak or soup with short ribs (macaroni and tomato added to soup) fry bread, cake, sweet rolls, coffee or tea.

Customary Uses Within Food Groups

Animal Sources

Meat is usually eaten regularly. The quantity tends to increase when Indians raise their own animals and when game is available.

Meat (beef or venison) may be dried in thin strips called jerky. When such meat is pulverized by pounding and mixed with acid fruits (such as choke cherries or buffalo berries), fat and sugar, and molded into small patties, it is called pemmican or wasna. This mixture may be stored for future use. Modern wasna is made with corn meal as a substitute for some or all of the meat.

Soup or stew meat and ground beef are forms bought especially by those with limited means. Soup is a popular main dish; it is often made with short ribs or dried meat, potatoes, rice, or macaroni and canned mixed vegetables.

Bologna, pork chops, chicken, liver, kidney, tripe and heart are also used.

Fresh milk, eggs, and cheese are available in grocery stores, but are not used universally except by families on the federally funded food program WIC (Women, Infants, Children), which provides these and certain other designated foods.

Some use is made of evaporated milk. Nonfat dry milk, reconstituted as a beverage, is not generally well accepted.

Bread and Cereals

Dry breakfast foods and those to be cooked are consumed routinely.

White bread is eaten in quantity. Fry bread—a dough fried in fat— sweet rolls, and doughnuts are favorites. Homemakers sometimes use powdered milk mixed with flour in making dough for fry bread.

Wheat flour, rice, oatmeal and corn meal are the chief cereal forms. Plains Indians of Oklahoma customarily use more corn meal than those of the north.

Vegetables

Potatoes (in soups or fried) and onions are eaten in quantity. Canned corn, peas, green beans, tomatoes, canned pork and beans, fresh cabbage and carrots are used. Amounts of vegetables eaten vary widely with families. There is a general dislike for non-starchy vegetables and little use of them among the older generation of Indians.

Fruits

Wild choke cherries, plums, berries, and rose hips are still used by some to make wajapi. Raisins are used by others. The fruits are often ground and dried and later cooked with suet, sugar and flour or cornstarch to form a soft pudding, that is eaten with fry bread.

Apples, oranges and bananas are often available in stores. Canned peaches and fruit cocktail are popular. Watermelon is a favorite fruit.

Beverages   Coffee, tea, soft drinks and artificially-flavored sweetened drinks are consumed universally.

Sweets   All kinds of sweets are enjoyed and eaten in large amounts. Candy is a favorite with children. The demand for preserves, jams, jellies and pancake syrup is increasing.

Methods of Cooking

Foods, for the most part, are fried or boiled indoors on a stove or outdoors on an open fire.

Nutritive Values

There are numerous variables in the diets of Plains Indians due to personal taste, income, seasonal availability of food, reservation food programs and the availability of wild life (deer, fish, fowl) and wild fruits and vegetables.

In general, diets on the reservations have a base of meat, potatoes and bread. They are also high in fats, cereals, sugar and coffee; low in non-starchy vegetables, fruits and milk. They are high in meat, except when cost and availability prevent. Such diets are usually adequate in calories but can be inadequate or marginal in minerals and vitamins and sometimes in protein. Calcium, iron and vitamins A and C are probably the nutrients most often deficient.

The WIC Program has improved the intake of milk, fruit juices, eggs and enriched cereals in the families it serves. Improvement is undoubtedly due to increased nutritional counseling provided the families, as well as the foods supplied.

The Federal Government is moving from commodity-donated programs to Food Stamps, a step which should lead to diversity in food selection and perhaps to diets higher in nutritive values.

Woodlands Indians*

Basic Diet

Traditional foods of the Woodlands Indians were: game and fish, wild fruits and berries, greens and roots, wild rice and nuts. Some of these foods are still available but, for the most part, in reduced amounts. Even if an Indian family spent long hours in gathering, preserving and storing them, there would not be enough to cover all family needs.

Indians of the Woodlands areas have traditionally raised corn, beans and squash. Many still have small gardens where they grow a variety of vegetables. Some Indians can fruits and vegetables, rather than drying them as formerly. Some have freezers.

More and more Woodlands Indians have come to depend on the grocery store for their food supplies. The staples purchased most include: flour, salt, meat, potatoes, dry beans, oatmeal, shortening and baking powder.

---

* The following persons contributed information on the diets of Woodlands Indians: Carolyn Kay, Public Health Nutritionist, Bemidji Area Office, Indian Health Service; Father Peter Powell, Director, St. Augustine's Indian Center, Chicago; and Vahide Özbayer in her M.S. thesis "Food Intake and Dietary Patterns of the Winnebago Indians in Wood County, Wisconsin" (University of Wisconsin, Stevens Point), 1975.

Customary Uses within Food Groups

Animal Sources   Meat is an important article of the diet.

Beef, particularly in ground form and boiling beef are purchased most often.

Organ meats are well liked.

Canned beef and luncheon meats are also used.

Chicken, both fresh and canned, is a favorite.

Fresh fish are available in most lakes and streams. Canned fish is purchased.

Many families still add a bear or a deer to their winter larder, as well as smaller game animals and game birds.

Eggs are used; cheese is eaten to some extent.

Milk is consumed in limited amounts and in different forms, mostly as homogenized milk. Some evaporated milk is used; nonfat dry milk is better accepted than formerly.

Breads and Cereals

White Indian corn is raised and used for corn soup and hominy. Wild rice is gathered in sections where it is grown. Some is sold.

Oatmeal is used in quantity; dry breakfast cereals, macaroni and spaghetti are also staples.

Fry bread, johnny cakes, and pancakes, originally made with cornmeal, are now largely made with white enriched flour.

White bakery bread, sweet rolls, doughnuts and coffee cakes are purchased.

Vegetables

Most vegetables that are grown or available in the area are used in varying amounts: corn, squash, beets, peas, green beans, tomatoes, asparagus, lettuce, carrots, and cabbage, both raw and cooked.

Some wild greens, particularly kalsa, milk weed, wild onions, and Indian macaroni (young fern sprouts) are still used.

Potatoes are eaten two to three times a day.

Dry beans, dry peas and onions are used in quantity.

Fruits   Many wild berries and fruits that grow in the woodlands area can still be gathered for food: blueberries, raspberries, strawberries, cranberries, gooseberries, plums, cherries, and crab apples. Apples, rhubarb and other locally grown fruits are eaten in season. Canned fruits are largely purchased.

Nuts   Wild nuts and squash seeds are eaten roasted.

Fats   Shortening is the most common fat. Butter, margarine, and peanut butter are used as spreads.

Sweets   Sugar, honey, and maple syrup (local) are favorite sweets.

Beverages   Coffee, tea, soft drinks, and artificially-flavored sweetened drinks, are the principal beverages.

Methods of Cooking

Frying and boiling are the principal methods of cooking.

Nutritive Values

The Woodlands Indian diet, at its best, is probably nutritionally adequate or nearly so. Possibilities for inadequacy include: A calcium shortage due to low-to-moderate milk intake, especially low among adults; a vitamin A shortage when consumption of dark green leafy and deep yellow vegetables is low; and a deficiency of vitamin C at seasons of the year when fruits are not readily available. However, the daily intake of potatoes by Woodlands Indians should make a real vitamin C shortage unlikely. When the diet is low in lean meat *and* in greens, the iron intake could be inadequate.

II FOOD PROBLEMS OF AMERICAN INDIANS WHO MIGRATE FROM THE RESERVATIONS TO CITIES

Money Management and Buying Food

The major problem of migrating Indians, regardless of tribe or of region from which they originate, is learning how to spend their food money in large markets or in neighborhood stores in a city.

All foods must be purchased. For the first time, many families find they cannot fall back on home garden produce, game, fish or wild fruits and vegetables to supplement their purchases. They must shop often, which in itself is a hardship. They have little or no storage space in city apartments which would permit them to buy food in quantity, and sometimes they have inadequate refrigeration.

Migrants are frustrated when their customary foods are unavailable or are unduly expensive. A problem for Navajos, for example, is in obtaining mutton in city markets that sell chiefly lamb. Problems are doubly difficult when the amount of money for food is small in relation to need.

Adjusting Food Habits in a New Environment

From Reservation to City: American Indians migrate to cities with food habits that largely reflect the eating practices of the geographical areas from which they come, and a few traditional Indian food cutoms.

It is impossible to generalize on the adjustments required to make their diets nutritionally adequate in the new environment. It may be said, however, that the *Woodlands Indians,* who have followed the traditional food patterns of their home lands, would probably be required to make the fewest changes. The *Southwest Indians* would need to add to their diets: milk and cheese, dark green leafy and deep yellow vegetables (especially in the case of low chili consumption), and more inexpensive year-round sources of vitamin C. The *Plains Indians,* in most cases, need general upgrading of their diets with a balanced intake of all protective foods and fewer sweets, cereals and fats. Some migrants are flexible enough to adjust quickly to new conditions. This is usually true of children. But for many the change is a slow, difficult process.

Health Importance of Food Habit Changes

An immediate problem is how to provide professional guidance in helping Indians select foods from those available in the new environment that will meet reasonable nutritional goals, yet be acceptable and satisfying to them.

A long-range problem concerns helping Indians relate food habits to health—to place emphasis on the *kinds* of foods chosen rather than primarily on quantity. The difficulty is greater when funds are limited and the primary goal is satisfying taste and hunger.

Day-to-Day Problems

Some Indians follow eating customs and cooking practices that tend to lower the nutritional level of their diets. For example, they may reject nonfat dry milk as a beverage because of its flavor, a practice that can seriously reduce the calcium content of low cost diets, often already low in milk.

Unenriched white flour is preferred by some Indians to the enriched product for making high quality tortillas and fry bread, thus reducing the intake of B vitamins and iron.

Food Stamps. Failure of many Indians to take advantage of the Federal Food Stamp Program and other food assistance programs, for which they may be eligible, makes it more difficult for them to obtain the quantity and variety of foods they need in order to maintain an adequate diet.

III SUGGESTIONS FOR ADAPTING INDIAN FOOD PATTERNS TO CITY ENVIRONMENT

Provide nutritional guidance, particularly for homemakers responsible for family meals. Focus consultation on specific needs of families and their individual members, as far as possible. The reports of food habits on the reservations, outlined above, provide the consultant with background dietary information of a general character. It does not take the place of food habit histories, which will still be necessary if families and individuals are to receive effective help. The suggestions that follow, are therefore offered with the understanding that they apply overall, not necessarily in individual cases.

Base guidance on cultural patterns of migrant Indians when they enhance the nutritive values of the diets. Encourage Indians to retain the best features of these patterns.

For Indians from the *Southwest,* this means: continued use of chili peppers in quantities to which they are accustomed, unless cost prevents this practice. In that case, more of other vegetables would be needed, especially of dark leafy green and deep yellow varieties, and fruits and fruit juices, in least expensive forms; continued use also of dry beans as a staple, along with small amounts of economy cuts of lean meat. There should be increased consumption of milk in its various forms; consistent use of wholegrain or enriched cereal products; and decreased intake of fats, sweets, and non-nutritious beverages.

Migrant Plains Indians should diversify their diets to include more nonstarchy vegetables, fruits and milk. They should continue their consumption of potatoes in liberal amounts, of nutritious soups, of lean meat in moderate amounts, and of their traditional Indian dishes, particularly those made with enriched cereals containing fruits. The use of fats and sweets should be kept under control.

Migrant Woodlands Indians should be urged to continue their liberal use of fish of the varieties available at reasonable price; to select moderate amounts of lean meats and dry legumes, to alternate with the fish; to continue to eat potatoes regularly; to use whole-grain and enriched breakfast foods, breads and other cereals; to choose a variety of vegetables, including cultivated greens to replace their wild greens and garden products; to buy fruits and juices in their least expensive forms; and to use nonfat dry milk in their recipes and as a beverage to increase milk consumption.

Nutrition Counseling for Indian Families in the City

Regardless of their regional origin or tribal differences, most Indian families are confronted with similar problems of food selection, buying, and meal practices when they reach the city. Summarized here are a few guidelines that would aid in achieving dietary improvement for most migrant Indians.

Dietary Content

Diversify family meals to include representation from the major food groups.

Continue the use of wholesome, traditional Indian dishes.

More milk in all forms, including cheese. Demonstrations of uses of nonfat dry milk should include many applications as well as that of beverage. Reconstituted dry milk, lightly flavored, may be more acceptable than plain. Urge milk in meals, instead of soft drinks.

Moderate amounts of economical cuts of lean meat. More dry beans when meat or fish is limited, due to cost. Use organ meats. Demonstrate cuts of meat and cooking methods.

More fresh vegetables in season, as well as canned and frozen vegetables. Use white potatoes often. Use fresh or canned chili peppers or fresh bell peppers, in place of dried or powered forms, to increase vitamin C. Use red chili peppers for vitamin A.

More tomatoes and citrus fruits in season, or as canned or frozen concentrates, for vitamin C (especially important to Southwest tribes if raw red or green peppers are not available).

Substitute: dry legumes for some of pasta and rice; enriched flour for unenriched; whole-grain and fortified breakfast cereals for those less nutritious.

Curtail heavy use of fats, sweets, and nonnutritious beverages.

Build educational procedures, in the city, on the nutritional instruction already provided Indians on the reservations. Encourage families to continue such basic practices as adding nonfat dry milk in making fry bread and flour tortillas.

Urge migrants to apply for benefits of the Federal Food Stamp Program and other food assistance programs for which they may be eligible, in order to make available more protective foods and thus help to balance potentially inadequate diets.

Provide instructions and aid in selecting foods under the Food Stamp Program, to achieve maximum results.

Discourage use of convenience foods. The younger generation is cooking less and taking short cuts which can result in less nutritious meals which cost more.

Give special attention to the snack problem. Indians come to the city with well developed snacking habits. Recommend snacks which contribute to the nutrient content of the day's intake, such as cheese, peanut butter, milk, fruit, nuts. Discourage high-calorie, low-nutrient snacks such as: potato chips, cookies, candies; and popular beverages including soft drinks and artificially-flavored sweetened beverages.

Appendix F
Equivalents in Weights and Measures with Abbreviations

Metric System		Customary System
1 milliliter (ml)	=	0.03 fluid oz
1 kilogram (kg)	=	2.20 pounds (lb)
1 kg = 1000 g		
1 g = 1000 milligrams (mg)		
1 mg = 1000 micrograms (μ)		
1 millimeter (mm)	=	0.04 inch (in)
1 centimeter (cm)	=	0.40 inch
1 cubic centimeter (cc)	=	0.06 inch
1 kilojoule (kjoule)	=	0.24 kilocalorie (kcal)

Customary System		Metric System
1 teaspoon (tsp)	=	5 ml
1 tablespoon (tbsp); 3 tsp	=	15 ml
1 cup (16 tbsp)	=	237 ml
1 pint (2 cup)	=	474 ml
1 quart (2 pt)	=	0.95 liter (L)
1 fluid ounce	=	29.6 ml
1 ounce	=	28.4 g
1 pound (16 oz)	=	454 g
1 inch	=	2.54 cm
1 cubic inch	=	16.40 cc
1 kilocalorie (kcal)	=	4.184 kilojoules (kjoule)

Appendix G
Metric Conversion Table

When you know:	Multiply by:	To find:
length & distance		
inches	25.0	millimeters
feet	30.0	centimeters
yards	0.9	meters
millimeters	0.04	inches
centimeters	0.4	inches
meters	1.1	yards
volume and capacity		
ounces (fluid)	30.0	milliliters
pints	0.47	liters
quarts	0.95	liters
milliliters	0.034	ounces (fluid)
liters	2.1	pints
liters	1.06	quarts
weight and mass		
ounces	28.0	grams
pounds	0.45	kilograms
grams	0.035	ounces
kilograms	2.2	pounds
temperature		
degrees Fahrenheit	5/9 (after subtracting 32)	degrees Celsius
degrees Celsius	9/5 (then add 32)	degrees Fahrenheit

Appendix H
Calculation of Specimen Diet

Based on sample day's meals, Chapter 4*

Meals	Amount of foods	Kilo-calories	Pro-tein g	Fat g	Cal-cium mg	Iron mg	Vita-min A IU	Thia-min mg	Ribo-flavin mg	Nia-cin mg	Ascorbic acid mg
breakfast											
doughnut	1	98	1	5	10	0.4	20	0.04	0.04	0.3	tr
coffee	1 cup										
sugar	2 tsp	31	0	0	0	tr	0	0	0	0	0
breakfast totals		129	1	5	10	0.4	20	0.04	0.04	0.3	tr
lunch											
hamburger on a	3 oz	186	23	10	10	3.0	20	0.08	0.20	5.1	—
bun, enriched	1 bun	119	3	2	30	0.8	tr	0.11	0.07	0.9	tr
pickle relish	1 tbsp	21	tr	tr	3	0.1	—	—	—	—	—
catsup, tomato	1 tbsp	16	tr	tr	3	0.1	210	0.01	0.01	0.2	2
mustard	1 tsp	4	tr	tr	4	0.1	—	—	—	—	—
onions, raw	2 green	14	tr	tr	12	0.2	tr	0.02	0.01	0.1	8
milk, whole	1 cup	159	9	9	288	0.1	350	0.07	0.41	0.2	2
lunch totals		519	35	21	350	4.4	580	0.29	0.70	6.5	12
dinner											
pork chop	2.7 oz	305	19	25	9	2.7	(0)	0.75	0.22	4.5	—
potato, mashed	½ cup	99	2	5	25	0.4	180	0.09	0.06	1.1	10
corn, canned	½ cup	87	3	1	3	0.6	370	(0.03)	(0.07)	(1.2)	6
coleslaw	¼ cup	30	tr	2	13	0.1	45	0.02	0.02	0.1	9
rolls, enriched,	2	168	4	4	40	1.0	tr	0.14	0.12	1.2	tr
butter or											
margarine	1 tbsp	102	tr	12	3	0	470	—	—	—	0
ice cream	1 slice	127	3	7	96	tr	290	0.03	0.14	0.1	1
cookies, choco-late chip	2	103	1	6	7	0.4	20	0.02	0.02	0.2	tr
dinner totals		1021	32	62	196	5.2	1375	1.08	0.65	8.4	26
snacks											
potato chips	10 chips	114	1	8	8	0.4	tr	0.04	0.01	1.0	3
cola-type drink	12 oz	144	(0)	(0)	—	—	(0)	(0)	(0)	(0)	(0)
snack totals		258	1	8	8	0.4	(0)	0.04	0.01	1.0	3
grand totals for day		1927	69	96	564	10.4	1975	1.45	1.40	16.2	41

Compare the grand totals for energy and all nutrients on the specimen diet with the RDA values for your own sex-age group.

*See Appendices F and J for keys to abbreviations and markings for the diet calculation.

Appendix I
Specimen Weight Chart

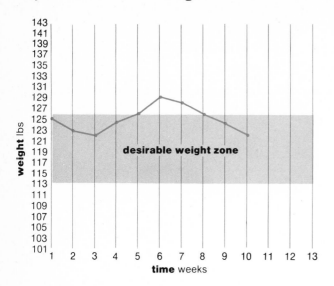

Appendix J
Background Material for Appendix K

Purpose, Source, Content, and Application of Food Values Table

Purpose of Table   Appendix K provides a tool for the study of nutrition. The table furnishes nutritive values for some 450 foods commonly eaten in the United States. Such values can be used in various ways indicated in the text, to evaluate the varied nutritive contributions of the foods listed.

Source of Data   The major source of composition data for Appendix K is the newly published official book:

> *Nutritive Value of American Foods In Common Units.* Agricultural Handbook, No. 456. Agricultural Research Service, U.S. Department of Agriculture, Washington, D.C. 1975.

The foods selected for Appendix K were largely taken from Table 1 of the handbook. Original nutritive values for foods in Handbook No. 456 were assembled by USDA from scientific laboratories throughout the United States, including those of the government.

Content of Table   Most of the wide variety of common foods in Appendix K are arranged in alphabetical order. Certain foods are grouped for easy reference, such as dark green leafy vegetables under "greens," various kinds of cookies under the general heading "cookies," and most alcoholic and nonalcoholic drinks under "beverages." Many items are cross-referenced to expedite the location of foods sought.

The first three columns (from the left) identify the foods. They give the weight of the unit, the amount, the form in which it is presented, and other descriptive information. Data for most foods are based on food ready for consumption: cooked meats, cooked vegetables, or raw fruits and vegetables if they are usually eaten that way. If foods are enriched or fortified, these facts are noted on the table. Ascorbic acid values given for canned fruit sauces, juices, and nectars are usually those naturally present in the fruit. (Manufacturers often add ascorbic acid to these products. Refer to labels on cans and bottles for information on individual products.)

Application of Table Contents

Items on the table consist of individual foods for menu use, simple and complex food combinations, ready-to-eat foods, and basic ingredients (such as flours) required in preparing other products. Data are given for food energy, protein, fat, carbohydrate, two minerals, and five vitamins.

The foods are chiefly in frequently-used household units such as cups and tablespoons, which can be used as bases for calculating values for smaller or larger units. For the reader's convenience, measures have further been adjusted to common serving sizes in many cases. For example, cooked vegetables are presented in ½-cup servings and cooked cereals in ⅔-cup servings.

Key to Abbreviations and Symbols on Table

tr   = trace
dia = diameter
med = medium

All other abbreviations used in the table, as well as weight and measure equivalents, are listed in Appendix F.

Values in parentheses ( ) denote imputed values, usually from another form of the food or from a similar food.

Zeros in parentheses (0) indicate that the amount of a constituent, if present, is probably too small to be measured.

Dashes — denote lack of reliable data for a constituent believed to be present in a measurable amount.

Appendix K
Nutritive Values of Foods in Household Measures

Foods Largely in Forms Ready to Eat

Food	Weight g	Approximate measure and description	Food energy kilocal	Pro-tein g	Fat g	Carbo-hydrate g	Cal-cium mg	Iron mg	Vitamin A Activity IU	Thia-min mg	Ribo-flavin mg	Nia-cin mg	Ascorbic acid mg
Anchovies, pickled	220	5 anchovies, rolled, ½ to ¾ in dia, ½ in thick	35	4	2	tr	34	—	—	—	—	—	—
Apples, raw	150	1 apple, 2¾ in dia (3 per lb)	80	tr	1	20	10	0.4	120	0.04	0.03	0.1	6
Apple brown betty	108	½ cup (enriched bread)	163	2	4	32	20	0.7	110	0.07	0.05	0.5	1
Apple butter	18	1 tbsp	33	tr	tr	8	2	0.1	0	tr	tr	tr	tr
Apple pie (see pies)													
Apple juice (sweet cider)	124	½ cup (small glass)	59	tr	tr	15	8	0.8	—	0.01	0.03	0.1	1
Applesauce	128	½ cup, sweetened	116	tr	tr	30	5	0.7	50	0.03	0.04	tr	2
Apricots, raw	114	3 apricots	55	1	tr	14	18	0.5	2800	0.03	0.04	0.6	11
Apricots, dried, stewed	150	½ cup, med fruit, liquid, sugar added	169	2	tr	46	30	2.0	4200	tr	0.03	1.2	3
Apricot nectar	126	½ cup (small glass)	72	tr	tr	18	12	0.3	1190	0.02	0.02	0.3	4
Artichokes, cooked	250	1 bud	26	3	tr	10	51	1.1	150	0.07	0.04	0.7	8
Asparagus, green, canned	118	½ cup drained, cut spears	25	3	tr	4	23	2.3	940	0.07	0.12	1.0	18
Avocado, raw (as purchased)	125	½ (10-oz fruit), all varieties	188	2	19	7	11	0.7	330	0.12	0.23	1.8	16
Bacon, broiled or fried	15	2 med slices, drained (20 slices per lb)	86	4	8	1	2	0.5	(0)	0.08	0.05	0.8	—
Bamboo shoots, raw	76	½ cup, 1 in pieces	20	2	tr	4	10	0.4	15	0.11	0.05	0.5	3
Bananas, raw (as purchased)	175	1 med banana (8¾ x 1½ in)	101	1	tr	26	10	0.8	230	0.06	0.07	0.8	12
Barbecue sauce	63	¼ cup	57	1	4	5	13	0.5	225	0.01	0.01	0.2	3
Barley, pearled, raw	50	¼ cup Scotch barley	174	5	1	39	17	1.4	0	0.11	0.04	1.9	(0)
Bass, oven fried	200	1 fillet, 8¾ x 4½ x ⅝ in	392	43	17	13	—	—	—	—	—	—	—
Beans, lima, canned	85	½ cup, drained (immature seeds)	82	5	tr	16	24	2.1	160	0.03	0.05	0.5	5
Beans, lima, dry, cooked	143	¾ cup, drained	197	12	1	37	41	4.4	—	0.19	0.08	1.0	—
Beans, pinto, dry, raw	48	¼ cup, red beans	166	11	1	30	64	3.1	—	0.40	0.10	1.1	—
Beans, red kidney, dry, canned	191	¾ cup	173	11	1	31	56	3.5	8	0.10	0.08	1.1	—
Beans, snap, green, boiled	63	½ cup, brief cooking, drained	16	1	tr	3	32	0.4	340	0.05	0.06	0.3	8
Beans, sprouts, cooked	63	½ cup mung, drained	18	2	tr	3	11	0.6	15	0.06	0.07	0.5	4

Food	Measure	Weight (g)	Food energy	Protein (g)	Fat (g)	Carbohydrate (g)	Calcium (mg)	Iron (mg)	Vitamin A (IU)	Thiamine (mg)	Riboflavin (mg)	Niacin (mg)	Ascorbic acid (mg)
Beans, wax (yellow), cooked	1/2 cup, 1- to 2-in lengths, drained	63	14	1	tr	3	32	0.4	145	0.05	0.06	0.3	8
Beans, white, navy, cooked	3/4 cup, drained	143	168	11	1	31	71	3.8	0	0.20	0.10	1.0	0
Beans, white dry, canned	3/4 cup, with pork and tomato sauce	191	233	12	5	36	104	3.5	248	0.15	0.06	1.1	4
Beans and frankfurters, canned	3/4 cup	191	275	15	14	24	71	3.6	248	0.14	0.11	2.5	tr
Beef, corned, canned	1 slice, 3 x 2 x 3/8 in	40	86	10	5	0	8	1.7	—	0.01	0.10	1.4	0
Beef, corned hash, canned	1/2 cup	110	199	10	12	12	15	2.2	—	0.01	0.10	2.3	—
Beef, dried or chipped	1 oz	28	58	10	2	0	6	1.4	—	(0.02)	(0.09)	(1.1)	—
Beef, hamburger, broiled	3-oz patty, 3 x 5/8 in	85	186	23	10	0	10	3.0	20	0.08	0.20	5.1	—
Beef, heart, braized	3 oz	84	159	27	5	1	6	5.1	30	0.21	1.05	6.6	tr
Beef, lean, chuck, cooked	3-oz piece, 4 1/8 x 2 1/4 x 1/2 in (fat trimmed)	85	212	25	12	0	11	3.1	20	0.05	0.19	3.8	—
Beef liver (see liver)													
Beef loaf (see meat loaf)													
Beef potpie, baked	1/6 of pie, 9 in dia	105	259	11	15	20	15	1.9	860	0.12	0.13	2.1	3
Beef, pot roast, cooked	2 pieces (3-oz), each 4 1/8 x 2 1/4 x 1/4 in	85	295	20	23	0	9	2.6	40	0.05	0.15	3.7	—
Beef roast, rib, cooked	2 pieces (3-oz), each 4 1/8 x 2 1/4 x 1/4 in	85	205	24	11	0	10	3.1	20	0.06	0.18	4.3	—
Beef, round steak, cooked	3-oz piece, 4 1/8 x 2 1/4 x 1/2 in	85	222	24	13	0	10	3.0	20	0.07	0.19	4.8	—
Beef, sirloin, broiled	3-oz piece, 3 1/2 x 2 x 3/4 in	85	329	20	27	0	9	2.5	50	0.05	0.15	4.0	—
Beef and vegetable stew	3/4 cup (lean chuck)	184	164	12	8	11	22	2.2	1800	0.11	0.13	3.5	13
Beets, canned	1/2 cup diced or sliced, drained	85	32	1	tr	8	16	0.6	15	0.01	0.03	0.1	3
Beverages, alcoholic, beer	12 fluid oz, 3.6% alcohol by weight	360	151	1	0	14	18	tr	—	0.01	0.11	2.2	—
Beverages, alcoholic, 90-proof	1 1/2 fluid oz (1 jigger), 37.9% alcohol by weight (gin, rum, vodka, whiskey)	42	110	—	—	tr	—	—	—	—	—	—	—
Beverages, alcoholic, wines (dessert)	3 1/2 fluid oz (1 wine glass), 15.3% alcohol by weight port, muscatel, sherry, tokay)	103	141	tr	0	8	8	—	—	0.01	0.02	0.2	—
Beverages, alcoholic, wines (table)	3 1/2 fluid oz (1 wine glass), 9.9% alcohol by weight (chablis, claret, Rhine wine, sauterne)	102	87	tr	0	4	9	0.4	—	tr	0.01	0.1	—
Beverages, carbonated, cream sodas	12 fluid oz	371	160	(0)	(0)	41	—	—	(0)	(0)	(0)	(0)	(0)
Beverages, carbonated, dietary drinks	12 fluid oz (with artificial sweetener)	355	—	(0)	(0)	—	—	—	(0)	(0)	(0)	(0)	(0)
Beverages, carbonated, fruit-flavored sodas	12 fluid oz, 10 to 13% sugar (citrus, cherry, grape, other)	372	171	(0)	(0)	45	—	—	(0)	(0)	(0)	(0)	(0)

Food	Wt. g	Approximate measure and description	Food Energy kilocal	Protein g	Fat g	Carbohydrate g	Calcium mg	Iron mg	Vitamin A Activity IU	Thiamin mg	Riboflavin mg	Niacin mg	Ascorbic acid mg
Beverages, carbonated, ginger ale	366	12 fluid oz	113	(0)	(0)	29	—	—	(0)	(0)	(0)	(0)	(0)
Beverages, carbonated, root beer	370	12 fluid oz	152	(0)	(0)	39	—	—	(0)	(0)	(0)	(0)	(0)
Beverages, carbonated waters, sweetened	366	12 fluid oz (quinine sodas)	113	(0)	(0)	29	—	—	(0)	(0)	(0)	(0)	(0)
Beverages, carbonated waters, unsweetened	355	12 fluid oz (club sodas)	0	(0)	(0)	0	—	—	(0)	(0)	(0)	(0)	(0)
Beverages, cola type	369	12 fluid oz (carbonated)	144	(0)	(0)	37	—	—	(0)	(0)	(0)	(0)	(0)
Biscuit, baking powder	28	1 biscuit, 2 in dia (enriched flour)	103	2	5	13	34	0.4	tr	0.06	0.06	0.5	tr
Blackberries, raw	72	½ cup	42	tr	tr	9	23	0.7	145	0.02	0.03	0.3	15
Blueberries, raw	73	½ cup	45	1	tr	11	11	0.8	75	0.02	0.05	0.4	10
Bluefish, baked or broiled	155	1 fillet, 7¾ x 3⅞ x ⅜ in	246	41	8	0	45	1.1	80	0.17	0.16	2.9	—
Bologna, luncheon meat	26	2 slices, 3 in dia, each ⅛ in thick	80	3	7	tr	2	0.4	—	0.04	0.06	0.6	—
Bouillon cubes	4	1 cube, approx ½ in	5	1	tr	tr	—	—	—	—	—	—	—
Bran cereal, ready-to-eat	40	⅔ cup, added sugar, salt, malt extract, vitamins	96	5	1	30	33	3.9	(0) value without added vit. A	(*)	(*)	(*)	(*)
Bran flakes (40% bran)	26	¾ cup, added sugar, salt, iron, vitamins	80	3	1	21	14	9.3	1238	0.31	0.37	3.1	9
Bread, cracked wheat	25	1 slice, 4 x 4¼ x ½ in	66	2	1	13	22	0.3	tr	0.03	0.02	0.3	tr
Bread, French	15	1 slice, 2½ x 2 x ½ in (enriched)	44	1	1	8	6	0.3	tr	0.04	0.03	0.4	tr
Bread, Italian	30	1 slice, 4½ x 3¼ x ¾ in (enriched)	83	3	tr	17	5	0.7	(0)	0.09	0.06	0.8	(0)
Bread, pumpernickel, (dark rye)	7	1 slice, snack size, 2½ x 2 x ¼ in)	17	1	tr	4	6	0.2	(0)	0.02	0.01	0.1	(0)
Bread, raisin	25	1 slice, 3¾ x 3⅝ x ½ in	66	2	1	13	18	0.3	tr	0.01	0.02	0.2	tr
Bread, rye (American)	25	1 slice, 4¾ x 3¾ x ½ in	61	2	tr	13	19	0.4	(0)	0.05	0.02	0.4	(0)
Bread sticks	20	2 sticks, each 4¼ x ½ in	77	2	1	15	6	0.2	tr	0.01	0.01	0.2	tr
Bread, Vienna	25	1 slice, 4¾ x 4 x ½ in, (enriched)	73	2	1	14	11	0.6	tr	0.07	0.06	0.6	tr
Bread, white	28	1 slice, 4⅜ x 4 x ½ in (enriched)	76	2	1	14	24	0.7	tr	0.07	0.06	0.7	tr
Bread, white	28	1 slice, 4⅜ x 4 x ½ in (unenriched)	76	2	1	14	24	0.2	tr	0.02	0.03	0.3	tr
Bread, white, toasted	24	1 slice, 4⅜ x 4 x ½ in (enriched)	76	2	1	14	24	0.2	tr	(0.02)	0.02	0.3	tr
Bread, whole wheat	28	1 slice, 4⅛ x 3⅝ x ½ in	67	3	1	14	24	0.8	tr	0.09	0.03	0.8	tr

* See nutrition label on package for values.

Food	Measure	Grams	Food energy (cal)	Protein (g)	Fat (g)	Carbohydrate (g)	Calcium (mg)	Iron (mg)	Vitamin A (IU)	Thiamin (mg)	Riboflavin (mg)	Niacin (mg)	Ascorbic acid (mg)
Breadcrumbs, dry	½ cup, enriched bread	50	196	6	2	37	61	1.8	tr	0.11	0.15	1.8	tr
Bread stuffing, mix	1 cup, coarse crumbs	70	260	9	3	51	87	2.2	tr	0.15	0.18	2.2	tr
Broccoli, cooked	½ cup, ½-in pieces	78	20	2	tr	4	68	0.6	1940	0.07	0.16	0.6	70
Brown bread, Boston	1 piece, round, 3¼ in dia, ½ in thick	45	95	3	1	21	41	0.9	0	0.05	0.03	0.5	0
Brussels sprouts, cooked	½ cup, drained (from frozen)	78	26	3	tr	5	17	0.6	440	0.06	0.08	0.5	63
Bulgur, dry (parboiled wheat)	¼ cup, from red winter wheat	43	151	5	tr	32	12	1.6	0	0.12	0.06	1.9	(0)
Buns, or rolls	1 long bun, 6 x 2 x 1½ in or round, 3½ x 1½ in (enriched)	40	119	3	2	21	30	0.8	tr	0.11	0.07	0.9	tr
Butter or margarine	1 tbsp or ⅛ stick (margarine fortified with vitamin A)	14	102	tr	12	tr	3	0	470	—	—	—	0
Buttermilk (skim milk)	1 cup, cultured	245	88	9	tr	13	296	0.1	10	0.10	0.44	0.2	2
Cabbage, cooked	½ cup drained, brief cooking	73	15	1	tr	3	32	0.2	95	0.03	0.03	0.2	24
Cabbage, raw	½ cup, finely chopped	45	11	1	tr	3	22	0.2	60	0.03	0.03	0.3	21
Cake, angel food	1 piece (mix), 1⅞-in arc, 1/16 cake, 9¾ in dia	40	104	2	tr	24	38	0.1	0	tr	0.04	tr	0
Cake, Boston cream pie	1 piece, 3⅛-in arc, ⅛ cake, 8 in dia	103	311	5	10	51	69	0.5	220	0.03	0.11	0.2	tr
Cake, devil's food, frosted	1 piece (mix) 1⅝-in arc, 1/16 cake, 8 in dia, with chocolate icing	69	234	3	9	40	41	0.6	100	0.02	0.06	0.2	tr
Cake, fruitcake, dark	1 slice, 2 x 1½ x ¼ in 1/30 of 1-lb loaf	15	57	1	2	9	11	0.4	20	0.02	0.02	0.1	tr
Cake, plain cupcake	1 cupcake (mix) 2½ dia without icing	25	88	1	3	14	40	0.1	40	0.01	0.03	0.1	tr
Cake, plain cupcake, frosted	1 cupcake (mix) 2½ in dia with chocolate icing	36	129	2	5	21	47	0.3	60	0.01	0.04	0.1	tr
Cake, pound	1 slice (home recipe) 3½ x 3 x ½ in, 1/17 of loaf	30	142	2	9	14	6	0.2	80	0.01	0.03	tr	0
Cake, sponge	1 wedge, 1⅞-in arc, 1/16 cake, 9¾ in dia	49	146	4	3	27	15	0.6	220	0.02	0.07	0.1	tr
Cake, white frosted	1 piece (home recipe) 2-layer, 3 in high, 1⅝-in arc, 1/16 cake 8 in dia, with uncooked white icing	61	229	2	8	38	29	0.1	70	0.01	0.04	0.1	tr
Cake, yellow frosted	1 piece (home recipe) 2-layer, 1⅝-in arc, 1/16 cake 8 in dia, with chocolate icing	59	215	3	8	36	40	0.4	90	0.01	0.05	0.1	tr
Candy, caramels	1 oz (plain or chocolate)	28	113	1	3	22	42	0.4	tr	0.01	0.05	0.1	tr
Candy, chocolate, fudge, plain	1 cubic in	21	84	1	3	16	16	0.2	tr	tr	0.02	tr	tr
Candy, chocolate fudge, nuts	1 cubic in	21	89	1	4	15	17	0.3	tr	0.01	0.02	0.1	tr
Candy, gum drops	1 oz (10 small, cone-shaped)	28	98	tr	tr	25	2	0.1	0	0	tr	tr	0
Candy, hard	1 oz (5 balls, ea 2½ in circum)	28	109	0	tr	28	6	0.5	0	0	0	0	0

Food	Wt. g	Approximate measure and description	Food Energy kilocal	Pro-tein g	Fat g	Carbo-hydrate g	Cal-cium mg	Iron mg	Vitamin A Activity IU	Thia-min mg	Ribo-flavin mg	Nia-cin mg	Ascorbic acid mg
Candy, milk chocolate, with almonds	28	1 oz	151	3	10	15	65	0.5	70	0.02	0.12	0.2	tr
Candy, mints, chocolate-coated	11	1 mint, 1⅜ in dia	45	tr	1	9	6	0.1	tr	tr	0.01	tr	tr
Candy, nougat & caramel	28	1 oz	118	1	4	21	36	0.5	10	0.02	0.05	0.1	tr
Candy, peanut brittle	28	1 oz	119	2	3	23	10	0.7	0	0.05	0.01	1.0	0
Candy, vanilla creams	28	1 oz	123	1	5	20	36	0.2	tr	0.01	0.02	tr	tr
Carrots, cooked	73	½ cup, diced, drained	23	1	tr	5	24	0.5	7615	0.04	0.04	0.4	5
Carrots, raw	81	1 carrot, 7½ x 1⅛ in	30	1	tr	7	27	0.5	7930	0.04	0.04	0.4	6
Carrots, raw	55	½ cup, grated or shredded	23	1	tr	5	21	0.4	6050	0.04	0.03	0.4	5
Catsup, tomato (See tomato)													
Cauliflower, cooked	63	½ cup drained	14	1	tr	3	13	0.5	40	0.06	0.05	0.4	35
Caviar, sturgeon	16	1 tbsp granular	42	4	2	1	44	1.9	—	—	—	—	—
Celery, raw	60	½ cup diced	10	1	tr	2	24	0.2	160	0.02	0.02	0.2	6
Celery, raw, stalk	50	3 inner stalks, 5 x ¾ in	9	1	tr	2	20	0.2	140	0.02	0.02	0.2	5
Cheese, blue	17	1 cubic in cheese (Roquefort type)	64	4	5	tr	54	(0.1)	(210)	tr	0.11	0.2	(0)
Cheese, cheddar	28	1 oz	113	7	9	1	213	0.3	(370)	0.01	0.13	tr	(0)
Cheese, cheddar, shredded	57	½ cup (½ package)	225	14	18	1	424	0.6	(740)	0.02	0.26	0.1	(0)
Cheese, cottage, creamed	61	¼ cup, packed (4.2% fat)	65	8	3	2	58	0.2	105	0.02	0.15	0.1	(0)
Cheese, cottage, dry curd	50	¼ cup, packed (0.3% fat)	43	9	tr	1	45	0.2	(5)	0.02	0.14	(0.1)	(0)
Cheese, cream	16	1 cubic in	60	1	6	tr	10	tr	(250)	tr	0.04	tr	(0)
Cheese, food	14	1 tbsp	45	3	3	1	80	(0.1)	(140)	tr	0.08	tr	(0)
Cheese, processed	17	1 cubic in	65	4	5	tr	122	0.2	(210)	tr	0.07	tr	(0)
Cheese soufflé	110	1 portion, 3¼ x 3¼ x 2 in	240	11	19	7	221	1.1	880	0.06	0.26	0.2	tr
Cheese spread	14	1 tbsp	40	2	3	1	79	(0.1)	120	tr	0.08	tr	(0)
Cheese straws	30	5 straws, each 5 x ⅜ in	136	3	9	10	78	0.2	115	0.01	0.05	0.1	0
Cheese, Swiss	14	1 slice, 2 x 2 x ¼ in	52	4	4	tr	130	0.1	(160)	(tr)	(0.06)	tr	(0)
Cherries, acerola, raw	100	10 cherries (West Indian) 1 in dia	23	tr	tr	6	10	0.2	—	0.02	0.05	0.3	1066
Cherries, sweet, raw	75	10 cherries	47	1	tr	12	15	0.3	70	0.03	0.04	0.3	7
Chestnuts, in shell	90	10 nuts	141	2	1	31	20	1.2	—	0.16	0.16	0.4	—
Chewing gum	2	1 piece, candy-coated	5	—	—	2	—	—	—	(0)	(0)	(0)	(0)
Chicken à la king, cooked	184	¾ cup	351	21	26	9	95	1.9	848	0.08	0.32	4.1	9
Chicken, creamed*	99	½ cup (chicken in ¼ cup white sauce)	222	20	12	6	84	1.1	445	0.04	0.20	—	1

* One-half cup of a creamed dish calls for ¼ cup white sauce and about ⅓ cup of any one of a variety of meats, vegetables, or other foods that may be combined suitably (see eggs, creamed and fish, creamed).

Food	Measure	Grams	Calories	Protein	Fat	Carbohydrate	Calcium	Iron	Vitamin A	Thiamin	Riboflavin	Niacin	Vitamin C
Chicken, drumstick, fried	1 drumstick	56	88	12	4	tr	6	0.9	50	0.03	0.15	2.7	—
Chicken, fried	½ breast	94	160	26	5	1	9	1.3	70	0.04	0.17	11.6	—
Chicken, meat only, canned	½ cup	103	203	22	12	0	22	1.6	235	0.04	0.13	4.5	4
Chicken and noodles, cooked	¾ cup	180	275	17	14	19	20	1.7	323	0.04	0.13	3.2	tr
Chicken potpie, baked	⅙ pie, 9 in dia	116	273	12	16	21	35	1.5	1545	0.13	0.13	2.1	3
Chicken, roasted	2 pieces, each 2½ x 1⅞ x ¼ in	50	83	16	2	0	6	0.7	30	0.02	0.05	5.8	—
Chickpeas (garbanzos) dry, raw	½ cup	100	360	21	5	61	150	7.0	50	0.31	0.15	2.0	—
Chicory	1 cup, ½-in pieces	90	14	1	tr	3	16	0.5	tr	—	tr	tr	—
Chili con carne, canned	¾ cup, with beans	191	254	14	12	23	62	3.2	113	0.06	0.14	2.5	—
Chili peppers, hot, canned sauce (green)	¼ cup (from immature green peppers)	61	12	tr	tr	3	3	0.3	373	0.02	0.02	0.4	42
Chili peppers, hot, canned sauce (red)	¼ cup (from mature red peppers)	61	13	1	tr	2	6	0.3	5875	0.01	0.06	0.4	19
Chili powder, dried	1 tsp. (from hot mature, red peppers)	2	7	tr	tr	1	5	0.3	1300	tr	0.02	0.2	tr
Chives, raw	1 tbsp, chopped	3	1	tr	tr	tr	2	0.1	170	tr	tr	tr	2
Chocolate, baking	1 oz, 1 square	28	143	3	15	8	22	1.9	20	0.01	0.07	0.4	0
Chocolate candy (see candy)													
Chocolate milk	1 cup, made with skim milk, 2% butterfat added	250	190	8	6	27	270	0.5	210	0.10	0.40	0.3	3
Chocolate morsels	¼ cup, approx 90 pieces, semi-sweet	43	216	2	15	24	13	1.1	8	tr	0.04	0.2	0
Chocolate, syrup, fudge	¼ cup, topping	75	248	4	10	41	95	1.0	113	0.03	0.17	0.3	tr
Chocolate syrup, thin	¼ cup, topping	75	184	2	2	47	13	1.2	tr	0.02	0.05	0.3	0
Chop suey, cooked	¾ cup, with meat	188	225	20	13	10	45	3.6	450	0.21	0.29	3.8	25
Chow mein, chicken, cooked	¾ cup, without noodles	188	191	23	8	8	44	1.9	210	0.06	0.17	3.2	8
Clams, raw	4 cherry stones or 5 little necks	70	56	8	1	4	48	5.3	—	tr	tr	—	—
Cocoa, beverage	1 cup, homemade, with milk	250	243	10	12	27	295	1.0	400	0.10	0.45	0.5	3
Cocoa powder, with nonfat dry milk	1 oz or 4 heaping tsp	28	102	5	1	20	167	0.5	10	0.04	0.21	0.2	1
Coconut cream	1 tbsp (liquid expressed from fresh grated coconut)	15	50	1	5	1	2	0.3	0	tr	tr	0.1	tr
Coconut, meat	1 piece, 2 x 2 x ½ in	45	156	2	16	4	6	0.8	0	0.02	tr	0.2	1
Coconut milk	1 cup expressed from grated coconut meat and coconut water	240	605	8	60	13	38	3.8	0	0.07	tr	1.9	5
Coconut, shredded fresh	¼ cup, not packed	20	69	1	7	2	3	0.4	0	0.01	tr	0.1	1
Codfish, broiled	1 fillet, 5 x 2½ x ⅞ in	65	111	19	3	0	20	0.7	120	0.05	0.07	2.0	0
Coffee cake	1 piece, frosted, 3 x 3 x 1¼ in	79	260	4	11	37	25	1.0	477	0.12	0.13	—	0
Coffee, dry powder	1 tsp freeze-fried	1	1	tr	tr	tr	2	0.1	—	0	tr	0.3	0
Coleslaw	¼ cup, made with mayonnaise-type dressing	30	30	tr	tr	2	13	0.1	45	0.02	0.02	0.1	9

503

Food	Wt. g	Approximate measure and description	Food Energy kilocal	Protein g	Fat g	Carbohydrate g	Calcium mg	Iron mg	Vitamin A Activity IU	Thiamin mg	Riboflavin mg	Niacin mg	Ascorbic acid mg
Cookies, brownies	20	1 brownie, 1¾ x 1¾ x ⅞ in (with nuts, enriched flour)	97	1	6	10	8	0.4	40	0.04	0.02	0.1	tr
Cookies, chocolate chip	40	4 cookies (home recipe) 2½ in dia (enriched flour)	206	2	12	24	14	0.8	40	0.04	0.04	0.4	tr
Cookies, coconut bars	45	5 cookies, 3 x 1¼ x ¼ in	223	3	11	29	33	0.7	70	0.02	0.03	0.2	0
Cookies, fig bars	56	4 cookies, 1½ x 1¾ x ½ in	200	2	3	42	44	0.6	60	0.02	0.04	0.2	tr
Cookies, ginger snaps	35	5 cookies, 2 in dia x ¼ in	147	2	3	28	26	0.8	25	0.02	0.02	0.2	tr
Cookies, macaroons	38	2 cookies, 2¾ in dia x ¼ in	181	2	9	25	10	0.3	0	0.02	0.06	0.2	0
Cookies, molasses	33	1 cookie, 3⅝ in dia x ¾ in	137	2	3	25	17	0.7	30	0.01	0.02	0.2	0
Cookies, oatmeal with raisins	52	4 cookies, 2⅝ in dia x ¼ in	235	3	8	38	11	1.5	30	0.06	0.04	0.3	tr
Cookies, sandwich type	40	4 cookies, 1¾ in dia x ⅜ in (chocolate or vanilla)	198	2	9	28	10	0.3	0	0.02	0.02	0.2	0
Cookies, sugar	40	5 cookies, 2¼ in dia x ¼ in	178	2	7	27	31	0.6	45	0.07	0.07	0.5	tr
Cookies, vanilla wafers	15	5 cookies, 1⅜ x ¼ in	70	1	2	11	6	tr	20	tr	0.01	0.1	0
Corn, sweet, boiled	140	1 ear, 5 x 1¾ in	70	3	1	16	2	0.5	310 (yellow corn)	0.09	0.08	1.1	7
Corn, sweet, canned	105	½ cup, whole kernel	87	3	1	22	3	0.6	370 (yellow corn)	(0.03)	(0.07)	(1.2)	6
Cornflakes, plain	25	1 cup, added sugar, salt, iron, vitamins	97	2	tr	21	tr	0.6	1180 (yellow corn)	0.29	0.35	2.9	9
Corn fritters, cooked	35	1 fritter, 2 in x 1½ in	132	3	8	14	22	0.6	140 (yellow corn)	0.06	0.07	0.6	1
Corn grits, cooked	163	⅔ cup grits (enriched)	83	2	tr	18	1	0.5	100 (yellow corn)	0.07	0.05	0.7	(0)
Corn muffins (see muffins)													
Corn pone	60	⅛ pone, 3½ in arc, whole ground meal	122	3	3	22	37	0.7	tr (white corn)	0.09	0.03	0.5	0
Corn pudding, cooked	123	½ cup	128	5	6	16	81	0.6	320	0.04	0.16	0.5	3
Cornstarch	8	1 tbsp	29	tr	tr	7	(0)	(0)	(0)	(0)	(0)	(0)	(0)
Corned beef (see beef)													
Corned beef hash (see beef)													
Cow peas (blackeye) dry, cooked	124	¾ cup	134	10	1	22	30	2.6	435	0.37	0.14	1.7	21
Crabmeat, canned	63	½ cup flaked	58	11	1	tr	27	0.5	1355	0.10	0.05	1.8	1
Crackers, butter	17	5 crackers, round, 1¾ in dia	76	1	3	11	25	0.1	35	tr	0.01	0.2	(0)
Crackers, graham	14	2 square crackers, 2½ in	55	1	1	10	6	0.2	(0)	0.01	0.03	0.2	(0)
Crackers, saltines (see saltines)													
Cranberry juice, sweetened	127	½ cup (small glass)	82	tr	tr	21	7	0.4	tr	0.02	0.02	0.1	20
Cranberry sauce, sweetened	69	¼ cup, strained	101	tr	tr	26	4	0.2	15	0.01	0.01	tr	2
Cranberry-orange relish, raw	69	¼ cup	123	tr	tr	31	13	0.3	48	0.02	0.02	0.1	13

Cream, half-and-half	15	1 tbsp fluid, 12% fat	20	1	2	1	16	tr	70	tr	0.02	tr	tr
Cream, heavy, whipping	15	1 tbsp	53	tr	6	1	11	tr	230	tr	0.02	tr	tr
Cream, light, coffee	15	1 tbsp	32	1	3	1	15	tr	130	tr	0.02	tr	tr
Cream puffs	130	1 puff, custard filling, 3½ in dia x 2 in	303	9	18	27	105	0.9	460	0.05	0.22	0.1	tr
Creamer, coffee (powdered)	2	1 tsp artificial cream (vegetable fat)	10	tr	1	1	1	tr	tr	—	—	—	—
Cucumber, raw	28	6½ slices, 2½ in dia	4	tr	tr	1	5	0.1	tr	0.01	0.01	0.1	3
Custard, baked	133	½ cup	153	7	7	15	149	0.6	465	0.06	0.25	0.2	1
Dates, pitted	40	5 dates	110	1	tr	29	24	1.2	20	0.04	0.04	0.9	0
Doughnuts, plain	25	1 doughnut, 3½ in dia enriched flour	98	1	5	13	10	0.4	20	0.04	0.04	0.3	tr
Dessert topping (see topping, whipped)													
Eclairs, custard filling, chocolate icing	100	1 eclair, 5 x 2 x 1¾ in	239	6	14	23	80	0.7	340	0.04	0.16	0.1	tr
Egg plant, boiled	100	½ cup, diced, drained	19	1	tr	4	11	0.6	10	0.05	0.04	0.5	3
Egg white, raw	29	1 white (med egg)	15	3	tr	tr	3	tr	0	tr	0.08	tr	0
Egg yolk, raw	15	1 yolk (med egg)	52	2	5	tr	21	0.8	510	0.03	0.07	tr	0
Eggs, creamed*	113	½ cup (1 egg in ½ cup white sauce)	190	9	14	7	103	1.2	928	0.07	0.25	—	tr
Eggs, raw, boiled, poached	50	1 med egg	72	6	5	tr	24	1.0	520	0.05	0.13	tr	0
Eggs, scrambled	56	prepared with 1 med egg	97	6	7	1	45	1.0	600	0.04	0.16	tr	0
Endive, curly, raw	25	½ cup, small pieces (also escarole)	5	tr	tr	1	21	0.5	825	0.02	0.04	0.2	3
Farina, cooked (Cream of Wheat)	163	⅔ cup (enriched)	69	2	tr	14	7	8.5	(0)	0.07	0.05	0.7	(0)
Fats, cooking (see oils)													
Figs, whole, raw	50	1 med, 2¼ in dia	40	1	tr	10	18	0.3	40	0.03	0.03	0.2	1
Filberts (see nuts)													
Fish (see various kinds)													
Fish, creamed*	136	½ cup, (tuna, salmon, other in white sauce)	220	20	13	8	81	0.9	385	0.05	0.18	—	tr
Fish loaf, cooked	150	1 slice, 4⅛ x 2½ x 1 in	186	21	6	11	—	—	—	—	—	—	—
Fish sticks, breaded, cooked	28	1 fish stick (1 oz)	50	5	3	2	3	0.1	0	0.01	0.02	0.5	—
Fishcakes, fried	60	1 cake, 3 in dia ⅝ in thick	103	9	5	6	—	—	—	—	—	—	—
Flounder, baked	57	1 fillet, 6 x 2½ x ¼ in	115	17	5	0	13	0.8	—	0.04	0.05	1.4	1
Flour, wheat, white	115	1 cup, sifted (unenriched)	419	12	1	88	18	0.9	(0)	0.07	0.06	1.0	(0)
Flour, wheat, white	115	1 cup, sifted (enriched)	419	12	1	88	18	3.3	(0)	0.51	0.30	4.0	(0)
Frankfurters (hot dogs, wieners)	45	1 frankfurter, 5 x ¾ in (10 per lb)	139	6	12	1	3	0.9	—	0.07	0.09	1.2	—
Fruit cocktail, canned	128	½ cup, syrup pack	97	1	tr	25	12	1.0	180	0.03	0.02	0.5	3
Fruit salad, canned	123	½ cup water pack	43	1	tr	11	10	0.4	575	0.01	0.04	0.8	4

* One-half cup of a creamed dish calls for ¼ cup of white sauce and about ⅓ cup of any one of a variety of meats, vegetables, or other foods that may be combined suitably.

Food	Wt. g	Approximate measure and description	Food Energy kilocal	Protein g	Fat g	Carbohydrate g	Calcium mg	Iron mg	Vitamin A Activity IU	Thiamin mg	Riboflavin mg	Niacin mg	Ascorbic acid mg
Garlic, raw	3	1 clove	4	tr	tr	1	1	tr	tr	0.01	tr	tr	tr
Gelatin dessert, plain	120	½ cup, ready-to-eat	71	2	0	17	—	—	—	—	—	—	—
Gelatin, dry	7	1 envelope (1 tbsp)	23	6	tr	0	—	—	—	—	—	—	—
Giblets, turkey, cooked	145	1 cup, chopped or diced	338	30	22	2	—	—	—	—	3.94	—	—
Gingerbread	117	1 piece, 3 x 3 x 2 in (enriched flour)	371	4	13	61	80	2.7	110	0.14	0.13	1.1	0
Ginger root, crystalized	28	1 oz (3 pieces, each 1½ x ¼ in)	96	tr	tr	25	—	—	—	—	—	—	—
Goose, roasted, flesh only	85	2½ pieces (3 oz) each piece 3½ x 3 x ¼ in	198	29	8	0	(12)	(1.4)	—	(0.09)	(0.14)	(7.9)	—
Gooseberries, raw	75	½ cup	30	1	tr	7	14	0.4	220	—	—	—	25
Grapefruit, canned in syrup	127	½ cup, solids, liquid	89	2	tr	23	17	0.4	15	0.04	0.03	0.3	38
Grapefruit juice	124	½ cup (small glass) unsweetened	51	1	tr	12	10	0.5	10	0.04	0.03	0.3	42
Grapefruit peel, candied	28	1 oz	90	tr	tr	23	—	—	635	—	—	—	—
Grapefruit, pink, raw	301	½ med 4¼ in dia	55	1	tr	13	13	0.3	635	0.06	0.03	0.3	57
Grapefruit, white, raw	241	½ grapefruit, 4¼ in dia	46	1	tr	12	19	0.5	10	0.05	0.02	0.2	44
Grapes, raw	40	10 grapes, American type, as Concord	18	tr	tr	4	4	0.1	30	(0.01)	(0.01)	(0.1)	1
Grapes, seedless	50	10 grapes, European type, as Thompson	34	tr	tr	9	6	0.2	(50)	0.03	0.02	0.2	2
Grapejuice, canned	127	½ cup (small glass)	84	tr	tr	21	14	0.4	—	0.05	0.03	0.3	tr
Greens, beet tops, cooked	73	½ cup, drained	13	1	tr	2	72*	1.4	3700	0.05	0.11	0.2	11
Greens, collards, cooked	95	½ cup, drained, (cooked in little water)	32	3	1	5	179	0.8	7410	0.11	0.19	1.2	72
Greens, dandelion, cooked	53	½ cup drained	18	1	tr	3	74	1.0	6145	0.07	0.09	—	10
Greens, kale, cooked	55	½ cup drained	22	(3)	(tr)	3	103	0.9	4565	0.06	0.10	0.9	51
Greens, mustard, cooked	70	½ cup drained	16	2	tr	3	97	1.3	4060	0.06	0.10	0.4	34
Greens, spinach, frozen, cooked	103	½ cup drained	24	3	tr	4	116*	2.2	8100	0.07	0.16	0.4	20
Greens, turnip tops, cooked	73	½ cup, drained, cooked short time, little water	15	2	tr	3	134	0.8	4570	0.11	0.18	0.5	50
Guavas, raw	82	1 guava	50	1	tr	12	21	0.5	180	0.05	0.03	—	212
Haddock, fried	110	1 fillet, 2¾ x 2½ x ⅞ in	182	22	7	6	44	1.3	—	0.04	0.08	3.5	2
Halibut, broiled	125	1 fillet, 6½ x 2¾ x ⅝ in	214	32	9	0	20	1.0	850	0.06	0.09	10.4	—
Ham, baked (cured)	85	2 pieces, each 4⅛ x 2¼ x ¼ in, lean with fat	246	18	19	0	8	2.2	(0)	0.40	0.15	3.1	—
Ham, boiled	28	1 slice, 6¼ x 4 x 1/16 in (1 oz)	66	5	5	0	3	0.8	(0)	0.12	0.04	0.7	—

* Unavailable

Food	g	Measure	Food energy (cal)	Protein (g)	Fat (g)	Carbohydrate (g)	Calcium (mg)	Iron (mg)	Vitamin A (I.U.)	Thiamin (mg)	Riboflavin (mg)	Niacin (mg)	Ascorbic acid (mg)
Ham, deviled, canned	13	1 tbsp	46	2	4	0	1	0.3	(0)	0.02	0.01	0.2	—
Hamburger (see beef, hamburger)													
Heart (see beef, heart; veal, heart)													
Herring, pickled	50	1 herring, 7 x 1½ x ½ in	112	10	8	0	—	—	—	—	—	—	tr
Honey, strained	21	1 tbsp	64	tr	0	17	1	0.1	0	tr	0.01	0.1	—
Hot dog (see frankfurters)													
Horseradish, prepared	5	1 tsp	2	tr	tr	1	3	tr	—	—	—	—	1
Ice cream, plain	66	1 slice, ⅛ qt, 10% fat	127	3	7	14	96	tr	290	0.03	0.14	0.1	1
Ice cream, plain, rich	74	½ cup, 16% fat	165	2	12	13	58	tr	490	0.02	0.08	0.1	1
Ice milk	66	½ cup, frozen dessert, 5.1%fat	100	3	3	15	102	0.1	140	0.04	0.15	0.1	1
Ices, water (lime)	97	½ cup, frozen dessert	124	tr	tr	31	tr	tr	tr	tr	tr	tr	tr
Jams, preserves	20	1 tbsp	54	tr	tr	14	4	0.2	tr	tr	0.01	tr	tr
Jellies	18	1 tbsp	49	tr	tr	13	4	0.3	tr	tr	0.01	tr	1
Kale (see greens)													
Kohlrabi, cooked	83	½ cup, diced, drained	20	1	tr	4	27	0.3	15	0.05	0.03	0.2	36
Lamb chop, broiled	71	1 loin chop, 4 per lb	255	16	21	0	6	0.9	—	0.09	0.16	3.6	—
Lamb, leg, roasted	85	2 pieces (3 oz), each 4⅛ x 2¼ x ¼ in	237	22	16	0	9	1.4	—	0.13	0.23	4.7	—
Lemon juice, raw	15	1 tbsp	4	tr	tr	1	1	tr	tr	tr	tr	tr	7
Lemons, wedges	18	1 wedge, ⅙ med fruit	3	tr	tr	1	3	0.1	tr	tr	tr	tr	6
Lemonade	185	6 oz (made from frozen concentrate, diluted with 4½ parts water by volume)	81	tr	tr	21	2	0.1	10	0.01	0.01	0.1	13
Lentils, dry, cooked	150	¾ cup	159	12	tr	29	38	3.2	30	0.11	0.09	0.9	0
Lettuce, head	75	1 cup, small chunks	10	1	tr	2	15	0.4	250	0.05	0.05	0.2	5
Lettuce, head	135	¼ head, wedge	18	1	tr	4	27	0.7	450	0.08	0.08	0.4	8
Lettuce, loose leaf	55	1 cup, chopped or shredded	10	1	tr	2	37	0.8	1050	0.03	0.04	0.2	10
Lime juice, raw	15	1 tbsp	4	tr	tr	1	1	tr	tr	tr	tr	tr	5
Liver, beef, fried	57	2-oz slice	130	15	6	3	6	5.0	30,260	0.15	2.37	9.3	15
Liver, calf, fried	57	2-oz slice	148	17	8	2	7	8.1	18,533	0.13	2.36	9.3	21
Liver, chicken, cooked	75	3 livers, each 2 x 2 x ⅝ in	123	20	3	2	9	6.3	9,240	0.12	2.01	8.7	12
Liver, pork, fried	57	2-oz slice	137	17	7	1	9	16.5	8,447	0.19	2.47	12.7	13
Liverwurst, fresh	57	2 oz	174	9	15	1	5	3.1	3,600	0.11	0.74	3.2	—
Lobster, cooked	73	½ cup, bite-size cubes	69	14	1	tr	47	0.6	—	0.08	0.05	—	—
Lobster (see salad)													
Macaroni, cooked	105	¾ cup, enriched	116	4	tr	24	8	1.0	(0)	0.15	0.08	1.1	(0)
Macaroni and cheese, baked	150	¾ cup, enriched macaroni	322	13	17	30	272	1.4	645	0.15	0.30	1.4	tr
Mackerel, broiled	105	1 fillet, 8½ x 2½ x ½ in	248	23	17	0	6	1.3	(560)	0.16	0.28	8.0	—
Mangos, raw	83	½ cup, diced or sliced	55	1	tr	14	9	0.4	3960	0.04	0.04	0.9	29
Margarine	14	1 tbsp, ⅛ stick (fortified vit. A)	102	tr	12	tr	3	0	470	—	—	—	0
Marshmallows	7	1 large, 1⅛ dia x ¾ in	23	tr	tr	6	1	0.1	0	0	tr	tr	0
Mayonnaise (see salad dressing)													
Meat loaf, baked	91	1 slice, 3.2 oz	91	14	12	3	8	1.6	—	0.12	0.20	2.2	—
Melon, casaba, raw	245	1 wedge, 7¾ in x 2 in, at base	38	2	tr	9	(20)	(0.6)	40	(0.06)	(0.04)	(0.8)	18
Melon, honeydew	226	1 wedge, 7 in x 2 in, at base	49	1	tr	12	21	0.6	60	0.06	0.04	0.9	34

Food	Wt. g	Food Energy kilocal	Protein g	Fat g	Carbohydrate g	Calcium mg	Iron mg	Vitamin A Activity IU	Thiamin mg	Riboflavin mg	Niacin mg	Ascorbic acid mg
Milk, chocolate (see chocolate milk)												
Milk, dry skim	¼ cup, nonfat, instant	26	93	9	tr	13	336	0.2	8 (unfortified)	0.09	0.46	0.2	2
Milk evaporated, canned	½ cup undiluted, unsweetened	126	173	9	10	12	318	0.2	405	0.05	0.43	0.3	2
Milk, fluid, skim* or buttermilk	1 cup (½ pt)	245	88	9	tr	13	296	0.1	10* (unfortified)	0.09	0.44	0.2	2
Milk, fluid, whole	1 cup (½ pt) 3.5% butterfat	244	159	9	9	12	288	0.1	350	0.07	0.41	0.2	2
Milk, goat	1 cup, fluid milk	244	163	8	10	11	315	0.2	(390)	0.10	0.27	0.7	2
Milk, low-fat	1 cup, fluid, skim, with 2% nonfat milk solids added	246	145	10	5	15	352	0.1	200	0.10	0.52	0.2	2
Milk, malted, plain beverage	1 fountain-size glass (about 1½ cups)	353	368	17	15	42	476	1.1	885	0.21	0.74	—	3
Milkshake, chocolate	1 fountain-size glass	342	420	11	18	58	363	0.9	687	0.12	0.55	—	4
Molasses, blackstrap	1 tbsp	20	43	—	—	11	137	3.2	—	0.02	0.04	0.4	—
Molasses, light	1 tbsp	20	50	—	—	13	33	0.9	—	0.01	0.01	tr	—
Muffins, blueberry	1 muffin, 2⅜ in dia (enriched flour)	40	112	3	4	17	34	0.6	90	0.06	0.08	0.5	tr
Muffins, bran	1 muffin, 2⅝ in dia (enriched flour)	40	104	3	4	17	57	1.5	90	0.06	0.10	1.6	tr
Muffins, corn	1 muffin, 2⅜ in dia (mix, egg, milk)	40	130	3	4	20	96	0.6	100	0.07	0.08	0.6	tr
Muffins, plain	1 muffin, 3 in dia at top (enriched flour)	40	118	3	4	17	42	0.6	40	0.07	0.09	0.6	tr
Mushrooms, raw	½ cup, sliced or chopped	35	10	1	tr	2	2	0.3	tr	0.04	0.16	1.5	1
Muskmelons, as purchased	½ melon, 5 in dia (with orange-colored flesh)	477	82	2	tr	20	38	1.1	9240	0.11	0.08	1.6	90
Mustard, prepared, yellow	1 tsp or individual pouch	5	4	tr	tr	tr	4	0.1	—	—	—	—	—
Nectarines, raw	1 nectarine, 2½ in dia	150	88	1	tr	24	6	0.7	2280	—	—	—	18
Noodles, cooked	½ cup, egg noodles, enriched	80	100	33	1	19	8	0.7	55	0.11	0.07	1.0	(0)
Nuts, almonds, shelled	¼ cup, whole	36	212	7	19	7	83	1.7	0	0.09	0.33	1.3	tr
Nuts, Brazil, shelled	1 oz, 6 to 8 kernels	28	185	4	19	3	53	1.0	tr	0.27	0.03	0.5	—
Nuts, cashew, shelled	1 oz, 18 medium kernels	28	159	5	13	8	11	1.1	30	0.12	0.07	0.5	tr
Nuts, filberts (hazelnuts), shelled	1 oz, approximately 20 nuts	28	180	4	18	5	59	1.0	—	0.13	—	0.3	tr
Nuts, peanuts, roasted, salted	10 large or 20 small, whole nuts (1 tbsp chopped)	9	53	2	5	2	7	0.2	—	0.03	0.01	1.5	—
Nuts, pecans, shelled	10 halves, large	9	62	1	6	1	7	0.2	10	0.08	0.01	0.1	tr
Nuts, walnuts, English	¼ cup halves (about 12)	25	163	4	16	4	25	0.8	8	0.08	0.03	0.2	1

* It is mandatory in the United States that fluid skim milk be fortified with not less than 2000 IU of Vitamin A per quart. (This does not apply to buttermilk.)

Food, approximate measure	Weight (g)	Food energy (cal)	Protein (g)	Fat (g)	Carbohydrate (g)	Calcium (mg)	Iron (mg)	Vitamin A (IU)	Thiamin (mg)	Riboflavin (mg)	Niacin (mg)	Vitamin C (mg)
Oatmeal, cooked — ⅔ cup, regular or instant	160	87	3	2	16	15	0.9	(0)	0.13	0.03	0.1	(0)
Oils, salad or cooking — 1 tbsp, corn, cottonseed, soybean, other oils	14	120	0	14	0	0	0	0	0	0	0	0
Okra, cooked — ½ cup, crosscut slices, drained	80	23	2	tr	5	74	0.4	390	(0.11)	(0.15)	(0.7)	16
Olives, green — 5 olives, large, ¾ in dia	23	23	tr	2	tr	12	0.3	60	—	—	—	—
Olives, ripe — 5 olives, extra large, 1 in dia	28	31	tr	3	1	20	0.4	15	tr	tr	—	—
Onions, boiled — ½ cup, whole or sliced, drained	105	31	1	tr	7	25	0.4	40	0.03	0.03	0.2	8
Onions, young green, raw — 2 med or 6 small	30	14	tr	tr	3	12	0.2	tr	0.02	0.01	0.1	8
Orange juice — ½ cup (small glass), from frozen concentrate	125	61	1	tr	14	13	0.1	270	0.12	0.02	0.5	60
Oranges, raw — 1 orange, 2⅝ in dia, all varieties	180	64	1	tr	16	54	0.5	260	0.13	0.05	0.5	66
Oysters, raw — 2 med or 3 small	28	19	2	1	1	27	1.6	90	0.04	0.05	0.7	—
Oyster stew (see soup)												
Pancakes, plain — 1 cake, 6 x ½ in (mix, egg, milk)	73	164	5	5	24	157	0.9	180	0.11	0.18	0.6	tr
Papayas, raw — ½ cup, cubed	70	28	tr	tr	7	14	0.2	1225	0.03	0.03	0.2	39
Parsley — 1 tbsp, chopped	4	2	tr	tr	tr	7	0.2	300	tr	0.01	tr	6
Parsnips, cooked — ½ cup, 2-in lengths, or diced, drained	78	51	1	tr	12	35	0.5	25	0.06	0.07	0.1	8
Peach nectar — ½ cup (small glass)	125	60	tr	tr	16	5	0.3	535 (yellow flesh)	0.01	0.03	0.5	tr
Peaches, canned — ½ cup with syrup, halved or sliced	128	100	1	tr	26	5	0.4	550 (yellow flesh)	0.02	0.03	0.8	4
Peaches, raw — 1 fruit, 2½ in dia	115	33	1	tr	9	8	0.4	1160 (yellow flesh)	0.02	0.03	0.9	6
Peanut butter — 2 tbsp	32	188	8	16	6	18	0.6	—	0.04	0.04	4.8	0
Peanuts (see nuts)												
Pears, canned — ½ cup, with syrup, halved or sliced	128	97	tr	tr	25	7	0.3	5	0.02	0.04	0.2	2
Pears, raw — 1 pear, 2½ in dia x 3½ in	180	100	1	1	25	13	0.5	30	0.03	0.07	0.2	7
Peas, green, canned — ½ cup, drained solids	85	75	4	tr	14	22	1.6	585	0.08	0.05	0.7	7
Peas, green, frozen, cooked — ½ cup, drained solids	80	55	4	tr	9	15	1.5	480	0.22	0.07	1.4	11
Peas, cowpeas, dry, cooked — ½ cup, blackeye peas or frijoles	124	95	7	1	17	21	1.6	10	0.21	0.06	—	tr
Peas, pigeon, dry, raw — 6 tbsp (gandules)	99	310	22	2	50	140	4.0	169	0.45	0.34	—	0
Peas, split, dry, cooked — ½ cup	115	115	8	tr	21	11	1.7	40	0.15	0.09	0.9	—
Pecans (see nuts)												
Peppers, green, sweet, cooked — 1 pepper, 2¾ x 2½ in (garden variety, immature)	73	13	1	tr	3	7	0.4	310	0.05	0.05	0.4	70
Peppers, green, sweet, raw — ½ med pepper, 2¾ x 2½ in	45	8	tr	tr	2	4	0.3	155	0.03	0.03	0.3	47
Peppers, green, sweet, stuffed — 1 pepper, stuffed, with beef and crumbs	185	315	24	10	31	78	3.9	520	0.17	0.81	4.6	74

Food	Wt. g	Approximate measure and description	Food Energy kilocal	Protein g	Fat g	Carbohydrate g	Calcium mg	Iron mg	Vitamin A Activity IU	Thiamin mg	Riboflavin mg	Niacin mg	Ascorbic acid mg
Peppers, red, sweet raw	90	1 pepper, 2¾ x 2½ in (garden variety, mature)	23	1	tr	5	10	0.4	3280	(0.06)	(0.06)	(0.4)	151
Perch, breaded, fried	88	1 fillet 6¾ x 1¾ x ⅝ in	281	17	17	15	—	—	—	—	—	—	—
Persimmons, raw	30	1 persimmon (native)	31	tr	tr	8	7	0.6	—	—	—	—	16
Pickles, cucumber, dill	65	1 med pickle, 3¾ x 1¼ in	7	1	tr	1	17	0.7	70	tr	0.01	tr	4
Pickles, cucumber, sweet	35	1 pickle, 3 x 1 in	51	tr	tr	13	4	0.4	30	tr	0.01	tr	2
Pickle relish, sweet	15	1 tbsp finely cut or chopped	21	tr	tr	5	3	0.1	—	—	—	—	—
Pies, apple	118	1 sector, 3½-in arc (⅛ pie, 9 in dia)	302	3	13	45	9	0.4	40	0.02	0.02	0.5	1
Pies, cherry	118	1 sector, 3½-in arc (⅛ pie, 9 in dia)	308	3	13	45	17	0.4	520	0.02	0.02	0.6	tr
Pies, lemon meringue	105	1 sector, 3½-in arc (⅛ pie, 9 in dia)	268	4	11	40	15	0.5	180	0.03	0.08	0.2	3
Pies, mince	118	1 sector, 3½-in arc (⅛ pie, 9 in dia)	320	3	14	49	33	1.2	tr	0.08	0.05	0.5	1
Pies, pumpkin	114	1 sector, 3½-in arc, (⅛ pie, 9 in dia)	241	5	13	28	58	0.6	2810	0.03	0.11	0.6	tr
Pies, strawberry	93	1 sector, 3½-in arc, (⅛ pie, 9 in dia)	184	2	7	29	15	0.7	40	0.02	0.04	0.4	23
Piecrust, baked	180	1 pie shell, enriched flour	900	11	60	79	25	3.1	0	0.36	0.25	3.2	0
Pineapple, canned	123	½ cup, pieces 1¼ x ½ in, with liquid, (water pack)	48	tr	tr	13	15	0.4	60	0.10	0.03	0.3	9
Pineapple juice, canned	125	½ cup (small glass) unsweetened	69	1	tr	17	19	0.4	65	0.07	0.03	0.3	12
Pineapple, raw	84	1 slice, 3½ x ¾ in	44	tr	tr	12	14	0.4	60	0.08	0.03	0.2	14
Pizza, cheese topping, baked	65	1 sector, 5⅓-in arc, ⅛ pie, 14 in dia	153	8	5	18	144	0.7	410	0.04	0.13	0.7	5
Pizza, sausage topping, baked	67	1 sector, 5⅓-in arc, ⅛ pie, 14 in dia	157	5	6	20	11	0.8	380	0.06	0.08	1.0	6
Plantain, green, raw	365	1 banana, 11 x 1⅞ in	313	3	1	82	18	1.8	—	0.16	0.11	1.6	37
Plums, canned	136	½ cup, fruit in liquid, syrup pack	107	1	tr	29	12	1.2	1565	0.03	0.03	0.5	3
Plums, raw	55	5 Damson plums, 1 in dia	33	tr	tr	9	9	0.3	(150)	0.04	0.02	0.3	—
Popcorn, popped, plain	6	1 cup, large kernel	23	1	tr	5	(1)	(0.2)	—	—	(0.01)	(0.1)	(0)
Popcorn, sugar coated	35	1 cup	134	2	1	30	2	0.5	—	—	0.02	0.4	0
Popcorn, with oil and salt	9	1 cup, large kernel	41	1	2	5	1	0.2	—	—	0.01	0.2	0
Popovers	40	1 popover, 2¾ in dia (enriched flour)	90	4	4	10	38	0.6	130	0.06	0.10	0.4	tr
Pork loin chop, broiled	78	2.7-oz chop (3 per lb)	305	19	25	0	9	2.7	(0)	0.75	0.22	4.5	—
Pork loin chop, broiled	58	2-oz chop (4 per lb)	227	14	18	0	7	2.0	(0)	0.56	0.16	3.4	—
Pork loin, roasted	85	3-oz piece, 2½ x 2½ x ¾ in	308	21	24	0	9	2.7	(0)	0.78	0.22	4.8	—
Potato chips	20	10 chips, 2½ x 1¾ in	114	1	8	10	8	0.4	tr	0.04	0.01	1.0	3
Potato salad (see salad)													

Potatoes, baked	202	1 potato, 4¾ x 2⅓ in	145	4	tr	33	14	1.1	tr	0.15	0.07	2.7	31
Potatoes, french fried	50	10 strips, 2 to 3½ in	137	2	7	18	8	0.7	tr	0.07	0.04	1.6	11
Potatoes, hashed brown, cooked	78	½ cup	178	2	9	23	10	0.7	tr	0.06	0.04	1.7	7
Potatoes, mashed, cooked	105	½ cup, milk, fat, added	99	2	5	13	25	0.4	180	0.09	0.06	1.1	10
Potatoes, white, boiled	188	1 potato, long type, 4¾ x 2⅓ in, pared (raw)	122	4	tr	27	11	0.9	tr	0.17	0.07	2.3	30
Potatoes, white, boiled	135	1 med potato, round type, 2½ in dia, pared (raw)	88	3	tr	20	8	0.7	tr	0.12	(0.05)	1.6	22
Pretzels, twisted type	16	1 pretzel, 2¾ x 2⅝ x ⅝ in	62	2	1	12	4	0.2	(0)	tr	tr	0.1	(0)
Prune juice, canned	128	½ cup (small glass)	99	1	tr	24	18	5.3	—	0.02	0.02	0.5	3
Prune whip, baked	65	½ cup, served cold	102	3	tr	24	15	0.9	300	0.02	0.09	0.4	2
Prunes, dried, cooked	140	½ cup, with juice, added sugar	205	1	tr	54	23	1.8	715	0.03	0.07	0.7	1
Puddings, bread, raisins	133	½ cup, enriched bread	248	7	8	38	145	1.5	400	0.08	0.25	0.7	2
Puddings, chocolate	130	½ cup, starch base	193	4	6	33	125	0.7	195	0.03	0.18	0.2	1
Puddings, rice	133	½ cup, with raisins	194	5	4	35	130	0.6	145	0.04	0.19	0.3	tr
Puddings, tapioca cream	83	½ cup	111	4	4	14	87	0.4	240	0.04	0.20	0.1	1
Puddings, vanilla	128	½ cup, starch base	142	4	5	20	149	tr	205	0.04	0.21	0.2	1
Pumpkin, canned	123	½ cup	41	1	tr	10	31	0.5	7840	0.04	0.06	0.8	6
Rabbit, cooked	70	5 med, ¾ cup diced meat	151	21	7	0	15	1.1	—	0.04	0.05	7.9	—
Radishes, raw	25	5 med, ¾ to 1 in dia	4	tr	tr	1	7	0.3	tr	tr	tr	0.1	6
Raisins, uncooked	36	¼ cup, seedless	105	1	tr	28	23	1.3	8	0.04	0.03	0.2	tr
Raspberries, black, raw	105	½ cup	49	1	1	11	20	0.6	tr	(0.02)	(0.06)	(0.6)	12
Rhubarb, frozen, cooked	67	½ cup, sugar added	191	1	tr	49	106	0.8	110	(0.03)	(0.07)	(0.4)	8
Rice, brown, cooked	135	⅔ cup, long grain	155	3	1	33	15	0.7	(0)	0.12	0.03	1.8	(0)
Rice, puffed	15	1 cup, without salt and sugar; added iron, thiamin, niacin	60	1	tr	13	3	0.3	(0)	0.07	0.01	0.7	(0)
Rice, white, cooked	154	¾ cup, enriched, except riboflavin	167	3	tr	37	16	1.4	(0)	0.17	0.02	1.6	(0)
Rolls (see buns)													
Rolls, white, "brown and serve"	28	1 roll, pan or dinner, 2 x 2 x 2 in (enriched)	84	2	2	14	20	0.5	tr	0.07	0.06	0.6	tr
Rolls, white, hard	25	1 roll, 3¾ x 2½ x 1¾ in (enriched)	78	3	1	15	12	0.6	tr	0.07	0.06	0.7	tr
Rutabagas, cooked	120	½ cup, mashed	42	1	tr	10	71	0.4	660	0.07	0.07	1.0	31
Rye wafers	7	1 wafer, 3½ x 1⅞ x ¼ in (whole-grain)	22	1	tr	5	3	0.3	(0)	0.02	0.02	0.1	(0)

Salads*

* Only a few common types of salads are listed here. The calorie and nutritive values of any combination of foods in a salad are easily estimated. The ½ cup servings of salads using mayonnaise in this table were made with ⅓ cup of the main ingredient, such as chicken, plus 2 tablespoons of a crisp vegetable, such as celery, plus 1 tablespoon of mayonnaise. One tablespoon of French dressing was used in the fruit and lettuce salads. The total calorie yield of a salad may vary greatly depending on the kind and amount of salad dressing added.

Food	Wt. g	Approximate measure and description	Food Energy kilocal	Protein g	Fat g	Carbohydrate g	Calcium mg	Iron mg	Vitamin A Activity IU	Thiamin mg	Riboflavin mg	Niacin mg	Ascorbic acid mg
Salad, chicken	125	½ cup, with mayonnaise	280	25	19	1	20	1.7	200	0.04	0.15	—	1
Salad, fresh fruit	125	½ cup, with french dressing	130	—	6	21	25	0.6	154	0.06	0.05	—	22
Salad, lettuce	130	½ solid head, french dressing	80	1	6	5	28	0.7	618	0.05	0.10	—	9
Salad, lobster	260	½ cup, (1 salad), with mayonnaise	286	26	17	6	94	2.3	—	0.23	0.21	—	47
Salad, potato	125	½ cup, with cooked dressing	124	3	4	20	40	0.8	175	0.10	0.09	1.4	14
Salad, tuna	103	½ cup, with mayonnaise	175	15	11	4	21	1.4	295	0.04	0.12	5.2	1
Salad dressing, blue or Roquefort cheese	15	1 tbsp regular, commercial (low-fat, 15 cal per tbsp)	76	1	8	1	12	tr	30	tr	0.02	tr	tr
Salad dressing, french	16	1 tbsp regular (low-fat, 15 cal per tbsp)	66	tr	6	3	2	0.1	—	—	—	—	—
Salad dressing, home cooked	16	1 tbsp	26	1	2	2	14	0.1	80	0.01	0.03	tr	tr
Salad dressing, Italian	15	1 tbsp regular (low-calorie, 6 cal per tbsp)	83	tr	9	1	2	tr	tr	tr	tr	tr	—
Salad dressing, mayonnaise	14	1 tbsp	101	tr	11	tr	3	0.1	40	tr	0.01	tr	—
Salad dressing, mayonnaise type	15	1 tbsp regular (low-calorie, 24 cal per tbsp)	65	tr	6	2	2	tr	30	tr	tr	tr	—
Salad dressing, Russian	15	1 tbsp	74	tr	8	2	3	0.1	100	0.01	0.01	0.1	1
Salad dressing, thousand island	16	1 tbsp regular (low-calorie, 30 cal per tbsp)	80	tr	8	3	2	0.1	50	tr	tr	tr	tr
Salami, sausage, cooked	28	1 slice, 4½ in dia (1 oz)	88	5	7	tr	3	0.7	—	0.07	0.07	1.2	—
Salmon, broiled or bkd	145	1 fillet, 6¾ x 2½ x 1 in	232	35	9	0	—	1.5	200	0.20	0.08	12.5	—
Salmon, pink, canned	110	½ cup, drained solids, with bones	155	23	7	0	216	0.9	75	0.04	0.20	8.8	—
Salmon rice, loaf	174	1 piece, 3¾ x 2½ x 1½ in	212	21	8	13	—	—	—	—	—	—	—
Salmon, smoked	84	3 oz	150	18	8	0	12	—	—	—	—	—	—
Saltines, crackers	11	1 packet, 4 saltines 1⅛ in sq	48	1	1	8	2	0.1	(0)	tr	tr	0.1	(0)
Sandwiches*													
Sandwich spread	15	1 tbsp (with chopped pickle)	57	tr	5	2	2	0.1	40	tr	tr	tr	1
Sardines, canned	12	1 fish, 3 x 1 x ½ in	24	3	1	—	52	0.3	30	tr	0.02	0.6	—
Sauces (see various kinds)													
Sauerkraut, canned	118	½ cup, solids and liquid	21	1	tr	5	43	0.6	60	0.04	0.05	0.3	17

* Sandwiches, as such, are not included in this list, but the "makings" are available for any type desired. For example, a simple sandwich might consist of two slices of enriched bread, 1 tablespoon butter, one slice boiled ham, 1 tablespoon mayonnaise, plus two leaves of lettuce. The sum of the calories and of the nutrients gives the total contribution of the sandwich. For salad sandwiches, the procedure is essentially the same. Chicken, egg, or tuna salads, in the measures given in this table, provide the amount of filling needed for a sandwich made with a large bun or two slices of bread.

Food		Measure											
Sauerkraut, juice (canned)	121	½ cup (small glass)	12	1	tr	3	45	1.4	—	0.04	0.05	0.3	22
Sausage, bologna	56	2 slices (2 oz), 4½ in dia	172	7	16	1	4	1.0	—	0.10	0.12	1.4	—
Sausage, brown and serve, browned	23	1 patty	97	4	9	1	—	—	—	—	—	—	—
Scallops, breaded, fried	25	1 scallop (15 to 20 per lb)	49	5	2	3	—	—	—	—	—	—	—
Scrapple	25	1 slice, 2¾ x 2⅛ x ¼ in	54	2	3	4	1	0.3	—	0.05	0.02	0.5	2
Sherbet, orange	97	½ cup, frozen dessert	130	1	1	30	16	tr	60	0.01	0.03	tr	—
Shrimp, canned	32	10 med, 2½ in long	37	8	tr	tr	37	1.0	20	tr	0.01	0.6	—
Syrups, table blends	21	1 tbsp	59	0	0	15	9	0.8	0	0	0	0	0
Soup, beans with pork	250	1 cup, ready-to-serve, from canned, condensed, reconstituted with water	168	8	6	22	63	2.3	650	0.13	0.08	1.0	3
Soup, beef bouillon, (consommé)	240	1 cup, ready-to-serve, from canned, condensed, reconstituted with water	31	5	0	3	tr	0.5	tr	tr	0.02	1.2	—
Soup, chicken noodle	240	1 cup, ready-to-serve, from canned, condensed, reconstituted with water	62	3	2	8	10	0.5	50	0.02	0.02	0.7	tr
Soup, clam chowder	245	1 cup, ready-to-serve, from canned, condensed, reconstituted with milk	81	2	3	12	34	1.0	880	0.02	0.02	1.0	—
Soup, cream of asparagus	245	1 cup, ready-to-serve, from canned, condensed, reconstituted with water	147	7	6	17	176	0.7	490	0.07	0.29	0.7	tr
Soup, cream of chicken	245	1 cup, ready-to-serve, from canned, condensed, reconstituted with water	179	7	10	15	172	0.5	610	0.05	0.27	0.7	2
Soup, cream of mushroom	245	1 cup, ready-to-serve, from canned, condensed, reconstituted with milk	216	7	14	16	191	0.5	250	0.05	0.34	0.7	1
Soup, cream of tomato	250	1 cup, ready-to-serve, from canned, condensed, reconstituted with milk	173	7	7	23	168	0.8	1200	0.10	0.25	1.3	15
Soup, minestrone	245	1 cup, ready-to-serve, from canned, condensed, reconstituted with water	105	5	3	14	37	1.0	2350	0.07	0.05	1.0	—
Soup, onion	240	1 cup, ready-to-serve, from canned, condensed, reconstituted with water	65	5	2	5	29	0.5	tr	tr	0.02	tr	—
Soup, oyster stew	240	1 cup, 4 med oysters (1 part oysters, 3 parts milk)	206	12	13	11	281	3.4	670	0.14	0.43	1.7	—
Soup, split pea	245	1 cup, ready-to-serve from canned, condensed, reconstituted with water	145	9	3	21	29	1.5	440	0.25	0.15	1.5	1
Soup, vegetable, with beef broth	245	1 cup, ready-to-serve, from canned, condensed, reconstituted with water	78	3	2	14	20	0.7	3190	0.05	0.02	1.2	—

Food	Wt. g	Approximate measure and description	Food Energy kilocal	Protein g	Fat g	Carbohydrate g	Calcium mg	Iron mg	Vitamin A Activity IU	Thiamin mg	Riboflavin mg	Niacin mg	Ascorbic acid mg
Soup, vegetarian vegetable	245	1 cup, ready-to-serve, from canned, condensed, reconstituted with water	78	2	2	13	20	1.0	2940	0.05	0.05	1.0	—
Soybean curd	120	1 piece, 2½ x 2¾ x 1 in	86	9	5	3	154	2.3	0	0.07	0.04	0.1	0
Soybeans, dry, cooked	135	¾ cup	175	15	8	15	98	3.7	38	0.29	0.12	0.8	0
Soy sauce	18	1 tbsp	12	1	tr	2	15	0.9	0	tr	0.05	0.1	0
Spaghetti in tomato sauce with cheese, canned	188	¾ cup, spaghetti enriched	143	4	1	29	30	2.1	698	0.26	0.21	3.4	8
Spaghetti with meat balls and tomato sauce, canned	188	¾ cup, spaghetti enriched	194	9	8	21	40	2.5	750	0.11	0.14	1.7	4
Spinach (see greens)													
Squash, summer, cooked	90	½ cup, sliced, drained (all varieties)	13	1	tr	3	23	0.4	350	0.05	0.07	0.7	9
Squash, winter, baked	103	½ cup, mashed	65	2	tr	16	29	0.8	4305	0.05	0.14	0.7	14
Strawberries, raw	75	½ cup, whole	28	1	tr	6	16	0.8	45	0.02	0.05	0.5	44
Sturgeon, cooked	84	3 oz	135	22	5	0	33	1.8	—	—	—	—	—
Sugar, white, granulated	12	1 tbsp, beet or cane	46	0	0	12	0	tr	0	0	0	0	0
Sunflower seeds, dry	36	¼ cup kernels	203	9	17	7	44	2.6	18	0.71	0.08	2.0	—
Sweet potatoes, boiled	180	1 potato, 5 x 2 in	172	3	1	40	48	1.1	11,940	0.14	0.09	0.9	26
Tangerines, raw	116	1 med, 2⅜ in dia	39	1	tr	10	34	0.3	360	0.05	0.02	0.1	27
Toast (see bread, white, toasted)													
Tartar sauce	14	1 tbsp	74	tr	8	1	3	0.1	30	tr	tr	tr	tr
Tomato catsup	15	1 tbsp, canned or bottled	16	tr	tr	4	3	0.1	210	0.01	0.01	0.2	2
Tomato chili sauce	15	1 tbsp, bottled	16	tr	tr	4	3	(0.1)	(210)	(0.01)	(0.01)	(0.2)	(2)
Tomato juice, canned	122	½ cup (small glass)	23	1	tr	5	9	1.1	970	0.06	0.04	1.0	20
Tomato paste	66	¼ cup, canned	54	2	tr	12	18	2.3	2163	0.13	0.08	2.0	32
Tomatoes, canned	121	½ cup, solids, liquid	26	1	tr	5	7	0.6	1085	0.06	0.04	0.9	21
Tomatoes, raw	100	1 tomato, 2⅔ in dia	20	1	tr	4	12	0.5	820	0.05	0.04	0.6	21
Tongue, beef, cooked	20	1 slice, 3 x 2 x ⅛ in	49	4	3	tr	1	0.4	—	0.01	0.06	0.7	—
Topping, whipped, pressurized	4	1 tbsp, artificial cream (vegetable fat)	10	tr	1	tr	tr	—	20	—	0	—	—
Tortillas	20	1 tortilla, 5 in dia	50	1	1	10	22	0.4	40 (yellow corn)	0.04	0.01	—	—
Tuna salad (see salad)													
Tunafish, canned	80	½ cup, drained solids	158	23	7	0	(7)	1.5	65	0.04	0.10	9.5	—
Turkey giblets (see giblets)													
Turkey, roasted	85	3 pieces, dark and white, meat only (3 oz)	162	27	5	0	7	1.5	—	0.04	0.15	6.5	—
Turnip greens (see greens, turnip tops)													
Turnips, boiled	78	½ cup, cubed	18	1	tr	4	27	0.3	tr	0.03	0.04	0.3	17
Veal, cutlets, cooked	85	1 piece, 4⅛ x 2¼ x ½ in (3 oz)	184	23	9	0	9	2.7	—	0.06	0.21	4.6	—

Food	(g)	Measure											
Veal heart, cooked	84	3 oz	177	24	8	2	3	3.6	30	0.24	1.23	6.9	tr
Veal, roasted	85	2 pieces, each 4⅛ x 2¼ x ¼ in (3 oz)	229	23	14	0	10	2.9	—	0.11	0.26	6.6	—
Vegetable juice cocktail, canned	121	½ cup (small glass)	21	1	tr	4	15	0.6	845	0.06	0.04	1.0	11
Vinegar, cider	15	1 tbsp	2	tr	(0)	1	(1)	(0.1)	—	—	—	—	—
Waffles	34	1 waffle, prebaked, 4⅝ x 3¾ in frozen (enriched flour)	86	2	2	14	41	0.6	40	0.06	0.05	0.4	tr
Walnuts (see nuts)													
Watermelon, raw	926	1 wedge, 4 in	111	2	1	27	30	2.1	2510	0.13	0.13	0.9	30
Welsh rarebit	174	¾ cup	311	14	24	11	437	0.5	923	0.07	0.40	0.2	tr
Wheat flour (see flour, wheat)													
Wheat flakes	30	1 cup	106	3	1	24	12	( )	1410	0.35	0.42	3.5	11
Wheat germ	6	1 tbsp, without salt and sugar, toasted	23	2	1	3	3	0.5	10	0.11	0.05	0.3	1
Wheat puffed	15	1 cup, without sugar, salt; added iron, thiamin, niacin	54	2	tr	12	4	0.6	(0)	0.08	0.03	1.2	(0)
Wheat, shredded	25	1 oblong biscut, without added ingredients	89	3	1	20	11	0.9	(0)	0.06	0.03	1.1	(0)
Whitefish, cooked, stuffed	84	3 oz	183	13	12	5	—	0.3	1710	0.09	0.09	2.1	tr
White sauce	125	½ cup, medium	203	5	16	11	144	0.3	575	0.05	0.22	0.3	1
Wild rice, raw	80	½ cup	283	11	1	60	15	3.3	(0)	0.36	0.51	5.0	(0)
Yeast, bakers	18	1 package, 1¼-in sq x ¾ in	15	(2)	tr	2	2	0.9	tr	0.13	0.30	2.0	tr
Yeast, brewers, dry	8	1 tbsp	25	3	tr	3	17	1.4	tr	1.25	0.34	—	tr
Yogurt, plain	123	½ cup, from partially skimmed milk	62	4	2	6	147	0.1	85	0.05	0.22	0.1	1

Index

Figures and tables in the book are indicated in the Index by the letters F (for figure) and T (for table). The table of Recommended Dietary Allowances found on the inside back cover is indicated by the letters RDAT.

Few individual foods appear in the index. Appendix K (pp. 498–515) carries a complete alphabetical list of foods with their nutritive values.

prevention measures in, 397
use of weight chart in, 396, 496F
weights and measures, equivalents in, 493
whey, 171–172, 305
White House Conference on Food, Nutrition and
Health
recommendations for the United States:
for a national nutrition policy, 441–442
for a comprehensive nutrition education
program, 442–443
for continuous surveillance of nutritional
status, 443–444
for conducting a household dietary survey
every five years, 444
for giving special consideration to vulnerable
groups, 444
for providing food of maximum nutritive
value, 444–445
WIC (Special Supplemental Food Program for
Women, Infants and Children)
educational program of, 337–338F

food distribution to by USDA, 337
medical evaluation of, 337–338
purpose and procedures, 337
vulnerable groups served by, 337, 444
work capacity, 76, 77F, 78
world nutrition problems
conservation of food and, 424F–425
family planning and, 425–426F, 427
local food production and, 423–424F
new sources of nutrients and, 425
nutrient inadequacies and, 422
population control and, 425, 426F, 427FT, 428F,
429F
where food is plentiful, 428–433
where food is scarce, 421–428

xerophthalmia, 233

yogurt, 19, 193

zinc, 221, 222F, 223

Acknowledgments

Figure 1.4   Redrawn from Bogert, *et al., Nutrition and Physical Fitness,* 9th Edition, copyright 1973, W. B. Saunders Company, Philedelphia.

Figure 3.2   From Fawcett, *The Cell,* copyright 1966, W. B. Saunders Company, Philadelphia.

Figure 3.3   From "Earlier Maturation in Man," Tanner, J. M., copyright Jan. 1968 by Scientific American, Inc. All rights reserved.

Figure 3.9   Reproduced with permission of *Nutrition Today* magazine, 101 Ridgely Avenue, Annapolis, Maryland 21404, copyright Spring, 1969.

Figure 3.10   Nevin S. Scrimshaw, "Infant Malnutrition and Adult Learning," *Saturday Review,* March 16, 1968.

Figure 5.1   From *Health for Effective Living* by Johns, *et al.,* copyright 1966. Used with permission of McGraw-Hill Book Company.

Figure 8.2   From Homans, John, *A Textbook of Surgery,* 6th ed., 1945. Courtesy of Charles C. Thomas, Publisher, Springfield, Illinois.

Figure 11.4   Courtesy of the Mayor's Office for Senior Citizens and Handicapped—City of Chicago.

Figure 12.6   Lutheran General Hospital and Lutheran General's Service League. Photograph by Ernest Tisil.